Diseases of the Salivary Glands

Diseases of the Salivary Glands

Pathology – Diagnosis – Treatment – Facial Nerve Surgery

G. Seifert, A. Miehlke, J. Haubrich
and R. Chilla

Translated by Philip M. Stell

630 Illustrations, partly in color
39 Tables

1986
Georg Thieme Verlag Thieme Inc.
Stuttgart · New York New York

Prof. Dr. G. SEIFERT
Director of the Institute of Pathology
University of Hamburg
Martinistraße 52
D-2000 Hamburg 20, F.R.G.

Prof. Dr. A. MIEHLKE
Director of the Ear-, Nose- and Throat-Clinics
University of Göttingen
Geiststraße 10
D-3400 Göttingen, F.R.G.

Prof. Dr. J. HAUBRICH
Director of the Ear-, Nose- and Throat-Clinics
of the Community Hospital Krefeld
Lutherplatz 40
D-4150 Krefeld, F.R.G.

Prof. Dr. R. CHILLA
Director of the Ear-, Nose- and Throat-Clinics
Community Hospital
St.-Jürgen-Straße
D-2800 Bremen, F.R.G.

Prof. P. M. STELL, CH. M., F.R.C.S.
Head of Department of Oto-Rhino-Laryngology
Royal Liverpool Hospital
Prescot Street
Liverpool L 69 3 BX, G.B.

Library of Congress Cataloging-in-Publication Data

Speicheldrüsenkrankheiten. English.
Diseases of the salivary glands.

Translation of: Speicheldrüsenkrankheiten.
Includes bibliographies and index.
1. Salivary glands--Diseases. I. Seifert, Gerhard, 1921- . II. Title. [DNLM: 1. Salivary Gland Diseases. WI 230 S7415]
RC815.5.S7313 1986 616.3'16 86-14445
ISBN 0-86577-229-0 (U.S.)

This book is an authorized translation from the German edition published and copyrighted 1984 by Georg Thieme Verlag, Stuttgart, Germany. Title of the German edition: Speicheldrüsenkrankheiten.

Important Note: Medicine is an ever-changing science. Research and clinical experience are continually broadening our knowledge, in particular our knowledge of proper treatment and drug therapy. Insofar as this book mentions any dosage or application, readers may rest assured that the authors, editors and publishers have made every effort to ensure that such references are strictly in accordance with the state of knowledge at the time of production of the book. Nevertheless, every user is requested to carefully examine the manufacturers' leaflets accompanying each drug to check on his own responsibility whether the dosage schedules recommended therein or the contraindications stated by the manufacturers differ from the statements made in the present book. Such examination is particularly important with drugs which are either rarely used or have been newly released on the market.

Printed in Germany.
Typesetting by Druckhaus Dörr, D-7140 Ludwigsburg on Linotype System 5, Linotron 202
Printed by Gutmann & Co., D-7100 Heilbronn, FRG

ISBN 3-13-689101-5 (Georg Thieme Verlag, Stuttgart)
ISBN 0-86577-229-0 (Thieme Inc., New York)

Dedicated in gratitude to
Dr. Dr. h. c. JOHN J. CONLEY
who paved the way for modern head and neck surgery and into the miraculous world of salivary gland pathology

Preface

Since the appearance of Rauch's book in 1959, interdisciplinary research has contributed to great advances in the understanding of salivary gland diseases. New methods of investigation have been developed, and much basic work has been done on the physiology of salivary secretion, the biochemistry of the saliva, and the ultrastructure, cytochemistry, and immunology of the salivary glands.

The *clinical diagnosis of salivary gland disease* is based on a wide range of methods that ensure optimal treatment based on precise identification of the disease. Preoperative diagnosis of tumors is of particular significance for the planning of an operation utilizing modern methods of surgery of the facial nerve. The correct diagnosis is usually based on critical analysis of the clinical, radiologic, laboratory, and pathologic findings.

Numerous aspects must be taken into account in the *classification of salivary gland diseases,* including clinical findings, disordered physiology, etiologic factors, and pathologic anatomy. The main themes of this book are, firstly, a pathologic classification differentiating between neoplastic and non-neoplastic diseases, such as congenital anomalies, disorders of secretion, calculus formation, cysts, and inflammation; secondly, the association between salivary gland diseases and other systems; thirdly, the peculiarities of salivary disorders in childhood; and finally, the differential diagnosis of salivary gland swellings.

New criteria for classification of *salivary gland tumors* have been established by international cooperation: they form the basis of accurate diagnosis and treatment. The WHO classification of salivary gland tumors (Thackray and Sobin, 1972) has now been accepted by numerous centers (The Armed Forces Institute of Pathology in Washington, the Salivary Gland Register at the Pathological Institute of the University of Hamburg), and its application has become established in practice. Classical methods of histopathologic examination have been supplemented in recent years by aspiration cytology and immunohistologic methods. The diagnosis can be further refined by the use of tumor markers, investigation of the stromal immunologic reaction, cytochemistry, and electron microscopy. The transplantation of human cells to the athymic nude mouse, and the assay of human tumor cells in tissue culture against therapeutic agents hold promise for the future.

Modern facial nerve surgery is required both for the treatment of tumors and the management of trauma. The increase in severe traffic accidents poses a problem in the correct management of deep injuries of the face, with destruction of the salivary parenchyma and laceration of the duct system or the facial nerve.

Interesting aspects for the explanation of human salivary disorders follow from the *phylogenetic development* of the salivary gland (Rauch, 1959). The salivary glands are widely distributed throughout the entire animal kingdom, being found in most, if not all, invertebrates and vertebrates. The salivary glands are converted into poisonous glands in some species of snake, which do not masticate their prey. The size of the salivary glands in the vertebrates is related to the type of food they eat: herbivores who eat food rich in carbohydrate have better developed salivary glands than carnivores. The salivary glands are thus maximally developed in the ruminants, such as the cow and the horse, which produce 50–60 liters of saliva per day. The weight of the entire salivary tissue in the average human attains 35 g. The human daily salivary production 1–1.5 liters.

Accurate knowledge of the *human salivary gland* has only been acquired relatively recently. Thomas Wharton (1614–1673) dissected the submandibular glands of man, and Nikolaus Steno (1639–1686) dissected the parotid gland and its ducts. Both investigators spoke out strongly against the view held at that time that the saliva originated from a branch of the thoracic duct. In the second half of the 19th century and the beginning of this century Claude Bernard, Heidenhain, Bayliss, and Langley used the human salivary glands as a model for the investigation of secretory gland activity. Pavlov and other members of his school also extended knowledge of the secretory pattern of the salivary glands.

It is difficult to assess the results of research into the function of the salivary glands, because their function is so labile, and definition of resting autonomic activity is difficult. Research into the biochemistry of the human saliva is therefore difficult, but rewarding. An up-to-date review of this subject can be found in Arglebe's monograph (1981).

This book is designed as a synopsis of salivary diseases; considerations of pathology are followed by clinical aspects and these by treatment of the individual disorders. Particular stress is laid on treatment, including surgery of the facial nerve. The book is profusely illustrated to assist comprehension and it is hoped will extend the knowledge of all those physicians who treat salivary gland disorders. This book is intended as a "state of the art" report. Unsolved questions and future directions for research are outlined in numerous parts of the book.

Hamburg, Göttingen, Krefeld and Bremen,
Summer 1984

G. Seifert, A. Miehlke,
J. Haubrich and R. Chilla

Arglebe, Ch.: Biochemistry of Human Saliva. In Pfaltz, C. R., R. Chilla: Advances in ORL, Vol. 26. Karger, Basel 1981

Rauch, S.: Die Speicheldrüsen des Menschen. Thieme, Stuttgart 1959

Thackray, A. C., L. H. Sobin: Histological Typing of Salivary Gland Tumors. World Health Organization, Genève 1972

Contents

1. Topographic Anatomy

This chapter will be limited to the points of surgical importance.

Parotid Gland

The parotid gland is lobular and shaped like a pyramid standing on its apex. Anteriorly, it lies on the masseter muscle; superiorly, it reaches the zygoma; and posteriorly, it is limited by the tragus. Inferiorly, the parotid gland borders on the anterior face of the mastoid process, it overlies the anterior border of the sternocleidomastoid muscle in its upper part, and it sinks into the retromandibular fossa. Processes of parotid tissue extend from the latter site into the parapharyngeal space.

The duct system of the gland leaves at its anterior border and consists of the confluence of the tributaries arising within the body of the gland. The duct continues over the masseter muscle, curves, and then sinks through the buccinator muscle and through the tissues of the cheek to open in the mouth at the parotid papilla opposite the second upper molar tooth. The course of the duct is indicated by an imaginary line running from the base of the ear lobe to the vermillion border of the upper lip. This fact may occasionally help the surgeon to find the buccal branches of the facial nerve by dissecting backward along the duct (see Chapter 22). As it passes across the surface of the masseter muscle, the parotid duct is often accompanied by a small accessory gland. Tumors may occasionally arise from this accessory gland (see Chapter 6), and tumors arising from the ducts themselves have also been described (Kleinsasser et al 1968).

That part of the parotid gland that extends over the horizontal ramus of the mandible is covered by fibers of the platysma. Thiel (1969) described the parotidomasseteric fascia that covers the gland and the masseter muscle anterior to it.

This fascia is important from a surgical point of view, since the overlying skin with the subcuticular layer can be freed by dissecting along it. This fascia has an interesting property: fine connective tissue septae pass from it between the individual lobules of the parotid gland so that the gland cannot be dissected out bluntly, as can the submandibular gland. The parotid gland also adheres relatively tightly to the masseter muscle beneath it, whereas it can be easily freed from the anterior edge of the sternocleidomastoid muscle, the stylohyoid muscle, and the posterior belly of the digastric muscle.

Because of its firm attachment to its surroundings, the parotid gland has little opportunity to expand. Swelling of the gland, in mumps, for example, therefore leads to marked tension on the investing fascia and causes considerable pain.

The parotid gland occasionally develops processes extending toward the pharynx. The internal jugular vein and the glossopharyngeal nerve are the most lateral of the structures in the parapharyngeal space and they therefore lie closest to the parotid gland. The internal carotid artery lies more medially at a distance from the parotid. The relationships are particularly close in tumors of the salivary glands, especially the dumbbell tumor, and the structures may then be displaced in a dangerous manner.

The vessels and nerves that run through the body of the gland are of particular importance. These are the auriculotemporal nerve running superiorly, anterior to the tragal cartilage, and the superficial temporal artery, which arises from the external carotid artery lying close to the nerve. The course of the facial nerve as it runs through the parotid gland will be discussed later. The great auricular nerve arises from the cervical plexus and reaches the posteroinferior part of the gland to break up there into several branches. The small transverse facial artery runs in the anterior part of the parotid region close to the parotid duct.

The primary consideration of the surgeon during any operation on the parotid gland, for whatever indication, is preservation of the function of the facial nerve.

Operations on the parotid gland and on the extratemporal course of the facial nerve require a detailed knowledge of the relationships between the facial nerve and its peripheral branches to the parotid gland and its lobes. The question whether the nerve penetrates the parenchyma of the parotid gland or whether it divides the gland into two lobes from which it is separable is also important. The answer to this question considerably simplifies the operation and forms the basis of all modern parotid surgery.

In 1859, Triquet and Bruns showed that the facial nerve does not penetrate the substance of the parotid gland, but lies in a groove in the gland completely separate from it and enclosed in loose connective tissue. Luschka in his book "Anatomie des Menschen" (1862 and 1867) confirmed the observation that the facial nerve and its branches divide the parotid gland into two portions, the medial of which is smaller than the lateral. Henle (1873) came to the same conclusion, noting that the parotid gland is divided into a large external and a small internal part by the trunk and main branches of the facial nerve. Nicoladoni summarized the situation as follows: the entire nerve lies in a groove pointing upward formed by the parotid doubling back on itself around the nerve. Kermauner (1899) carried out his own investigations and came to the same conclusion as his teacher Nicoladoni.

Gregoire (1912) dissected a large number of parotid glands of man (both adult and fetus), apes, rabbits, dogs, and guinea pigs. In all his dissections, apart from those on dogs and guinea pigs, he found that the parotid gland was divided into a superficial and a deep lobe. The facial nerve is embedded between the two parts. Gregoire demonstrated an isthmus of glandular tissue joining both parts of the parotid, which according to him lies above the trunk of the facial nerve. He stressed that this important relationship is due to the development of the gland. In a 3-month old human fetus (length, 8 cm), he observed that the entire part of the superficial lobe present at that time covered the facial nerve.

The deep lobe only begins to develop in the sixth or seventh fetal month.

McWhorter (1917) dissected 66 human parotid specimens and confirmed the presence of a large superficial lobe and a separate deep lobe each with its own duct system. He confirmed that the facial nerve lies in a groove between these two lobes from which it can be easily separated. Furthermore, the two lobes are joined by an isthmus. According to McWhorter, this isthmus does not lie superior to the trunk, but in the middle of the gland, *anterior to the division* of the facial nerve into its end branches. Rouvière and Cordier (1934) carried out investigations on the fetus and came to the conclusion that both points of view about the position of the isthmus are correct.

Cody (1954) examined 24 fetuses at the ages of 8,16, and 21 weeks. He came to the same basic conclusions: in the eighth week a small glandular bundle is present lateral to the facial nerve from which it can be separated with ease (Fig. 1.**1a**). In the 16th week the gland parenchyma expands medially and above, so that the facial nerve and its branches are now surrounded by glandular tissue. This forms a small deep lobe (Fig. 1.**1b**). The parotid gland is developed in its entirety in the 21-week-old fetus and has now completely surrounded the facial nerve. The deep lobe forms only one fifth of the whole, and the main part of the gland lies lateral to the facial nerve and its branches (Fig. 1.**1c**). Cody emphasizes that the nerve and its branches lie loosely in the cleft within the gland.

Becker and Brünner (1958) came to the same conclusions based on dissections of the human as did Dargent and Duroux (1946) and McCormack et al (1945). The latter investigators also mentioned that the deep lobe varies in size from that of a cherrystone to almost the same volume as the superficial lobe.

In summary, these investigations show the following points of clinical importance. The facial nerve divides the parotid gland into two parts, a superficial lobe and a deep lobe that are joined by an isthmus anterior to the bifurcation of the facial nerve. However, there is no *connective tissue* separating these two layers.

Bailey (1947) remarked with humor and accuracy that "the facial nerve should be looked upon as the meat within a parotid sandwich."

It is to the credit of Becker and Brünner (1958) that they reaffirmed and drew attention to these forgotten anatomic relationships. Becker showed that the branches of the facial nerve always run in one layer parallel to the inner surface of the superficial lobe. This fact ensures safety, elegance, and speed in surgical dissection.

Thus, it is clear that the facial nerve is the landmark for surgery of the parotid region. The facial nerve may be exposed in greater safety by dissecting along it, opening up the two lobes of the parotid gland, and, if necessary, removing them successively. In this way the fibers of the facial nerve may be demonstrated in their entirety.

These facts are the basis of all successful surgery on the parotid gland, and also the key for surgery of the extratemporal course of the facial nerve, whether or not it must be preserved or sacrificed and replaced in some cases.

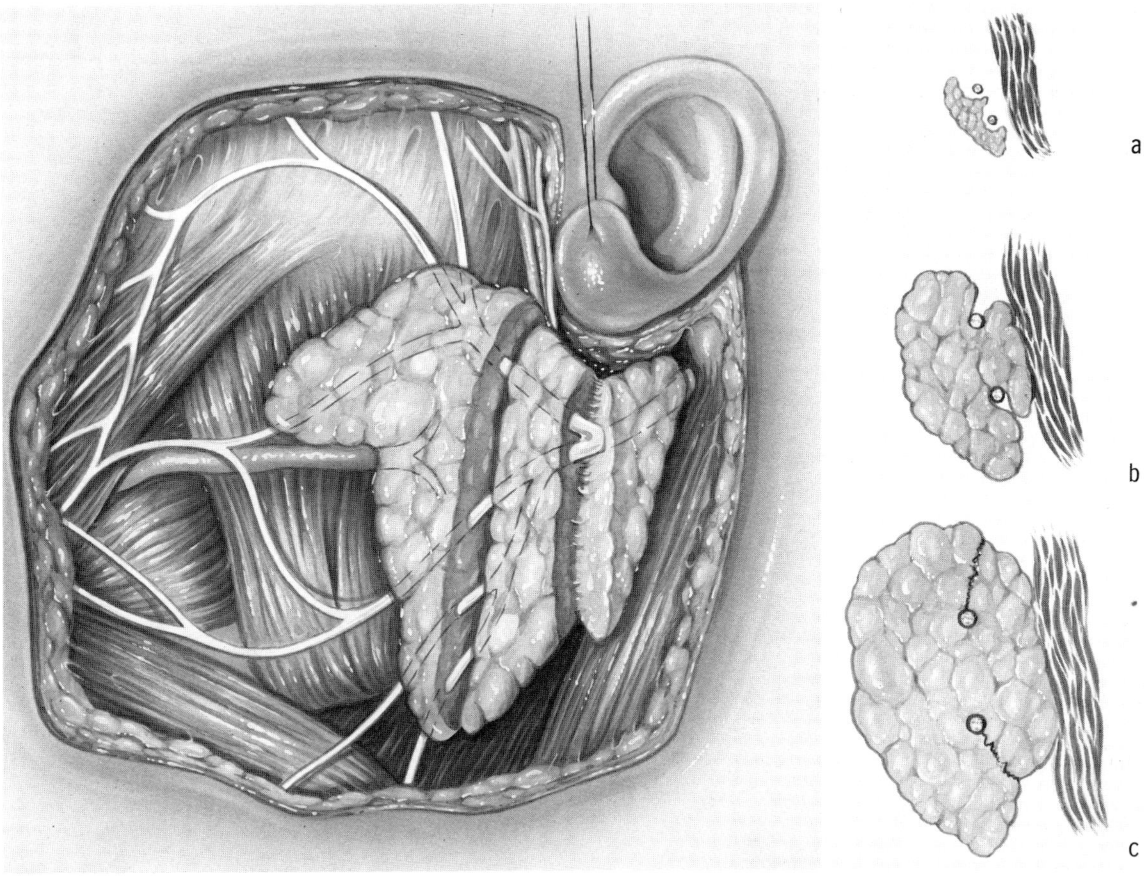

Figure 1.1 The course of the facial nerve in the parotid gland. **a–c** Progressive embedding of the facial nerve in the parotid gland during development. (McWhorter, Martin, Cody)

Even if the surgeon makes great efforts to identify and preserve all branches of the facial nerve, one or more branches may occasionally be damaged or deliberately removed. They should then be replaced immediately, if this appears to be desirable. It is therefore important to know the type of branches of the facial nerve fibers because lost fibers may often be compensated for by anastomoses within the plexus. The more peripheral a lesion of the branches of the facial nerve lies, the less is the danger of persistent loss of mobility of the facial muscles.

The following classification of the fibers of the facial nerve is based on a study of 100 of our patients (Chilla 1979) (Fig. 1.**2**):

Type I (48%): no anastomoses between the facial nerve branches.

Type II (27%): anastomoses within the temporofacial part (the temporozygomatic and possibly buccal rami).

Type III (8%): anastomoses between the temporofacial and the cervicofacial division.

Type IV (4%): anastomoses within the cervicofacial part (marginal mandibular, cervical, and possibly buccal rami).

Type V (5%): anastomoses within the temporofacial part combined with anastomoses between the temporofacial and cervicofacial divisions.

Type VI (3%): anastomoses within the cervicofacial division combined with anastomoses between the temporofacial and cervicofacial divisions.

Type VII (3%): anastomoses within the temporofacial and cervicofacial divisions.

Type VIII (2%): anastomoses in the temporo- and cervicofacial divisions combined with anastomoses between the temporo- and cervicofacial divisions of the nerve.

The *arrangement of the buccal rami* can specifically be described as follows (Fig. 1.**3a–d**):

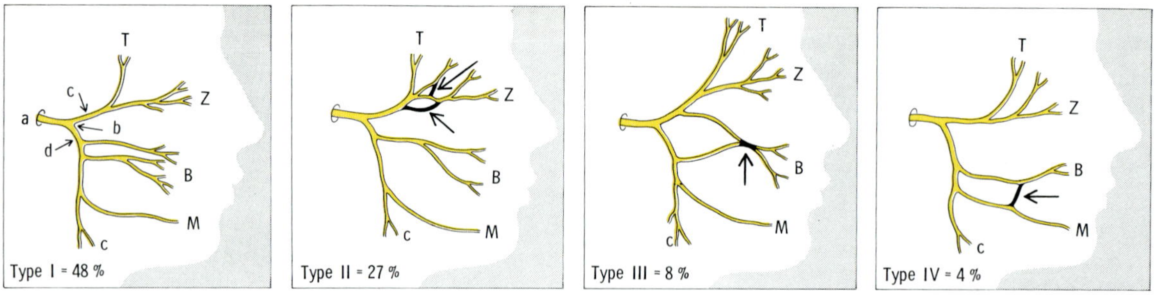

No anastomoses | Anastomoses within the temporofacial division | Anastomoses between the temporofacial and cervicofacial divisions | Anastomoses within the cervicofacial division

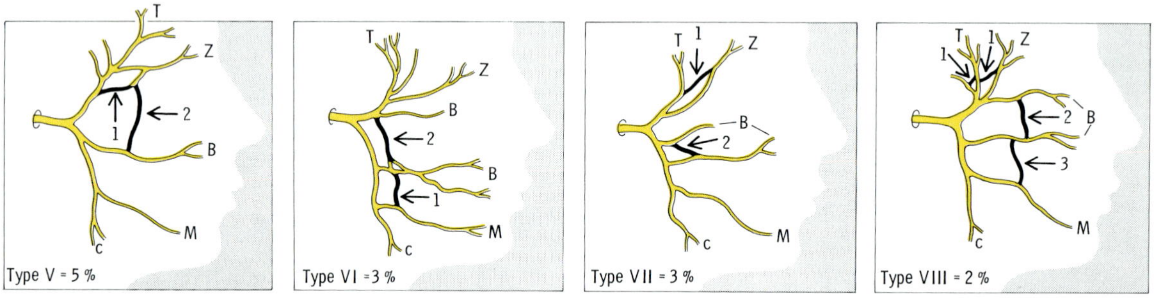

Anastomoses within the temporofacial division (1), and between the temporofacial and cervicofacial division (2)

Anastomoses within the cervicofacial division (1) and between the temporofacial and cervicofacial division (2)

Anastomoses within the temporofacial division (1) and in the cervicofacial division (2)

Anastomoses within the temporofacial division (1), between the temporofacial and the cervicofacial division (2) and the cervicofacial division (3)

Figure 1.**2** Classification of the extratemporal course of the facial nerve, depending on the type of anastomoses. B = buccal ramus, C = cervical ramus, M = marginal mandibular ramus, T = temporal ramus, Z = zygomatic ramus, a = stylomastoid foramen, b = bifurcation of the nerve, c = temporofacial ramus, d = cervicofacial ramus→ = anastomoses.

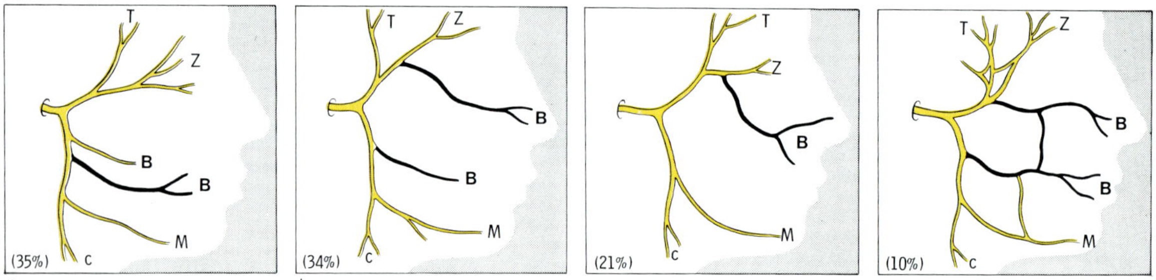

a b c d

Figure 1.**3a–d** Origin and position of the buccal ramus of the facial nerve. B = buccal ramus, C = cervical ramus, M = marginal mandibular ramus, T = temporal ramus, Z = zygomatic ramus.

35% arise from the cervicofacial division.
34% arise in the cervico- and temporofacial division.
21% arise from the temporofacial division.
10% arise from the temporofacial and cervicofacial divisions with additional anastomoses between the branches.

Most anastomoses (37%) occur in the temporofacial division (types II, V, VII, VIII). Fewer anastomoses (12%) lie in the cervicofacial part (types IV, VI, VII, VIII). Connections between the cervicofacial and the temporofacial area were present in only 18% of subjects (types III, V, VI, VIII). The overwhelming majority of these anastomoses (10%) run via the buccal rami (Fig. 1.**3**).

These data may be summarized for the guidance of the surgeon as follows: An anastomosis between the upper and lower areas of distribution of

Figure 1.4 Position of the submandibular gland. (von Lanz & Wachsmuth)
1 = sublingual process of the submandibular gland.
2 = submandibular duct.
3 = submandibular gland.

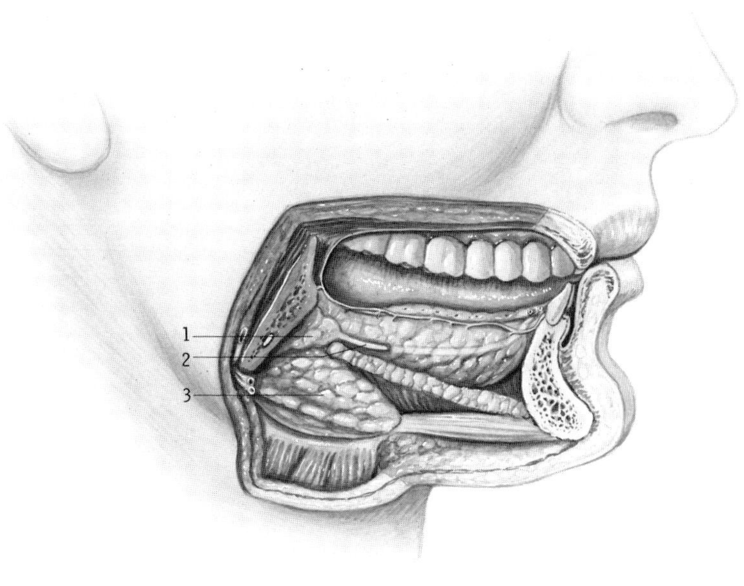

the facial nerve is only present in about 18% of cases. It is uncertain whether finer anastomoses lie in more peripheral areas, which we have not been able to demonstrate at parotidectomy. We mention this point particularly because Davis et al (1956) found a much higher rate of anastomoses (67%) between the upper and lower facial nerve divisions in their *cadaver dissections*.

Submandibular Gland

The submandibular gland lies on the hypoglossus muscle between the anterior and posterior bellies of the digastric muscle in a triangle open above. The inferior border of the body of the gland lies over the tendon, uniting the two bellies in the carotid triangle. The shape of the submandibular gland resembles that of a horseshoe open anteriorly enclosing the free edge of the mylohyoid muscle with its limbs (Fig. 1.**4**). The two limbs of the gland are not of equal size. The smaller inner part of the gland follows the duct as the sublingual process lying under the floor of the mouth, and thus is in direct relationship to the sublingual gland, which lies superior to the mylohyoid muscle in the floor of the mouth. The sublingual process of the mandibular gland may merge with the sublingual gland, but it may also be divided into several individual lobes. If the posterior part of the lobe is absent, the anterior part may compose a completely isolated group that forms an accessory submandibular gland. An individual case was described by Turner (1869) in which only the upper part of the gland was present, and this part was closely connected to the sublingual gland.

The submandibular duct follows a curious course determined by the horseshoe shape of the gland. The main part of the gland lies below the floor of the mouth beneath the mylohyoid muscle. Its saliva drains into tributary canaliculi that initially run backward to the submandibular duct. The duct then turns around the posterior edge of the mylohyoid muscle and runs in the opposite direction through the sublingual space on the medial side of the sublingual gland to the sublingual papilla.

The submandibular lymph nodes are arranged in a row in the space between the mandible and the body of the gland as the anterior, medial, and posterior submandibular lymph nodes.

In the submandibular triangle, the facial artery is covered by the submandibular gland. In contrast, the facial vein runs over the gland, so that the two vessels have the gland between them. The two vessels then come together above the edge of the mandible to supply the face. This relationship is important in surgery and will be discussed further in Chapter 22.

The hypoglossal nerve lies in the submandibular triangle medial to the gland and on the hypoglossus muscle. It runs anteriorly and then disappears at the posterior edge of the mylohyoid muscle. The end of the hypoglossal nerve spreads out in a fan shape to supply the individual muscles of the tongue.

The lingual nerve ascends on the medial side of the mandible in the depth of the submandibular triangle in a flat curve. Only a small segment is to be seen in the space, because it disappears rapidly at the posterior edge of the mylohyoid muscle. In

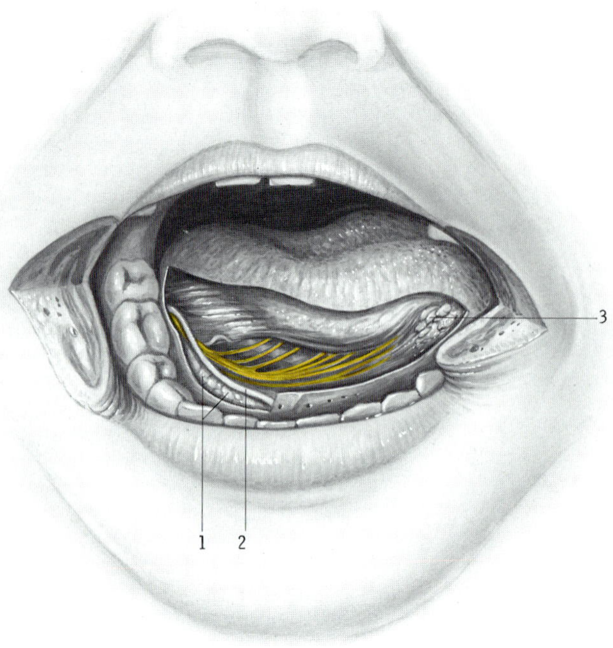

Figure 1.**5** Position of the sublingual gland with the lingual apical glands. (Hafferl)
1 = sublingual gland.
2 = submandibular gland.
3 = anterior lingual gland.

this short course under the submandibular gland, the lingual nerve gives off fine nerve fibers that form the afferent root of the submandibular ganglion. The course of the nerve must be a concern during operations on the submandibular gland.

Sublingual Gland

The sublingual gland lies in a hollow in the mandible, the sublingual fossa, beneath the mucosa of the floor of the mouth and anterior to the mylohyoid muscle. The gland is surrounded by loose connective tissue. It lies under the mucosa of the mouth, where it bulges to form the sublingual fold with the opening of the minor sublingual duct. The body of the sublingual gland is often close to the superior part of the submandibular gland. One or more of the minor sublingual ducts may open into the submandibular duct, which runs anteriorly on the medial side of the sublingual gland accompanied by the sublingual artery and vein. The lingual nerve approaches from the lateral side, passes under the submandibular duct, and then pierces the tongue from below as it divides into its end branches (see also Chapter 6).

Very small lingual apical glands or anterior lingual glands (Nuhn's glands) lie on the undersurface of the apex of the tongue next to the midline (Fig. 1.**5**).

References

Bailey, H.: Parotidectomy: indications and results. Brit. med. J. 1947/I, 404
Becker, W., H. Brünner: Über die makroskopische Struktur der Ohrspeicheldrüse. Z. Laryng. Rhinol. 37 (1958) 397
Chilla, R.: Types of facial nerve branching in the parotid plexus and their clinical significance. Clin. Plast. Surg. 6 (1979) 451
Cody, C. C.: Surgical anatomy of the facial nerve outside the skull. Arch. Otolaryng. 60 (1954) 291
Dargent, M., P. E. Duroux: Données anatomiques concernant la morphologise et certains rapports du facial intraparotidien. Presse med. 54 (1946) 523
Davis, R. A., B. J. Anson, J. M. Budinger, K. E. Kurth: Surgical anatomy of the facial nerve upon a study of 350 cervicofacial halves. Surg. 102 (1956) 384
Gregoire, R.: Le nerf facial et la parotide. J. Anat. (Paris) 48 (1912) 437
Henle, J.: Handbuch der systematischen Anatomie des Menschen, Bd. II. Braunschweig 1873
Kermauner, F.: Zur Kenntnis des makroskopischen Baues der Parotis. Arch. klin. Chirurg. 59 (1899) 805
Kleinsasser, O., H. J. Klein, G. Hübner: Speichelgangkarzinome. Arch. klin. exp. Ohr-, Nas.- u. Kehlk.-Heilk. 192 (1968) 100
Luschka, H.: Die Anatomie des Menschen, Bd. I und II. Tübingen 1862 und 1867
McCormack, W. J., E. W. Caldwell, B. J. Anson: The surgical anatomy of the facial nerve. Surg. 80 (1945) 620
McWorther, G. L.: The relations of the superficial and deep lobes of parotid gland to the ducts and facial nerve. Anat. Rec. 12 (1917) 149
Rouvière, H., G. Cordier: Sur le developement de la glande parotide etc. Ann. Anat. path. 11 (1934) 622
Thiel, W.: In A. Hafferl: Lehrbuch der Topographischen Anatomie, 3. Aufl. Springer, Berlin 1969
Triquet u. Bruns: Die chirurgische Pathologie und Therapie des Kau- und Geschmacksorgans, 1859; zit. nach Kermauner
Turner, J.: Anat. 4 (1869) 147; zit. nach T. v. Lanz, W. Wachsmuth: Praktische Anatomie (Hals), Springer, Berlin 1955

2. Histology and Ultrastructure

Histology

All the major and minor salivary glands are characterized by an acinar and a duct system (Fig. 2.**1**, Table 2.**1**) (Zimmermann 1927, Seifert 1964 and 1966, Schaetzle 1962, Donath 1976, Seifert & Donath 1976). The glands may be divided into three types: firstly, serous glands (the parotid gland and von Ebner's glands of the tongue); secondly, mucous glands lying in the palate, the tongue, the base and lateral border of the tongue; and thirdly, mixed glands. There are two mixed glands: firstly, the submandibular gland, consisting mainly of serous acini, intercalated ducts with serous end caps, well-formed striated ducts, and a vigorously branching duct system; secondly, the sublingual gland, consisting mainly of mucous acini, intercalated ducts, and short striated ducts. Finally, the minor salivary glands of the lip and cheek and the apical glands of the tongue are also mixed glands (Figs. 2.**2**–2.**4**).

Acinar System: The primary saliva is produced in the acini. That from the serous glands contains amylase and that from the mucous acini contains sialomucin (see Chapter 4). Nonspecific anti-

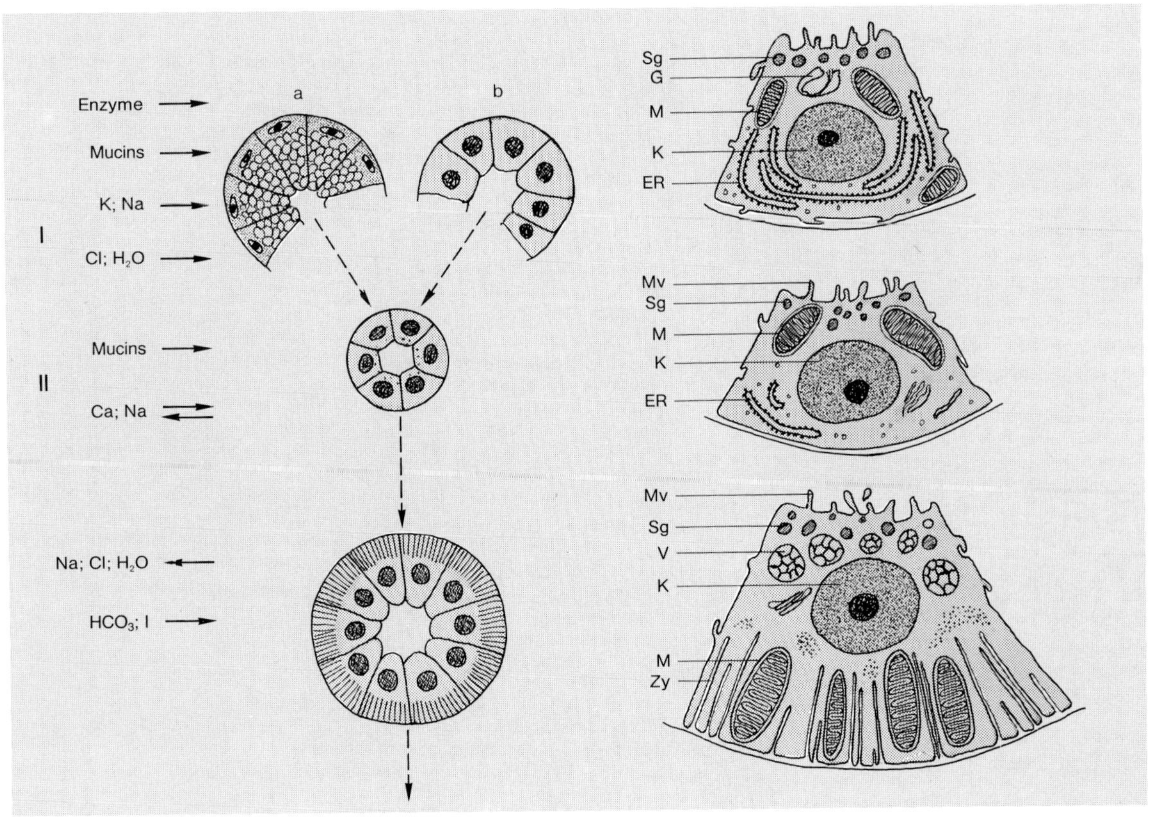

Figure 2.**1** Diagram of the functional classification of the salivary glands. I: mucous (a) or serous (b) acini. II: intercalated duct above and striated duct below. Secretion and resorption from the duct system on the left; ultrastructure of an acinus and an intercalated and a striated duct cell on the right.
Sg = secretory granule, G = Golgi apparatus, M = mitochondria, K = cell nuclei, ER = endoplasmic reticulum, Mv = microvilli, V = supranuclear vacuoles, Zy = cytomembrane. (Seifert, from Hals-Nasen-Ohren-Heilkunde in Praxis und Klinik, Vol. III, Ed. Berendes, J., Link, R. and Zoellner, F. Stuttgart, Thieme, 1978.)

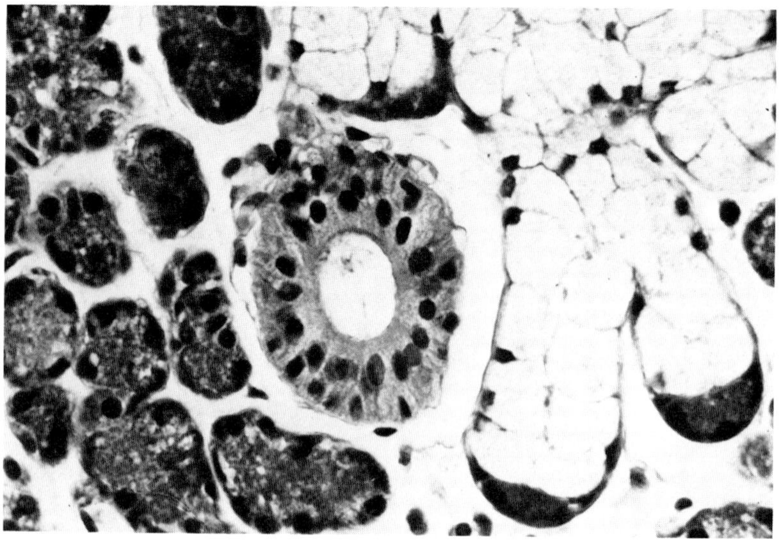

Figure 2.**2** Section of a normal submandibular gland showing serous acini with secretory granules (left), mucous acini with mucous vacuoles and serous end caps (right), a striated duct in the middle. H & E, 400×.

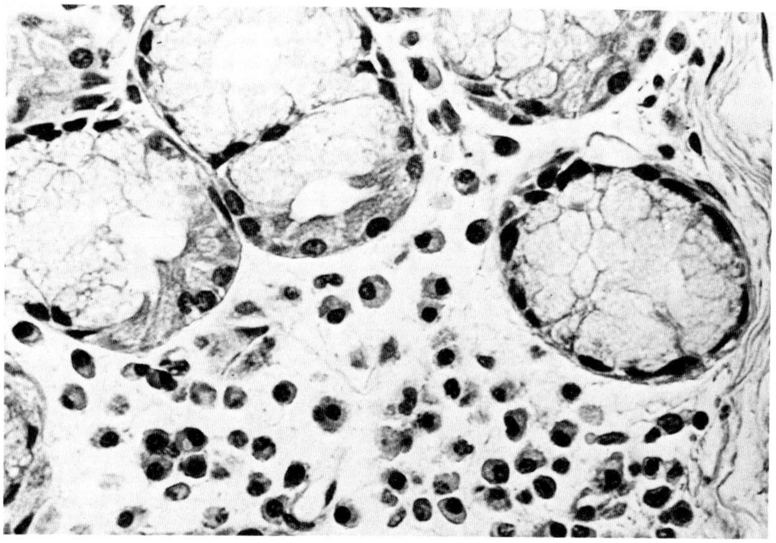

Figure 2.**3** Minor salivary gland of the lower lip showing mucous acini with mucous vacuoles and plasma cells in the interstitium. Astra blue, 400×.

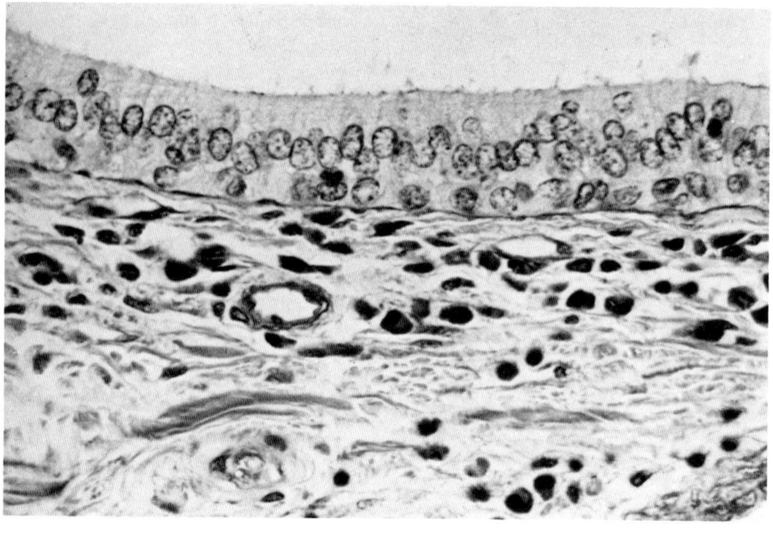

Figure 2.**4** Minor salivary glands from the lower lip showing a striated duct with stratified epithelium. Periductal collection of plasma cells. PAS, 400×.

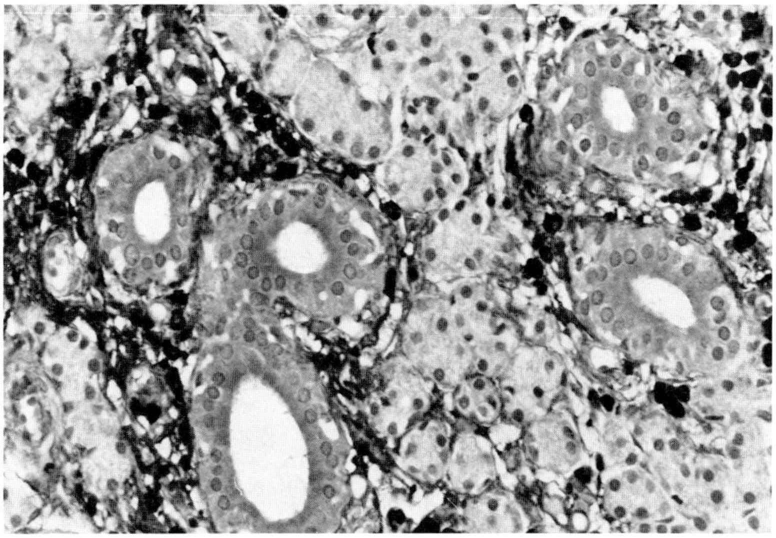

Figure 2.**11** Normal parotid gland with IgA forming plasma cells in periductal gland tissue. Immunoperoxidase, 400×.

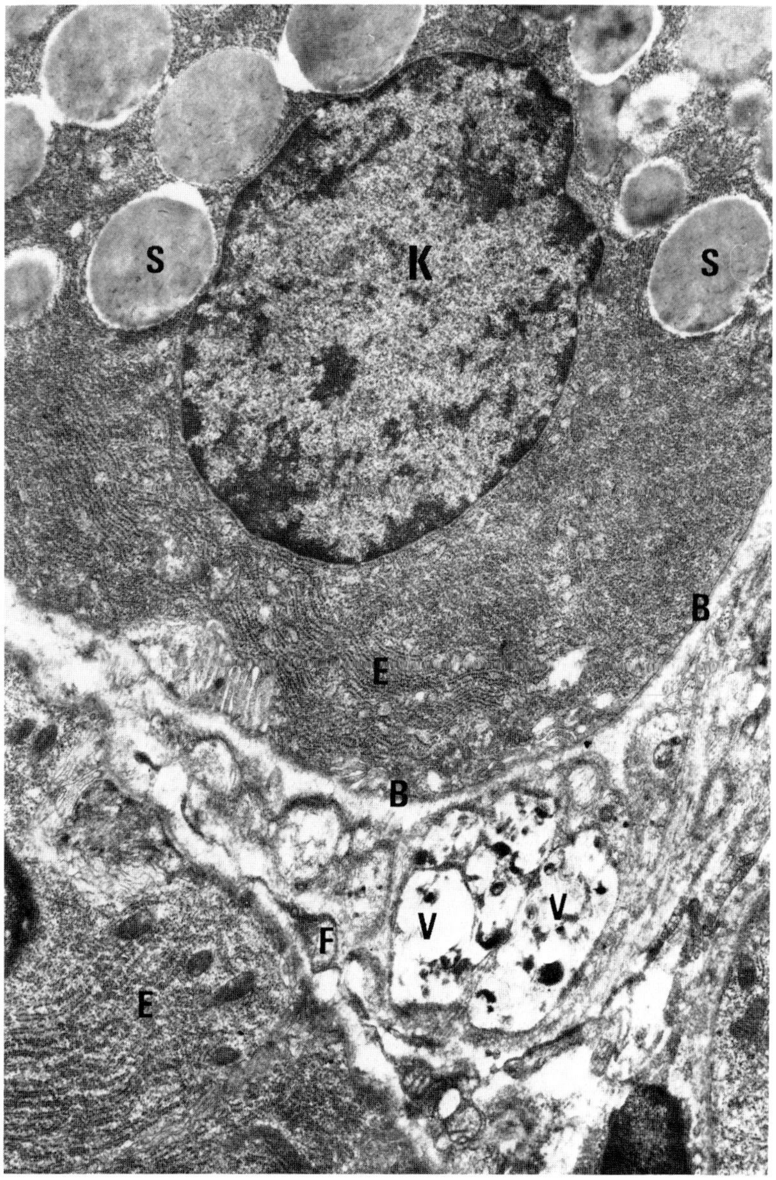

Figure 2.**12** Electron microscopic section of human parotid showing a serous acinus. E = endoplasmic reticulum, S = secretory granule, K = cell nucleus, B = basal cell membrane, V = varicosity of an altered autonomic fiber in the interstitium, F = fibroblastic offshoot, 10 400×. (Seifert & Donath 1976.)

Ultrastructure

Glandular Acini: The enzymes are produced in the *serous acini* (Figs. 2.**12**, 2.**13**). The latter possess mitochondria, Golgi vesicles, and secretory granules and a richly developed coarse endoplasmic reticulum identical to the basophilic ergastoplasm that can be identified with the light microscope. Intercellular secretory canaliculi run between individual gland cells. Adhesion of the glandular cells to form an acinar unit is ensured by the adhesive zone (zonula occludens, zonula adherens) near the lumen, and peripherally by desmosomes. The basal lamina separates the glandular cells from the interstitial cells. Cyclic AMP and calcium ions are particularly important in controlling secretion (see Chapter 4). Cyclic AMP is concentrated on the cell membrane and regulates transport into the cytoplasm. Calcium ions are also concentrated in the cell organelles (endoplasmic reticulum and mitochondria), which are important for the formation of secretion. The coupling of calcium ions to the secretory granules promotes transport into the intracellular secretory canaliculus and channelling by the cell membrane (Schaefer 1979, Westhofen et al 1984). The volume of the cell nucleus and the cytoplasmic organelles changes during the secretory cycle. During protein synthesis, the endoplasmic reticulum increases, the Golgi apparatus enlarges, and con-

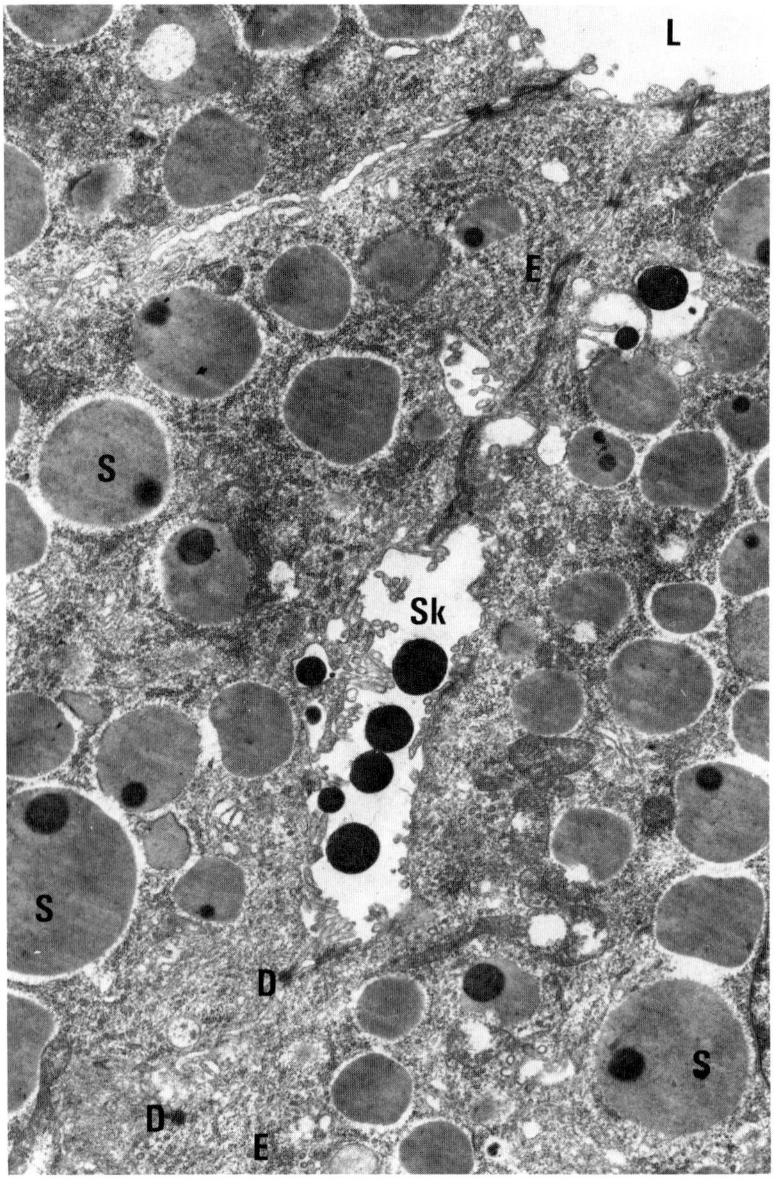

Figure 2.**13** Human parotid gland showing electron microscopic section of a serous acinus. L = lumen, Sk = intercellular secretory canaliculus with osmiophilic segments of secretory granules, S = immature secretory granule, D = desmosome, E = endoplasmic reticulum. 9100×. (Seifert & Donath 1976.)

densing vacuoles develop; during the formation of secretory granules, the granules mature, with an increase of osmiophilic substances. During discharge of the secretion, the volume of the individual acinar cells decreases and the membrane of the secretory granules merges with the cell membrane.

The *mucous acini* contain only a little coarse endoplasmic reticulum in the basal zone of cytoplasm. Mucous vacuoles in the cytoplasm and cisterns of the Golgi apparatus are characteristic. The precursors of various sialomucins are formed in the endoplasmic reticulum, transported via mucosal vacuoles to the Golgi apparatus and discharged into the lumen after further transformation and condensation.

The *myoepithelial cells* (Fig. 2.**14**) lie between the basal lamina of the acinar cells and the basal membrane of the acini. Myofilaments mainly arranged parallel to the cell base are characteristic. The myoepithelial cells contain glycogen granules and mitochondria. The pinocytic vesicles are an expression of an active transport between the extra- and intracellular space.

Duct System: The discharge and reabsorption of substances, particularly sodium, potassium, and chloride ions, into the duct system are active processes requiring energy. It is regulated by sev-

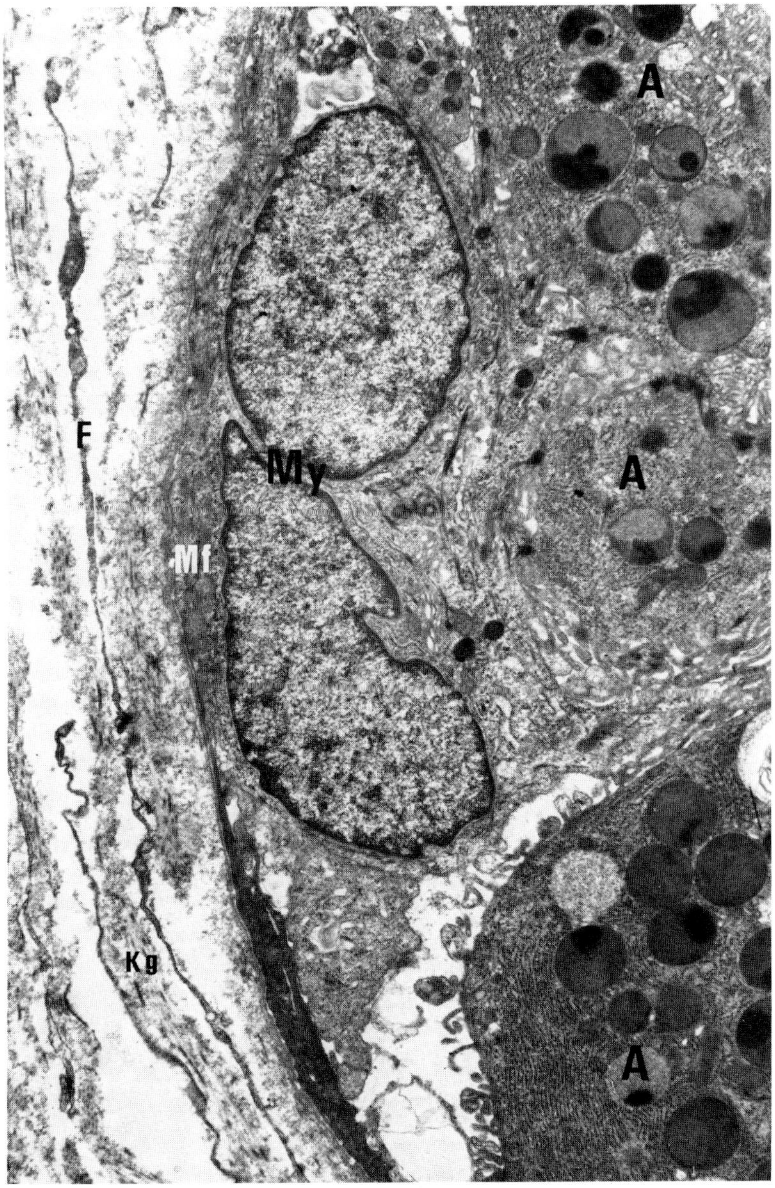

Figure 2.**14** Human parotid gland showing electron microscopic section of the base of an acinus with myoepithelial cells. A = three acinar cells with secretory granules of varying maturation, and endoplasmic reticulum, My = myoepithelial cell undergoing division with two cell nuclei, Mf = myofilaments, and interstitium with fibroblast offshoots (F) and collagen bundles (Kg). 7200×. (Seifert & Donath 1976.)

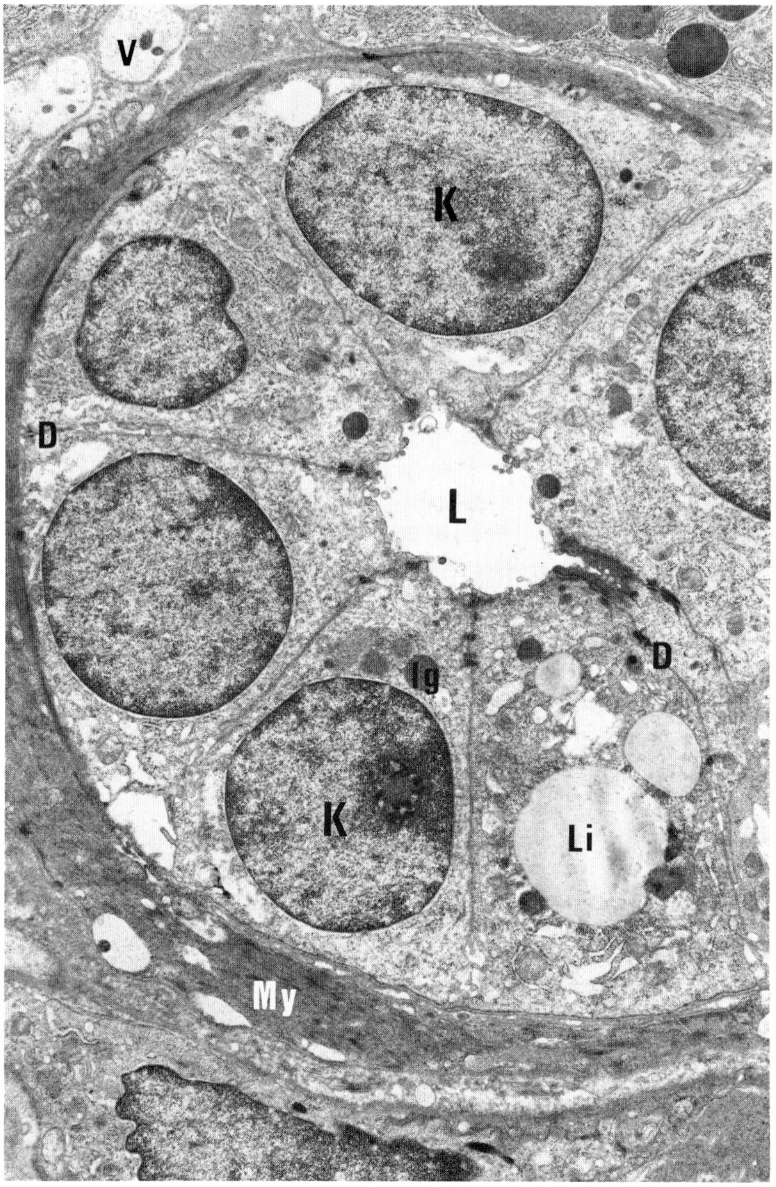

Figure 2.**15** Human parotid gland showing an electron microscopic section through an intercalated duct. L = lumen, K = cell nucleus, Ig = intracytoplasmic granule, Li = lipid droplet, My = myoepithelial cell, D = desmosome, V = varicosities of an autonomic nerve. 6900×. (Seifert & Donath 1976.)

eral factors, including the autonomic nervous system, the blood supply, the hydrostatic capillary pressure, and the ATP pump system. The epithelium of the *intercalated ducts* (Fig. 2.**15**) contains few cell organelles (mitochondria, granules, lipid droplets, and microvilli) and relatively large basal nuclei. Myoepithelial cells and varicosities of the autonomic nervous system lie on the external surface. The *striated ducts* (Fig. 2.**16**) possess a basal labyrinth consisting of fingerlike invaginations of the cell membrane and a porous filter for the active transport of osmolytes and water from the vascular system to the lumen of the duct. The potential energy is provided by ATPase on the cell membranes and by the mitochondrial enzymes arranged along the mitochondrial crest. A secretory stimulus leads to flattening of the luminal microvilli, and to formation of cytoplasmic blebs, which are transformed into large blisters and discharged by partial segmentation into the lumen.

Autonomic Nervous System: The preterminal nerve pathway consists of the clear Schwann cell and the infolded axons (Donath et al 1974, Donath 1976). The terminal axons lie only partially within the cytoplasmic processes of the Schwann cells and are surrounded externally by a basal membrane. The axons contain spindle-shaped varicosities with inclusions of neurotubules, neurofilaments, neurosecretory granules, and mitochondria. The varicosities of the terminal neural segments consist solely of

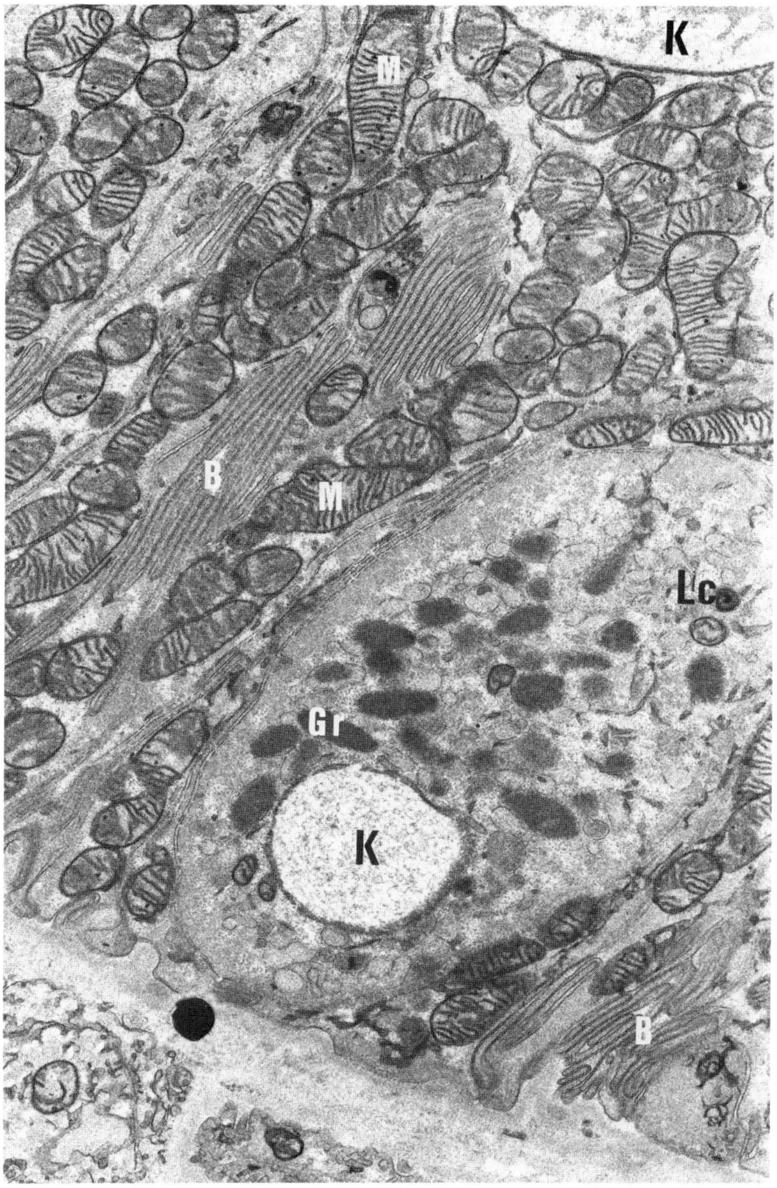

Figure 2.**16** Human parotid gland showing electron microscopic section through a striated duct of the parotid gland. B = basal labyrinth of the cell-limiting membrane with parallel arrangement of cytomembranes, M = mitochondria, Lc = interepithelial leukocytes, K = cell nucleus, Gr = granule. 13 100×. (Seifert & Donath 1976.)

neurosecretory granules and mitochondria. The spindle-shaped end swellings of the axons often contact the acinar cells and myoepithelium so that the basal membrane of the Schwann cell lies directly on the basal membrane of the effector cell. In addition, the acinar cells and intercalated duct cells possess direct synaptic contact for transmission of the stimulus. The terminal axon penetrates the basal membrane and lies in direct contact with the effector cell (Fig. 2.**17**). Two sorts of neurosecretory granules may be distinguished in the varicosities: the granular type with optically empty vesicles (the agranular vesicles) associated with the cholinergic system, and the granular type with optically dense nuclei (granular vesicles) associated with the adrenergic system.

Stimulation of the neuroreceptors by cholinergic or adrenergic impulses leads to characteristic changes in the granular structure (Donath 1976). Stimulation of the sympathetic system leads to rapid discharge of secretion and to protein synthesis characterized by swelling of the cell nucleus and nucleolus, an increase of the coarse endoplasmic reticulum, and formation of secretory granules. Parasympathetic stimulation leads to discharge of relatively small amounts of secretion and protein synthesis. Sympathetic paralysis leads to disorders of discharge of secretions and of protein synthesis, such as variation in size and optical density of the secretory granules and reduction of the protein-forming organelles, whereas paralysis of the parasympathetic system leads

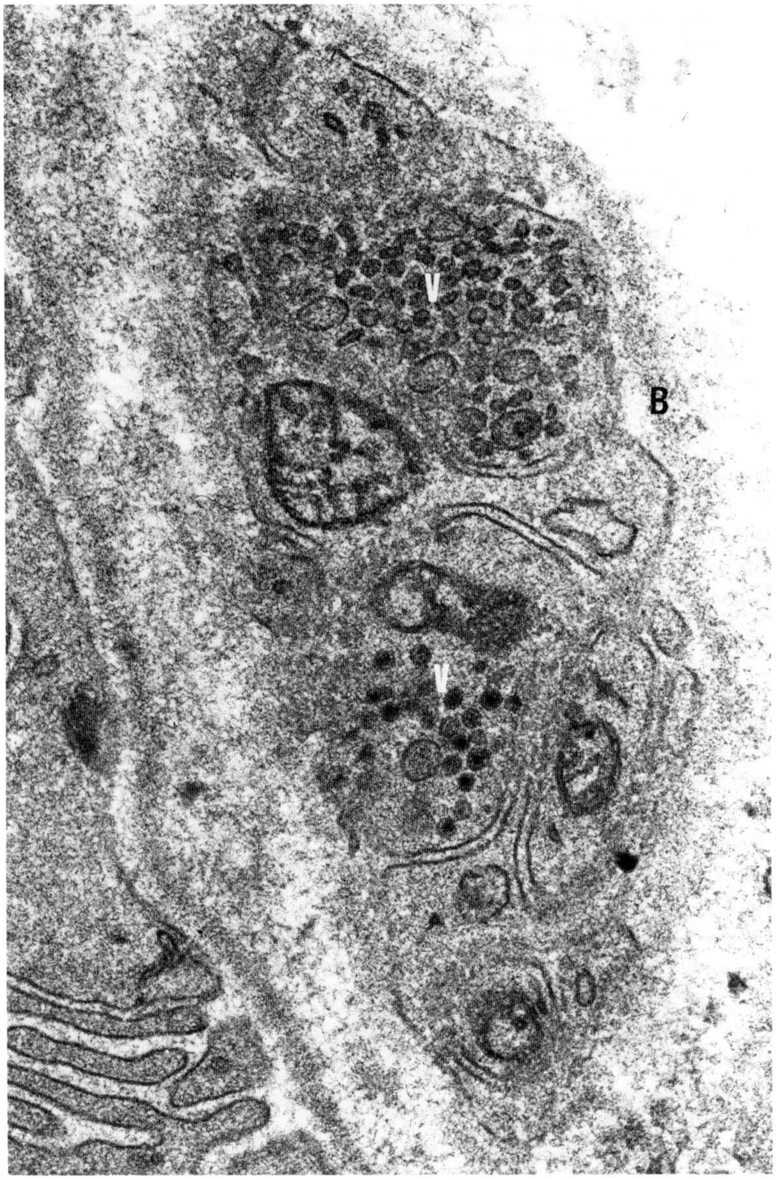

Figure 2.**17** Human parotid gland showing the ultrastructure of an autonomic nerve in the interstitium. B = basal membrane, V = varicosities of the preterminal axon with granular and agranular vesicles. 47 800×. (Seifert & Donath 1976.)

to disordered formation and discharge of secretions. An injury pattern also occurs on the terminal axons parallel to the changes in the glandular cells in sympathetic paralysis, leading to the loss of granular vesicles, destruction of mitochondria, disruption of the membrane, and formation of lysosomal bodies.

Clear Cells: Clear cytoplasm is the common, light microscopic hallmark of these salivary cells. Clear cells of this type occur in both normal salivary tissue and in salivary tumors (Seifert & Donath 1978). Analysis by cytochemistry and electron microscopy shows that these clear cells have a variable cytogenesis and functional significance.

In the *duct system* the clear cells are usually undifferentiated cells undergoing epithelial regeneration. The clear cytoplasm results from the slight provision of organelles (a sparse coarse endoplasmatic reticulum, few mitochondria, and few lysosomes). Cells resembling the clear cells may be formed in the intercalated ducts due to storage of glycogen granules, which are dissolved out during formol fixation. The other ultrastructural characteristics, such as the basal labyrinth and numerous mitochondria, resemble the structural elements of the intercalated ducts. Other clear cell forms of the duct system include myoepithelial cells, sebaceous cells (lipid vacuoles), and goblet cells (mucous vacuoles).

Modified clear acinar cells may be formed in the *glandular acini* by swelling and vacuolar transformation of the cytoplasm, particularly in sialadenosis and acinic cell tumors. Electron microscopy shows clear immature secretory granules in the cytoplasm.

Clear endocrine cells forming part of the disseminated endocrine cell system (Feyrter 1953, Pearse 1969, Carlsöö & Östberg 1976) with typical endocrine hormone granules are only rarely found in the intercalated ducts and acini of the human salivary glands (Donath & Seifert 1977). The question of partial endocrine function of the salivary glands requires further investigation. In some species of animals (in particular rodents, such as the mouse and rat) the submandibular gland shows sexual dimorphism. Furthermore, numerous pharmocologically active hormonelike substances, such as parotin, nerve growth factor, angiotensin, kallikrein, bradykinin, and salivogastrone, can be demonstrated. It is suspected that they are mainly formed in the duct system (Seifert 1960, 1964).

Regeneration of Salivary Tissue

The salivary glands belong to the stable tissues formed of reversible postmitotic cells. Under physiologic circumstances, these longlived cells demonstrate only a low regeneration rate for the replacement of lost cells, with a mitotic frequency less than 0.1%. Increased cell division similar to that in labile growth tissue may occur in certain circumstances, especially in the terminal ducts. Lost acini are usually not replaced, and the resulting space is much more likely to be filled by connective tissue and fat. Occasionally, the mitotic frequency of the acini increases to 3–4% under experimental conditions, such as exposure to isoproterenol (Seifert 1964).

The proliferative activity of the terminal duct system acquires a particular significance during development of the salivary glands. This regenerative potential persists after birth so that under certain pathologic conditions, such as inflammation, occlusion of the ducts, irradiation, and tumors, the terminal segment of the duct system (Fig. 2.**18**) may show regenerative hyperplasia (Langbein et al 1971, Donath et al 1973). Histologic examination shows ductular proliferation that can occasionally have an adenomatous arrangement and may also include cellular dysplasia. Parallel to this, the myoepithelial cells also show active increase initiated by formation of substances resembling the basal membrane. The intercalated ducts remain as an undifferentiated zone incapable of duct proliferation, but which may be regarded as the starting point of epithelial salivary gland tumors. Transplantation of human salivary cell tissue to the nude mouse is also accompanied by proliferation of the terminal ducts with ductal epithelium and myoepithelial cells and changes of the larger ducts similar to that found in obstructive sialadenitis (Sendler et al 1984).

Immunocytochemistry of the Salivary Glands

Recent developments in immunocytochemistry have allowed the demonstration of cell structures

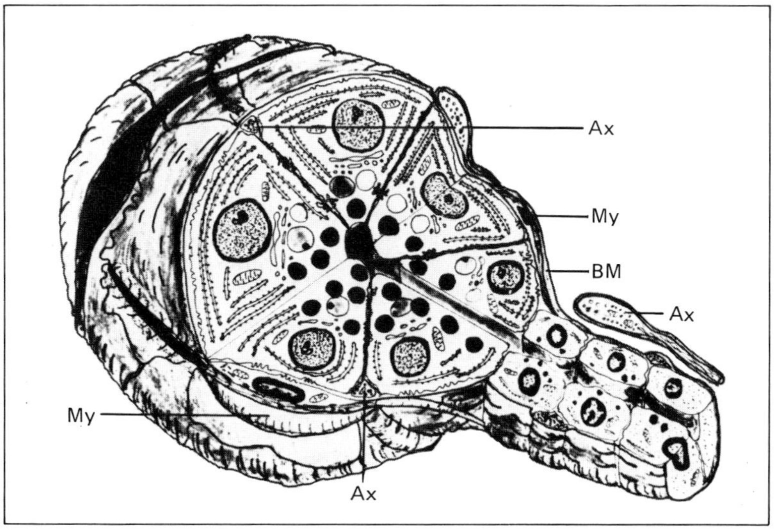

Figure 2.**18** Terminal duct with acinus: Axon (Ax) on the external surface of the intercalated segment and acinar cell. My = myoepithelial cell, BM = basal membrane. (Donath 1976.)

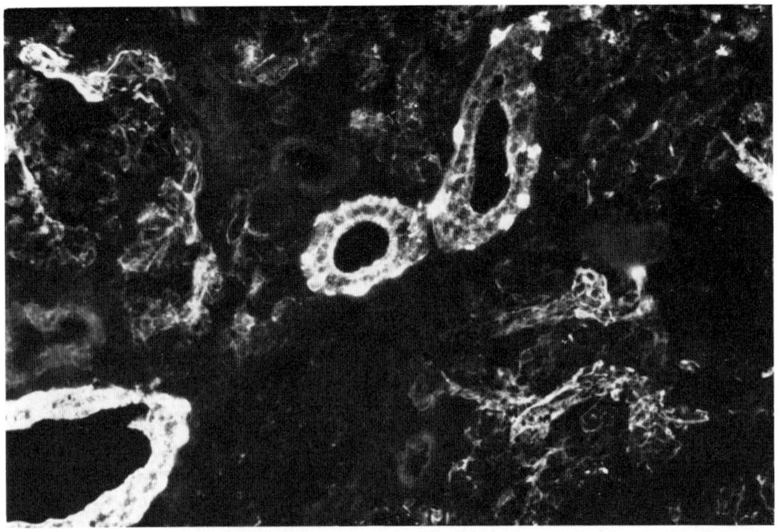

Figure 2.**19** Normal parotid gland demonstrating keratin in duct epithelium and myoepithelial cells. Immunofluorescence, 210 ×. (Caselitz et al 1982.)

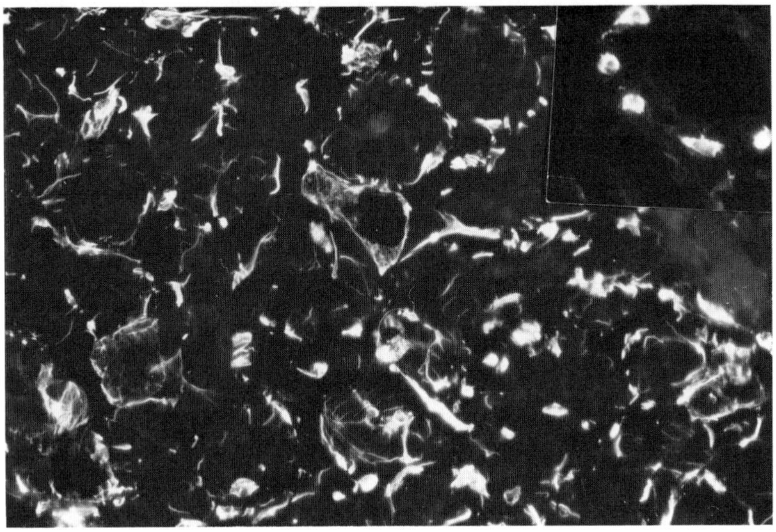

Figure 2.**20** Normal parotid showing vimentin in interstitial cells (fibroblasts and fibrocytes). Inset shows a positive demonstration of a periductal spindle-shaped myoepithelial cell. Immunoperoxidase, 20×. (Caselitz et al 1982.)

in tissue sections that occur in normal salivary gland tissue and also in tumors, and that can be used as tumor markers for the exact classification of poorly differentiated tumors (see page 173). Immunocytochemical reactions may be carried out on unfixed tissue and also on fixed tissue after paraffin embedding. The immunofluorescence technique and immunoperoxidase method may both be used (Heitz 1982, Sternberger 1979).

The components of the cytoskeleton, membrane-bound antigens, including lectin receptors, cytochemical cell products, cytochemically demonstrable immune phenomena, and viral reaction products may be demonstrated in a normal salivary gland with specific antisera (Seifert 1982).

The *components of the cytoskeleton* can be classified by their diameter into three groups: microfilaments, intermediate filaments, and microtubules. They are important for the various functions of the cell, such as the maintenance of the cell shape, participation in cellular transport processes, and cell movement. *Actin* is a contractile protein found in the duct epithelium, the myoepithelial cells, and the cells of the walls of blood vessels (Caselitz et al 1980, Caselitz & Löning 1981, Nilsen & Donath 1981). The *intermediate filaments* (Fig. 2.**19** and 2.**20**) include keratin, vimentin, and desmin. *Keratin,* one of the constituents of tonofilaments, can be demonstrated in duct epithelium and myoepithelial cells; vimentin occurs in mesenchymal cells, such as fibrocytes, endothelial cells, and smooth muscle cells; and desmin is found in muscle cells (Caselitz et al 1981c, 1981d, Seifert & Caselitz 1983, Löning et al 1982c). Spindle-shaped cells of the myoepithelial type contain both keratin and vimentin (Fig. 2.**20**.), a finding that requires further in-

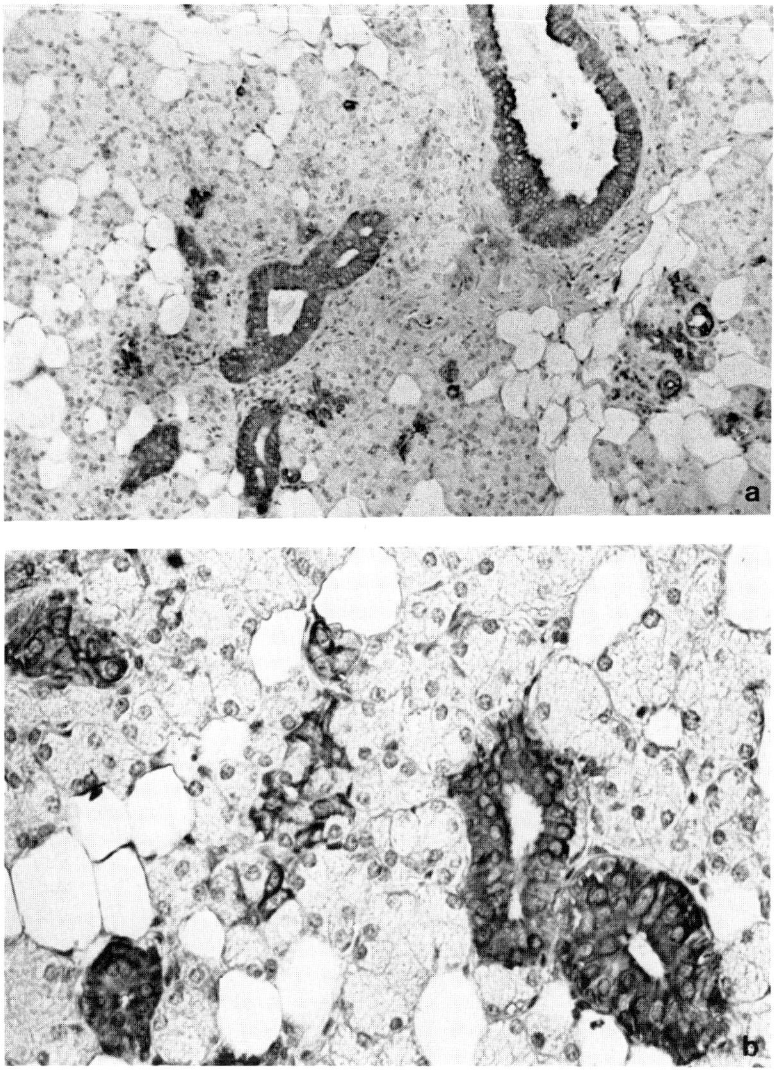

Figure 2.**21** Normal parotid gland showing Tissue Polypeptide Antigen. Immunoperoxidase. **a** 160×, **b** 400×.

terpretation in the light of the cytogenesis of the myoepithelial cell.

The main *cell membrane antigens* are the oncofetal antigen (carcinoembryonic antigen, [CEA]) and alpha-fetoprotein (AFP): AFP has not so far been demonstrated in the salivary glands, whereas CEA markers have been demonstrated on the apical pole of the acinar epithelium and intercalated duct cells (Caselitz et al 1981a). Tissue Polypeptide Antigen is a polypeptide localized to the cell membrane and the endoplasmic reticulum, especially of the terminal duct system (Fig. 2.**21a, b**). It is important in proliferation kinetics, for example, in ductular proliferation of the salivary gland (Caselitz et al 1983a).

Lectin receptors are found on the apical cell membrane (Fig. 2.**22**) of normal duct epithelium (Caselitz & Seifert 1981). Since lectins are glycoproteins that specifically bind to carbohydrates of the cell membrane, the properties of the cell surface may thus be investigated using these substances. Some lectins, such as peanut agglutinin (PNA), possess a particular affinity for blood group substances, for example, PNA lectin to the Thomsen-Friedenreich-antigen (the T antigen of the MN blood group system). A marked increase of reaction is produced by pretreatment with neuraminidase.

Enzymatic cell products provide an insight into the function of these cells. *Lactoferrin* is formed in the acinar and ductal epithelium (Caselitz et al 1981b) as is *lysozyme,* although with less intensity. *Amylase* may be demonstrated in the acini of the parotid especially (Caselitz et al 1983b, Morley et al 1983). The strength of the amylase reaction usually correlates with the granule content of the glandular cells (Fig. 2.**23**).

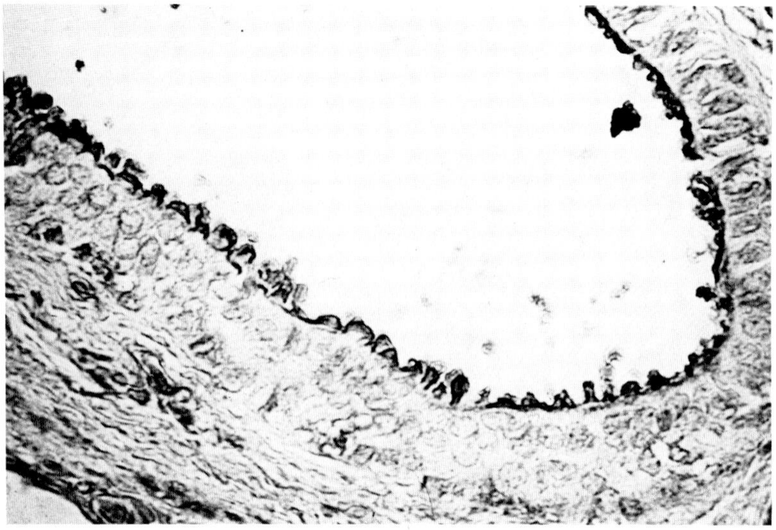

Figure 2.**22** Normal parotid with lectin (wheat germ agglutinin) on the apical cell membrane of a striated duct. Immunoperoxidase, 400×.

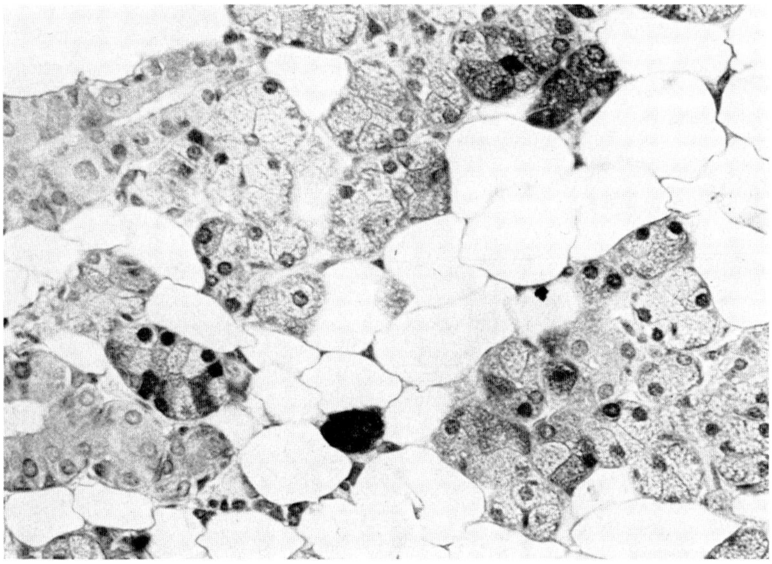

Figure 2.**23** Normal parotid gland showing amylase in individual acini. Immunoperoxidase, 400×.

The *cytochemical immune phenomena* include immunoglobulin synthesis by plasma cells (Löning 1977, Korsrud & Brandtzaeg 1982), differentiation of T lymphocytes by monoclonal antibodies (Caselitz et al 1983c), the demonstration of macrophages or Langerhans cells (Löning et al 1982b) and marking of the secretory component (Korsrud & Brandtzaeg 1982). The *virus-associated phenomena* are discussed in Chapter 12 under "Virus Sialadenitis."

References

Bennet, K. R., P. C. Reade: Salivary immunoglobulin A levels in normal subjects, tobacco smokers, and patients with minor aphthous ulceration. Oral Surg. 53 (1982) 461

Brandtzaeg, P.: Immunoglobulin systems of oral mucosa and saliva. In Dolby A. E.: Oral Mucosa in Health and Disease. Blackwell, Oxford 1976 (p. 137)

Carlsöö, B., Y. Östberg: On the occurrence of argyrophil cells in salivary glands. Cell Tiss. Res. 167 (1976) 341

Caselitz, J., Th. Löning: Specific demonstration of actin and keratin filaments in pleomorphic adenomas by means of immunoelectron microscopy. Virchows Arch. (Path. Anat.) 393 (1981) 153

Caselitz, J., G. Seifert: Immunhistologische Untersuchungen zum Verteilungsmuster von intrazytoplasmatischen Antigenen und Lektinrezeptoren bei Parotiskarzinomen. Verh. Dtsch. Ges. Path. 65 (1981) 378

Caselitz, J., G. Seifert: Das lokale Abwehr und Immunsystem der Speicheldrüsen unter physiologischen und pathologischen Bedingungen. Dtsch. Z. Mund-Kiefer-Gesichts-Chir. 6 (1982) 93

Caselitz, J., T. Jaup, G. Seifert: Presence of carcinoembryonic antigen in the normal and inflamed human parotid gland. J. Cancer Res. Clin. Oncol. 100 (1981a) 205

Caselitz, J., T. Jaup, G. Seifert: Lactoferrin and lysozyme in carcinomas of the parotid gland. A comparative immunocytochemical study with occurrence in normal and inflamed tissue. Virchows Arch. A. Path. Anat. 394 (1981b) 61

Caselitz, J., Th. Löning, G. Seifert: An approach to stain actin in parotid gland cells in paraffin-embedded material. – Staining by human anti-actin-antibodies using the indirect unlabelled immunoperoxidase technique. Virchows Arch. A. Path. Anat. Hist. 387 (1980) 301

Caselitz, J., A. Salfelder, G. Seifert: Cystadenolymphoma: An immunohistochemical study with monoclonal antibodies against lymphocyte antigens. J. oral Path. (1983c) im Druck
Caselitz, J., M. Osborn, G. Seifert, K. Weber: Intermediate-sized filament proteins (keratin, vimentin, desmin) in the normal parotid gland and parotid gland tumours. Virchows Arch. A. Path. Anat. Hist. 393 (1981d) 273
Caselitz, J., G. Seifert, B. Björklund, V. Björklund: Detection of tissue polypeptide antigen in salivary glands and salivary gland tumors. Appl. Pathol. 1 (1983a) 115
Caselitz, J., G. Seifert, G. Grenner, R. Schmidtberger: Amylase as an additional marker of salivary gland neoplasms. An immunoperoxidase study. Path. Res. Pract. 176 (1983b) 276
Caselitz, J., Th. Löning, M. J. Staquet, G. Seifert, J. Thivolet: Immunocytochemical demonstration of filamentous structures in the parotid gland. – Occurrence of keratin and actin in normal and tumoral parotid gland with special respect to the myoepithelial cells. J. Cancer Res. Clin. Oncol. 100 (1981c) 59
Crawford, J. M., M. A. Taubman, D. J. Smith: Minor salivary glands as a major source of secretory immunoglobulin A in the human oral cavity. Science 190 (1975) 1206
Donath, K.: Die Sialadenose der Parotis. Ultrastrukturelle, klinische und experimentelle Befunde zur Sekretionspathologie. Fischer, Stuttgart 1976
Donath, K., G. Seifert: Zur Problematik des "Helle-Zellen-Systems Feyrter" in der Parotis. – Ultrastrukturelle Untersuchungen. Verh. Dtsch. Ges. Path. 61 (1977) 108
Donath, K., G. Seifert: Immunologische und immunpathologische Reaktionen der Speicheldrüsen, Allergologie 4 (1981) 110
Donath, K., H.-U. Hirsch-Hoffmann, G. Seifert: Zur Pathogenese der Parotisatrophie nach experimenteller Gangunterbindung. Ultrastrukturelle Befunde am Drüsenparenchym der Rattenparotis. Virchows Arch. A. Path. Anat. Hist. 359 (1973) 31
Donath, K., M. Spillner, G. Seifert: The influence of the autonomic nervous system on the ultrastructure of the parotid acinar cells. Experimental contribution to the neurohormonal sialadenosis. Virchows Arch. A. Path. Anat. Hist. 364 (1974) 15
Eichner, E.: Die Bedeutung des Speichels für die Immunpathologie der Mundhöhle. Dtsch. Z. Mund-Kiefer-Gesichts-Chir. 6 (1982) 103
Feyrter, F.: Über die peripheren endokrinen (parakrinen) Drüsen des Menschen. Verlag Medizinische Wissenschaften, Wien 1953
Garrett, J. R., N. Emmelin: Activities of salivary myoepithelial cells: A review. Med. Biol. 57 (1979) 1
Gumberz, C. v., G. Seifert: Immunoglobulin containing plasma cells in chronic parotitis and malignant lymphomas of the parotid gland. Virchows Arch. A. Path. Anat. Hist. 389 (1980) 79
Heitz, Ph. U.: Immunocytochemistry. Theory and application. Acta histochem., Suppl. 25 (1982) 17
Hurliman, J.: Immunoglobulin synthesis and transport by human salivary glands. Curr. Top. Pathol. 55 (1971) 69
Korsrud, F. R., P. Brandtzaeg: Quantitative immunohistochemistry of immunoglobulin and J-chain-producing cells in human parotid and submandibular salivary glands. Immunology 39 (1980) 129
Korsrud, F. R., P. Brandtzaeg: Characterization of epithelial elements in human major salivary glands by functional markers: localization of amylase, lactoferrin, lysozyme, secretory component, and secretory immunoglobulins by paired immunofluorescence staining. J. Histochem. Cytochem. 30 (1982) 657
Langbein, H., S. Rauch, G. Seifert: Histochemische und autoradiographische Speicheldrüsenveränderungen nach partieller Speicheldrüsenresektion. Z. Laryng. Rhinol. 50 (1971) 672
Löning, Th.: Immunpathologie der Mundschleimhaut. Fischer, Stuttgart 1984
Löning, Th., A. Burkhardt, G. Seifert: Immunmorphologische Phänomene in der Mundhöhle. Dtsch. Z. Mund-Kiefer-Gesichts-Chir. 6 (1982a) 75
Löning, Th., J. Caselitz, G. Seifert, K. Weber, M. Osborn: Identification of Langerhans cells: simultaneous use of sera to intermediate filaments, T 6 and HLA-DR antigens on oral mucosa, human epidermis and their tumours. Virchows Arch. A. Path. Anat. Hist. 398 (1982b) 119
Löning, Th., J. Viac, J. Caselitz, J. Thivolet, H. F. Otto, G. Seifert: Comparative investigation of keratin filaments in normal tissues and tumours of skin, oral mucosa, salivary glands and thymus. Path. Res. Pract. 175 (1982c) 256
Morley, D. J., J. E. Hodes, J. Calland, M. E. Hodes: Immunohistochemical demonstration of ribonuclease and amylase in normal and neoplastic parotid glands. Human Path. 14 (1983) 969
Moro, I., S. Umemura, S. S. Crago, J. Mestecky: Immunohistochemical distribution of immunglobulins, lactoferrin, and lysozyme in human minor salivary glands. J. oral Path. 13 (1984) 97
Münzel, M.: Die Biochemie der menschlichen Speichelsekrete, Arch. Oto-Rhino-Laryng. 213 (1976) 209
Nilsen, R., K. Donath: Actin containing cells in normal human salivary glands. An immunohistochemical study. Virchows Arch. A. Path. Anat. Hist. 391 (1981) 315
Pearse, A. G. E.: The cytochemistry and ultrastructure of polypeptide hormone-producing cells of the APUD series and the embryologic, physiologic and pathologic implications of the concept. J. Histochem. Cytochem. 17 (1969) 303
Quintarelli, G.: Histochemical studies on human mucous-secreting salivary glands. Acta histochem. (Jena) 12 (1961) 1
Schäfer, Hj.: Zellkalzium und Zellfunktion. Fischer, Stuttgart 1979
Schätzle, W.: Histochemie der Speicheldrüsen. Acta histochem. (Jena) 13 (1962) 62
Seifert, G.: Über Spontanveränderungen der großen Kopfspeicheldrüsen bei Laboratoriumstieren. Beitr. path. Anat. 123 (1960) 299
Seifert, G.: Die Sekretionsstörungen (Dyschylien) der Speicheldrüsen. Ergebn. allg. Path. path. Anat. 44 (1964) 103
Seifert, G.: Mundhöhle, Mundspeicheldrüsen, Tonsillen und Rachen. In Doerr, W., E. Uehlinger: Spezielle pathologische Anatomie, Bd. I. Springer, Berlin 1966 (S. 1)
Seifert, G.: Der Einsatz von Tumormarkern bei der Diagnostik von Speicheldrüsentumoren. Wien. klin. Wschr. 94 (1982) 372
Seifert, G., J. Caselitz: Tumor markers in parotid gland carcinomas: Immunohistochemical investigations. Cancer Detect. Prev. 6 (1983) 119
Seifert, G., K. Donath: Die Morphologie der Speicheldrüsenerkrankungen. Arch. Oto-Rhino-Laryng. 213 (1976) 111
Seifert, G., K. Donath: Über das Vorkommen sog. heller Zellen in Speicheldrüsentumoren. Ultrastruktur und Differentialdiagnose. Z. Krebsforsch. 91 (1978) 165
Sendler, A., J. Caselitz, G. Seifert, P. Schmiegelow: Reaction pattern of xenografted human salivary glands in nude mice. Virchows Arch. (Path. Anat.) 403 (1984) 1
Sternberger, L. A.: Immunocytochemistry. Wiley, New York 1979
Tabak, L. A., M. J. Levine, I. D. Mandel, S. A. Ellison: Role of salivary mucins in the protection of the oral cavity. J. oral Pathol. 11 (1982) 1
Westhofen, M., H. Schäfer, G. Seifert: Calcium redistribution, calcification and stone formation in the parotid gland during experimental stimulation and hypercalcaemia. Cytochemical and X-ray microanalytical investigations. Virchows Arch. (Path. Anat.) 402 (1984) 425
Zimmermann, K. W.: Die Speicheldrüse der Mundhöhle und die Bauchspeicheldrüse. In: Handbuch der mikroskopischen Anatomie des Menschen, Bd. V/1. Springer, Berlin 1927

3. Development

The salivary glands are present from amphibia upward, but demonstrate varying differentiation in different species. Parotid glands are only present in mammals. All salivary glands arise from the ectoderm of the oral cavity and are thus comparable to other ectodermal derivatives, such as sweat, sebaceous, and mammary glands. The salivary glands originate from solid epithelial buds of the oral mucosa, with a variable growth potential. The anlage of the submandibular gland appears in the sixth embryonal week, that of the parotid in the seventh week, and that of the

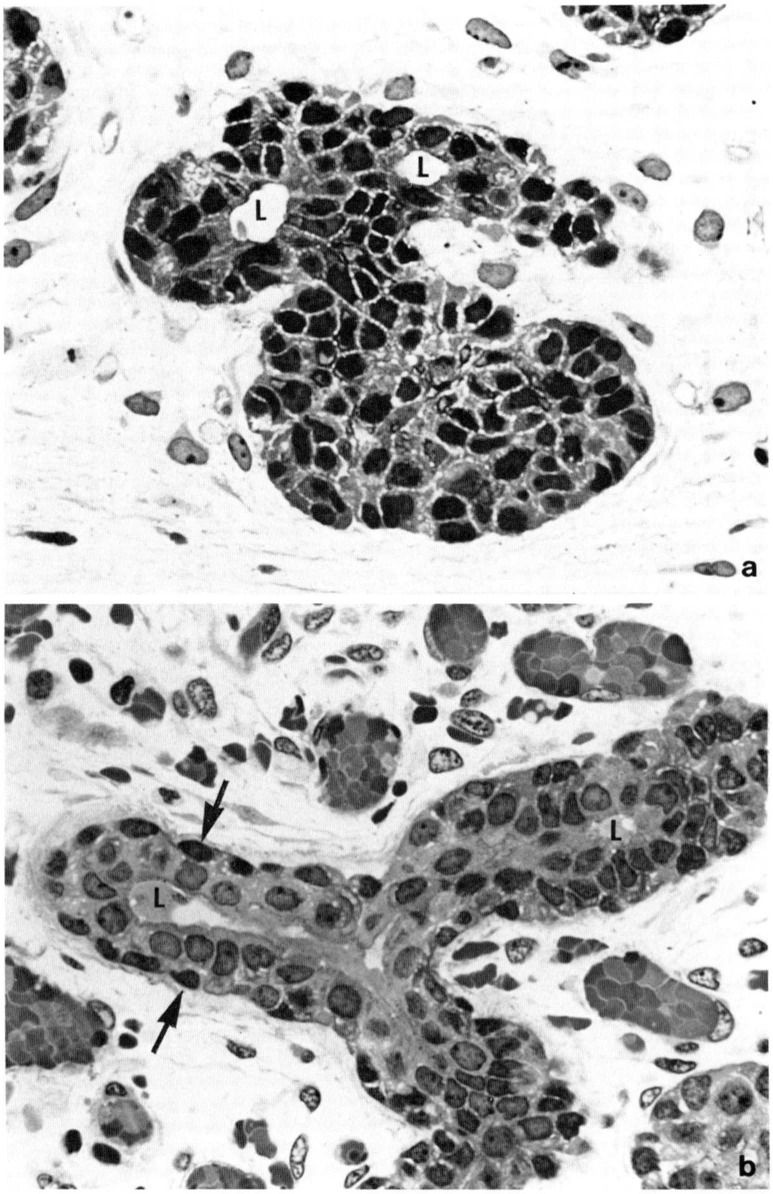

Figure 3.**1** Human fetal parotid at 20 weeks. **a** Primitive duct buds with narrow lumen (L) surrounded by loose mesenchyme. **b** Dichotomous duct bud with central lumen (L). Differentiation of an outer myoepithelial layer (arrows) with dark nuclei. Semithin section, toluidine blue. **a** 540×, **b** 700× (Seifert & Donath 1976.)

sublingual gland in the ninth week. The salivary glands have reached their final position at the end of the third embryonal month, at which time the parotid is the gland farthest removed from its point of origin in the mouth.

Three stages may be distinguished in the development of the salivary glands (Donath et al 1978). The first stage is characterized by the anlage and the development of the gland with dichotomic branched duct buds. The second stage shows further differentiation of the gland, with early formation of lobules and canalization of the ducts. This stage lasts until the seventh embryonal month and encompasses the period of formation of functional units. The third stage begins in the eighth embryonal month and leads to further structural maturation of the gland tissue, with differentiation of the acinar cells and intercalated ducts. The development of the glandular tissue is accompanied by reduction of the initially abundant interstitial connective tissue. The submandibular gland has a distinct capsule and is in an interfascial position, whereas the parotid gland develops in a niche of the subcutaneous tissue surrounded by connective tissue and it does not possess a distinct capsule (Becker et al 1978). The mobile sublingual gland lies in the sublingual connective tissue, which penetrates into the lobes of the gland so that a homogeneous capsule is not formed.

Detailed investigations are available of the special development of the human parotid glands (Bruenner 1962, Conley 1975, Gasser 1970, McKenzie 1948, Donath et al 1978). The primary anlage arises above the main trunk of the facial nerve between the temporofacial and cervicofacial divisions. The facial nerve divides the parotid into a superficial and a deep lobe.

In the first stage of the organ anlage (Fig. 3.**1a, b**) the duct buds possess two cell systems: embryonal ciliary epithelial cells that line the lumen, and myoepithelial cells that cover the external surface. In the second stage, dichotomic ramifications form new functional units of varying caliber, which are the forerunners of the later duct system. Myoepithelial cells are only found around the distal segment of the duct and the primitive acini. The first formation of coarse endoplasmic reticulum and supranuclear Golgi zones occurs in the glandular end pieces. In the third stage, a spherical distension of the glandular end units ensues. The caliber of the duct system matches that of the subsequent excretory duct, which does not yet show complete functional maturation. The striated ducts, in particular, cannot be recognized before birth. Secretion of saliva thus only occurs after birth under the influence of feeding. The early appearance of myoepithelial cells in the duct system indicates an ectodermal origin for this cell type. The number of myoepithelial cells decreases as the organ matures. After birth, new myoepithelial cells are formed by mitoses of these cells.

A further peculiarity of the development of the parotid is that an interstitium rich in lymphocytes is permeated by the buds of the glandular tissue. This explains the frequency of intraglandular lymph nodes with parenchymal inclusions in the parotid gland (Fig. 3.**2**), a finding rare in the

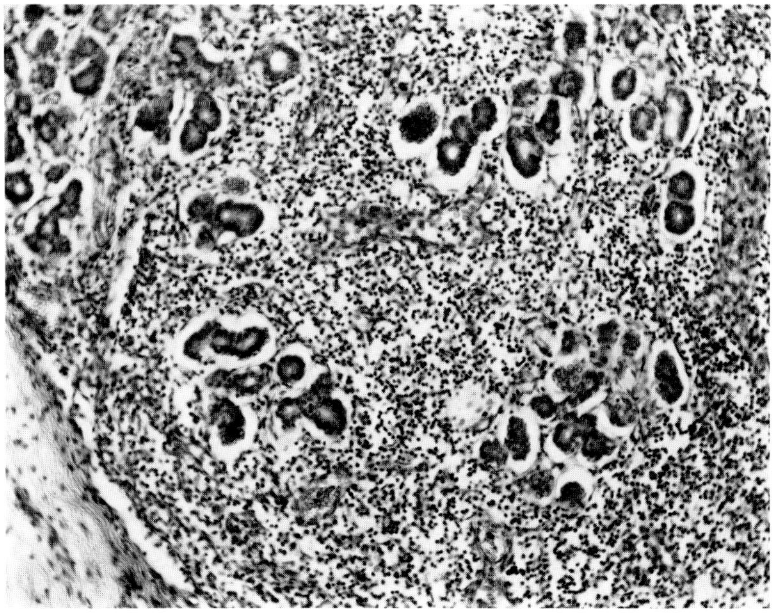

Figure 3.**2** Intraglandular parotid lymph nodes with duct inclusions (6-week-old baby). H & E, 160×.

submandibular gland and almost unknown in the sublingual gland (Seifert & Geiler 1956).

The human submandibular gland also develops through several stages (Gibson 1983). Initially, a network of primary ducts develops lined by a cell layer one or two cells thick. Electron microscopy shows that the cells have desmosomes and possess microvilli, glycogen granules are present in the cytoplasm, and secretory granules are found in the primitive acini, but their significance is as yet unknown. Myoepithelial cells lie on the external surface of the duct and on the glandular end pieces. The submandibular gland is relatively well differentiated at the time of birth.

The *Chievitz* (juxtaoral) organ develops from the epithelium of the masticatory pouch (Salzer & Zenker 1962) and is closely related to the buccal nerve. The epithelial cord formations are surrounded by connective tissue with inclusion of nerve fibers. In addition to their function as chemo- and pressure receptors, it is possible that they also have a paracrine secretory function. *Ackerknecht's organ* (Zorzoli 1949) lies close to the opening of the submandibular duct. It possesses a similar constitution to Chievitz's organ, and it is probably a receptor area.

References

Becker, W., J. Haubrich, G. Seifert: Krankheiten der Kopfspeicheldrüsen. In Berendes J., R. Link, F. Zöllner: Hals-Nasen-Ohren-Heilkunde in Praxis und Klinik, Bd. 3. Thieme, Stuttgart 1978 (S. 12.1)

Brünner, H.: Die embryonale Entwicklung der zweischichtigen Form der Glandula parotis. Anat. Anz. 111 (1962) 153

Conley, J.: Salivary Glands and the Facial Nerve. Thieme, Stuttgart 1975

Donath, K., H. Dietrich, G. Seifert: Entwicklung und ultrastrukturelle Cytodifferenzierung der Parotis des Menschen. Virchows Arch. A. Path. Anat. Hist. 378 (1978) 297

Gasser, R. F.: The early development of the parotid gland around the facial nerve and its branches in man. Anat. Rec. 167 (1970) 63

Gibson, M. H. L.: The prenatal human submandibular gland: a histological, histochemical and ultrastructural study. Anat. Anz. 153 (1983) 91

McKenzie, J.: The parotid gland in relation to the facial nerve. J. Anat. 82 (1948) 183

Salzer, G. M., W. Zenker: Das juxtaorale Organ (Chievitz'sches Organ). Bibl. anat. (Basel) 3 (1962) 1

Seifert, G., G. Geiler: Zur Pathologie der kindlichen Kopfspeicheldrüsen. Beitr. path. Anat. 116 (1956) 1

Zorzoli, G.: Ricerche e considerazioni sull'organo di Ackerknecht con particolare riferimento alla specie umano. Arch. ital. Anat. Embriol. 54 (1949) 144

4. Physiology and Biochemistry

The mouth is the first division of the human digestive tract. Its functions include assessment of the composition of food, preparation of food for digestion, and provision of defensive functions. A considerable part of this function is provided by the mixed saliva secreted by the major and minor salivary glands into the mouth. The production and control of saliva by autonomic reflexes have fascinated generations of physiologists during the last century. During the last two decades, modern methods of biochemistry and pharmocology have provided insight into the secretory process at a cellular level. The acinar cells of the parotid gland in particular have become a model for the investigation of the secretory mechanisms of exocrine glands.

Salivary Secretion

Innervation of the Salivary Glands

The stimulation experiments carried out on dogs in the last century by Bernard (1879), Loeb (1869), and Heidenhain (1878) still form the basis of the theory of innervation of salivary secretion. According to this theory, the parasympathetic system plays the central role in the secretory mechanism. The innervation of the parotid gland originates in the inferior salivatory nucleus with pathways via the glossopharyngeal nerve, the tympanic nerve, the tympanic plexus, and the lesser petrosal nerve. Pre- and postganglionic parasympathetic fibers synapse in the otic ganglion (Fig. 4.**1**). From there they follow the course of the auriculotemporal nerve to the parotid gland. The submandibular and sublingual glands derive their parasympathetic fibers from the superior salivatory nucleus via the nervus intermedius and the chorda tympani; the synapse is in the submandibular ganglion (Fig. 4.**2**). The rigid view that the nervus intermedius is the sole supply of the submandibular gland or the glossopharyngeal that of the parotid gland and that the parasympathetic is the salivary secretory nerve supply requires some modification.

There are probably many constant and inconstant anastomoses between the parasympathetic glossopharyngeal and intermedius fibers in man (Boyer & Gardner 1949, Chorobski 1951, Diamant & Wiberg 1965, Parisier et al 1978, Reichert & Poth 1932/1933, Vollrath et al 1980).

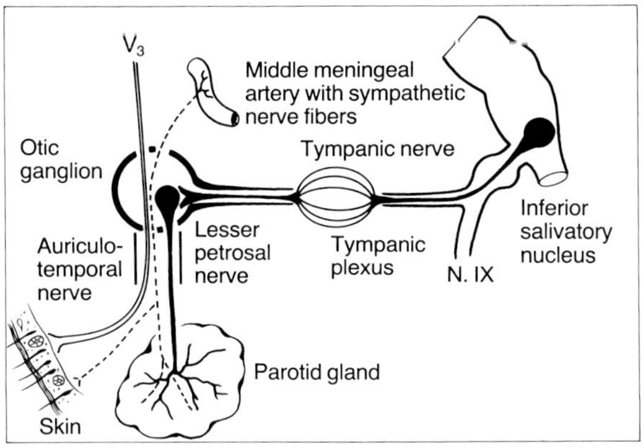

Figure 4.**1** Course of parasympathetic fibers to the otic ganglion. (Chilla.)
- - - - - - sympathetic fibers.
——— parasympathetic fibers.
═══ sensory fibers.

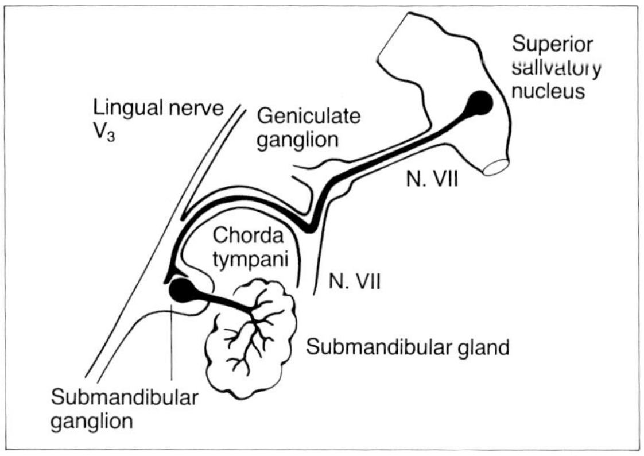

Figure 4.**2** Course of parasympathetic fibers to the submandibular gland. (Chilla.)
- - - - - - sympathetic fibers.
——— parasympathetic fibers.
═══ sensory fibers.

The possible significance of parasympathetic fibers of the chorda tympani for innervation of the parotid gland is of particular interest. The presence of such fibers has been challenged by many investigators (Diamant & Wiberg 1965, Reichert & Poth 1932/1933, Yannoulis & Manolidis 1958, Rauch 1959). Indeed, Ross (1970) could not produce parotid secretion by stimulation of the chorda tympani in the human middle ear.

Not all parasympathetic fibers reach the parotid gland via the auriculotemporal nerve, even in the dog, the classic animal for salivary secretion experiments (Holmberg 1971).

The *double innervation of the salivary glands* by the parasympathetic and sympathetic nerves was first suspected in 1851 by Ludwig based on sympathetic stimulation, but was later often interpreted as being due to the vascular effect of the sympathetic system. His suspicions were confirmed much later by histologic and electron microscopic examinations, which have shown that the human parotid gland is supplied equally by sympathetic and parasympathetic fibers (Eneroth et al 1969). Further confirmation was provided by the demonstration of secretory mechanisms and their disturbance by denervation (see Chapter 21).

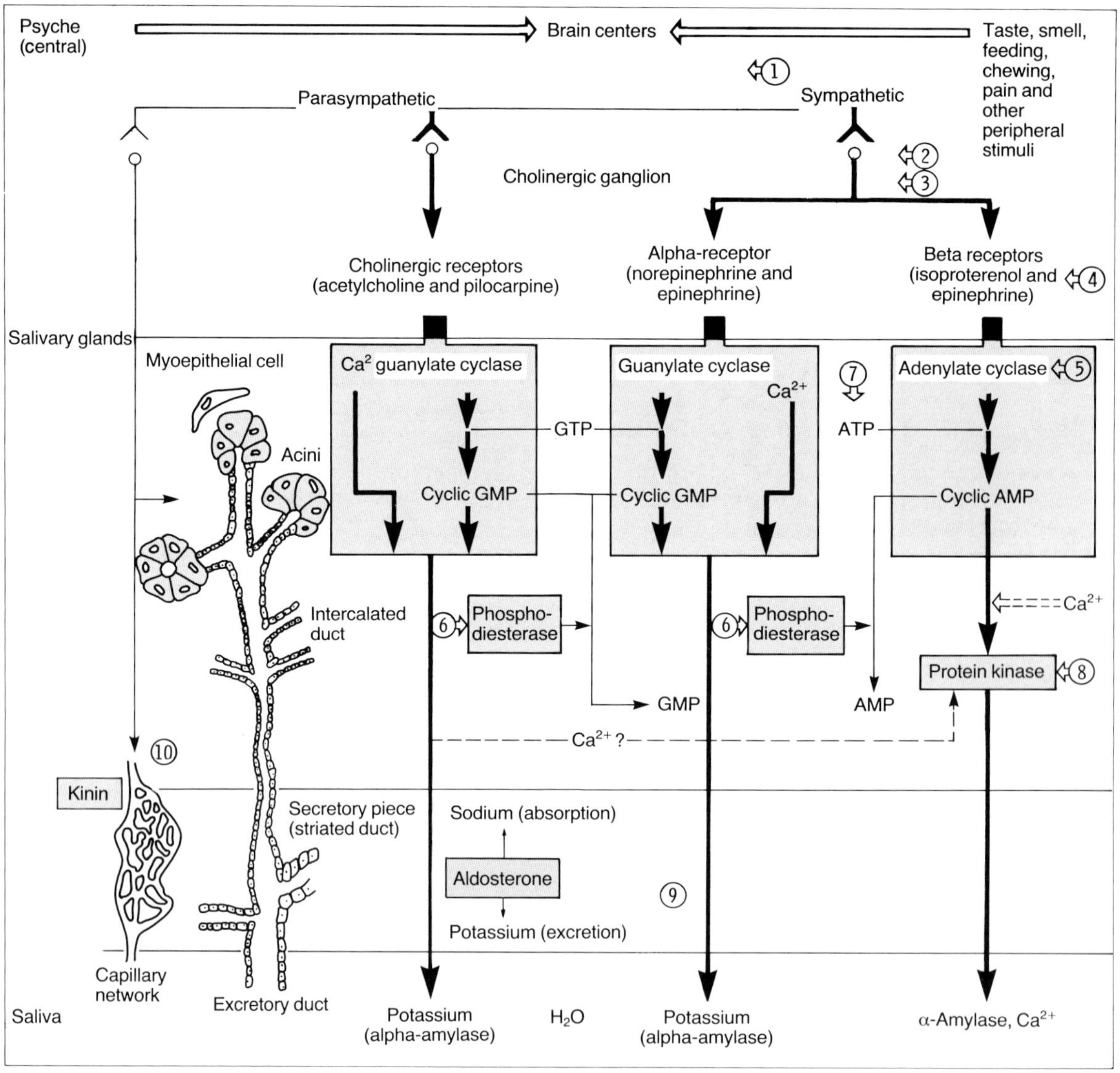

Figure 4.**3** A diagram of the secretory mechanisms in the parotid gland. Adrenergic and cholinergic receptors on the acinar cell and also on the myoepithelial cell are activated by several reflex arcs by which the gland is provided with postganglionic parasympathetic and sympathetic nerve fibers. The numbers indicate the point of action of the various pharmaceutic agents (see Table 4.**1**). (Chilla.)

Secretory Mechanism

A continuous resting secretion of saliva is excreted into the mouth without any external influence, and this is probably due to spontaneous activity of the salivatory nuclei in the brainstem. Increased quantities of saliva are secreted above this basal requirement in response to the stimulation of chewing, taste, and smell (Fig. 4.**3**). The minor salivary glands, the sublingual gland and the submandibular gland produce a mucous saliva (Table 4.**2**). The less viscous saliva, which is rich in digestive enzymes such as alpha-amylase, is mainly produced by the parotid gland (Mason & Chisholm 1975) (Table 4.**3**).

The impulses for salivary secretion arise in the cerebral centers and reach the acini via sympathetic and parasympathetic fibers. Indirect autonomic innervation is also possible by direct stimulation of the receptors by adrenergic and cholinergic substances circulating in the blood, but this hormone-dependent salivary secretion is of little significance.

The sympathetic system is the main regulator of protein secretion via the beta-adrenergic receptors. In contrast, the secretion of electrolytes is activated by alpha-adrenergic or cholinergic receptors (Chilla & Arold 1975). A reciprocal influence of these secretory mechanisms activated by three different receptors has been shown by repeated experiments (Gjoerstrup 1977, 1979). Thus, the amylase secretion released by adrenergic receptors is increased more than additively by simultaneous cholinergic stimulation: amylase is produced in small amounts by cholinergic receptors (Butcher et al 1976, Leslie et al 1976).

The intracellular mechanisms that lead to the secretion of electrolytes and water and to the discharge of zymogen granules are not yet completely explained. Cyclic AMP plays a decisive role for the beta receptor mechanism of protein secretion. Cyclic GMP could take over this role for the alpha-adrenergic and cholinergic receptors for whose function the exchange between extra- and intra-cellular calcium is important. A displacement of calcium between intracellular stores has been demonstrated for protein secretion via beta-adrenergic receptors (Putney et al 1977, Selinger 1975). The primary saliva produced by the acinus is isotonic with plasma, but becomes hypotonic in the striated ducts, which histologically resemble the distal tubules of the kidney. Sodium is resorbed and potassium is secreted at this site under the influence of aldosterone (Mangos & McSherry 1969, Shannon et al 1974).

Investigations into the changes of the saliva in the larger ducts have so far almost exclusively been carried out on the parotid duct (Laugesen et al 1976, Peterson 1970, Schneyer 1969). The secretory pressure in the duct system can be increased by contraction of the myoepithelial cells (Eneroth et al 1969, Garrett & Emmelin 1979, Shannon et al 1974).

Hormonal Influences on Salivary Secretion

Numerous investigations have been carried out on the influence of hormones and hormone-like substances on salivary secretion. Some of the results that are clinically important, or that could become so, will be summarized.

In the rat, thyroxine increases the sensitivity of the adrenergic beta-receptors to the neurogenic transmitters (Nelson & Stouffer 1972, Pointon & Banerjee 1979).

In man, synthetic calcitonin increases the amylase secretion of the parotid gland, but not that of the pancreas (Drack et al 1976).

Gastrointestinal hormones can influence salivary secretion (Malfertheiner et al 1980). Opinions vary about the effect of secretin and pancreozymin on the parotid secretion. Some investigations have shown that administration of secretin-pancreozymin has no influence on the parotid gland, in particular on its amylase secretion (Descos et al 1973, Drack et al 1976), whereas others claim to have shown such an influence (Grimmel et al 1976, Mulcahy et al 1972). Some peptides, such as physalaemin and eledoisin, stimulate the secretion of the salivary glands (Cantalamessa et al 1975, Thulin 1976). Receptors have even been demonstrated on the acinar cells for another peptide, substance P, which is formed mainly in neural tissue (Friedman & Selinger 1978, Liang & Cascieri 1979).

Influence of Drugs on Salivary Secretion

All drugs acting on the autonomic nervous system influence the parotid gland to a greater or lesser extent. These substances can act directly on the acinar cells, they may achieve their effect via the autonomic centers, or via the smooth musculature of the vascular system and the myoepithelial cells that regulate the blood flow through the gland and thus the metabolism and filtration processes of the gland. The drugs that influence the function of the salivary gland, and the point at which they do so are given in Table 4.**1**. In some cases the effect of these drugs has only been demonstrated experimentally and has no clinical relevance. A summary of the effect of some of the important, frequently used drugs follows.

Table 4.**1** Pharmaceutical Agents that Affect the Secretion of the Parotid Gland (Chilla & Arold)

Secretions Increased	Secretions Inhibited	Point of Action (see Fig. 4.**3**)	Reference
	Psychotropic drugs	1, 4	Fischbach 1973 Holmberg 1971 Kielholz 1966
	Antihypertensive drugs:		
	Clonidine	1, 10	Chilla et al 1975
	Methyldopa	1, 3, 10	Bock 1970
	Reserpine	1, 3, 10	Bock & Huep 1971
	Guanethidine	3, 10	
Nicotine in small doses	Nicotine in large doses	2	Volle 1966
	Ganglion blockers	2	Inoki et al 1971
Direct sympathomimetic drugs (for example, isoproterenol)		4, 10	Mandel & Katz 1968 Ansel 1974 Byrt 1966 Speirs et al 1974
Indirect sympathomimetic		4, 10	
Direct parasympathomimetic (for example, pilocarpine)		4	Currey & Patey 1964 Reinecke 1967
Indirect parasympathomimetic		4	
	parasympatholitic (for example, atropine)	4	Shannon et al 1969 Mandel & Katz 1968
	alpha receptor blockers (for example, phentolamine)	4	Arold & Schätzle 1973
	beta receptor blockers (for example, propranolol)	4	Schramm & Seliger 1974
Fluorides,		5	Schramm & Naim 1970
caffeine, theophylline		6	Kojima et al 1971
	Metabolic poisons:		
	dinitrophenol, oligomycin	7	Feinstein & Schramm 1970
	tolbutamide	8	Kanamori et al 1974
	aldosterone antagonists (for example, spironolactone)	9	Bartter 1960

Dryness of the mouth is a side effect of many *psychotropic drugs*, particularly the antidepressive agents such as the tricyclic thymoleptic drugs. They often cause troublesome dryness of the mouth that is ascribed to their atropine-like or anticholinergic effects (Fischbach 1973).

Dryness of the mouth is also a well-known side effect of many *antihypertensive agents*, including clonidine, methyldopa, those containing reserpine, and the guanethidine group (Chilla & Arglebe 1975). The method of action of these drugs varies. All inhibit the sympathetic and, unlike the antidepressive agents, interfere with the sympathetic innervation of the salivary glands. Thus, guanethidine and methyldopa inhibit the postganglionic sympathetic stimulation (Kroneberg et al 1962), whereas clonidine is said to inhibit the parasympathetic innervation by the stimulation of central alpha-adrenergic receptors (Green et al 1979). Pain in the parotid gland is less common than dryness of the mouth but is also a more severe symptom that can be caused by antihypertensive drugs. It occurs in 10% of patients taking clonidine, in 5% taking methyldopa and guanethidine derivatives and after guanethidine, guanoxan and guanacline (Bock et al 1966, Bock 1968, 1970, Bock & Huep 1971, Pirsig et al 1973, Schneider 1973). This pain is most marked when the patient starts to chew and usually affects both salivary glands. It is caused by the stimulus of secretion so that the pain syndrome is produced particularly by those acid foods that stimulate parotid secretion. In many cases the pain begins to fade after a few seconds and disappears during the course of the meal, although it can persist at a lower intensity. Many patients attempt to reduce this pain by taking small bites (Bock & Huep 1971, Schneider 1973). The pain syndrome disappears after antihypertensive agents are withdrawn. Resistant cases only occur after guanacline (Bock & Huep 1971, Pirsig et al 1973).

The chronic use of sympathomimetics leads to a sialadenosis with noninflammatory swelling of the gland. This occurs quite often in chronic asthmatics who use sympathomimetic aerosols frequently (Borsanyi & Blanchard 1961). Hyperplasia and hypertrophy of the parotid gland due to chronic use of sympathomimetics such as isoproterenol has been known experimentally for a long time (Selye et al 1969). It may be prevented by taking beta receptor blockers (Arold & Schaetzle 1973).

The increase in salivary secretion caused by anethole trithione is used in the treatment of various forms of xerostomia. Little is known about the mechanism of this drug whose activity depends on the presence of salivary parenchyma capable of active secretion.

Salivary Glands and Hormones

In addition to the influence of hormones on salivary secretion, the salivary glands themselves may have an endocrine function. Such an endocrine function has certainly been demonstrated in many animals, such as the cow and the mouse, but not so far in man.

Japanese workers especially have isolated a protein hormone called *parotin* from the parotid glands of cows and pigs that has regulatory properties in protein synthesis and in the calcification of cartilage and that lowers the calcium level in the blood (Ito & Mizutani 1952, Mizutani et al 1976, Ogata et al 1944, Takizawa 1954, Tieche et al 1980). It has not yet clearly been demonstrated whether a similar hormone is formed in the human salivary glands. The relationship between the salivary glands and disorders of sugar metabolism is also not clear. *Glucagon*, a hormone that increase the blood sugar level, is synthesized in the submandibular gland of both mice (Kim et al 1979) and men (Lawrence et al 1977, Pérez-Castillo & Blasquez 1980).

Godlowski et al (1971) have demonstrated a *trypsin inhibitor* in the submandibular gland that is said to inhibit a proteinase that splits proinsulin into the active insulin. This inhibitor prevents the synthesis of an adequate amount of insulin. Definite improvement or even resolution of the disease may be achieved in diabetic dogs and man by removal of the salivary glands (Godlowski et al 1971). Others workers have been unable to confirm these results (Steinberg et al 1972).

It has been known for a long time that *renin* is produced in the submandibular gland in the mouse (Bing & Poulsen 1979, Werle et al 1957). This substance releases angiotensin, which increases the blood pressure, from angiotensinogen and is produced in the submandibular gland of the mouse (Bing & Poulsen 1979, Werle et al 1957). It could even explain the secretory mechanism via alpha-adrenergic receptors (Michelakis et al 1976). It is not known whether the human submandibular gland produces renin.

The enzyme *kallikrein* should also be mentioned among the hormones and hormonelike substances formed in the human salivary glands (Schachter 1964). This is a peptidyl-peptide-hydrolase that can release hormonelike substances from serum protein. The kallikrein of human saliva splits a kininogen to form kinins, which can relax smooth muscle and thus reduce the blood pressure. The dilation of the blood vessels in the submandibular gland after stimulation of the chorda tympani is said to be due to a kallikrein effect (Ellison 1967).

Vitamin D is not a vitamin but a hormone that is a precursor from which the body itself produces the active hormone. This is mainly effected in the kidney, but also in the parotid gland, at least in the rat, which possesses the necessary enzymes (Goodwin et al 1978).

Volume of Saliva and Physiologic Changes

It is often stated that the daily production of saliva is 1–1,5 liters (Rauch 1959), but estimates of 500–600 ml are more realistic (Mason & Chisholm 1975).

There are also varying estimates of the contribution of different salivary glands to the total secretion (Tables 4.**2**, 4.**3**). The highest values are found for the submandibular gland, since this

Table 4.**2** Contribution of Individual Salivary Glands to the Daily Salivary Secretion (Münzel)

Gland	Total Volume (%)
Parotid gland	25
Submandibular gland	71
Sublingual gland	3–4
Minor glands	Trace

Table 4.**3** Contribution of Individual Salivary Glands to the Entire Secretion under Varying Degrees of Stimulation (Kerr)

Stimulation	Submandibular Gland (%)	Parotid Gland (%)
Minimal	66.6	33.3
Half maximal	50.0	50.0
Maximal	33.3	66.6

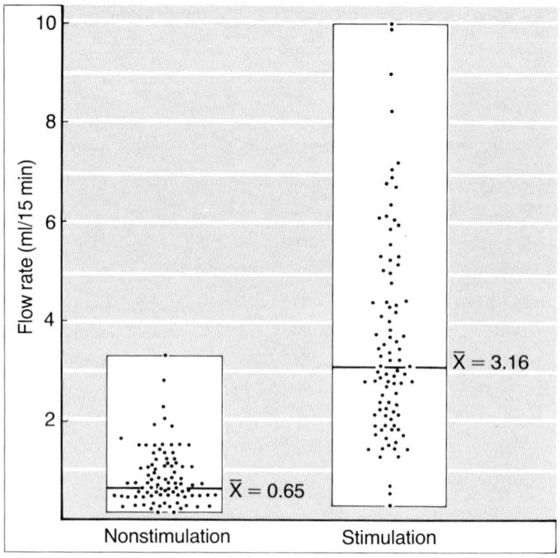

Figure 4.**4** Flow rate of stimulated and nonstimulated parotid saliva in 90 healthy subjects. X̄ = mean.

gland has the highest resting secretion. The volume of secretion of the parotid gland may exceed that of the submandibular gland in response to stimulation, for example, that of eating.

The contribution of the minor salivary glands is difficult to determine. It is thought to be slight (Muenzel 1976), with a value of 7–8% of the total (Dawes & Wood 1973).

The flow of saliva is subject to considerable physiologic changes, the most important being eating. The flow rate of stimulated saliva considerably exceeds the volume of the resting secretion. Figure 4.**4** shows the measurement of parotid secretion in 90 subjects. Eating was simulated by stimulation with citric acid.

Different but reproducible values are obtained if the secretion of saliva is measured at different times of the day at rest and also after stimulation. The many factors that influence the secretion of saliva include a *circadian rhythm* (Dawes & Ong 1973a, 1973b, Dawes 1974, Ferguson et al 1973, Ferguson & Botchway 1980), climate (Shannon 1966), ingestion of food (Behall et al 1973, Blumberger & Glatzel 1963, Dawes 1975, Kelsay et al 1972), the effect of light (Shannon & Feller 1974, Shannon et al 1975), age and sex (Vogt & Semmann 1970), and physical activity (Gilman et al 1979). These factors also affect the composition of the saliva. Correlation between the personality and the salivary flow rate has even been reported (Costa et al 1980).

It is difficult to deduce normal values for stimulated and resting secretion from the literature (Tables 4.**5**, 4.**6**) because of the different circumstances under which the saliva was obtained. The difficulties include: a small number of subjects (Dawes & Ong 1973, Kaiser et al 1974, Knauf & Froemter 1970), the selection of subjects, for example young men (Shannon et al 1974) or students (Benedek-Spät 1973a, 1973b), and finally quotes of variance without demonstrating that the data are normally distributed (Benedek-Spät 1973a, 1973b, Kreusser et al 1972, Shannon et al 1974). For these reasons, data about saliva vary considerably. Each investigator is advised to develop normal values using an accurately standardized method and taking the parameters just mentioned into account. This process is illustrated in Chapter 7: it allows comparison of abnormal values.

Composition of Saliva

Saliva is a watery solution of various substances of high and low molecular weight. Table 4.**4** provides an overview of the composition of the mixed saliva that, like parotid saliva, has been most analyzed. Electrolytes, proteins, and their solute water are the most important secretion products of the salivary glands independent of the site of production.

Electrolytes

Factors that influence the flow rate, just discussed also usually change the composition of the saliva. Thus, the electrolyte concentration shows a pronounced daily rhythm (Dawes & Ong 1973a, 1973b, Ferguson et al 1973, 1974). A 12-hour gap between the highest and the lowest values is typical, and the lowest values are about 40–50% of the maximum. The pH of saliva, the flow rate, and the content of inorganic phosphate show the same rhythm as the temperature in the mouth, with a minimum in the early morning (at 6 o'clock) and a peak value in the late afternoon (also at 6 o'clock). The sodium, iodine, and chloride ion concentrations show a reverse relationship, whereas the potassium ion concentration does not show this 12-hour rhythm (Ferguson et al 1974).

The *hydrogen ion concentration* (pH) of saliva varies around neutral (Table 4.**4**). The nonstimulated secretion of the parotid and submandibular glands have slightly acid pH values (Dawes 1969, Ferguson et al 1974), which become alkaline after stimulation. The increasing bicarbonate (HCO_3) content with increasing flow rate, which is accompanied by a decrease in dihydrogen phosphate (H_2PO_4) increases the pH of parotid saliva from 5.8–7.4 (Dawes 1969, Vogel et al 1965) H_2PO_4/

HPO_4 and H_2CO_3/HCO_3 are two buffer systems that along with proteins provide the saliva with a *buffer capacity*.

In unstimulated parotid secretion the *potassium ion concentration* is higher than the *sodium ion concentration* (Tables 4.**5**, 4.**6**). After stimulation, the ratio is inverted (Dawes 1969, Shannon 1973).

Calcium occurs in the saliva in an ionized and in a protein-bound form. The ratio is about 1 : 1. The total concentration (Dawes 1969, Dawes & Ong 1973a, 1973b, Ferguson et al 1974, Skurk et al 1973) is higher in nonstimulated submandibular saliva at 2–8 mmol/l than in unstimulated parotid secretion at 0.2–2.5 mmol/l and increases somewhat after stimulation.

The concentration of *chloride ion* in nonstimulated parotid and submandibular secretion follows the rhythm of the sodium ion concentration and lies between 17 and 22 mmol/l (Dawes 1969, Dawes & Ong 1973, Ferguson et al 1974). *Fluoride* is only found in traces in the saliva (about 5 µmol/l) (Ferguson 1975, Shannon et al 1974).

The large number of variables that can influence the electrolyte concentration in the saliva is reflected in the abundant data in the literature, and the impossibility of providing reliable ranges, as can be done for the serum electrolyte concentrations. A good summary of the electrolyte concentrations in the saliva at different flow rates and under the influence of various factors has been worked out by Shannon et al (1974). Table 4.**7** provides the values for the most important electrolytes from a selection of the available data.

Table 4.**4** Properties and Constituents of Human Saliva (Kolb)

pH	6.7 (5.6–7.6)
Density	1.01–1.02
Freezing point lowering	0.34–0.7
Resting secretion, ml/min.	0.6 (0.1–1.8)
Dry substances, g/dl	0.6 (0.1–1.0)
Ash content, g/dl	0.2
Mucin, mg/dl	270 (100–600)
Total nitrogen, mg/dl	90 (40–125)
Nonprotein nitrogen, mg/dl	35 (10–60)
Glucose, mg/dl	20 (1228)
Citrate, mg/dl	1.0 (0.2–3)
Cholesterol, mg/dl	8 (3–15)
Sodium, mg/dl	40 (15–55)
Potassium, mg/dl	55 (45–60)
Calcium, mg/dl	6 (4–10)
Inorganic phosphate, mg/dl	15 (7–20)
Total phosphate, mg/dl	19
Chloride, mg/dl	60 (40–70)

Table 4.**5** Constituents of Resting Saliva. Mean Values Vary, Depending on the Method of Obtaining the Saliva, and the Type and Number of Subjects (Chilla)

No. Subjects	Sodium Ion Concentration (mmol/l)	Potassium Ion Concentration (mmol/l)	Flow rate (ml/min)	Method of Collection	Remarks	References
513 527	2.65	25.4–46.3 (decreasing with increasing flow rate)	0.027 0.042		In summer In winter (in young men)	Shannon et al 1974
61	6.7	24		Sialography (using needle)		Brands 1972
	3.14 (n = 18)	29.7 (n = 29)	0.048 (n = 32)	Plastic tube	Students (in morning, fasting)	Benedek-Spät 1973a
			0.058	Capsule	Patients	Rauch & Khaksar 1966
			0.035	Plastic tube		
35	2–8	About 25	0.03–0.11	Plastic tube	Patients (18–35 yr)	Eichner et al 1975
71			3.1 drops/min, which equals 0.031 ml/min	Capsule		Enfors 1962
7	1.3	28.4		Capsule		Dawes & Ong 1973b

Table 4.**6** Constituents of Stimulated Saliva. Mean Values Vary Depending on the Type of Stimulus, Method of Obtaining the Saliva, and Number and Type

No. Subjects	Sodium Ion Concentration (mmol/l)	Potassium Ion Concentration (mmol/l)	Flow Rate (ml/min)	Method of Collection	Method of Stimulation	Remarks	Reference
125	64.41	18.15	1.18	Capsule	Lemon juice drops		Shannon et al 1974
26			0.75 ml/min × m^2	Capsule	Citric acid	Children	Schöni et al 1975
	21.1 (n = 18)	28.1 (n = 29)	0.57 (n = 32)	Plastic tube	2% citric acid	Students	Benedek-Spaet 1973b
6	Approx 22	8.0–10.5	Approx 1.1 ml/min × m^2 at maximal stimulation	Capsule	Citric acid	Children	Kaiser et al 1974
22	29.8	21.8		Capsule	2% citric acid	Children	Mandel et al 1965
35	8–40	About 25.0	0.2–0.5	Plastic tube	Ascorbic acid	Patients (18–35 yr)	Eichner et al 1975
23			24–142 drops/2 min	Capsule	6% citric acid	Patients (20–49 yr)	Enfors 1962
21	42.6	26.5	1.22	Capsule	Fruit acid		Ferguson et al 1973
11	41.4	13.3	1.0	Plastic tube	Pilocarpine	Students (20–27 yr)	Kreusser et al 1972
3(?)	50.4	45.3		Plastic tube	Pilocarpine	Students (20–26 yr)	Knauf & Froemter 1970

Proteins

The concentration of total protein in the saliva also depends on the type of subject investigated and the methods used (Table 4.**8**). It is composed of many different structured proteins whose functions are only partly known (see later).

Most salivary proteins are constituents of the zymogen granules and reach the saliva by exocytosis. These proteins include the digestive enzymes, such as alpha-amylase, and also many glycoproteins that are mainly responsible for the viscosity of the saliva. Other constituents, such as albumin and some immunoglobulins, follow a different pathway. Probably they diffuse from the serum into the primary saliva, depending on the concentration gradients.

The salivary proteins may be divided by their chemical composition into glycoproteins and sugar-free proteins, but they may also be classified by their function, for example, digestive enzymes, proteins for defence against infection, etc. The genetics of individual salivary proteins must be considered before this aspect is described.

Table 4.**7** Electrolyte Concentrations in Human Parotid Saliva: An Approximately Normal Range Collected from Different Series

	Without Stimulation (mmol/l)	After Stimulation (mmol/l)
Sodium	1–10	20–60
Potassium	20–50	10–30
Calcium	4–8	
Chloride	10–20	20–40
Bicarbonate	1– 5	5–30

Salivary Proteins and Genetics

The occurrence of some proteins in saliva is genetically determined (Tan & Teng 1979). These include glycoproteins that demonstrate an antigenicity similar to that of the blood groups of the AB0 system (Watkins 1972). The ability to secrete *blood group reactive substances* is inherited as a dominant factor independent of the AB0 system, so that the ability to secrete blood group reactive substances is only absent in recessive

Table 4.**8** Protein Content of Stimulated and Resting Parotid Saliva

No.Subjects	Protein Concentration (mmol/l)	Remarks	Method	References
35	2–10	Resting & stimulated secretion	Biuret*	Eichner et al 1975
75	2.28	Resting secretion in men	Amidoschwarz	Vogt & Semmann 1970
73	3.14	Resting secretion in women	Amidoschwarz	Vogt & Semmann 1970
30	2.56	Resting secretion	Lowry**	Benedek-Spät 1973a
30	2.36	Stimulated secretion	Lowry	Benedek-Spät 1973b
	2.53	Resting secretion	Biuret	Shannon et al 1974
7	2.72	Resting secretion	Lowry	Dawes & Ong 1973b
21	2.29	Stimulated secretion	Biuret	Ferguson et al 1973

* Beisenherz et al 1953.
** Lowry et al 1951.

homozygotes. This includes about 25% of the European population and has forensic significance.

The production of human *alpha-amylase* is determined by two genes. Amy_1 is the gene for salivary amylase, Amy_2 is that for pancreatic amylase. The most common Amy_1 allele is the allele A, whereas alleles B, C, K, and Rh are less common. Except for Rh they are dominant compared with A (Karn et al 1975, Merritt & Karn 1977). There are, however, racial differences (Merritt & Karn 1977). The primary product of the amylase gene Amy_1 is subject to post-translational modifications, mainly by enzymatic glycosylation, deglycosylation, and spontaneous deamination (Karn et al 1973, 1974, 1975) to form individual isoamylases. The high frequency of allele A in the white races leads to a predominance of homozygotes for the Amy_1 gene, so that 98,7% of the population have an isoamylase phenotype A (a basic pattern of six isoamylases) in the saliva (Merritt & Karn 1977).

A genetic polymorphism has been confirmed for other enzymes, such as *esterases* (Tan 1976) and for the peroxidases (Azen 1977, 1978) similar to that for alpha-amylase. The occurrence of some nonenzymatic active proteins in the saliva is also genetically determined and shows racial differences. These include the acid protein (Pa), the double-band protein (Db), the basic parotid protein (Pb), and the proline-rich proteins (Pr) (Friedman et al 1975, Azen & Denniston 1974).

These and other investigations of the inheritance of salivary proteins are not only of genetic interest, but they have forensic significance also (Burdett et al 1976).

Functional Significance of Salivary Constituents

The constituents of saliva carry several different functions. The specific function of many salivary components is not known, and indeed they may not have a specific function, because they reach the saliva by diffusion from the serum. This shows that a pure teleologic approach in the investigation of salivary composition is too biased. Therefore we ought to limit our investigations to functionally important constituents because a bewildering profusion of data is available. The extensive monograph of Arglebe (1981) provides further information about the chemical structure of the salivary proteins. The main function of the saliva is *digestion*. Substances are *excreted* in the saliva, but some constituents have a part to play in the *defence* mechanism of the mouth. Furthermore, in the absence of saliva the *dental apparatus* and the *oral mucosa* degenerate, the *sense of taste* is disordered, and *articulation* becomes more difficult.

Digestion

The digestive function of the saliva begins with the preparation of the food, which is broken up in the mouth preparatory to digestion in the gastrointestinal tract. Constituents of food are emulsified in saliva and dissolved. This process is a prerequisite for the sense of taste and for enzymatic digestion. The food is lubricated to decrease friction during *swallowing*. This lubricating function of the saliva rests especially on its content of *glycoproteins*. These are proteins that are bound to sugar molecules and that are included as a ground substance of mucus in any part of the body. They are present in higher concentration in the saliva of the minor salivary glands and

	Mixed Saliva	Parotid Saliva	Submandibular Saliva	Sublingual Saliva
Viscosity (centipoise)	2.9	1.5	3.4	13.4

Table 4.**9** Viscosity of Citrate-Stimulated Fractions of Saliva in One Person (Schneyder)

of the sublingual and submandibular glands than in the parotid gland. This explains the varying viscosity of the resting secretion (Table 4.**9**), which is also responsible for the smooth course of intraoral movement, for example the movement of the tongue during articulation.

The enzymatic digestion of food is also initiated by the saliva. Ribonuclease and oxyribonuclease, which split nucleic acid (Eichel et al 1964, Zoellner et al 1974), acid and alkaline phosphatases (Chauncey et al 1954, Eggers 1947, Mason & Chisholm 1975), nonspecific esterases (Chauncey 1961, Chauncey et al 1957, Lindqvist et al 1977, Robyt & French 1967), and also the peptide-splitting kallikreins (see before), have all been demonstrated in saliva. But their concentration in human saliva is not very high and their importance in digestion is probably slight. In particular, proteolytic activity has not been demonstrated to any great extent in human saliva. It is therefore incorrect to speak of a tissue-macerating property of the saliva, for example, in a parotid fistula, and to ascribe this to enzymatic effects. Comparisons cannot be drawn with the marked proteinase-containing pancreatic secretions (Rauch 1959) or with proteinases released in inflammatory diseases, as is suggested for pancreatitis. The salivary glands do not possess the appropriate secretory enzymes that can split proteins.

The main digestive enzyme of the saliva is alpha-amylase, previously called ptyalin or diastase, a starch-splitting enzyme that is produced in the parotid gland especially and that is released into the saliva via the zymogen granules.

Alpha-Amylase

Alpha-amylase hydrolyzes amylase, amylopectin, glycogen, and related polysaccharides, such as oligosaccharide. The alpha-D-(1→4) binding between the two glucose molecules is split, but not the 1→6 binding of amylopectin and glycogen. The reducing substances maltose and dextrins of different lengths of chains are thus produced as fission products (Robyt & French 1967). Under physiologic circumstances, glucose is not formed (Pazur 1965, Robyt & Whelan 1968). The amylase acts not only in the oral cavity, but also in the gastrointestinal tract where it is protected for some time from the gastric acid within the bolus of food. Active salivary amylase may even be demonstrated in duodenal secretions (Skude & Ihse 1976).

The animal and human amylases that have been investigated so far consist of single polypeptide chains with a molecular weight of 50 000–60 000 daltons (Keller et al 1971, Malacinski & Rutter 1969, Muus & Vnenchak 1964, Sanders & Rutter 1972). The salivary and the pancreatic amylase of man contain a sulfhydryl group (Stiefel & Keller 1973). The optimum pH of the enzyme lies at about 7 (Salt & Schenker 1976, Street & Close 1956). The alpha-amylases are calcium-metalloenzymes (Hsiu et al 1964), which can be inhibited by ethylene diaminetetraacetic acid (Mermall et al 1973). The chloride ion activates the alpha-amylase (Meur & De 1976). Inhibitory substances are derived from wheat extract (O'Donnell & McGeeney 1976, Silano et al 1975) and are formed by Streptomyces (Koba 1976). The inhibitors are partially active against salivary and pancreatic amylases and can thus be used for differentiation of these enzymes in human serum (O'Donnell et al 1976).

The parotid amylase of man is not a single enzyme. Electrophoresis has shown that alpha-amylase is composed of a number of isoenzymes (Meites & Rogols 1971, Rajasingham et al 1971). These show slight differences in their molecular weight and may be differentiated by their isoelectric points (Kauffman et al 1970, Rosenmund & Kaczmarek 1976).

Isoamylases have also been described in other tissues besides the parotid gland and the pancreas (Skude & Ihse 1976, Stiefel & Keller 1973, Thaysen et al 1964, Townes et al 1976), such as the submandibular gland (Kauffman et al 1973, Lamberts et al 1971), breast (Kuttner & Somogyi 1934), ovary (Skude et al 1976), lacrimal glands (von Haeringen et al 1975), liver (Bhutta & Rahman 1971), and lung (Heffernon et al 1976). The serum amylase has a half-life of about 3 hours (Ryan & Appert 1975) and may be demonstrated in the serum in the absence of any salivary disease. It consists of the isoamylases of the pancreas and of the salivary glands (Berk et al 1966, de la

Lande & Boettcher 1969, Meites & Rogols 1971, Otsuki et al 1976, Townes et al 1976).

The determination of the serum and urinary amylase with differentiation into the individual isoamylases is now very important in the diagnosis of pancreatic and parotid diseases, for example, acute and chronic sialadenitis, and for the demonstration of macroamylasemia. The latter is usually a harmless hyperamylasemia caused by high molecular weight amylases (Berk et al 1967, 1970, Berk & Fridhandler 1976, Goldberg & Spooner 1975, Lehrner et al 1976, Salt & Schenker 1976). The hydrolysis of starch by the enzyme (amyloclastic method) is now preferred for estimation of alpha-amylase activity. The decrease of color intensity of an iodine starch complex (Street & Close 1956) or the release of a dye bound to starch (Ceska et al 1969, Foot & Wiener 1979, Wiener & Foot 1977) are used as parameters. Table 4.**10** gives an overview of the amylase concentrations measured in both parotid and mixed saliva.

Excretion

The salivary glands have an excretory function, as do the pancreas and the gastric glands. The saliva is usually not lost to the metabolism, since it is reabsorbed in the gastrointestinal tract, apart from a slight loss due to evaporation.

All low molecular weight serum constituents can be demonstrated in the saliva, usually in low concentrations, but also in concentrations as high as or higher than in serum. This fact has led to attempts to replace serum investigations by the less invasive salivary examination, for example, in the assessment of electrolytes and also drug concentrations in the saliva (page 52).

Infective agents circulating in the blood may also reach the saliva without the glands themselves being diseased. This is especially true of viruses, such as hepatitis B (Irwin et al 1975, Villarejos et al 1974), which can render the saliva infectious.

Nitrates originating from the food (Tannenbaum et al 1976) reach the saliva and are then reduced by several microorganisms to nitrites (Eisenbrand et al 1980). They are said to be important in carcinogenesis.

Defense and Protective Mechanisms

The saliva contains several substances that provide a specific resistance against infection. They are said to protect the mouth, the primary portal of entry of many organisms in the food or in the air, or by direct contact with infected material (page 11).

Such substances include *immunoglobulins,* a heterogeneous group of glycoproteins whose structure will not be discussed further here (Arglebe 1981). The IgG and IgM content of saliva is small and is partly due to an admixture of serum immunoglobulins. The content of IgA in parotid secretion is up to 100 times higher (Chodirker & Tomasi 1963). This is mainly secretory IgA (sIgA), which is formed in plasma cells of the interstitial connective tissue. Secretion is carried out via epithelial cells in which the IgA is bound to a further protein (the secretory component). The sIgA is very important in local mucosal immunity: its formation is stimulated by bacteria and viruses reaching the mucosa (Brandtzaeg et al 1970). Local immunity can provide better protection against rhinoviruses and influenza viruses than systemic immunization (Tomasi 1972). The viruses are probably destroyed by a joint action between the secretory antibodies and the phagocytosis system. Patients who lack sIgA are not immune to viruses that cause superficial mucosal diseases (Tomasi 1972).

Bacteriolysis by salivary immunoglobulins has not so far been demonstrated, although the aggregation of bacteria in the saliva by immunoglobulins has been known for a long time and has been well investigated (Bratthall & Carlen 1978, Bratthall et al 1978, Kleinberg et al 1979, Mirth et al 1979). It plays a part in the etiology of dental caries and facilitates the phagocytosis of bacteria.

The salivary content of IgA can be reduced in deficiency diseases (McMurray et al 1977). It can be influenced either positively or negatively by taking antiepileptic drugs, such as phenytoin, for many years (Aarli 1976, Smith et al 1979). It is not clear whether there is a causative correlation with the known changes of the oral mucosa, particularly the gingiva, due to phenytoin medication.

The enzyme *lysozyme,* or *muraminidase,* is present in large amounts in the saliva. It has a protective function. The salivary lysozyme is a basic protein (pI greater than 10) consisting of single polypeptide chains of molecular weight 15 000 (Balekjian et al 1969, Petit & Jolles 1963). Lysozyme probably hydrolyzes the beta-1, 4-bond between N-acetylmuraminic acid and 2-acetylaminodesoxy-D-glucose remnants in mucopolysaccharides or mucopolypeptides of the cell walls of gram-positive bacteria.

Peroxidase is an enzyme that oxydizes substrates with the help of hydrogen peroxide. Peroxidase is synthesized in large amounts and actively secreted in the salivary glands (Arglebe 1981). In the hu-

Table 4.**10** Amylase Concentration in Human Parotid and Mixed Saliva (Arglebe et al)

No. Subjects	Method of Collection	Amylase Concentration	Remarks	References
17	Parotid saliva Catheter Resting saliva	178.2 ± 84.5 U/ml	Pankreas, healthy (18–76 yr old)	Grimmel et al 1976
?	Mixed saliva Resting saliva	119 ± 21 Lagerhof units/15 min	Healthy	Descos et al 1973
109	Parotid saliva Capsule Stimulated saliva (vitamin c)	14.7–21.6–31.9 AU/min Mean ± SD after logarithmic transformation	Healthy	Skurk et al 1975
29	Parotid saliva Catheter Resting saliva Stimulated saliva	164.6 ± 13.9 163.7 ± 13.7 mg of starch cleaved by 0.1 ml saliva in 5 min	Students (19–23 yr old)	Benedek-Spät 1973a & b
7	Parotid saliva Capsule 2 hr after drinking water	3000 ± 166 Somogyi U/ml	Women (20–26 yr old)	Behall et al 1973
32	Mixed saliva	101 ± 30.8 U	Healthy Europeans	Benedek-Spät 1973b
60	Parotid saliva Catheter Resting saliva Stimulated saliva (lemon juice)	M: 4571.64 ± 1835.21 F: 4435.03 ± 2368.2 M: 2591.7 ± 1432.77 F: 2264.67 ± 1130.18	M: 30, F: 30 Healthy (20–40 yr old)	Meyer & Nürn- berger 1974
74	Mixed saliva Stimulated saliva (citrate)	Median values from 5–190 U/ml	Aged up to 12 yr	Rossiter et al 1974
10	Daily	180 U/ml	Adults	
98	Parotid saliva Capsule Stimulated saliva (pilocarpine)	1650 ± 661 U/kg body weight	Patients without pancretic disorders (16 healthy)	Kakizaki et al 1976
90	Parotid saliva Catheter Resting saliva Stimulated saliva (citrate)	Mean of log normal distribution 402.9 U/ml 240.9 U/ml	45 men & 45 women with healthy salivary glands	Arglebe et al 1979 Chilla et al 1977
16	Parotid saliva Capsule Resting saliva	1.03 ± 0.11 mg amylase/ml	Healthy men (20–30 yr old)	Schneyer 1956
11	Stimulated saliva (acetic acid)	0.95 ± 0.15 mg amylase/ml	Healthy men (20–30 yr old)	Schneyer 1956

man, this applies to lactoperoxidases, whereas the myeloperoxydase is more likely to be of bacterial origin.

The lactoperoxidases form a defence mechanism in saliva along with the thiocyanate ion (SCN^-) (Klebanoff & Luebke 1965, Slowey et al 1968), since hypothiocyanate ($OSCN^-$), the oxidation product of thiocyanate, has a bacteriostatic action (Morris 1979). This applies also to the myeloperoxidase system in which the oxidation products of iodine, bromine, and chlorine take on this function and even display a virucidal action (Belding & Klebanoff 1970).

Alpha-amylase is mainly a digestive enzyme (see before), but it also has a defensive action in the saliva. Thus, it attacks the polysaccharide in the cell walls of gonococci (Mellersh et al 1979) and is an active inhibitory agent of the gonococcus in saliva.

The salivary constitutents assume a *blood coagulating function* after injuries or operations in the mouth. The lipoprotein thromboplastin (Factor III) can be demonstrated in human saliva (Zacharski & Rosenstein 1979), but it originates from cells or from cell segments. This probably applies also to other blood-coagulating factors, such as Factors VII, VIII, and IX (Ferguson 1975).

An antifibrinolytic activity similar to that of epsilon-aminocaproic acid can be demonstrated in the parotid saliva (Haze et al 1980). A fibrinolysis-promoting activity of the saliva has also been reported (Schulte 1964).

Maintenance of the Teeth and Mucosal Protection

The oral mucosa and the teeth become diseased if insufficient saliva is produced. This atrophy is caused by drying of the mucosa. Absence of the specific salivary protective mechanisms favors infection of the oral mucosa. This *xerostomia* renders eating and speaking difficult.

A possible correlation between *dental caries* and changes in the constitution of the saliva has been the subject of many investigations (Kleinberg et al 1979). It is well known that several acid salivary proteins, that is, proteins with a low isoelectric point, have a high affinity for hydroxylapatite. This is the form in which calcium mainly occurs in dental enamel (Hay 1973, 1975, Nawrot et al 1976). At physiologic pH values of saliva around neutral, the proteins are negatively charged and are attracted by positively charged calcium ions in the hydroxylapatite. This produces a protective protein film around the dental enamel. This must be continuously renewed, since it is destroyed by bacteria and disturbed by intraoral movements, such as chewing. A lower salivary pH reduces the dissociation of acid groups in the salivary protein, reduces its negative charge, and thus its ability to be laid down on the dental enamel. This effect can be produced by acid metabolic products of sugar-fermenting bacteria.

Several proteins in the saliva, such as the calcium precipitable protein of the submandibular gland have a high affinity for calcium and can also prevent the precipitation of calcium phosphate in a supersaturated solution (Hay 1973, 1975, Hay & Moreno 1979). In this way, protein-bound calcium salts may be laid down in the dental enamel if they are a constituent part of its protective protein film.

References

Aarli, J. A.: Phenytoin-induced depression of salivary IgA. Acta oto-laryng. 82 (1976) 199

Ansel, D. G.: Rat salivary glands after long-term isoproterenol administration. Arch. Otolaryng. 100 (1974) 256

Arglebe, C.: Biochemistry of human saliva. In Pfaltz, C. R., R. Chilla: Sialadenosis and Sialadenitis. Karger, Basel 1981

Arglebe, C., M. Opaitz, R. Chilla: Amylaseaktivität im unstimulierten Parotisspeichel des Menschen unter Berücksichtigung von Flußrate und Proteinkonzentration. Z. Laryng. Rhinol. 58 (1979) 700

Arold, R., W. Schätzle: Die "Experimentelle Sialadenose" und ihre Beeinflussung durch β-Receptoren-Blocker. Arch. klin. exp. Ohr.-, Nas.- u. Kehlk.-Heilk. 203 (1973) 274

Azen, E. A.: Salivary peroxidase (SAPX): genetic modification and relationship to the proline-rich (Pr) and acidic (Pa) proteins. Biochem. Genet. 15 (1977) 9

Azen, E. A.: Salivary peroxidase activity and thiocyanate concentration in human subjects with genetic variants of salivary peroxidase. Arch. oral Biol. 23 (1978) 801

Azen, E. A., C. L. Denniston: Genetic polymorphism of human salivary proline-rich proteins: further genetic analysis. Biochem. Genet. 12 (1974) 109

Balekjian, A. Y., K. C. Hoerman, V. J. Berzinskas: Lysozyme of the human parotid gland secretion: its purification and physicochemical properties. Biochem. biophys. Res. Comm. 35 (1969) 887

Bartter, F. C.: The Clinical Use of Aldosterone Antagonists. Thomas, Springfield 1960

Behall, K. M., I. L. Kelsay, I. M. Holden, W. M. Clark: Amylase and protein in parotid saliva after load doses of different dietary carbohydrates. Amer. J. clin. Nutrition 26 (1973) 17

Beisenherz, G., H. J. Boltze, T. Bücher, R. Czok, K. H. Garbade, E. Meyer-Arendt, G. Pfleiderer: Diphosphofructose-Aldolase, Phosphoglycerinaldehyd-Dehydrogenase, Milchsäuredehydrogenase und Pyruvatkinase aus Kaninchenmuskel in einem Arbeitsgang. Z. Naturforsch. 8b (1953) 555

Belding, M. E., S. J. Klebanoff, C. G. Ray: Peroxidase-mediated virucidal systems. Science 167 (1970) 195

Benedek-Spät, E.: The composition of unstimulated human parotid saliva. Arch. oral Biol. 18 (1973a) 39

Benedek-Spät, E.: The composition of stimulated human parotid saliva. Arch. oral Biol. 18 (1973b) 1091

Berk, J. E., L. Fridhandler: Pursuit of the elusive: adventure in quest of a specific test for pancreatic amylase. Mount Sinai J. Med. 43 (1976) 321

Berk, J. E., S. Hayashi, R. L. Searcy, N. Hightower: Differentiation of parotid and pancreatic amylase in human serum. Amer. J. Digest. Dis. 11 (1966) 695

Berk, J. E., H. Kizu, S. Take, L. Fridhandler: Macroamylasemia: serum and urine amylase characteristics. Amer. J. Gastroenterol. 53 (1970) 223

Berk, J. E., H. Kizu, P. Wilding, R. L. Searcy: Macroamylasemia: a newly recognized cause for elevated serum amylase activity. New Engl. J. Med. 277 (1967) 941

Bernard, C.: Leçons de physiologie opératoire. Baillière, Paris 1879

Bhutta, I. H., M. A. Rahman: Serum amylase activity in liver disease. Clin. Chem. 17 (1971) 1147

Bing, J., K. Poulsen: The renin system in mice. Acta Pathol. Microbiol. Scand. 79 (1971) 134

Blumberger, W., H. Glatzel: Über Variabilität von Speichelsekretion und Speichelbeschaffenheit des gesunden Menschen und ihre Beziehungen zur Kostform. Dtsch. Z. Verdau.- u. Stoffwechselkr. 23 (1963) 210

Bock, K. D.: Vermeidbare und unvermeidbare Komplikationen der Langzeittherapie mit Antihypertonika. Therapiewoche 18 (1968) 1102

Bock, K. D.: Gefahren der modernen antihypertensiven Therapie. Z. Allgemeinmed. 46 (1970) 1287
Bock, K. D., W. W. Huep: Irreversibler Parotisschmerz nach Verabreichung von Guanaclin. Dtsch. med. Wschr. 96 (1971) 1649–1650
Bock, K. D., V. Heimsoth, P. Merguet, J. Schönermark: Klinische und klinisch-experimentelle Untersuchungen mit einer neuen blutdrucksenkenden Substanz: Dichlorphenylaminoimidazolin. Dtsch. med. Wschr. 91 (1966) 1761
Borsanyi, S. J., C. L. Blanchard: Asymptomatic enlargement of the parotid glands due to the use of isoproterenol. Maryland State med. J. 10 (1961) 572
Boyer, F. C., W. J. Gardner: Paroxysmal lacrimation (syndrome of crocodile tears) and its surgical treatment. Arch. Neurol. Psychiat. 61 (1949) 56
Brands, T.: Diagnostik der Speicheldrüsenerkrankungen. Z. Laryng. Rhinol. 51 (1972) 639
Brandtzaeg, P., I. Fjellanger, S. T. Gjeruldsen: Human secretory immunoglobulins. I. Salivary secretions from individuals with normal or low levels of serum immunoglobulins. Scand. J. Haematol., Suppl. 12 (1970) 1
Bratthall, D., A. Carlen: Salivary agglutinin and secretory IgA reactions with oral streptococci. Scand. J. dent. Res. 86 (1978) 430
Bratthall, D., L. Gahnberg, B. Krasse: Method for detecting IgA antibodies to Streptococcus mutans serotypes in parotid saliva. Arch. oral Biol. 23 (1978) 843
Burdett, P. E., A. E. Kipps, P. H. Whitehead: A rapid technique for the detection of amylase isoenzymes using an enzyme sensitive "testpaper". Analyt. Biochem. 72 (1976) 315
Butcher, F. R., P. A. Mc Bridge, L. Rudich: Cholinergic regulation of cyclic nucleotide levels, amylase release, and K^+-efflux from rat parotid glands. Mol. cell. Endocrinol. 5 (1976) 243
Byrt, P.: Secretion and synthesis of amylase in the rat parotid gland after isoprenaline. Nature 212 (1966) 1212
Cantalamessa, F., G. de Caro, M. Perfumi: Effects of chronic administration of eledoisin or physalaemin on the rat salivary glands. Pharmacol. Res. Comm. 7 (1975) 259
Ceska, M., B. Brown, K. Birath: Ranges of α-amylase activities in human serum and urine and correlations with some other α-amylase methods. Clin. chim. Acta 26 (1969) 445
Chauncey, H. H.: Salivary enzymes. J. Amer. dent. Ass. 63 (1961) 360
Chauncey, H. H., F. Lionetti, V. F. Lisanti: Enzymes of human saliva. II. Parotid saliva total esterases. J. dent. Res. 36 (1957) 713
Chauncey, H. H., F. Lionetti, R. A. Winer, V. F. Lisanti: Enzymes of human saliva. I. The determination, distribution, and origin of whole saliva enzymes. J. dent. Res. 33 (1954) 321
Chilla, R.: Chirurgie der Nerven im HNO-Bereich: Vegetative Hirnnervenstrukturen. Arch. Oto-Rhino-Laryng. 231 (1981) 353
Chilla, R., C. Arglebe: Pharmakotherapie der Hypertonie und ihre Bedeutung für die Funktion der Kopfspeicheldrüsen. Münch. med. Wschr. 117 (1975) 1425
Chilla, R., R. Arold: Über Sekretionsmechanismen der Ohrspeicheldrüse und deren medikamentöse Beeinflussung. HNO 23 (1975) 229
Chilla, R., R. Kropp, C. Arglebe: Amylaseaktivität und Isoamylasenmuster im Parotisspeichel des Menschen. Z. Laryng. Rhinol. 56 (1977) 912
Chilla, R., M. Opaitz, C. Arglebe: Flußrate, Amylase- und Proteingehalt des Parotisspeichels bei Sialadenose. Z. Laryng. Rhinol. 57 (1978) 274
Chilla, R., R. Arold, K. H. Flucke, C. Arglebe: The effect of clonidine treatment on the salivary glands of the rat. Results of biochemical and histological investigations. Arch. Oto-Rhino-Laryng. 209 (1975) 47
Chodirker, W. B., T. B. Tomasi: Gamma globulins: quantitative relationships in human serum and non-vascular fluids. Science 142 (1963) 1080
Chorobski, J.: A syndrome of crocodile tears. Arch. Neurol. Psychiat. 65 (1951) 299
Costa, P. T., H. H. Chauncey, C. L. Rose, K. K. Kapur: Relationship of parotid saliva flow rate and composition with personality traits in healthy men. Oral. Surg. 50 (1980) 416
Curry, R. C., D. H. Patey: A clinical test for parotid function. Brit. J. Surg. 51 (1964) 891
Dawes, C.: The effects of flow rate and duration of stimulation on the concentrations of protein and the main electrolytes in human parotid saliva. Arch. oral Biol. 14 (1969) 277
Dawes, C.: Rhythmus in salivary flow rate and composition. Int. J. Chronobiol. 2 (1974) 253
Dawes, C.: The effect of food deprivation on the circadian rhythms in flow rate and protein concentration in human parotid saliva. Arch. oral Biol. 20 (1975) 547
Dawes, C., B. Y. Ong: Circadian rhythms in the flow rate and proportional contribution of parotid to whole saliva volume in man. Arch. oral Biol. 18 (1973a) 1145
Dawes, C., B. Y. Ong: Circadian rhythms in the concentrations of protein and the main electrolytes in human unstimulated parotid saliva. Arch. oral. Biol. 18 (1973b) 1233
Dawes, C., C. M. Wood: The contribution of oral minor mucous gland secretions to the volume of whole saliva in man. Arch. oral Biol. 18 (1973) 337
Descos, F., R. Lambert, Y. Minaire: Comparison of human salivary secretion in health and chronic pancreatitis. Digestion 9 (1973) 76
Descos, L., F. Andre, R. Lambert, C. Andre: Influence of secretin on salivary mucous secretion in man. Digestion 9 (1973) 199
Diamant, H., A. Wiberg: Does the chorda tympani in man contain secretory fibres for the parotid gland? Acta Otolaryng. 60 (1965) 255
Drack, G. T., H. R. Koelz, A. L. Blum: Human calcitonin stimulates salivary amylase output in man. Gut 17 (1976) 620
Eggers Lura, H.: Investigations on the salivary phosphates and phosphatases. J. dent. Res. 26 (1947) 203
Eichel, H. J., H. Conger, W. S. Chernick: Acid and alkaline ribonucleases of human parotid, submaxillary and whole saliva. Arch. Biochem. Biophys. 107 (1964) 197
Eichner, H., M. Münzel, G. Bretzel: Vergleichende Untersuchungen von Flußraten, Elektrolyt- und Gesamteiweißkonzentrationen und diskeletrophoretische Auftrennung des Sekretes an fraktioniert gewonnenem menschlichen Parotissekret. Z. Laryng. Rhinol. 54 (1975) 19
Eisenbrand, G., B. Spiegelhalder, R. Preussmann: Nitrate and nitrite in saliva. Oncology 37 (1980) 227
Ellison, S. A.: Proteins and glycoproteins of saliva. In: Code, Handbook of Physiology, sect. 6, vol. 2. American Physiological Society, Washington 1967 (p. 531)
Eneroth, C.-M., T. Hökfelt, K.-A. Norberg: The role of parasympathetic and sympathetic innervation for the secretion of human parotid and submandibular gland. Acta Otolaryng. 68 (1969) 369
Enfors, B.: The parotid and submandibular secretion in man. Acta Otolaryng., Suppl. 172 (1962) 1
Feinstein, H., M. Schramm: Energy production in rat parotid gland. Relation to enzyme secretion and effects of calcium. Eur. J. Biochem. 13 (1970) 158
Ferguson, D. B.: Salivary glands and saliva. In Lavell: Applied Physiology of the Mouth. Wright, Bristol 1975 (p. 145)
Ferguson, D. B., C. A. Botchway: Circadian variations in the flow rate and composition of whole saliva stimulated by mastication. Arch. oral Biol. 24 (1979) 877
Ferguson, D. B., A. Fort, A. L. Elliott, A. J. Potts: Circadian rhythms in human parotid saliva flow rate and composition. Arch. oral Biol. 18 (1973) 1155
Ferguson, D. B., A. Fort, A. L. Elliott, A. J. Potts: Circadian variations in human resting submandibular saliva flow rate and composition. Arch. oral Biol. 19 (1974) 47
Fischbach, R.: Die vegetativen Effekte der Antidepressiva im Bereich des Gastro-Intestinaltraktes. Wien. med. Wschr., Suppl. 5 (1973) 1
Foot, C. H., K. Wiener: Phadebas amylase test kits. Clin. Chem. 25 (1979) 818
Friedman, R. D., A. D. Merritt, M. L. Rivas: Genetic studies on human acidic salivary protein (Pa). Amer. J. hum. Genet. 27 (1975) 292
Friedman, Z. Y., Z. Selinger: A transient release of potassium mediated by the action of substance P on rat parotid slices. J. Physiol. 278 (1978) 461
Garrett, J. R., N. Emmelin: Activities of salivary myoepithelial cells: a review. Med. Biol. 57 (1979) 1
Gilman, S., R. Thornton, D. Miller, R. Biersner: Effects of exercise stress on parotid gland secretion. Horm. Metab. Res. 11 (1979) 454
Gjörstrup, P.: Effects of sympathetic nerve stimulation on the presence of a slow parasympathetic secretion in the parotid and maxillary glands of the rabbit. Acta Physiol. Scand. 101 (1977) 211
Gjörstrup, P.: Amylase secretion in the rabbit parotid gland when stimulating the sympathetic nerves during parasympathetic activity. J. Physiol. 296 (1979) 443

Godlowski, Z., M. Gazda, B. T. Withers: Ablation of salivary glands as initial step in the management of selected forms of diabetes mellitus. Laryngoscope 81 (1971) 1337

Goldberg, D. M., R. J. Spooner: Amylase, isoamylase, and macroamylase. Digestion 13 (1975) 56

Goodwin, D., D. Noff, S. Edelstein: The parotid gland: a new target organ for vitamin D action. Biochim. biophys. Acta 539 (1978) 249

Green, G. J., H. Wilson, M. S. Yates: The effect of clonidine on centrally and peripherally evoked submaxillary salivation. Eur. J. Pharmacol. 53 (1979) 297

Grimmel, K., G. Rossbach, H. Kasper: Amylase activity of parotid saliva in acute and chronic pancreatitis. Acta Hepato-Gastr. 23 (1976) 334

van Haeringen, N. J., F. Ensink, E. Glasius: Amylase in human tear fluid: origin and characteristics, compared with salivary and urinary amylases. Exp. Eve Res. 21 (1975) 395

Hay, D. I.: The interaction of human parotid salivary proteins with hydroxyapatite. Arch. oral Biol. 18 (1973) 1517

Hay, D. I.: Fractionation of human parotid salivary proteins and the isolation of a histidine-rich acidic peptide which shows high affinity for hydroxyapatite surfaces. Arch. oral Biol. 20 (1975) 553

Hay, D. I., E. C. Moreno: Macromolecular inhibitors of calcium phosphate precipitation in human saliva. Their roles in providing a protective environment for the teeth. In Kleinberg, I., S. A. Ellison, I. D. Mandel: Saliva and Dental Caries. Microbiology Abstracts, Suppl. Information Retrieval, New York 1979 (p. 45)

Haze, H., A. Eldor, A. A. Garfunkel: Antifibrinolytic activity of human saliva components. Thromb. Res. 17 (1980) 737

Heffernon, J. J., W. R. Smith, J. E. Berk, L. Fridhandler, F. L. Glauser, K. A. Montgomery: Hyperamylasemia in heroin addicts. Amer. J. Gastroent. 66 (1976) 17

Heidenhain, R.: Über sekretorische und trophische Drüsennerven. Pflügers Arch. 17 (1878) 1

Holmberg, J.: On the nerves to the parotid gland. In Emmelin, N., Y. Zotterman: Oral Physiology. Pergamon Press, Oxford 1971

Hsiu, J., E. H. Fischer, E. A. Stein: Alpha-amylases as calcium-metalloenzymes. II. Calcium and the catalytic activity. Biochemistry 3 (1964) 61

Inoki, R., S. Kojima, Y. Tamari, I. Yamamoto: Effects of nicotine in salivary amylase secretion from rabbit parotid gland. Brit. J. Pharmacol. 41 (1971) 285

Irwin, G. R., A. M. Allen, W. H. Bancroft, J. J. Karwacki, H. L. Brown, R. H. Pinderton, M. Willnight, F. H. Top jr.: Hepatitis B-antigen in saliva, urine and stool. Infect. Immun. 11 (1975) 142

Ito, Y., A. Mizutani: Studies on the salivary gland hormones. XIII: Purification of parotin. Jap. Pharmacol. 72 (1952) 239

Kaiser, D., M. Schöni, E. Drack: Anionen- und Kationenausscheidung der Parotis in Abhängigkeit von der Fließrate bei Mukoviszidosepatienten und Gesunden. Helv. paediat. Acta 29 (1974) 145

Kakizaki, G., T. Saito, T. Soeno, M. Sasahara: A new diagnostic test for pancreatic disorders by examination of parotid saliva. Amer. J. Gastroent. 65 (1976) 437

Kanamori, T., T. Hayakawa, T. Nagatsu: Adenosine 3', 5'-monophosphate-dependent protein kinase and amylase secretion from rat parotid gland. Biochem. biophys. Res. Comm. 57 (1974) 394

Karn, R. C., B. B. Rosenblum, J. C. Ward, A. D. Merritt: Genetic and post-translational mechanisms determining human amylase isozyme heterogeneity. In Markert: Isozymes IV, Genetics and Evolution, Academic Press, New York 1975 (p. 745)

Karn, R. C., J. D. Shulkin, A. D. Merritt, R. C. Newell: Evidence for post-transscriptional modification of human salivary amylase (Amy_1) isozymes. Biochem. Genet. 10 (1973) 341

Karn, R. C., B. B. Rosenblum, J. C. Ward, A. D. Merritt, J. D. Shulkin: Immunological relationships and posttranslational modifications of human salivary amylase (Amy_1) and pancreatic amylase (Amy_2) isozymes. Biochem. Genet. 12 (1974) 485

Kauffman, D. L., S. Watanabe, J. R. Evans, P. J. Keller: The existence of glycosylated and non-glycosylated forms of human submandibular amylase. Arch. oral Biol. 18 (1973) 1105

Kauffman, D. L., N. I. Zager, E. Cohen, P. J. Keller: The isoenzymes of human parotid amylase. Archs. Biochem. Biophys. 137 (1970) 325

Keller, P. J., D. L. Kauffman, B. J. Allan, B. L. Williams: Further studies on the structural differences between the isoenzymes of human parotid α-amylase. Biochemistry 10 (1971) 4867

Kelsay, J. L., K. E. McCague, J. M. Holden: Variations in flow rate, metabolites and enzyme activities of fasting human parotid saliva. Arch. oral Biol. 17 (1972) 439

Kerr, A. C.: The Physiological Regulation of Salivary Secretion in Man. Int. Series of Monographs on Oral Biology. Pergamon Press, Oxford 1961

Kielholz, P.: Der heutige Stand der medikamentösen Depressionsbehandlung. Nervenarzt 37 (1966) 118

Kim, Y. T., K. Hoshino, T. Hyodo, H. G. Friesen, L. J. Nahynybida: Hyperglycemic factor in submandibular glands and its etiological relations to diabetes mellitus in mice. Endocr. Jap. 26 (1979) 487

Klebanoff, S. J., R. G. Luebke: The antilactobacillus system of saliva. Role of salivary peroxidase. Proc. Soc. exp. Biol. Med. 118 (1965) 483

Kleinberg, I., S. A. Ellison, I. D. Mandel: Saliva and Dental Caries. Microbiology Abstracts, Suppl. Information Retrieval, New York 1979

Knauf, H., E. Frömter: Die Kationenausscheidung der großen Speicheldrüsen des Menschen. Pflügers Arch. Physiol. 316 (1970) 213

Koba, Y., M. Najima, S. Ueda: Further purification of amylase inhibitor produced by streptomyces sp. Agr. Biol. Chem. 40 (1976) 1167

Kojima, S., M. Ikeda, A. Tsujimoto: Effect of theophylline and 3', 5'-cyclic adenosine monophosphate on the salivary amylase secretion from rabbit parotid gland. Jap. J. Pharmacol. 21 (1971) 199

Kolb, E.: Körper- und Zellbestandteile. I. D.: Die Verdauungssekrete. In Rauen: Biochemisches Taschenbuch, Bd. II. Springer, Berlin 1964 (S. 365)

Kreusser, W., A. Heidland, H. Hennemann, M. E. Wigand, H. Knauf: Mono- and divalent electrolyte patterns, pCO_2 and pH in relation to flow in normal human parotid saliva. Eur. J. clin. Invest. 2 (1972) 398

Kroneberg, G., H. J. Schümann, A. Eckhardt: Untersuchungen zum Wirkungsmechanismus des Guanethidins. Naunyn-Schmiedeberg's Arch. exp. Path. Pharmak. 243 (1962) 16

Kuttner, M., M. Somogyi: Diastase in milk. Proc. Soc. exp. Biol. 32 (1934) 564

Lamberts, B. L., T. S. Meyer, R. M. Osborne: A comparative study of human parotid and submaxillary amylase. Arch. oral Biol. 16 (1971) 517

de la Lande, F. A., B. Boettcher: Electrophoretic examination of human serum amylase isoenzymes. Enzymologia 37 (1969) 335

Laugesen, L. P., J. O. D. Nielsen, J. H. Poulsen: Partial dissociation between salivary secretion and active potassium transport in the perfused cat submandibular gland. Pflüger's Arch. Eur. J. Physiol. 364 (1976) 167

Lawrence, A. M., S. Tan, S. Hojvat, L. Kirsteins: Salivary gland hyperglycemic factor: an extrapancreatic source of glucagon-like material. Science 195 (1977) 70

Lehrner, L. M., J. C. Ward, R. C. Karn, C. E. Ehrlich, A. D. Merritt: An evaluation of the usefulness of amylase isoenzyme differentiation in patients with hyperamylasemia. Amer. J. clin. Pathol. 66 (1976) 576

Leslie, B. A., J. W. Putney jr., J. M. Sherman: α-Adrenergic, β-adrenergic and cholinergic mechanisms for amylase secretion by rat parotid gland in vitro. J. Physiol. 260 (1976) 351

Liang, T., A. Cascieri: Substance P stimulation of amylase release by isolated parotid cells and inhibition of substance P induction of salivation by vasoactive peptides. Mol. cell. Endocrin. 15 (1979) 151

Lindqvist, L., C.-E. Nord, P.-Ö. Söder: Origin of esterases in human whole saliva. Enzyme 22 (1977) 166

Loeb, L.: Über die Sekretionsnerven der Parotis und über Salivation nach Verletzung des Bodens des vierten Ventrikels. Z. Anat. Physiol. 5 (1869) 1

Lowry, O. H., N. J. Rosebrough, A. L. Farr, R. J. Randall: Protein measurement with the Folin phenol reagent. J. biol. Chem. 193 (1951) 265

Ludwig, C.: Neue Versuche über Beihilfe der Nerven zur Speichelabsonderung. Z. rat. Med. 1 (1851) 255

Malacinski, G. M., W. J. Rutter: Multiple molecular forms of α-amylase from the rabbit. Biochemistry 8 (1969) 4382

Malfertheiner, P., R. Fußgänger, H. Minne, H. Ditschuneit: Influence of gastrointestinal hormones on human salivary secretion. Horm. Metab. Res. 12 (1980) 485

Mandel, I. D., R. Katz: The effect of pharmacologic agents on the salivary secretion and composition. 2. Isoproterenol, alpha- and beta-adrenergic blockers. J. oral Therap. Pharmac. 4 (1968) 260

Mandel, I. D., R. H. Thompson, S. Wotman, M. Taubman, A. H. Kutscher, E. V. Zegarelli, C. R. Denning, J. T. Botwick, B. S.

Fahn: Parotid saliva in cystic fibrosis. Amer. J. Dis. Child. 110 (1965) 646
Mangos, J. A., N. R. McSherry: Micropuncture study of sodium and potassium excretion in rat parotid saliva: role of aldosterone. Proc. Soc. exp. Biol. Med. 132 (1969) 797
Mason, D. K., D. M. Chisholm: Salivary Glands in Health and Disease. Saunders, London 1975
McMurray, D. N., H. Rey, L. J. Casazza, R. R. Watson: Effect of moderate malnutrition on concentrations of immunglobulins and enzymes in tears and saliva of young Columbian children. Amer. J. clin. Nutr. 30 (1977) 1944
Meites, S., S. Rogols: Amylase isoenzymes. Critical Rev. Clin. Lab. Sci. 2 (1971) 103
Mellersh, A., A. Clark, S. Hafiz: Inhibition of Neisseria gonorrhoeae by normal human saliva. Brit. J. vener. Dis. 55 (1979) 20
Mermall, H. L., M. O. Hanhila jr., W. M. Reeves: Effects of cations on the activation of salivary amylase. I. Na^+, K^+, Ca^{2+}, and Mg^{2+}. J. dent. Res. 52 (1973) 1148
Merritt, A. D., R. C. Karn: The human α-amylases. In Harris, Hirschhorn: Advances in Human Genetics, vol. 8. Plenum Press, New York 1977 (p. 135)
Meur, S. K., K. B. De: Anionic activation of human salivary amylase. Experientia 32 (1976) 1133
Meyer, P., E. Nürnberger: Zur Sekretion von Amylase und saurer Phosphatase durch die Parotis des Menschen vor und nach gustatorischer Stimulation unter Berücksichtigung der Enzymkonzentration und der Enzymsekretionsrate. Z. Laryng. Rhinol. 53 (1974) 222
Michelakis, A. M., J. W. Menzie, H. Yoshida: Sympathetic nervous system and renin release from submaxillary glands in vitro. Amer. J. Physiol. 231 (1976) 551
Mirth, D. B., C. J. Miller, A. Kingman, W. H. Bowen: Inhibition of saliva-induced aggregation of Streptococcus mutans by wheat germ agglutinin. Caries Res. 13 (1979) 121
Mizutani, A., A. Okano, Y. Isobe, T. Mizutani, Y. Matsushita, H. Goto: Purification and characterization of hypocalcemic protein from porcine parotid gland. Chem. Pharm. Bull (Tokyo) 74 (1976) 2391
Morris, J. G.: Oxygen and growth of the oral bacteria. In Kleinberg, I., S. A. Ellison, I. D. Mandel: Saliva and Dental Caries. Microbiology Abstracts, Suppl. Information Retrieval, New York 1979 (p. 293)
Münzel, M.: Die Biochemie der menschlichen Speicheldrüsensekrete. Arch. Oto-Rhino-Laryng. 213 (1976) 209
Mulcahy, H., O. Fitzgerald, K. F. McGeeney: Secretion and pancreozymin effect on salivary amylase concentration in man. Gut 13 (1972) 850
Muus, J., J. M. Vnenchak: Isozymes of salivary amylase. Nature 204 (1964) 283
Nawrot, C. F., D. J. Campbell, J. K. Schroeder, M. van Valkenburg: Dental phosphoprotein-induced formation of hydroxylapatite during in vitro synthesis of amorphous calcium phosphate. Biochemistry 15 (1976) 3445
Nelson, T. E., J. E. Stouffer: Thyroxine modulation of epinephrine stimulated secretion of rat parotid α-amylase. Biochem. biophys. Res. Comm. 48 (1972) 480
O'Donnell, M. D., K. F. McGeeney: Purification and properties of an α-amylase inhibitor from wheat. Biochim. biophys. Acta 422 (1976) 159
O'Donnell, M. D., O. Fitzgerald, K. F. McGeeney: A new method for detecting pancreatic and salivary gland malfunction. Irish J. Med. Sci. 145 (1976) 267
Ogata, A., Y. Ho, N. Nozaki: On the parotid gland hormone. Med. Biol. 5 (1944) 253
Otsuki, M., S. Saeki, H. Yuu, M. Maeda, S. Baba: Electrophoretic pattern of amylase isoenzymes in serum and urine of normal persons. Clin. Chem. 22 (1976) 439
Parisier, S. C., W. J. Binder, A. Blitzer, W. H. Friedman, W. F. Marovitz: Evaluation of tympanic neurectomy and chorda tympanectomy for gustatory sweating and benign salivary gland disease. Ear Nose Throat J. 57 (1978) 213
Pazur, J. H.: Enzymes in synthesis and hydrolysis of starch. In Whistler, R. I., E. F. Paschall: Starch, Chemistry and Technology, vol. 1. Academic Press, New York 1965
Pérez-Castillo, A., E. Blásquez: Synthesis and release of glucagon by human salivary glands. Diabetologia 19 (1980) 123
Peterson, O. H.: The effect of dinitrophenol on secretory potentials, secretion and potassium accumulation in the perfused cat submandibular gland. Acta physiol. scand. 80 (1970) 117
Petit, J. F., P. Jolles: Purification and analysis of human saliva lysozyme. Nature 200 (1963) 168
Pirsig, W., H.-J. Proescher, K. Donath: Zur Ultrastruktur geschädigter Nerven in der Parotis bei Guanacline-therapierten Hypertonikern: morphologische Substrate zum Parotisschmerz. Arch. Ohr.-, Nas.- u. Kehlk.-Heilk. 205 (1973) 103
Pointon, S. E., S. P. Banerjee: β-Adrenergic and muscarinic cholinergic receptors in rat submaxillary glands. Effects of thyroidectomy. Biochim. biophys. Acta 583 (1979) 129
Putney, J. W. jr., S. J. Weiss, B. A. Leslie, S. H. Marier: Is calcium the final mediator of exocytosis in the rat parotid gland? J. Pharmacol. exp. Ther. 203 (1977) 144
Rajasingham, R., J. L. Bell, D. N. Baron: A comparative study of the isoenzymes of mammalian α-amylase. Enzyme 12 (1971) 180
Rauch, S.: Die Speicheldrüsen des Menschen. Anatomie, Physiologie und klinische Pathologie. Thieme, Stuttgart 1959
Rauch, S., A. Khaksar: Prüfung der Speicheldrüsenfunktion. HNO 14 (1966) 120
Reichert, F. L., E. J. Poth: Pathways for the secretory fibers of the salivary glands in man. Proc. Soc. exp. Biol. 30 (1932/33) 973
Reinecke, M.: Sekretionsstudien an den Azinuszellen der Parotis des Meerschweinchens im normalen Zustand, im Hunger und nach Pilocarpingabe. Arch. klin. exp. Ohr.-, Nas.- u. Kehlk.-Heilk. 189 (1967) 168
Robyt, J. F., D. French: Multiple attack hypothesis of α-amylase action: Action of porcine pancreatic, human salivary, and aspergillus oryzae α-amylases. Archs. Biochem. Biophys. 122 (1967) 8
Robyt, J. F., W. J. Whelan: The α-amylases. In Radley, J. A.: Starch and its Derivatives. Chapman & Hall, London 1968
Rosenmund, H., M. J. Kaczmarek: Isolation and characterization of isoenzymes of human salivary and pancreatic α-amylase. Clin. chim. Acta 71 (1976) 185
Ross, J. A. T.: The function of the tympanic plexus as related to Frey's syndrome. Laryngoscope 80 (1970) 1816
Rossiter, M. A., J. A. Barrowman, A. Dand, B. A. Wharton: Amylase content of mixed saliva in children. Acta paediat. scand. 63 (1974) 389
Ryan, J., H. Appert: Circulatory turnover of pancreatic amylase. Proc. Soc. exp. Biol. Med. 149 (1975) 921
Salt, W. B., S. Schenker: Amylase – its clinical significance: A review of the literature. Medicine 55 (1976) 269
Sanders, T. G., W. J. Rutter: Molecular properties of rat pancreatic and parotid α-amylase. Biochemistry 11 (1972) 130
Schachter, M.: Kinins – a group of active peptides. Ann. Rev. Pharmacol. 4 (1964) 281
Schneider, K. W.: Ätiologie und Therapie des Parotissyndroms. Münch. med. Wschr. 115 (1973) 795
Schneyer, L. H.: Method for the collection of separate submaxillary and sublingual salivas in man. J. dent. Res. 34 (1955) 257
Schneyer, L. H.: Amylase content of separate salivary gland secretions of man. J. appl. Physiol. 9 (1956) 453
Schneyer, L. H.: Secretion of potassium by perfused excretory duct of rat submaxillary gland. Amer. J. Physiol. 217 (1969) 1324
Schöni, M., D. Kaiser, E. Drack, U. Axmacher: Excretion of trypsin-like activity, electrolytes and protein in mixed and parotid saliva of patients with cystic fibrosis of the pancreas. Eur. J. Clin. Invest. 5 (1975) 153
Schramm, M., E. Naim: Adenyl cyclase in rat parotid gland. Activation by fluoride and norepinephrine. J. biol. Chem. 245 (1970) 3225
Schramm, M., Z. Selinger: The function of α-and β-adrenergic receptors and a cholinergic receptor in the secretory cell of rat parotid gland. In Ceccarelli, B., F. Clementi, J. Meldolesi: Advances in Cytopharmacology, vol. 2. Raven Press, New York 1974
Schulte, W.: Speichel und Blutgerinnung. Dtsch. zahnärztl. Z. 19 (1964) 193
Selinger, Z.: Diverse functions of calcium in the rat parotid acinar cell. In Carafoli, E.: Calcium Transport in Contraction and Secretion. North Holland Publishing Amsterdam 1975
Selye, H., R. Veilleux, M. Cantin: Excessive stimulation of salivary gland growth by isoproterenol. Science 133 (1961) 44
Shannon, I. L.: Climatological effects of human parotid gland function. Arch. oral Biol. 11 (1966) 451
Shannon, I. L.: Reference table for human parotid saliva collected at varying levels of exogenous stimulation. J. dent. Res. 52 (1973) 1157
Shannon, I. L., R. P. Feller: Effects of lights of specific spectral characteristics on human resting parotid gland function. Arch. oral Biol. 19 (1974) 1077
Shannon, I. L., R. P. Suddick, H. H. Chauncey: Effect of atropineinduced flow rate depression on the composition of unstimulated human parotid fluid. Arch. oral Biol. 14 (1969) 761

Shannon, I. L., R. P. Suddick, F. J. Dowd: Saliva: Composition and Secretion. Karger, Basel 1974
Shannon, I. L., R. P. Feller, W. B. Wescott: Environmental lighting and human salivary gland function. Proc. Soc. exp. Biol. Med. 148 (1975) 758
Silano, V., M. Furia, L. Gianfreda, A. Macri, R. Palescandolo, A. Rab, V. Scardi, E. Stella, F. Valfre: Inhibition of amylases from different origins by albumins from the wheat kernel. Biochim. biophys. Acta 391 (1975) 170
Skude, G., I. Ihse: Salivary amylase in duodenal aspirates. Scand. J. Gastroent. 11 (1976) 17
Skude, G., P.-A. Mårdh, L. Westrom: Amylases of genital tract. 1. Isoamylases of genital tract tissue homogenates and peritoneal fluid. Amer. J. Obstet. Gynec. 126 (1976) 652
Skurk, A., D. Fritsche, K. Fendel: Variation in the amylase isoenzymes of human parotid saliva in health and disease. Arch. oral Biol. 20 (1975) 429
Skurk, A., K. Winnefeld, H.-J. Tiedt, A. Schmidt, K. Fendel: Spurenelemente in Speichelsteinen. Die Bestimmung von Ca, Mg, Fe, Cu, Zn, Mn und P. Z. Laryng. Rhinol. 52 (1973) 822
Slowey, R. R., S. Eidelman, S. J. Klebanoff: Antibacterial activity of the purified peroxidase from human parotid saliva. J. Bact. 96 (1968) 575
Smith, Q. T., M. J. Hamilton, M. H. Biros, B. L. Pihlstrom: Salivary and plasma IgA of seizure subjects receiving phenytoin. Epilepsia 20 (1979) 17
Speirs, R. L., J. Herring, W. D. Cooper, C. C. Hardy, C. R. K. Hind: The influence of sympathetic activity and isoprenaline on the secretion of amylase from the human parotid gland. Arch. oral Biol. 19 (1974) 747
Steinberg, T., V. Passy, G. Gwinup: Effect of submaxillary gland extirpation on glucose and insulin tolerance in dogs. Diabetes 21 (1972) 722
Stiefel, D. J., P. J. Keller: Preparation and some properties of human pancreatic amylase including a comparison with parotid amylase. Biochim. biophys. Acta 302 (1973) 345
Street, H. V., J. R. Close: Determination of amylase activity in biological fluids. Clin. chim. Acta 1 (1956) 256
Takizawa, N.: A pathological research on the internal secretion of the salivary glands. Acta Pathol. Jap. 4 (1954) 229
Tan, S. G.: Human saliva esterases: genetic studies. Hum. Hered. 26 (1976) 207
Tan, S. G., Y. S. Teng: Human saliva as a source of biochemical genetic markers. I. Techniques. Hum. Hered. 29 (1979) 69
Tannenbaum, S. R., M. Wiesman, D. Fett: The effect of nitrate intake on nitrite formation in human saliva. Food Cosmet. Toxicol. 14 (1976) 549
Thaysen, E. H., S. Müllertz, H. Worning, H. O. Bang: Amylase concentration of duodenal aspirates after stimulation of the pancreas by a standard meal. Gastroenterology 46 (1964) 23
Thulin, A.: Secretory and motor effects in the submaxillary gland of the rat on intraarterial administration of some polypeptides and autonomic drugs. Acta Physiol. scand. 97 (1976) 343
Tieche, J.-M., J. Leonora, R. R. Steinmann: Isolation and partial characterization of a porcine parotid hormone that stimulates dentinal fluid transport. Endocrinology 106 (1980) 1994
Tomasi, T. B.: Secretory immunoglobulins. New Engl. J. Med. 287 (1972) 500
Townes, P. L., W. D. Moore, M. R. White: Amylase polymorphism: Studies of sera and duodenal aspirates in normal individuals and in cystic fibrosis. Amer. J. hum. Genet. 28 (1976) 378
Villarejos, V. M., K. A. Visoná, A. D. Gutiérrez, A. Rodriguez: Saliva and feces as transmittors of type B hepatitis. New Engl. J. Med. 291 (1974) 1375
Vogel, J. J., R. Naujoks, F. Brudevold: The effective concentrations of calcium and inorganic phosphate in salivary secretions. Arch. oral Biol. 10 (1965) 523
Vogt, K., W. M. Semmann: Zur physiologischen Beeinflussung der Gesamtproteinsekretion der großen Kopfspeicheldrüsen durch Tageszeit, Alter und Geschlecht. Z. Laryng. Rhinol. 49 (1970) 611
Volle, R. L.: Modifications by drugs of synaptic mechanisms in autonomic ganglia. Pharmacol. Rev. 18 (1966) 839
Vollrath, M., M. Brüner, C. Arglebe, R. Chilla: Der N. facialis als Träger sekretorischer Parotisfasern. Arch. Oto-Rhino-Laryng. 228 (1980) 57
Watkins, W. M.: Blood-group specific substances. In Gottschalk: Glycoproteins; their Composition, Structure and Function. B. B. A. Library, vol. 5, part B. Elsevier, Amsterdam 1972 (p. 830)
Werle, E., R. Vogel, L. F. Goldel: Über ein blutdrucksteigerndes Prinzip in Extrakten aus der Gl. submaxillaris der weissen Maus. Arch. exp. Path. Pharm. 230 (1957) 236
Wiener, K., C. H. Foot: A study of some factors affecting the Phadebas amylase test. Clin. chim. Acta 75 (1977) 177
Yannoulis, G., L. Manolidis: Über den Speichelausfluß der Parotis nach Radikaloperation und Lempertoperation. Arch. klin. exp. Ohr.-, Nas.- u. Kehlk.-Heilk. 173 (1958) 380
Zacharski, L. R., R. Rosenstein: Reduction of salivary tissue factor (thromboplastin) activity by warfarin therapy. Blood 53 (1979) 366
Zöllner, E. J., D. M. Klepsch, R. K. Zahn, R. Knepper: Deoxyribonucleases in human parotid saliva. Enzyme 19 (1974) 60

5. Methods of Investigation

Clinical Findings

A careful history is essential for the diagnosis of salivary gland diseases. Questions about generalized diseases, particularly metabolic diseases, and the use of medicines, such as antihypertensive and psychotropic agents, are of particular importance.

The age and sex of the patient are crucial: tumors of the parotid gland in the newborn and young children are almost always hemangiomas or lymphangiomas, or rare congenital cystic duct ectasia. In school children, virus infections predominate, whereas the sialadenoses occur mainly in middle age, and malignant tumors in patients beyond the age of 45 years. A bilateral tumor in a man is almost always a cystadenolymphoma. The size, consistency, mobility, and tenderness of the gland is assessed by examination. An experienced examiner can differentiate neoplastic from non-neoplastic disease by simple clinical examination.

Careful examination of the oral cavity, including assessment of the salivary ducts and the tonsillar region, is also essential. Pressure on the gland provides a rough estimate of the quantity and quality of the saliva. Parotid tumors may extend into the parapharyngeal space, bulging the pharyngeal wall. This finding is very important in planning the operation. If inflammatory disease can be excluded, tenderness almost always indicates malignancy, as does a facial paralysis.

Sialography

Undesirable side effects must be considered in the choice of the contrast medium. Oily contrast medium has been used for a long time: its advantages are that it does not mix with saliva, and it is retained for a long period in the duct system, providing a good contrast. But if the contrast medium penetrates the parenchyma of the gland, a severe infection is set up that often requires surgical treatment. The oily contrast medium may be extravasated by injury to the duct during dilation or by the use of too much medium.

Brands (1972) therefore recommends that oily contrast medium should only be injected under visual control using the image intensifier.

A water-contrast medium, for example, triiodinated Conray 80, should preferably be used for the first sialogram. If the required contrast is not achieved, an oily contrast medium can be used later, but in most cases this is not necessary, if good radiologic equipment is available. If manipulation under the x-ray screen is prolonged, contrast medium flows rapidly into the mouth so that assessment is no longer possible. The value of the contrast medium depends on its iodine content. The examiner must therefore be well informed about the qualitative composition of the contrast medium used (Pfeiffer 1968).

A watery crystal suspension (Hytrast) was used by Kempfle (1970) and by Herberhold and Müller (1971). One advantage of this preparation compared with a pure water-contrast medium is its long period of retention in the duct system, providing good contrast.

According to Brands (1972), this preparation has the same side effects as the oily substances. The patient may experience considerable symptoms if the contrast medium is long retained in the duct system: these are probably to be explained by the fact that the water content of the preparation is absorbed by the duct epithelium, whereas the crystalline content remains in the duct lumen and produces a retention effect. Parotitis has been reported after the use of Hytrast for sialography by Lenz (1971), but Herberhold and Müller (1971) did not observe this complication in any of their patients.

The duct system is filled with contrast as follows: The patient is placed in the sitting position. The papilla of the duct is dilated without premedication or local anesthesia and is then catheterized with a small plastic tube. Quantitative and qualitative investigations of the saliva must, of course, be carried out before sialography is undertaken. The contrast medium is then injected into the duct system via a small polyethylene tube, ensuring that no air is present in the tube. The contrast medium is injected under slight pressure until a

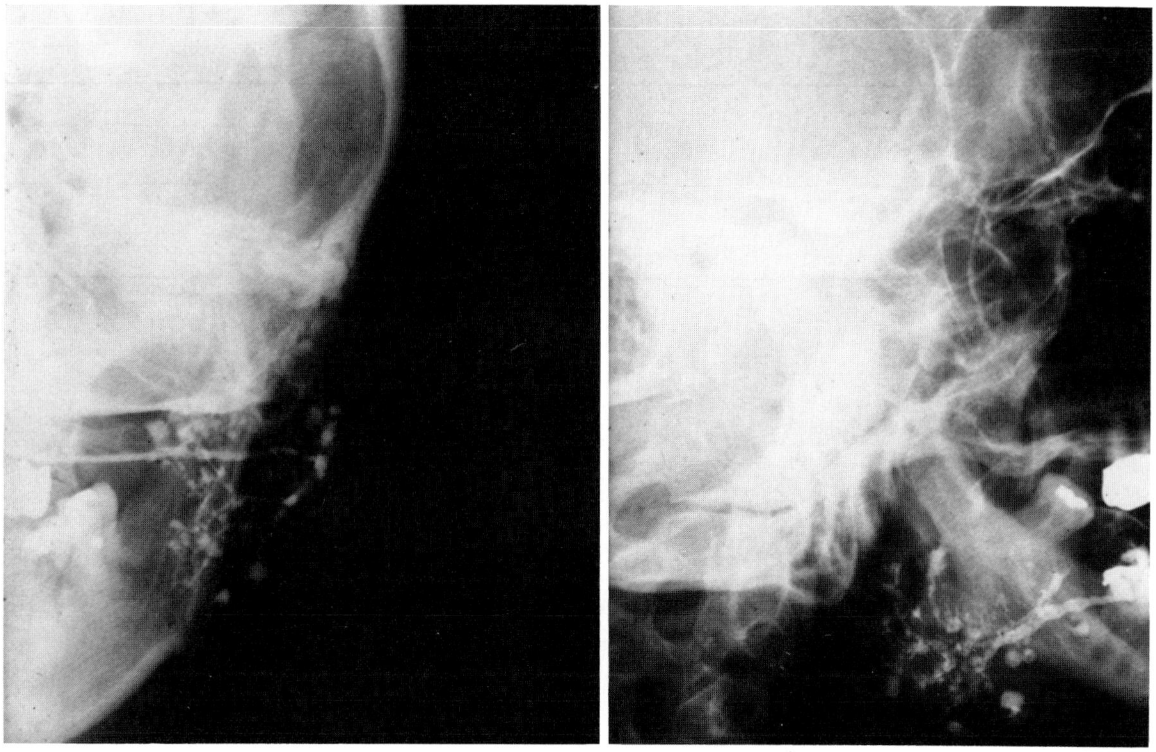

Figure 5.**1** Sialogram in chronic recurrent parotitis: **a** Diffuse spherical duct ectasia.

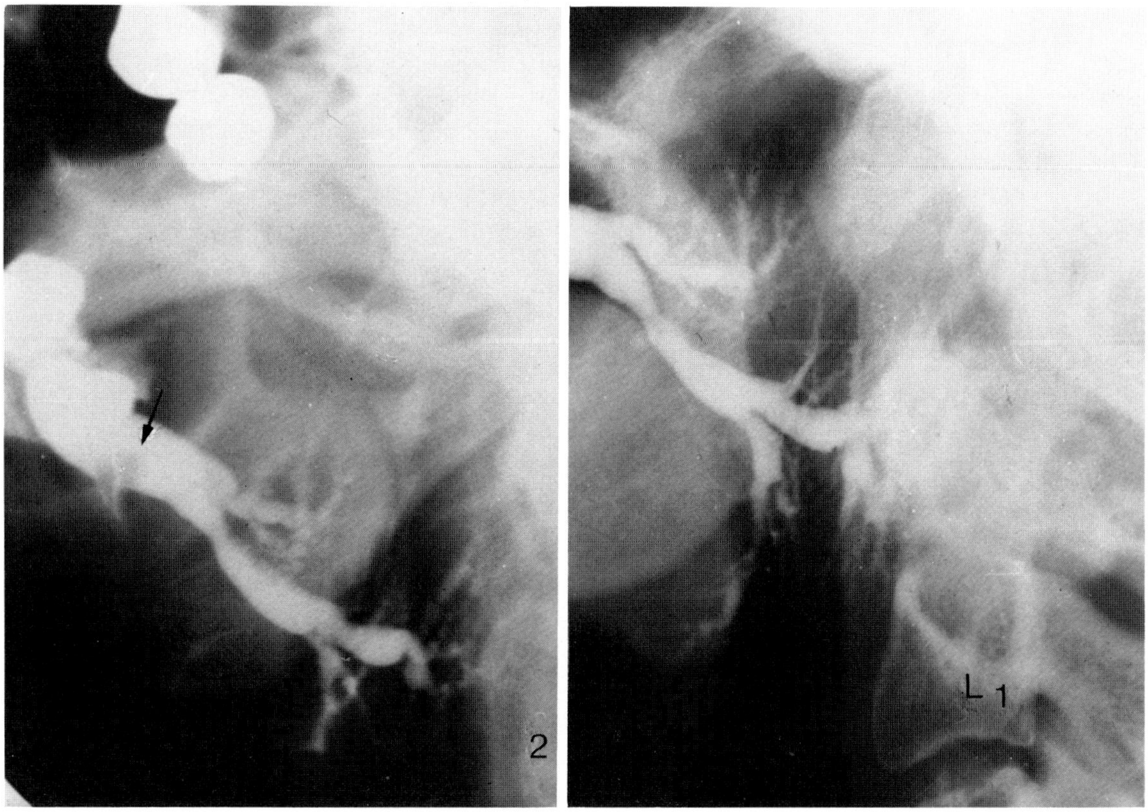

5.**1b** Grossly dilated duct in advanced chronic recurrent parotitis.

rapidly increasing feeling of tension becomes painful, albeit tolerable. Depending on the size of the parotid gland, 0.7–2 ml may be injected.

Approximately the same amount may be injected into the duct system of the submandibular gland. The patient presses his lips lightly together to fix the tube. Radiographs in the anteroposterior and lateral position are then taken (Fig. 5.**1a**, **b**).

Injection of too much contrast medium ruptures the duct, allowing the contrast medium to escape into the parenchyma. On the other hand, injection of insufficient contrast medium may cause a filling defect, leading to an incorrect diagnosis. Iodine sensitivity is a contraindication to sialography using iodine-containing contrast medium, and a barium-containing medium may then be used. Normally, the contrast medium is excreted after 15 minutes to 2 hours. This may be used as the basis of a functional test by assessing the excretion of the contrast medium after giving atropine to suppress the salivary secretion. The subcutaneous injection of 0.02 g of pilocarpine then follows to reverse the action of atropine (Kempfle 1970).

Brands (1969, 1972) described fractionated sialography in which the contrast medium is injected gradually under closed circuit television control. The individual filling phases can be well demonstrated and recorded by this method.

Scintiscanning

Scintiscanning provides information about the size, position, and contour of an organ and about uptake of radionuclides by that organ.

Dynamic imaging of the salivary glands provides an assessment of the uptake and excretion of radionuclides, with an early phase representing vascular perfusion.

Static imaging is also of considerable importance (Börner et al 1965, Kessler & Theuring 1975). In this type of imaging there is little change in the radionuclide concentration in the organ under investigation. Static imaging provides mainly morphologic data. The combination of dynamic and static images is very useful and increases the value of nuclear medicine (Glaubitt & Haubrich 1980). Quantification of a salivary scan is useful using the ratio of impulse to image elements.

In our practice dynamic imaging is performed in the anterior projection immediately after intravenous injection of ^{99m}Tc-pertechnetate (1.0 MBq/kg body weight) to assess the blood supply and the initial uptake of the technetium in the salivary glands. Occasionally, dynamic imaging in the posterior projection is necessary. Sequential imaging in the anterior, posterior, right lateral, and left lateral planes will record the position and shape of the organ, the extent of the uptake, and also any deviation from normal. This phase of the investigation is therefore mainly of morphologic significance.

Dynamic imaging to assess salivary secretion is performed after instillation of 2.0 ml of fresh lemon juice into the oral cavity. Views are taken at intervals from 8 minutes before to 12 minutes after stimulation, allowing an estimate of function in the whole salivary gland, and, if necessary, in specific areas (Haubrich & Glaubitt 1982). This

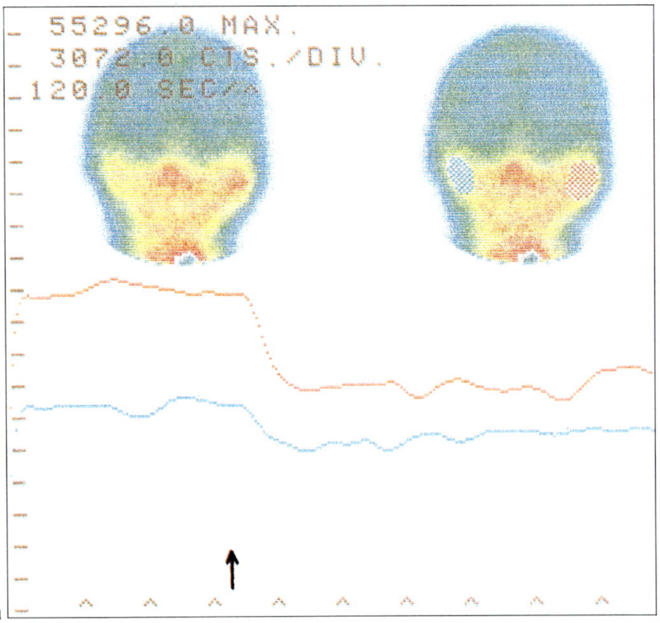

a

Figure 5.**2** Functional imaging of the parotid gland in the occipital plane: **a** A 74-year-old patient with a pleomorphic adenoma of the parotid gland. After stimulation of parotid secretion (↑), radioactive technetium is released freely from the right parotid gland, but in smaller amounts from the left parotid gland, although still within the normal range.

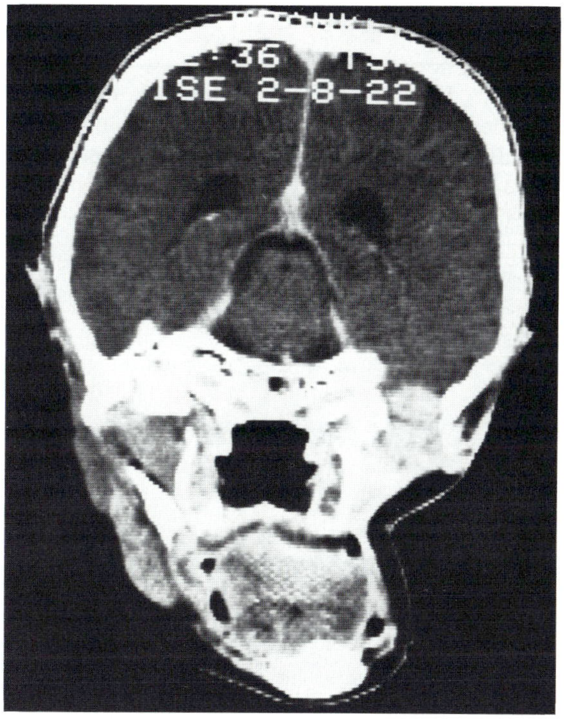

Figure 5.**4** Computed tomogram of a 61-year-old woman: situation after operation for a duct carcinoma with resection of the left cheek and a segment of the upper jaw, followed by recurrence. The CT scan shows the posterosuperior extent of the tumor toward the skull base, with destruction of the temporal bone, and intracerebral extension of the tumor.

sialadenitis who experienced a marked increase in size of the parotid gland. A repeat biopsy showed a malignant non-Hodgkin's lymphoma, a malignant transformation that may occur during chronic myoepithelial sialadentis. A B-ultrasound scan showed the echo-poor zones of lymph nodes and the echogenic areas of parotid tissue.

The advantages of ultrasound include the absence of radiation exposure of the patient and the surgeon, the speed of the examination (5 to 10 minutes), and the lower costs (Mann 1977). Ultrasound, like CT, provides no conclusions about the pathologic process, but it does demonstrate nonhomogeneity of tissue and bone destruction due to a malignant tumor. More experience is needed to assess the place of ultrasound in the diagnosis of salivary disorders.

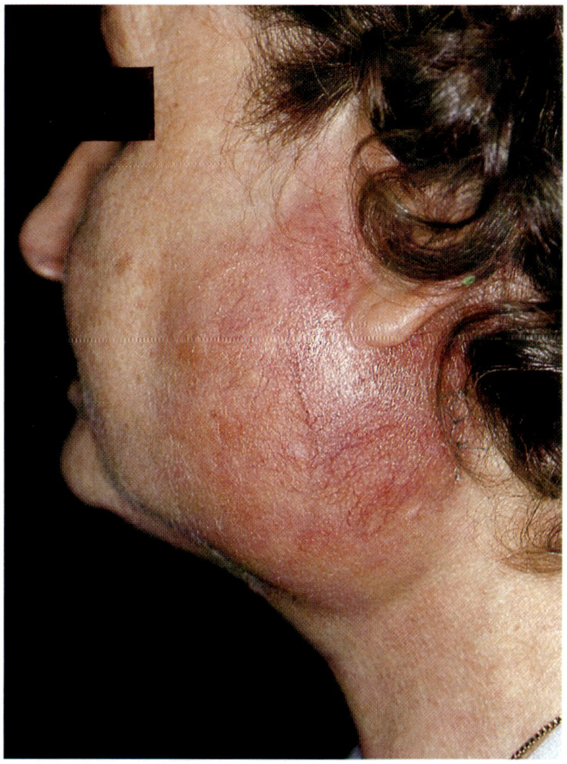

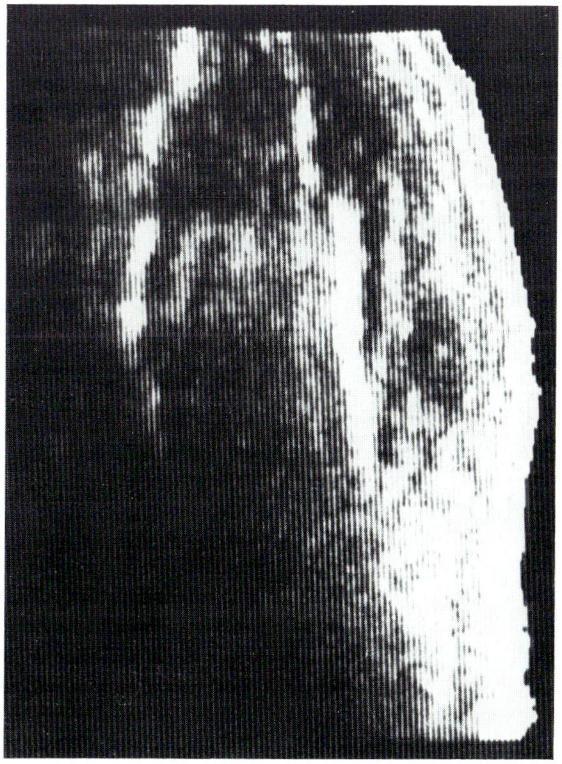

Figure 5.**5a** A 58-year-old patient with a chronic myoepithelial sialadenitis with malignant transformation to a non-Hodgkin's lymphoma.

b B-ultrasound scan.

Needle Biopsy

This diagnostic method may supplement other methods of investigations, as does needle biopsy of other organs, such as the liver, the pancreas, and the lungs (Wolf 1982). There are two prerequisites: firstly, expertise, allowing the acquisition of a representative cylinder of tissue, and secondly, an appropriate indication. The needle used is similar in caliber to that used for urologic prostate punch biopsies. A cylinder of tissue 1–2 cm long is obtained that is processed and analyzed after paraffin embedding, cutting, and staining (Figs. 5.**6**–5.**10**).

Needle biopsy has not yet achieved much place in the diagnosis of salivary diseases, although at its best it is as good as open biopsy. The salivary glands are readily accessible for biopsy (see later), if this is necessary. This has the advantage that a facial nerve paralysis is very unlikely to occur if certain rules are observed. On the other hand, needle biopsy has considerable disadvantages compared with aspiration cytology, so that it is not really possible to compare the two methods.

The material obtained by aspiration is examined by cytology, whereas that obtained by needle biopsy is examined by routine histologic methods. Aspiration is not expensive and causes little pain, so that local anesthesia is superfluous. In more than 1000 aspiration biopsies obtained from salivary glands, we have not seen any of the possible complications, such as spillage of tumor cells or facial nerve paralysis, and we have seen only one reactionary hemorrhage. The risk of complications is considerably greater after needle biopsy.

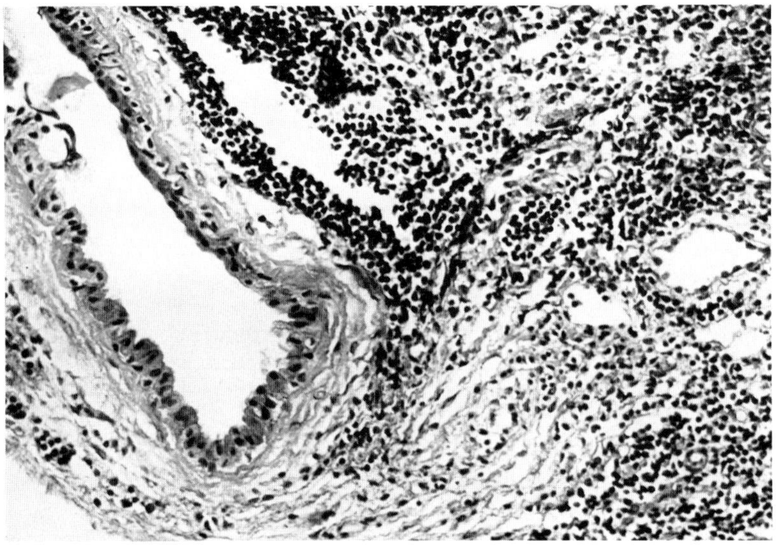

Figure 5.**6** Needle biopsy from the parotid gland showing chronic sialectasis. H & E, 160×.

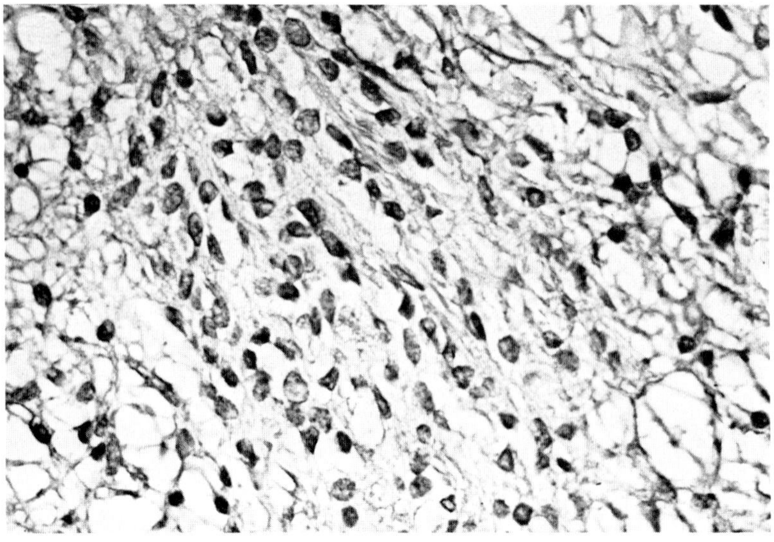

Figure 5.**7** Pleomorphic parotid adenoma: needle biopsy. Astra blue, 400×.

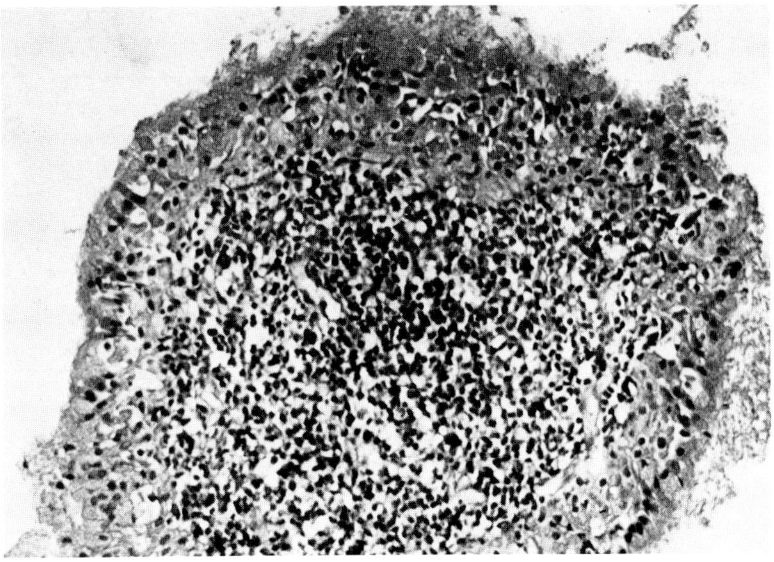

Figure 5.**8** Needle biopsy from a cystadenolymphoma with oncocytic tumor cells and lymphoid stroma. H & E, 400×.

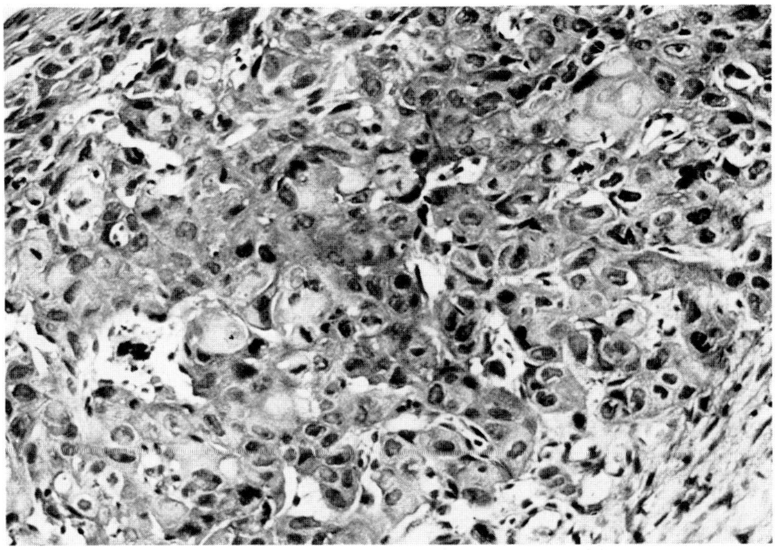

Figure 5.**9** Needle biopsy from a squamous cell carcinoma of the parotid gland. H & E, 160×.

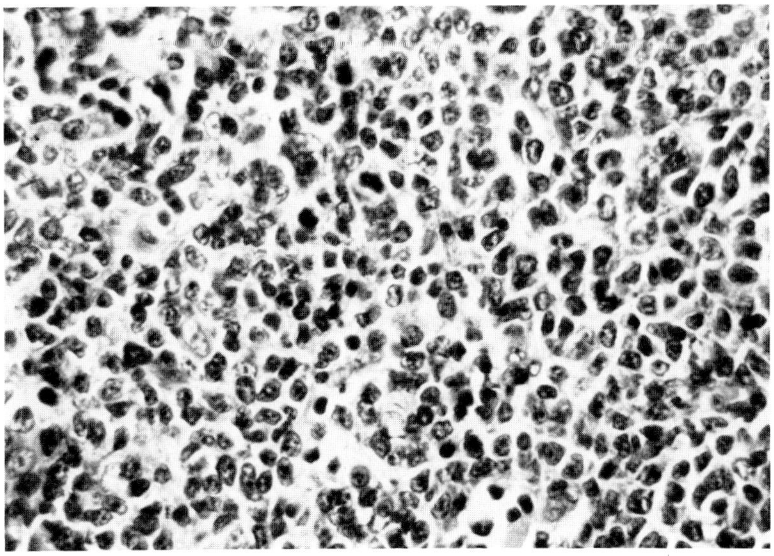

Figure 5.**10** Needle biopsy from a malignant lymphoma (immunocytoma of the parotid). H & E, 400×.

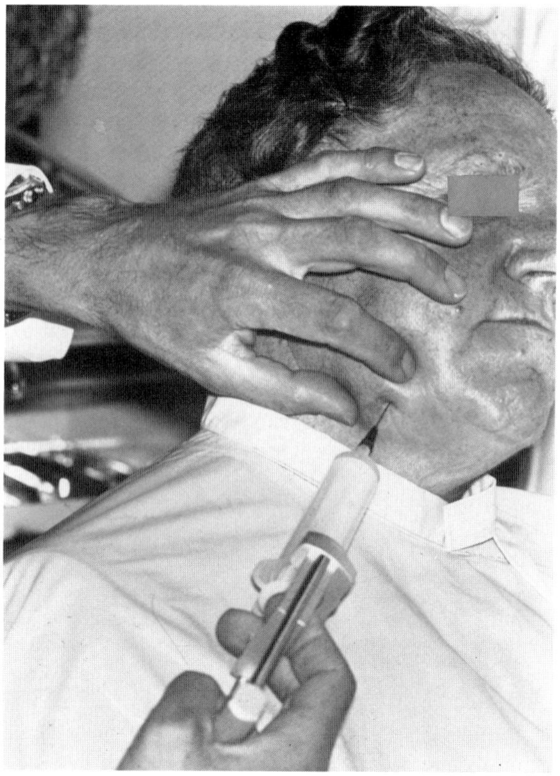

Figure 5.**11** Fine needle aspiration of the submandibular gland.

Fine Needle Aspiration Cytology

Fine needle aspiration followed by cytologic examination of the aspirate was first used for the investigation of salivary diseases at the Radiumhemmet in Stockholm in 1953 (Eneroth et al 1967a, 1967b, Mavec et al 1964). The widespread use of aspiration cytology in the diagnosis of salivary diseases was placed on a firm footing by several investigations in which the findings of cytology and histopathology were compared (Droese et al 1977 and 1978, Lindenberg & Akerman 1976, Persson & Zettergren 1973, Hagelqvist 1978, Zajicek 1974, Bremer et al 1982). The establishment of reproducible diagnostic criteria was of even greater significance. The most comprehensive study carried out is that of 600 cases reported by Droese in 1980. Morphometric and flow-through cytophotometric analyses were also carried out in addition to analyses of the cell appearance (Eneroth & Zetterberg 1974).

The fine needle aspirate is obtained by the method introduced by Franzén et al (1960) (Fig. 5.**11**). A disposable number 17 needle and a disposable 20 ml syringe are used. A special hand grip (Fig. 5.**12**) allows the syringe to be manipulated with one hand so that the other hand can be used to fix the test area (Fig. 5.**13**). The needle is introduced through the skin and is then pushed in different directions into the tumor under continuous aspiration. The low pressure in the syringe is released before removing the needle so that the material obtained is not sucked from the needle into the syringe. The material is then squirted onto a slide, maintaining continuous contact between the needle and the slide. The tissue is smeared on the slide, dried in air, and stained by the May-Grünwald-Giemsa method. The usual cytologic criteria are used, including cell type, cell differentiation, arrangement of the cells in the smear, and assessment of noncellular elements (Figs. 5.**14**–5.**17**).

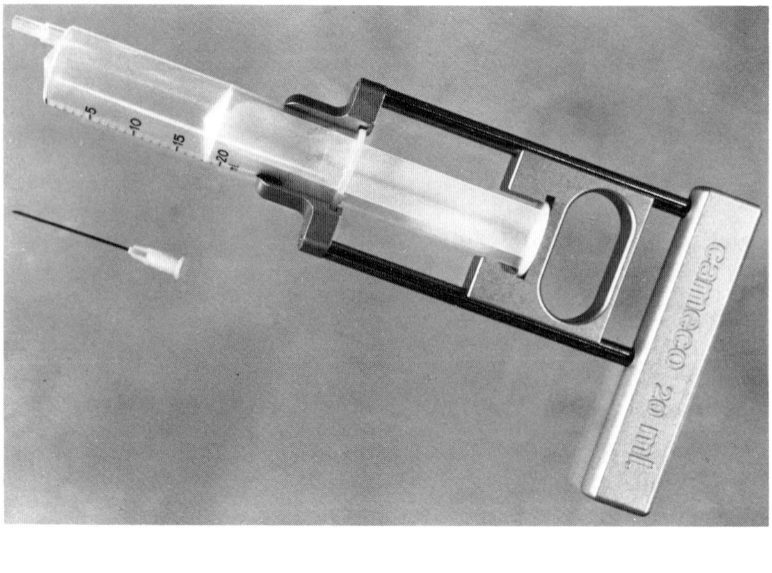

Figure 5.**12** Apparatus for fine needle aspiration: a 20 ml disposable syringe fixed in a distal hand grip (made by the Swedish firm Chemico), to permit one-handed use (Fig. 5.**13**). A number 17 or 18 needle is used.

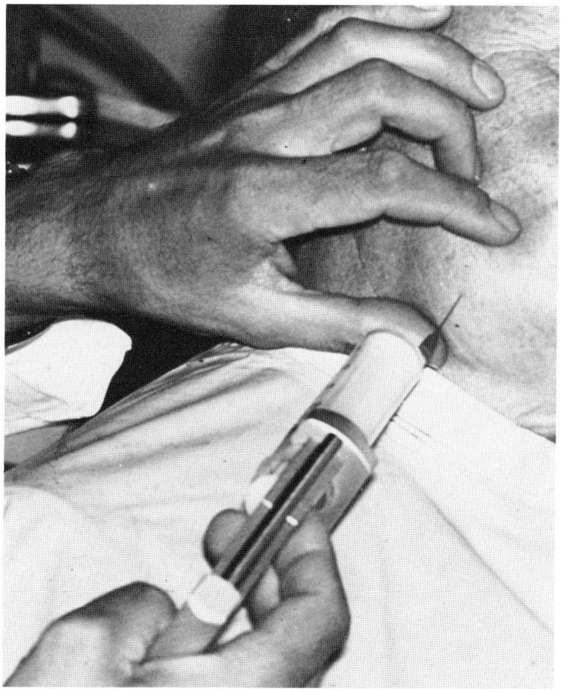

Figure 5.**13** Fine needle aspiration biopsy of a submandibular tumor. Usually any tumor is punctured twice in different directions (Fig. 5.**11**). The aspirated material is immediately smeared on a slide.

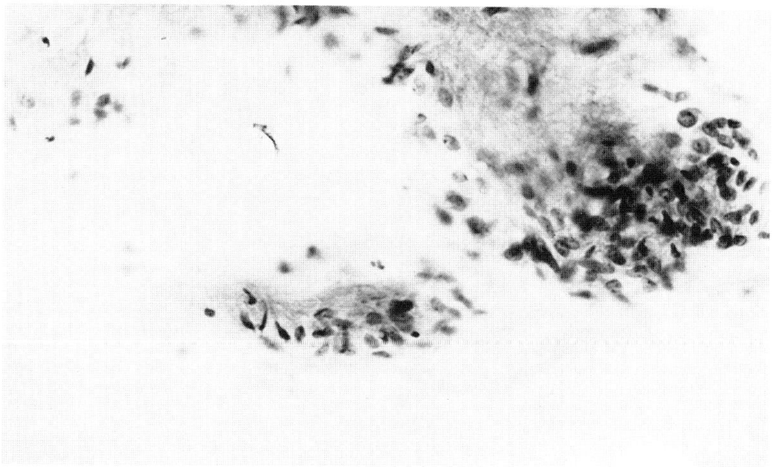

Figure 5.**14** Pleomorphic adenoma showing aspiration cytology of spindle-shaped cells and mucoid substances. 160×.

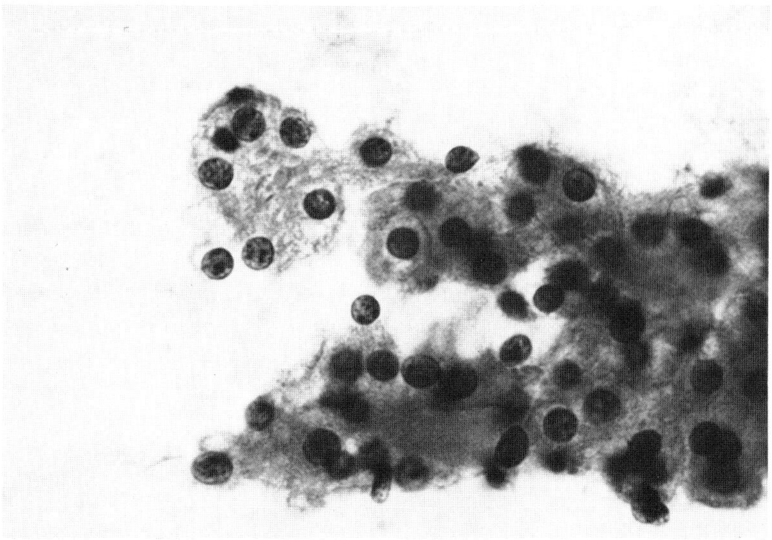

Figure 5.**15** Acinic cell tumor of the parotid gland showing acinar arrangement of cells with granular cytoplasm. 400×.

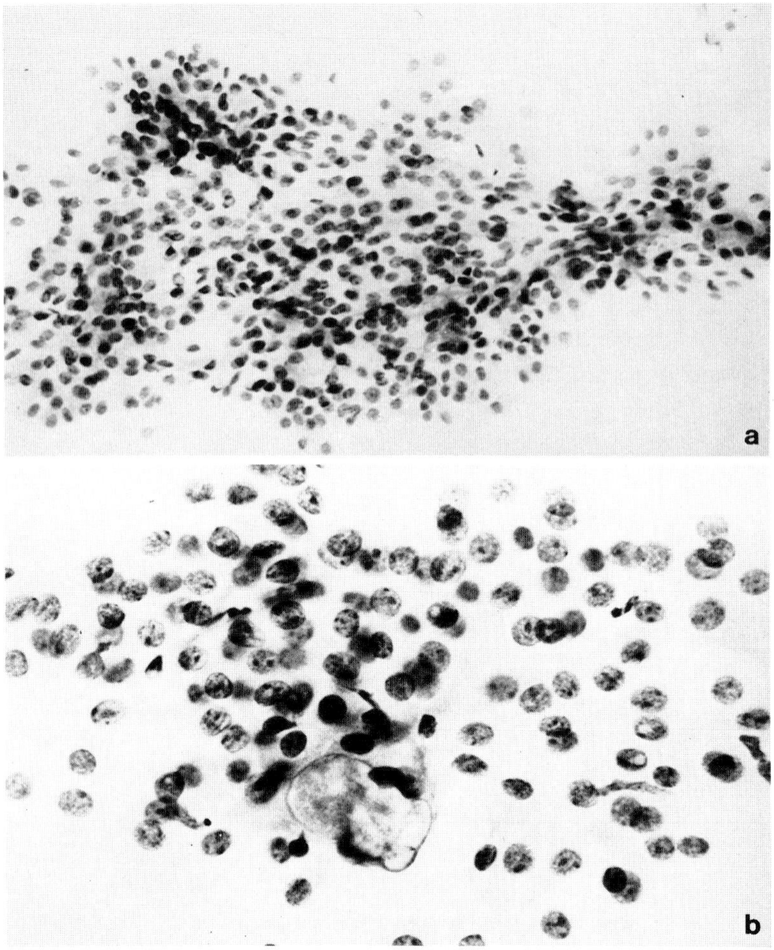

Figure 5.**16** Mucoepidermoid tumor of the parotid gland. Epidermoid cell groups with inclusion of mucous-forming vacular cells. **a** 160×, **b** 400×.

A histologic diagnosis of a salivary tumor can be made before operation in a high proportion of patients using this procedure (Eneroth & Zajicek 1965, Eneroth et al 1967b, Persson & Zettergren 1973, Webb 1973, Zajicek 1974, Droese et al 1978, Droese 1980). Non-neoplastic lesions are considerably more difficult to diagnose. In our experience, the differentiation of the tumor can be determined in 95% of cases (Droese et al 1978). Difficulties only arise with cystadenolymphomas in which degenerative oncocytes or metaplastic squamous cells from the tissue surrounding the tumor are incorrectly diagnosed as tumor cells. The type of tumor can be correctly determined in 90% of cases. The diagnostic success rate for malignant tumors (74.3%) is clearly worse than that for benign tumors (96.5%). Difficulties arise, particularly in differentiating poorly differentiated mucoepidermoid tumors from poorly differentiated acinic cell tumors. The success rate is particularly high in pleomorphic adenomas and adenoid cystic carcinomas (Droese et al 1978). The method of investigation is easy for the clinician to carry out, but the cytologic assessment of the aspirate is difficult. The success rate is determined largely by the experience of the histopathologist.

Cytology and histology are not competing diagnostic methods, but rather complementary. Aspiration cytology in the preoperative diagnosis of salivary gland diseases is a very useful step that allows the details of the operation to be explained to the patient. Furthermore, it is useful in the follow-up of the patient who has already undergone an operation and is suspected of having a recurrence of the tumor. The final diagnosis is confirmed by histopathologic examination of the surgical specimen. There is no doubt that histology is more reliable than aspiration cytology. The question also arises as to which method permits the simplest and safest method of assessing the pathologic features of a salivary gland disease. A biopsy of a tumor is contraindicated for several reasons, so that the surgeon should resort to fine needle biopsy in planning an operation, particularly because the success rate in the hands of a practiced cytologist is very high.

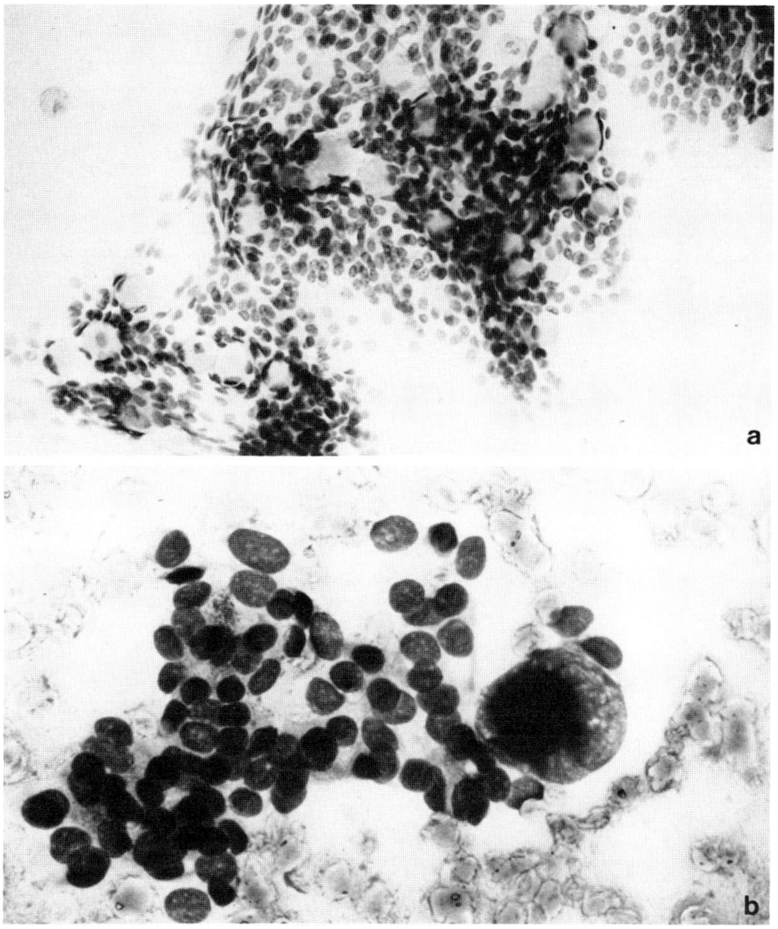

Figure 5.**17** Adenoid cystic carcinoma showing trabecular arrangement of duct epithelium with cylindrical inclusions **a** 160×, **b** 400×.

If the cytologic findings are suggestive of or positive for tumor, the finding must be verified by histologic examination. This is particularly true when a tumor is not suspected on clinical grounds, since in our experience false-positives results are found in 2.2% of patients. Negative cytologic findings must also agree with the clinical picture; otherwise, further procedures must be carried out. The risk of false-negative findings arises, particularly in cystic tumors (Eneroth et al 1967b).

Biopsy

Removal of tissue by a biopsy requires accurate knowledge of the course of the facial nerve (Kleinsasser 1976, Conley 1975). There is an extensive literature on the indications for biopsy and its possible dangers (Beck, 1971, Boehme 1966, Conley 1975, Eneroth 1976, Haubrich 1976, Jasper 1969, Kleinsasser 1976, von Westernhagen 1966). If the biopsy is too superficial, there is danger of an incorrect diagnosis, because representative material is not available for examination. Damage to the tumor capsule leads to spillage and implantation of tumor into the surrounding tissue. Furthermore, the success of a radical procedure is compromised. A biopsy is justifiable if the specimen can be examined by frozen section, which can be followed immediately by surgery if indicated. The material obtained by biopsy can also be analyzed by the usual staining of paraffin sections after embedding. A biopsy of a tumor should not be carried out, if the necessary operation cannot proceed immediately.

The indications for biopsy are therefore nonneoplastic lesions of the salivary glands, for example, chronic inflammation. In myoepithelial sialadenitis particularly, a fine needle biopsy often fails to differentiate other inflammatory lesions or lymphocytic tumors. A biopsy is only indicated if good cytology is not available or the results of cytology are equivocal. The position can be summarized as follows:

a) A *biopsy* is contraindicated for all clinically *benign tumors*. A superficial parotidectomy is the correct diagnostic procedure. This procedure is based on the behavior of a pleomorphic

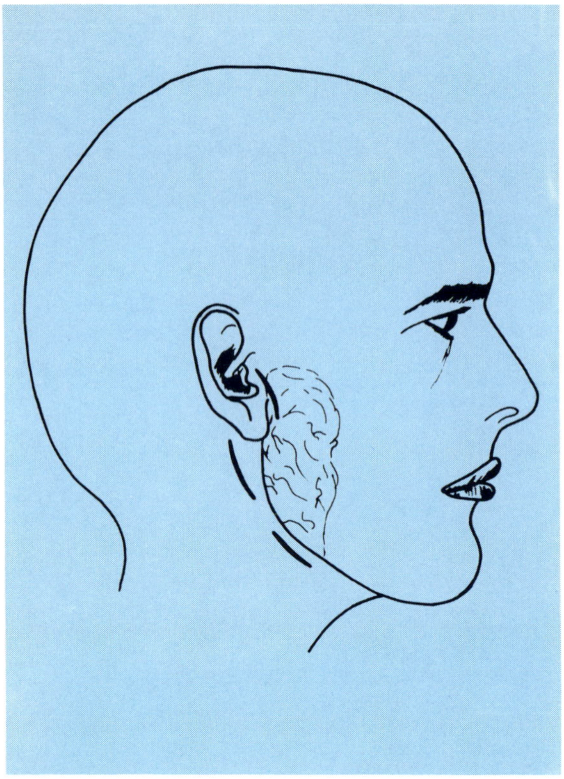

a

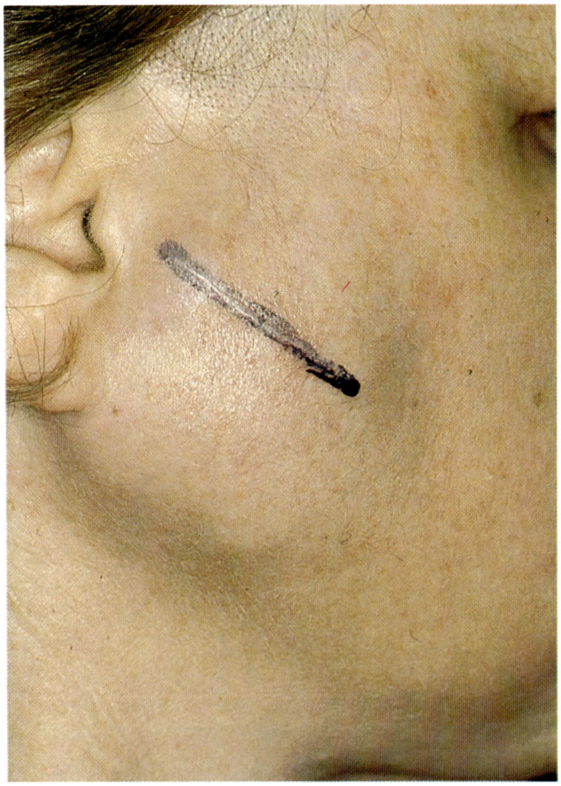

b

Figure 5.**18** Incision for taking a biopsy of the parotid gland: **a** correct, **b** incorrect.

adenoma: opening the tumor capsule carries the risk of local recurrence of tumor, even if the operation is carried out immediately.

b) A biopsy should be carried out immediately before the operation, if a *malignant tumor* (page 222ff) is suspected, firstly, to establish the diagnosis before operation, and secondly, to improve planning of the operation, for example, whether it is necessary to resect and reconstruct the facial nerve (page 278ff). The biopsy is then supplemented by intraoperative frozen sections.

The incision for biopsy runs immediately anterior to the ear 1–2 cm from the anterior meatal wall. Sufficient salivary tissue can be removed easily from this area without injuring the facial nerve. If the diseased area lies more in the retromandibular space, the incision must lie over the most pronounced part of the swelling, even if the danger of damage to the facial nerve is greater at this site than in the preauricular area (Fig. 5.**18a, b**). Without such a biopsy, sialosis, chronic myoepithelial sialadenitis, and chronic recurrent parotitis cannot be diagnosed with certainty. For this reason, it is the most important step in the diagnosis of salivary gland disease.

References

Allars, H. M., J. Blomfield, A. R. Rush, J. M. Brown: Colloid and crystal formation in parotid saliva of cystic fibrosis patients and non-cystic fibrosis subjects. I. Physiochemistry. Pediat. Res. 10 (1976a) 578

Allars, H. M., D. J. H. Cockayne, J. Blomfield, A. R. Rush, E. W. van Lennep, J. M. Brown: Colloid and crystal formation in parotid saliva of cystic fibrosis patients and non-cystic fibrosis subjects. II. Electron microscopy and electrophoresis. Pediat. Res. 10 (1976b) 584

Anavekar, S. N., R. H. Saunders, W. M. Wardell, I. Shoulson, F. G. Emmings, C. E. Cook, A. J. Gringeri: Parotid and whole saliva in the prediction of serum total and free phenytoin concentrations. Clin. Pharmacol. Ther. 24 (1978) 629

Arglebe, C.: Biochemistry of human saliva. In Pfaltz, C. R., R. Chilla: Sialadenosis and Sialadenitis. Karger, Basel 1981

Arglebe, C., M. Opaitz, R. Chilla: Amylaseaktivität im unstimulierten Parotisspeichel des Menschen unter Berücksichtigung von Flußrate und Proteinkonzentration. Z. Laryngol. Rhinol. 58 (1979) 700

Bannet, J., J. Avni, E. Weissenberg, R. P. Ebstein, R. H. Belmaker: Salivary lithium. Brit. J. Psychiat. 134 (1979) 446

Bardon, A., D. Shugar: Properties of purified salivary ribonuclease, and salivary ribonuclease levels in children with cystic fibrosis and in heterozygous carriers. Clin. chim. Acta 101 (1980) 17

Beck, C.: Zur Frage der Probeexzision aus der Ohrspeicheldrüse. Arch. klin. exp. Ohr.-, Nas.- u. Kehlk.-Heilk. 197 (1971) 327

Becker, W., J. Haubrich, G. Seifert: Krankheiten der Speicheldrüsen. In Berendes, J., R. Link, F. Zöllner: Hals-Nasen-Ohren-Heilkunde in Praxis und Klinik, Bd. 3. Thieme, Stuttgart 1978

Ben-Aryeh, H.: Salivary phosphate as an indicator of hormonal status of women. J. dent. Res. 55 (1976) D 168

Bertram, U.: Xerostomia. Acta Odont. Scand., Suppl. 49 (1967) 1

Bhoola, K. D., R. W. Matthews, F. Roberts: A survey of salivary kallikrein and amylase in a population of schoolgirls, throughout the menstrual cycle. Clin. Sci. mol. Med. 55 (1978) 561

Blomfield, J., A. R. Rush, H. M. Allars, J. M. Brown: Parotid gland function in children with cystic fibrosis and child control subjects. Pediat. Res. 10 (1976) 574

Blomfield, J., E. W. van Lennep, C. D. Shorey, A. S. Malin, J. Dascalu, J. M. Brown: Ultrastructure of the in vitro formation of hydroxyapatite in submandibular saliva of children with cystic fibrosis. Arch. oral Biol. 19 (1974) 1153

Böhme, P.: Die Parotischirurgie und ihre morphologischen Grundlagen. Thieme, Stuttgart 1966

Börner, W., H. Grünberg, E. Moll: Die szintigraphische Darstellung der Kopfspeicheldrüsen mit Technetium 99^{m}. Med. Welt (1965) 2378

Brands, Th.: Die röntgenologische Untersuchung der Speicheldrüsen unter besonderer Berücksichtigung der gezielten fraktionierten Sialographie. Z. Laryng. Rhinol. 48 (1969) 124

Brands, Th.: Diagnose und Klinik der Erkrankungen der großen Kopfspeicheldrüsen. Urban & Schwarzenberg, München 1972

Bremer, W., I. F. Herrmann, P. H. Wuensch: Die Feinnadelpunktion zur Tumordiagnostik im Kopfhalsbereich. Eine Methode für die Praxis. HNO (Berl.) 30 (1982) 447

Bunting, R. W., U. G. Rickert: Dental caries. J. nat. dent. Ass. 2 (1915) 247

Carlson, A. J., A. L. Crittenden: The relation of ptyalin concentration to the diet and to the rate of secretion of the saliva. Amer. J. Physiol. 26 (1910) 169

Chilla, R., T. Kropp, C. Arglebe: Amylaseaktivität und Isoamylasenmuster im Parotisspeichel des Menschen. Z. Laryng. Rhinol. 56 (1977) 912

Cole, C. H., G. Sella: Inhibition of ouabain-sensitive ATPase by the saliva of patients with cystic fibrosis of the pancreas. Pediat. Res. 9 (1975) 763

Conley, J.: Salivary Glands and the Facial Nerve. Thieme, Stuttgart 1975

Dawes, C., G. N. Jenkins: The effects of different stimuli on the composition of saliva in man. J. Physiol. (Lond.) 170 (1964) 86

Doggett, R. G., G. M. Harrison: Cystic fibrosis: reversal of ciliary inhibitor in serum and saliva by heparin. Tex. Rep. Biol. Med. 31 (1973) 685

Droese, M.: Punktionszytologie der Speicheldrüsenerkrankungen. Habil.-Schrift, Göttingen 1980

Droese, M.: Cytological diagnosis of sialadenosis, sialadenitis and parotid cysts by fine-needle aspiration biopsy. Adv. Oto-Rhino-Laryng. 26 (1981) 49

Droese, M., J. Haubrich, M. Tutz: Stellenwert der Punktionscytologie in der Diagnostik der Speicheldrüsentumoren. Schweiz. med. Wschr. 198 (1978) 933

Droese, M., M. Tutz, J. Haubrich: Punktionszytologie der Speicheldrüsentumoren. Z. Laryng. Rhinol. 56 (1977) 703

Eichner, H., G. Bretzel, K. Hochstrasser: Biochemische Veränderungen der Sekretzusammensetzung von menschlichen Ohrspeicheldrüsen mit malignen Tumoren, chronischen Entzündungen und Sialadenosen. Immunglobulin-A-, Lysozym-, Flußraten- und Gesamteiweißbestimmungen. Z. Laryngol. Rhinol. 56 (1977) 32

Eichner, H., G. Bretzel, M. Münzel, K. Hochstrasser: Über die Proteinzusammensetzung des menschlichen Parotissekrets bei akuten und chronischen Entzündungen. Quantitative densitometrische Bestimmung der einzelnen Proteinfraktionen im Vergleich zu normalen Drüsensekreten. Z. Laryngol. Rhinol. 55 (1976a) 499

Eichner, H., V. Eichner, F. Fiedler, K. Hochstrasser: Zum Sekretionsverhalten der BAEE-Esterase (Kallikrein) im gesunden menschlichen Parotissekret unter fraktionierter Abnahme bei Ruhe und Reiz. Z. Laryngol. Rhinol. 55 (1976b) 239

Eichner, H., V. Eichner, M. Münzel, K. Hochstrasser: Simultanbestimmungen von Lysozym- und Immunglobulin-A-Gehalt von menschlichem Parotissekret im Vergleich zu Flußrate und Gesamtproteinausscheidung bei fraktionierter Ruhe- und Reizabnahme. Z. Laryngol. Rhinol. 54 (1975) 554

Eneroth, C.-M.: Die Klinik der Kopfspeicheldrüsentumoren. Arch. Oto-Rhino-Laryng. 213 (1976) 61

Eneroth, C.-M., J. Zajicek: Aspiration biopsy of salivary gland tumors. II. Morphologic studies on smears and histological sections from oncocytic tumors. Acta cytol. 9 (1965) 355

Eneroth, C.-M., A. Zetterberg: Microspectrophotometric DNA analysis of malignant salivary gland tumors. Acta otolaryng. 77 (1974) 289

Eneroth, C.-M., S. Franzén, J. Zajicek: Aspiration biopsy of salivary gland tumors: A critical review of 910 biopsies. Acta cytol. 11 (1967a) 470

Eneroth, C.-M., S. Franzén, J. Zajicek: Cytologic diagnosis on aspirates from 1000 salivary-gland tumors. Acta oto-laryng. (Stockh.), Suppl. 224 (1967b) 168

Ericson, S.: The variability of the human parotid flow rate on stimulation with citric acid, with special reference to taste. Arch. oral Biol. 16 (1971) 9

Franzén, S., G. Giertz, J. Zajicek: Cytological diagnosis of prostatic tumours by transrectal aspiration biopsy. A preliminary report. Brit. J. Urol. 32 (1960) 193

Gillard, B. K., H. C. Markman, S. A. Feig: Direct spectrophotometric determination of α-amylase activity in saliva, with p-nitrophenyl α-maltoside as substrate. Clin. Chem. 23 (1977) 2279

Glaubitt, D., J. Haubrich: Functional scintigraphy of parotid glands affected by tumor, inflammation or sialosis. IV. Congress of the European Nuclear Medicine Society, Barcelona 1980. Eur. J. nucl. Med. (1980) 5 A 12

Hagelqvist, E.: Light and electron microscopic studies on material obtained by fine needle biopsy. Acta oto-laryngol. (Stockh.), Suppl. 354 (1978) 1

Haubrich, J.: Klinik der nichttumorbedingten Erkrankungen der Speicheldrüsen. Arch. Oto-Rhino-Laryng. 213 (1976) 1

Haubrich, J., D. Glaubitt: Quantitative Scintigraphy of the Salivary Glands. In: Proceedings of the 29th Annual Meeting of the Society of Nuclear Medicine. Schattauer, Stuttgart 1982 (p. 89)

Herberhold, C., G. Müller: Sialographie mit Hytrast. Arch. klin. exp. Ohr.-, Nas.- u. Kehlk.-Heilk. 199 (1971) 623

Jasper, A.: Parotidektomie und die Frage der Probeexzision. Arch. klin. exp. Ohr.-, Nas.- u. Kehlk.-Heilk. 194 (1969) 313

Jones, A. W.: Distribution of ethanol between saliva and blood in man. Clin. exp. Pharmacol. Physiol. 6 (1979) 53

Kakizaki, G., N. Noto, T. Onuma, T. Saito, S. Izumi: Experimental study on the correlation between pancreas and parotid gland. Tohoku J. Exp. Med. 105 (1971) 223

Kakizaki, G., T. Saito, T. Soeno, M. Sasahara, J. Fujiwara: A new diagnostic test for pancreatic disorders by examination of parotid saliva. Amer. J. Gastroent. 65 (1976) 437

Kakizaki, G., N. Noto, T. Saito, J. Fujiwara, T. Ohizumi, T. Soeno, T. Ishidate: Laboratory diagnostic test for pancreatic disorders by examination of parotid saliva. Tohoku J. Exp. Med. 109 (1973) 121

Kempfle, B.: Füllungen der Speicheldrüsen mit einem mikrokristallinen Röntgenkontrastmittel. Radiologe 10 (1970) 259

Kerr, A. C.: The Physiological Regulation of Salivary Secretion in Man. Int. Series Monographs Oral Biol. Pergamon Press, Oxford 1961

Kessler, L., F. Theuring: Kopfspeicheldrüsen. Szintigraphische und autoradiographische Untersuchungen. Hals-Nasen-Ohrenheilkunde. Zwanglose Schriftenreihe, hrsg. von A. Herrmann, München; J. Jacobi, Halle/S. Barth, Leipzig 1975 (S. 24).

Kleinsasser, O.: Nervus facialis und Glandula parotis. HNO (Berl.) 24 (1976) 116

Kutscher, A. H., I. D. Mandel, E. V. Zegarelli, C. Denning, A. Eriv, L. Ruiz, K. Ellgood, J. Phalen: A technique for collecting the secretion of minor salivary glands: use of capillary tubes. J. oral Ther. Pharm. 3 (1967) 391

Lankisch, P. G., R. Chilla, K. Luerssen, H. Koop, C. Arglebe, W. Creutzfeldt: Parotid saliva test in the diagnosis of chronic pancreatitis. Digestion 19 (1979) 52

Lashley, K. S.: Reflex secretion of the human parotid gland. J. exp. Psychol. 1 (1916) 461

Lenz, H.: Diskussionsbemerkung. Arch. klin. exp. Ohr.-, Nas.- u. Kehlk.-Heilk. 199 (1971) 628

Lindenberg, L. G., M. Akerman: Aspiration cytology of salivary gland tumors: diagnostic experience from six years of routine laboratory work. Laryngoscope 86 (1976) 584

Lohkamp, F., C. Claussen: Die Bedeutung der Computertomographie für die TNM-Klassifikation der Gesichtsschädelmalignome im Bereich der Nasennebenhöhlen, des Nasopharynx und der Parotis. Z. Laryng. Rhinol. 56 (1977) 740

Lohkamp, F., C. Claussen, H. Spenneberg: Computertomographie der Parotis. Z. Laryng. Rhinol. 56 (1977) 104

Maier, H., M. T. Coroneo, A. Heidland, M. E. Wigand: Ionisiertes Calcium und Totalcalcium im Parotisspeichel bei Normalpersonen und essentiellen Hypertonikern. Z. Laryngol. Rhinol. 57 (1978) 1013

Maier, H., M. Geissler, A. Heidland, J. G. Schindler, M. E. Wigand: Beeinflussung speichelchemischer Parameter in Abhängigkeit vom Menstruationszyklus. Z. Laryngol. Rhinol. 58 (1979) 706

Mann, W.: Neue Möglichkeiten der Nasennebenhöhlendiagnostik. Habil.-Schrift, Freiburg 1977

Mann, W.: Diagnostik entzündlicher Nasennebenhöhlenerkrankungen. Arch. Oto-Rhino-Laryng. 235 (1982) 41

Marmar, J., G. J. Barbero, M. S. Sibinga: The pattern of parotid gland secretion in cystic fibrosis of the pancreas. Gastroenterology 50 (1966) 551

Mason, D. K., D. M. Chisholm: Salivary Glands in Health and Disease. Saunders, London 1975

Mavec, P., C.-M. Eneroth, S. Franzén, G. Moberger, J. Zajicek: Aspiration biopsy of salivary gland tumors. I. Correlation of cytologic reports from 652 aspiration biopsies with clinical and histological findings. Acta oto-laryng. 58 (1964) 471

Mayo, J. M., W. M. Wallace, L. W. Matthews, D. M. Carlson: Quantitation of submandibular proteins resolved from normal individuals and children with cystic fibrosis. Arch. Biochem. Biophys. 175 (1976) 507

McColl, K. E. L., M. J. Brodie, R. White-Smith, T. J. Thomson: Parotid gland function in patients with pancreatic disease. Gut 18 (1977) 960

McColl, K. E. L., B. Whiting, M. R. Moore, A. Goldberg: Correlation of ethanol concentrations in blood and saliva. Clin. Sci. 56 (1979) 283

Mucklow, J. G., M. R. Bending, G. C. Kahn, C. T. Dollery: Drug concentration in saliva. Clin. Pharmacol. Ther. 24 (1978) 563

Münzel, M.: Zur szintigraphischen Diagnostik der Speicheldrüsenerkrankungen. II. International Symposion on Nuclear Medicine. Karlovy Vary 1971

Nacchiero, M., D. A. Dreiling: The parotid and the pancreas. I. The effects of secretion, CCK-PZ, and prostaglandin E on canine parotid secretion. Mount Sinai J. Med. 45 (1978) 187

Nacchiero, M., M. Addler, P. Pieroni, T. Takeshima, D. A. Dreiling: The parotid and the pancreas. II. Parotid secretion in canine chronic pancreatitis. Mount Sinai J. Med. 45 (1978a) 192

Nacchiero, M., M. Addler, P. Pieroni, T. Takeshima, J. Rudick, D. A. Dreiling: The parotid and the pancreas. III. Correlation of the parotid gland and pancreatic secretion after radiation-induced chronic pancreatitis. Amer. J. Gastroent. 70 (1978b) 151

Nishihara, K., K. Uchino, Y. Saitoh, Y. Honda, F. Nakagawa, Z. Tamura: Estimation of plasma unbound phenobarbital concentration by using mixed saliva. Epilepsia 20 (1979) 37

Peck, R. E.: The S. H. P. test – an aid in the detection and measurement of depression. Arch. General. Psychiat. 1 (1959) 35

Persson, P. S., L. Zettergren: Cytologic diagnosis of salivary gland tumors by aspiration biopsy. Acta cytol. 17 (1973) 351

Pfeiffer, K.: Die Röntgendiagnostik der Speicheldrüsen und ihrer Ausführungsgänge. In: Handbuch der Medizinischen Radiologie, Bd. VI. Springer, Berlin 1968

Posti, J.: Arzneimittelkonzentrationen im Plasma und im Speichel. – Physiologische und pharmakokinetische Betrachtungen. Pharm. Acta Helv. 54 (1979) 191

Puskulian, L.: Salivary electrolyte changes during the normal menstrual cycle. J. dent. Res. 51 (1972) 1212

di Sant'Agnese, P. A., R. C. Darling, G. A. Perera, E. Shea: Abnormal electrolyte composition of sweat in cystic fibrosis of the pancreas. Pediatrics 12 (1953) 549

Schaefer, M. E., M. Rhodes, S. Prince, S. M. Michalek, J. R. McGheo: A plastic intraoral device for the collection of human parotid saliva. J. dent. Res. 56 (1977) 728

Schätzle, W.: Diskussionsbemerkung. Arch. Klin. exp. Ohr.-, Nas.- u. Kehlk.-Heilk. 199 (1971) 619

Schmidt, G., K. Hempel, L. Fricke, H. Wernze, A. Heidland: Erhöhte cAMP-Konzentration im Parotisspeichel des Menschen bei arterieller Hypertonie. Dtsch. med. Wschr. 100 (1975) 1435

Schneyer, L. H.: Method for the collection of separate submaxillary and sublingual salivas in man. J. dent. Res. 34 (1955) 257

Schneyer, L. H.: Amylase content of separate salivary gland secretions of man. J. appl. Physiol. 9 (1956) 453

Seifert, G.: Die Sekretionsstörungen (Dyschylien) der Speicheldrüsen. In Cohrs, P., W. Giese, H. Meessen: Ergebnisse der allgemeinen Pathologie und pathologischen Anatomie, Bd. 44. Springer, Berlin 1964

Seifert, G., K. Donath: Die Morphologie der Speicheldrüsenerkrankungen. Arch. Oto-Rhino-Laryng. 213 (1976) 111 u. 371

Shannon, I. L.: Reference table for human parotid saliva collected at varying levels of exogenous stimulation. J. dent. Res. 52 (1973) 1157

Shannon, I. L., H. H. Chauncey: A parotid fluid collection device with improve stability characteristics. J. oral Therap. Pharmacol. 4 (1967) 93

Skurk, A., S. Krebs, J. Rehberg: Flow rate, amylase, lysozyme and kallikrein of human parotid saliva in health and disease. Arch. oral Biol. 24 (1979) 739

Stephen, K. W., C. F. Speirs: Methods for collecting individual components of mixed saliva: The relevance to clinical pharmacology. Brit. J. clin. Pharmacol. 3 (1976) 315

Stephen, K. W., J. McCrossan, D. Mackenzie: Factors determining the passage of drugs from blood into saliva. Brit. J. clin. Pharmacol. 9 (1980) 51

Truelove, E. L., D. Bixler, A. D. Merritt: Simplified method for collection of pure submandibular saliva in large volumes. J. dent. Res. 46 (1967) 1400

Varletzidis, E., D. Ikkos, G. Paleologou, P. Pantazopoulos, K. Miras, G. Adamopoulos: Salivary amylase activity in diabetes mellitus. Panminerva med. 20 (1978) 255

Vogt, K., W. M. Semmann: Zur physiologischen Beeinflussung der Gesamtproteinsekretion der großen Kopfspeicheldrüsen durch Tageszeit, Alter und Geschlecht. Z. Laryng. Rhinol. 49 (1970) 611

Webb, A. J.: Cytologic diagnosis of salivary gland lesions in adult and pediatric surgical patients. Acta cytol. 17 (1973) 51

Westernhagen, B. von: Aspirationsbiopsie oder Probeexzision zur Diagnostik von Parotistumoren. HNO (Berl.) 14 (1966) 142

Wolf, G.: Die Menghini-Nadelbiopsie. Ein wertvolles Hilfsmittel zur Diagnose von Parotistumoren. Arch. Oto-Rhino-Laryng. 236 (1982) 257

Zajicek, J.: Aspiration biopsy cytology. Part 1: Cytology of supradiaphragmatic organs. Monographs in Cytology. Vol 4. Karger, Basel 1974

6. Congenital Anomalies

Aplasia, Hypoplasia, and Duct Atresia

Congenital *aplasia* of the salivary glands is very rare (Seifert 1966, Becker et al 1978). Complete aplasia of all salivary glands causes xerostomia and widespread loss of teeth. Aplasia of the salivary tissue may also accompany other congenital anomalies of the head and neck; a few cases of unilateral aplasia of the parotid gland have been reported. *Hypoplasia* of one salivary gland is generally compensated for by the remaining normal glands.

Duct atresia is also relatively rare, but examples arising in the submandibular gland have been reported. A duct cyst may develop due to obstruction to the flow of secretion in a normal gland.

Ectopia

This is a normal gland in an abnormal position. For example, the parotid gland may lie at the anterior border of the masseter muscle with a shortened duct system. Ectopia of the ducts of the salivary glands is ascribed to displacement of the opening of the duct bud from the oral epithelium. Opening of the submandibular duct on the palate or of a parotid duct in the angle of the mouth are described.

Accessory Salivary Glands

An accessory salivary gland consists of ectopic salivary tissue, which possesses its own duct system and is thus capable of functioning. An accessory duct may open either into the main duct or into a subsidiary duct of the main gland. An aberrant salivary gland also lies in an abnormal position but does not possess ducts and thus does not function.

An accessory parotid gland is particularly common. It lies anterior to the parotid capsule, either on the masseter muscle or within the fatty tissue of the cheek (Polayes & Rankow 1979). The gland consists of lobules that open by a small subsidiary duct into the main duct of the parotid gland. Systematic examination of the parotid demonstrates accessory parotid glands in 20% of subjects (Polayes & Rankow 1979). The secondary duct system of an accessory parotid may be demonstrated before operation by sialography. There is no histologic difference between accessory and normal parotid tissue. Furthermore, the same diseases can develop in the accessory parotid as in the main gland. These include chronic inflammation (Ferguson & MacDonald 1978) and cysts and benign or malignant tumors (Johnson & Spiro 1979). The accessory parotid must be removed when dealing with a parotid tumor, observing the main points of facial nerve surgery to prevent recurrence of the tumor (Frommer 1977).

Aberrant Salivary Glands

Aberrant salivary glands are defined as heterotopic salivary anlages without their own duct system. They therefore do not secrete during eating, but they may form a fistula from which saliva is secreted in response to eating. The occurrence of aberrant salivary tissue in the lateral part of the neck, in the pharynx, and middle ear is due to the complicated development of the branchial system, particularly the close spatial relationships of the first and second branchial arches to the individual cranial nerves, including the facial nerve.

Aberrant salivary tissue may be found in the lateral part of the neck (Frommer 1977, Mair et al 1977, Polayes & Rankow 1979, Singer et al 1979, Youngs & Scofield 1967), in the middle ear (Abadir & Pease 1978, Bruner 1970, Mischke et al 1977, Hociota & Ataman 1975, Saeger et al 1982, Wine & Metcalf 1977), on the gingiva (Moskow & Baden 1964, Ide et al 1983, Moss-Salentijn & Applebaum 1972, Ritchey & Orban 1953, Traeger 1961, Wilson & MacEntee 1974), in the pituitary gland and cerebollepontine regions (Curry et al 1982, Schochet et al 1974), in the base of the tongue and the mandible (Hayashi et al 1984), and finally in the tonsillar fossa (Seifert 1966).

Branches of the facial nerve are enveloped by the lesion especially in heterotopia of the middle ear. This can result in a facial palsy or conductive deafness of uncertain cause. In addition, bony and other anomalies, such as congenital cholesteatoma, may occur (Saeger et al 1982).

Aberrant salivary tissue is formed of mucous and serous acini, between which salivary ducts are arranged. Fatty tissue may also develop within the salivary lobules.

Heterotopia is often first discovered because of complications, such as the development of a mucocele, a salivary fistula, or inflammation.

Salivary tumors may also develop in aberrant salivary tissue, and the following have been described: pleomorphic adenomas (Hulbert 1973, Mair et al 1978, Pesavento & Ferlito 1976, Saeed & Bassis 1971, Worthington 1982, Cotelingam & Gerberi 1983) and mucoepidermoid tumors (Zajtchuk et al 1982). An acinic cell tumor or oncocytoma is very rare (Yacoub et al 1981, Zajtchuk et al 1982). A salivary gland choristoma is not a true tumor, but a heterotopic salivary gland lying in the middle ear or gingiva.

Dysgenetic Salivary Gland Cysts

Primary dysgenetic cysts must be differentiated from secondary acquired cysts which have many different causes, such as abstruction of the duct, inflammation, and tumors. The details are described in Chapter 10.

Polycystic Parotid Gland

This very rare disorder resembles cystic anomalies of other organs, such as kidney, liver, pancreas, and lung. It may occur on one or both sides (Seifert et al 1981). Two cystic parotid glands are recorded in the material of the Salivary Gland Register from a total of 8000 salivary gland disorders (end of 1982).

The cysts vary in size and are lined by duct epithelium of varying differentiation (Figs. 6.**1**, 6.**2**). Their structure resembles partly that of the intercalated or striated ducts and partly also that of the primitive duct buds of the embryonal period. The duct lumen contains secretion and in places crystalline spheroliths (Fig. 6.**3a, b**) and microliths. Occasionally, the cyst epithelium shows degenerative changes with desquamation into the lumen (Fig. 6.**4**). Remnants of gland tissue with acini can be recognized between the cysts, but inflammatory changes are absent. The pathogenesis of a cystic parotid must rest on early embryonal disturbance of ramification and canalization of the duct system, during the second stage of the development of the salivary gland extending up to the end of the seventh embryonal month (see Chapter 3).

The spur-shaped incomplete septa (Fig. 6.**5**) or hourglass constrictions of the cyst wall (Fig. 6.**6**) are also evidence of disordered differentiation.

Ranula

The term "ranula" is based on the resemblance of the cyst to the throat pouch of frogs. The mucus-

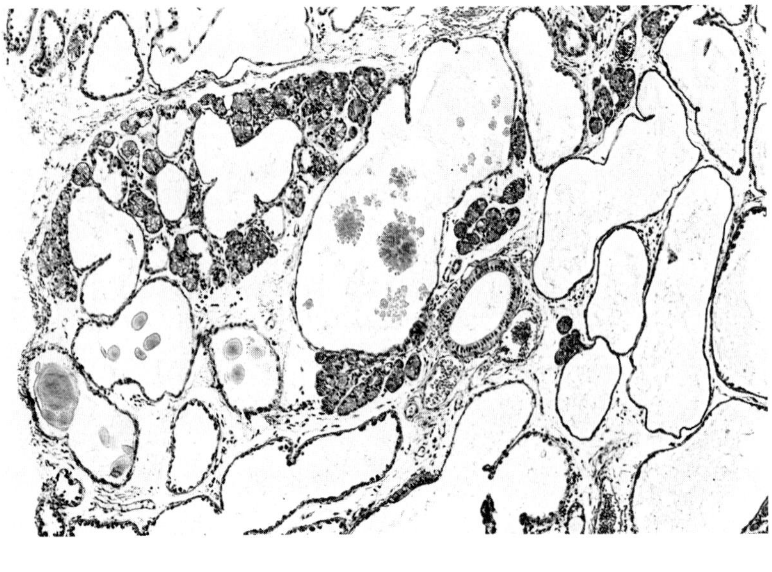

Figure 6.**1** Cystic parotid gland: permeation of the gland tissue by multiple duct cysts interspersed with remnants of parenchyma. H & E, 63×.

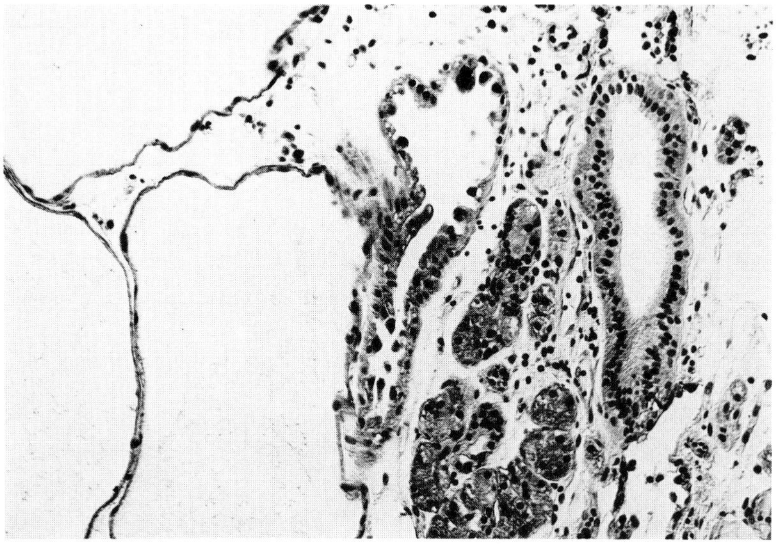

Figure 6.**2** Cystic parotid gland showing various types of epithelial lining of the cyst, (left) endothelioid flat cells; polypoid epithelium in the middle; normal striated duct on the right. Masson-Goldner, 160×.

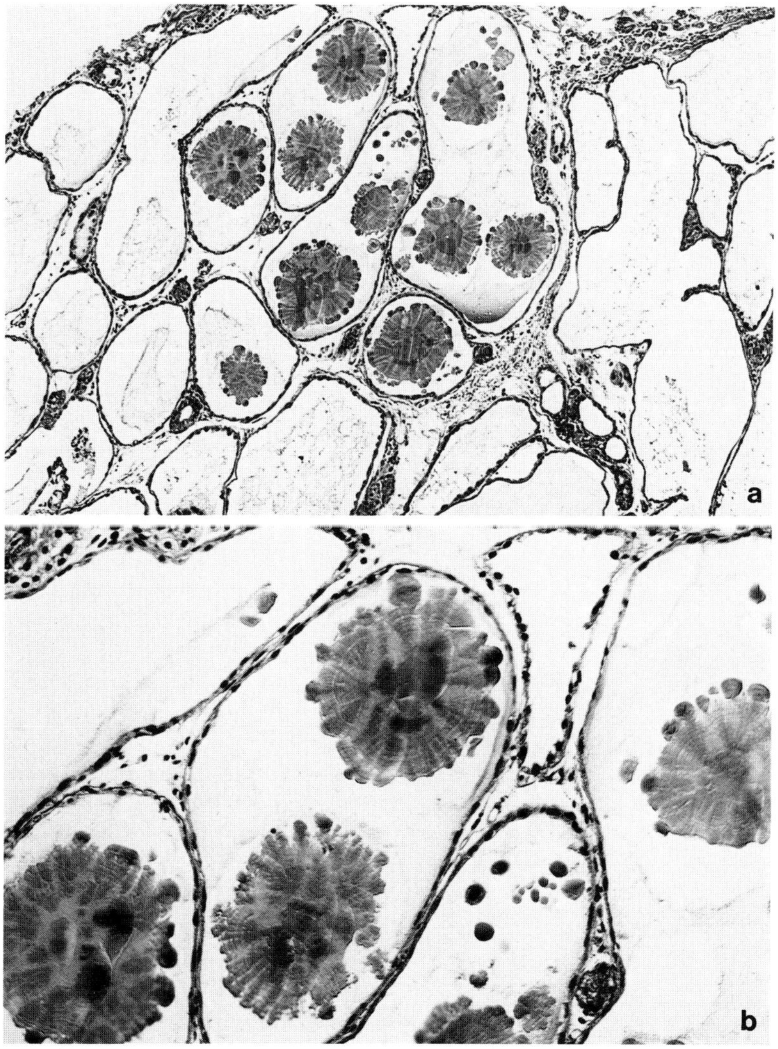

Figure 6.**3** Cystic parotid gland showing multiple spheroliths with radial and concentric stratification within the cysts. H & E. **a** 63×, **b** 160×.

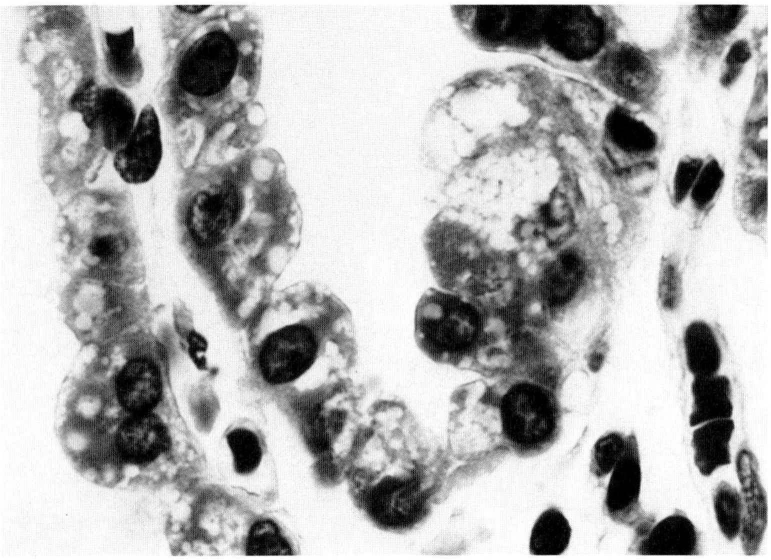

Figure 6.**4** Cystic parotid gland showing cyst epithelium with hydropic swelling, vacuolation of the cytoplasm and irregular nuclear forms. Masson-Goldner, 1000×.

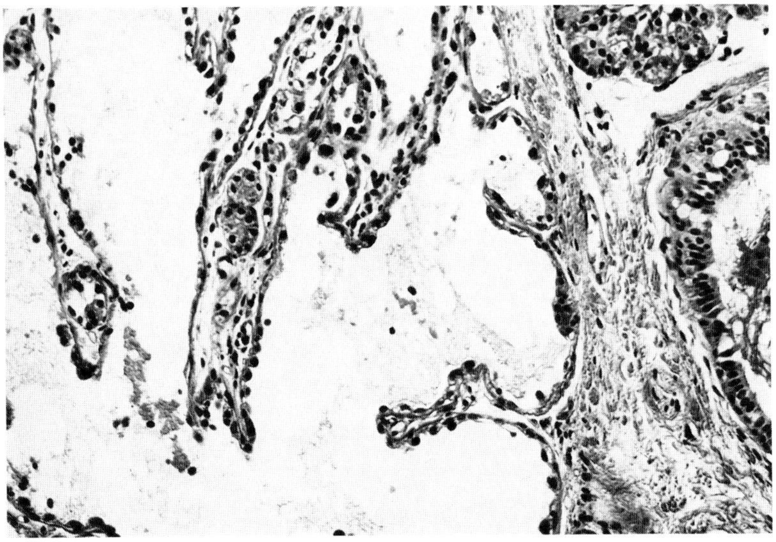

Figure 6.**5** Cystic parotid gland showing spurlike septae of individual cysts. H & E, 160×.

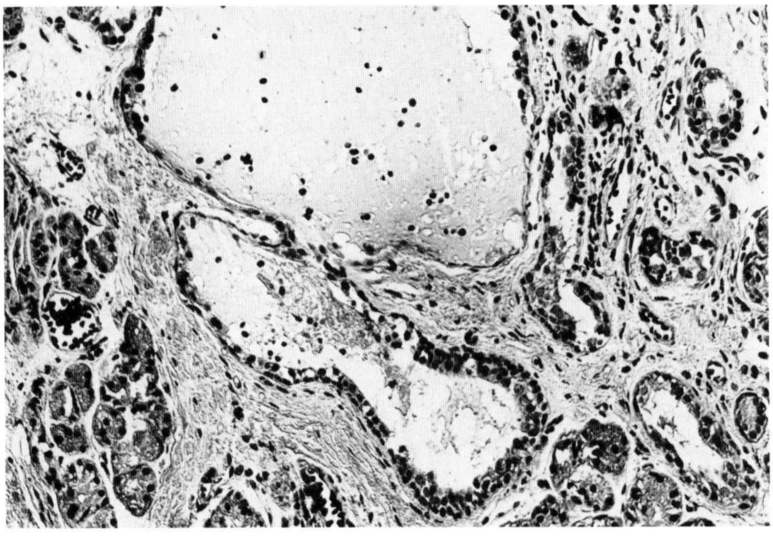

Figure 6.**6** Cystic parotid gland showing hourglass constriction of a cyst. Masson-Goldner, 160×.

filled cysts lie under the mucosa of the floor of the mouth, just lateral to the frenulum. The form that pierces the oral diaphragm and is constricted about its middle like an hourglass by the mylohyoid muscle is unusual. A plunging ranula lies mainly in the neck in the suprahyoid-inframylohyoid region (McClatchey et al 1984). The cysts may be uni- or multilocular and contain a secretion rich in mucus. Epithelial-lined retention cysts may be distinguished from pseudocysts lined with granulation tissue by histologic examination (Figs. 6.**7**–6.**9**). Squamous and sebaceous gland metaplasia may sometimes occur in epithelial cysts. The presence of inflammation and the appearance of the ranula before, during, or after puberty is evidence that two factors are important in the genesis of these cysts: firstly, dysgenetic disturbances of the differentiation of the duct system of the sublingual gland, and secondly, secondary inflammation and trauma causing extrusion of mucus from the duct system into the interstitial tissues. With increase in size, the ranula obstructs breathing and swallowing.

Congenital Sialectasis of the Parotid Gland

Globular duct ectasia may occur on one or both sides, and, in contrast to the cystic parotid gland, the ducts always have direct contact with an otherwise intact duct system (Becker et al 1960). The sialectasia (Figs. 6.**10**, 6.**11**) is lined by a single or multilayered epithelium and usually contains floccular secretions. Stagnation of secretions

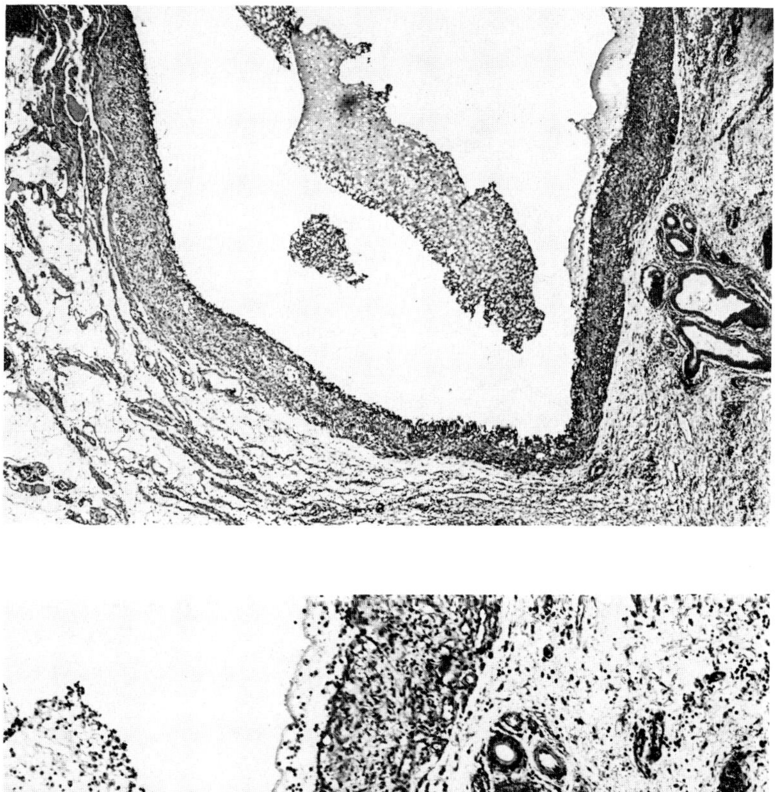

Figure 6.**7** Ranula of the sublingual gland showing a pseudocyst filled by mucus and limited by granulation tissue. H & E, 25×.

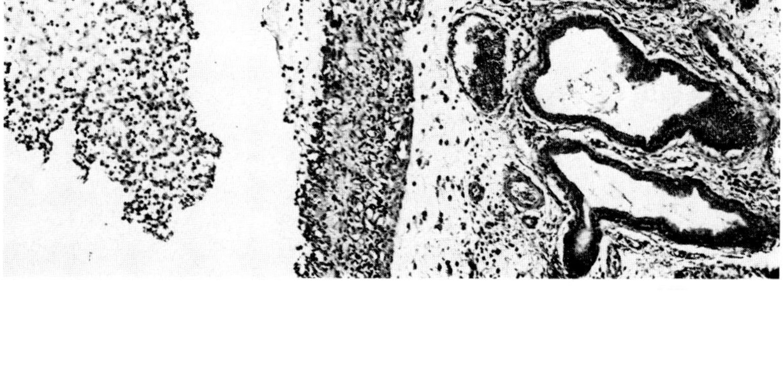

Figure 6.**8** Ranula of the sublingual gland showing a dilated duct in the region of a pseudocyst. H & E, 63×.

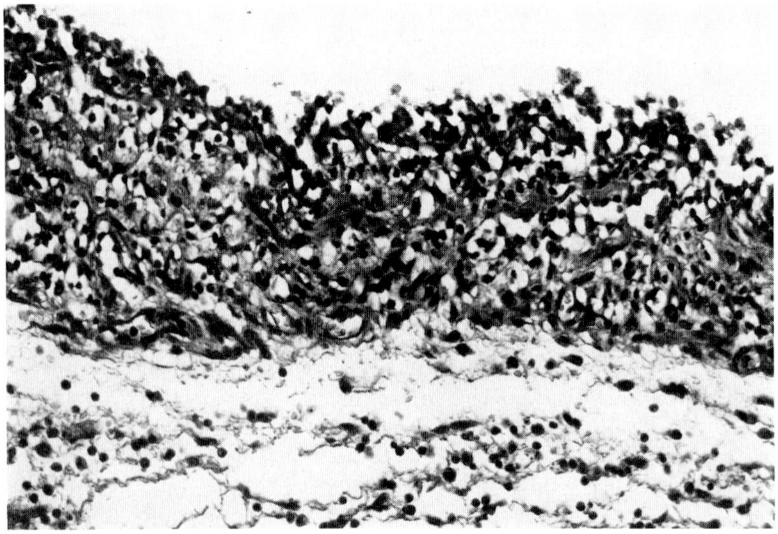

Figure 6.**9** Sublingual ranula showing formation of the pseudocyst wall from granulation tissue with foam cells, histiocytes, and leukocytes. H & E, 160×.

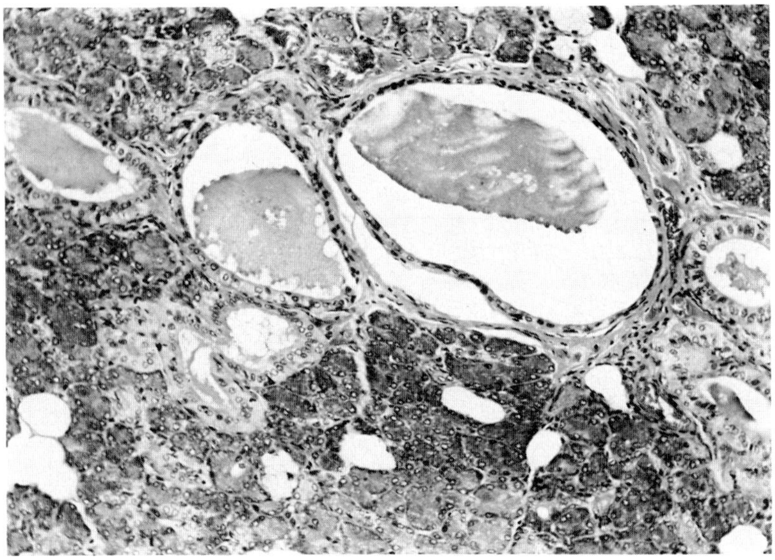

Figure 6.**10** Congenital sialectasis of the parotid gland in a 1-year-old boy, showing clumps of secretion in the lumen, but no inflammatory infiltrate. H & E, 160×.

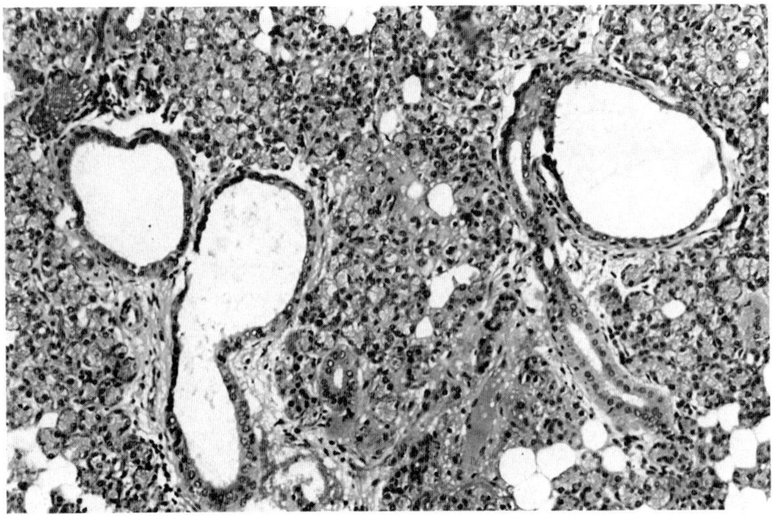

Figure 6.**11** Multiple sialectasis of the parotid gland in a 49-year-old woman showing no inflammatory changes. H & E, 100×.

Figure 6.**12** Merkel's cyst of the submandibular gland. H & E, 25×.

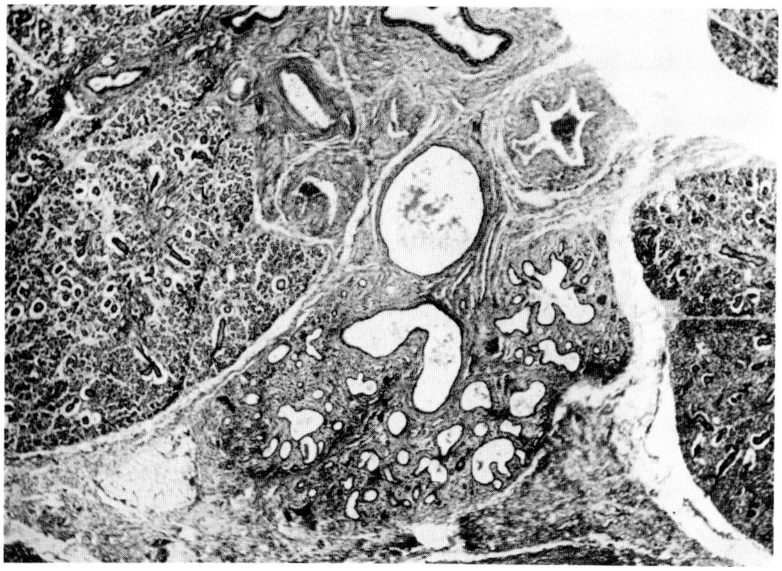

favors the development of recurrent sialadenitis. Acquired secondary duct ectasia can only be distinguished from chronic recurrent sialectatic parotitis with certainty in babies and young children. In our material, 5 of 360 (1.4%) non-neoplastic salivary gland cysts were observed with congenital bilateral sialectasis of the parotid gland.

Other Dysgenetic Cysts

Merkel's cysts of the submandibular gland are caused by distortion and segmentation of segments of the duct (Fig. 6.**12**). They are usually lined by flattened epithelium (Seifert & Geiler 1956). *Dermoid cysts of the floor of the mouth* are of ectodermal origin and, unlike the ranula, always lie in the midline (Fig. 6.**13**). They must be distinguished from *congenital teratomas* of the submandibular region, which may present with a well-demarcated, easily recognizable cyst (Rose & Howard 1982, Tang et al 1979). *Branchiogenic cysts* in the parotid area are discussed in the section on lymphoepithelial and salivary duct cysts (Chapter 10).

Other Anomalies

Congenital *hyperplasia* of the salivary glands is very rare and must be distinguished from pseudohypertrophy due to lipomatosis, tumors, or other diseases such as sialadenosis. *Nodular hyperplasia* of the minor *mucous salivary glands* has occassionally been described on the palate and in the retromolar region (Arafat et al 1981, Devildos & Langlois 1976, Giansanti et al 1971). Histologic examination shows focal hyperplasia of mucous gland acini arranged in lobules. It is not certain whether this lesion represents a reactive hyperplasia or a congenital hamartoma. It must be distinguished from a true tumor.

Congenital salivary fistulas may develop from both aberrant and accessory salivary glands (see before), and also in combined anomalies of the branchial cleft system (Weidauer 1971).

Epithelial metaplasia of the sebaceous glands, of goblet cells, and of islands of squamous epithelium is discussed in Chapter 11.

References

Abadir, W. F., W. S. Pease: Salivary gland choristoma of the middle ear. J. Laryngol. Otol. 92 (1978) 247

Arafat, A., R. B. Brannon, G. L. Ellis: Adenomatoid hyperplasia of the mucous salivary glands. Oral Surg. 52 (1981) 51

Becker, W., J. Haubrich, G. Seifert: Krankheiten der Kopfspeicheldrüsen. In Berendes J., R. Link, F. Zöllner: Hals-Nasen-Ohren-Heilkunde in Praxis und Klinik, Bd. 3. Thieme, Stuttgart 1978 (S. 12.1)

Becker, W., J. Matzker, J. Ruckes: Zur Morphologie der "diffusen kugelförmigen Gangektasien" in der Glandula parotis. Z. Laryng. Rhinol. 39 (1960) 479

Bruner, R. C.: Salivary gland choristoma of the middle ear. A case report. Arch. Otolaryng. 91 (1970) 303

Cotelingam, J. D., M. P. Gerberi: Parotid heterotopia with pleomorphic adenoma. Arch. Otolaryng. 109 (1983) 563

Curry, B., Ch. W. Taylor, W. F. Fisher: Salivary gland heterotopia. A unique cerebellopontine angle tumor. Arch. Pathol. Lab. Med. 106 (1982) 35

Devildos, L. R., C. C. Langlois: Minor salivary gland lesion presenting clinically as tumor. Oral Surg. 41 (1976) 657

Ferguson, M. M., D. G. MacDonald: Persistent sialadenitis in an accessory parotid gland. Oral Surg. 45 (1978) 696

Frommer, J.: The human accessory parotid gland: Its incidence, nature, and significance. Oral Surg. 43 (1977) 671

Giansanti, J. S., G. O. Baker, C. A. Waldron: Intraoral, mucinous, minor salivary gland lesions presenting clinically as tumors. Oral Surg. 32 (1971) 918

Hayashi, Y., Y. Kimura, M. Nagumo: Anterior lingual mandibular bone concavity. Report of a case. Oral Surg. 57 (1984) 139

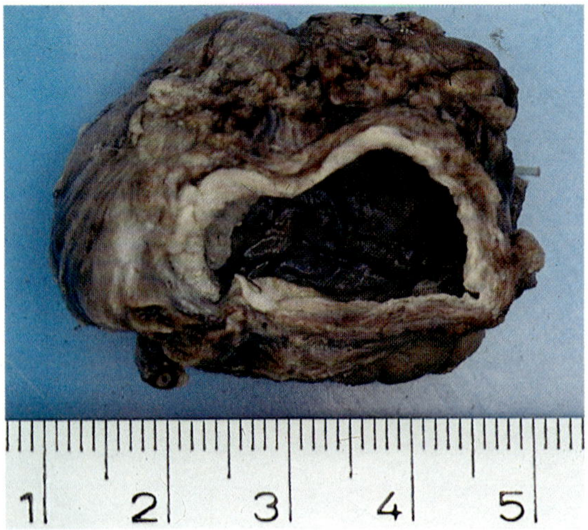

Figure 6.**13** Thick-walled dermoid cyst of the floor of the mouth lying close to the submandibular gland.

Hociota, D., T. Ataman: A case of salivary gland choristoma of the middle ear. J. Laryngol. Otol. 89 (1975) 1065

Hulbert, J. C.: Ectopic mixed salivary tumors in the neck. J. Laryngol. Otol. 92 (1973) 533

Ide, F., H. Shimura, I. Sato, Sh. Umemura: Gingival salivary gland choristoma: An extremely rare phenomenon. Oral Surg. 55 (1983) 169

Johnson, F. E., R. H. Spiro: Tumors arising in accessory parotid tissue. Amer. J. Surg. 138 (1979) 576

Mair, I. W., S. G. Borang, M. S. Kearney: Heterotopical cervical salivary glands. J. Laryng. Otol. (Lond.) 91 (1977) 35

Mair, I. W. S., H. H. Elverland, O. S. Knudsen: Heterotopic salivary pleomorphic adenoma. J. Otolaryngol. 7 (1978) 158

McClatchey, K. D., N. H. Appelblatt, R. J. Zarbo, D. M. Merrel: Plunging ranula. Oral Surg. 57 (1984) 408

Mischke, R. E., D. E. Brackmann, P. Gruskin: Salivary gland choristoma of the middle ear. Arch. Otolaryngol. 103 (1977) 432

Moskow, B. S., E. Baden: Gingival choristoma. Oral Surg. 18 (1964) 504

Moss-Salentijn, L., E. Applebaum: A minor salivary gland in human gingiva. Arch. oral Biol. 17 (1972) 1373

Pesavento, G., A. Ferlito: Benign mixed tumor of heterotopic salivary gland tissue in the upper neck: Report of case with a review of literature on heterotopic salivary gland tissue. J. Laryngol. Otol. 90 (1976) 577

Polayes, I. M., R. M. Rankow: Cysts, masses, and tumors of the accessory parotid gland. Plast. Reconstr. Surg. 64 (1979) 17

Ritchey, B., B. Orban: Cysts of the gingiva. Oral Surg. 6 (1953) 765

Rose, P. E., E. R. Howard: Congenital teratoma of the submandibular gland. J. Pediat. Surg. 17 (1982) 414

Saeed, Y. M., M. L. Bassis: Mixed tumor of the middle ear. Arch. Otolaryngol. 93 (1971) 433

Saeger, K. L., P. Gruskin, J. N. Carberry: Salivary gland choristoma of the middle ear. Arch. Pathol. Lab. Med. 106 (1982) 39

Schochet, J. R., W. F. McCormick, N. S. Halmi: Salivary gland rests in the human pituitary: Light and electron microscopic study. Arch. Pathol. Lab. Med. 98 (1974) 193

Seifert, G.: Mundhöhle, Mundspeicheldrüsen, Tonsillen und Rachen. In Doerr W., E. Uehlinger: Spezielle pathologische Anatomie, Bd. 1. Springer, Berlin 1966 (S. 1)

Seifert, G., G. Geiler: Zur Pathologie der kindlichen Kopfspeicheldrüsen. Beitr. path. Anat. 116 (1956) 1

Seifert, G., St. Thomsen, K. Donath: Bilateral dysgenetic polycystic parotid glands. Morphological analysis and differential diagnosis of a rare disease of the salivary glands. Virchows Arch. path. Anat. 390 (1981) 273

Singer, M. I., E. L. Applebaum, K. D. Loy: Heterotopic salivary tissue in the neck. Laryngoscope 89 (1979) 1772

Tang, T. T., M. Glicklich, K. A. Siegesmund, H. W. Oechler, S. R. McCreadie: Neonatal cystic choristoma in submandibular salivary gland simulating cystic hygroma. Arch. Path. Lab. med. 103 (1979) 537

Traeger, K. A.: Cyst of the gingiva (mucocele). Oral Surg. 14 (1961) 243

Weidauer, H.: Ein Beitrag zu den seltenen kongenitalen Mißbildungen der Glandula parotis und deren Ausführungsgang. Z. Laryng. Rhinol. 50 (1971) 686

Wilson, D. F., M. I. MacEntee: Cystadenoma of ectopic minor salivary gland origin. Oral Surg. 37 (1974) 915

Wine, C. J., J. E. Metcalf: Salivary gland choristoma of the middle ear and mastoid. Arch. Otolaryngol. 103 (1977) 435

Worthington, Ph.: Mischtumor im heterotopen Speicheldrüsengewebe des Halses. Dtsch. Z. Mund-Kiefer-Gesichts-Chir. 6 (1982) 381

Yacoub, U., P. H. Becher-Carstens, R. J. Biscopink, G. T. McMurry: Acinic-cell tumor in ectopic salivary gland tissue. Arch. Pathol. Lab. Med. 105 (1981) 500

Youngs, L. A., H. H. Scofield: Heterotopic salivary gland tissue in the lower neck. Arch. Pathol. Lab. Med. 83 (1967) 550

Zajtchuk, J. T., C. A. Patow, V. J. Hyams: Cervical heterotopic salivary gland neoplasms: A diagnostic dilemma. Otolaryngol. Head Neck Surg. 90 (1982) 178

7. Disorders of Secretion

Every *disease of the salivary glands* affects their function, mainly the production and secretion of saliva. Usually, the quantity of saliva is reduced and its composition changed (Chapter 4).

Diseases such as sialadenitis, sialolithiasis, and tumors usually cause nonspecific changes of salivary secretion and will be discussed elsewhere. Abnormal composition and secretion of the saliva are important features of *sialolithiasis,* but the *sialadenoses* (see Chapter 8) cause only a modest change of the amount and composition of the saliva (Chilla et al 1978). Diseases of organs, such as the *pancreas*, and *metabolic diseases,* such as cystic fibrosis and diabetes mellitus, have (or are said to have) effects on the function of the salivary glands (see page 51).

Abnormal function of the salivary glands affects the secretion of saliva as follows:

a) The salivary secretion may be reduced.
b) The salivary secretion may be increased.
c) The composition of the saliva may be changed at a reduced, increased, or normal flow rate.
d) The outflow of secretion may be abnormal.

There are several terms for these disorders. Their meaning is identical or overlapping, so that it is necessary first of all to define the terms that will be used. Disorders of salivary secretion and composition can in general be termed *dyschylia* a term derived from pathologic anatomy and originally coined by Seifert (1964). Increased secretion of saliva is termed *hypersalivation, ptyalism, sialorrhea,* or *hypersialia.* The terms for reduced or absent secretion of saliva include *hyposialia, hyposalivation,* or *asialia.* We will use the terms hypersalivation and hyposalivation. The term "asialia" will be used if practically no saliva is secreted (Table 7.**1**). The term *sialorrhea* should be restricted to the symptom complex consisting of involuntary flow of saliva from the mouth; this may also be called drooling.

Disordered secretion of saliva may be the most pressing of the patient's symptoms. This applies to *xerostomia* in which there is insufficient secretion of saliva and to sialorrhea, whose causes, clinical effects, and treatment will be discussed.

Table 7.**1** Salivary Gland Secretion, Rauch's Classification (1959)

Estimation	Nonstimulated Secretion (ml/min)	
	Parotid Gland	Submandibular Gland
Marked hyposalivation	Less than 0.01	Less than 0.03
Mild hyposalivation	0.01–0.03	0.03–0.08
Normal values	0.03–0.08–0.02	0.08–0.22–0.4
Hypersalivation	More than 0.2	More than 0.4

Xerostomia

Xerostomia is a symptom caused by lack of saliva in the oral cavity. The amount of saliva present at any one time depends on the balance between production and consumption (Fig. 7.**1**). If the production of saliva is low or its consumption is increased, the balance is negative. Inefficient irrigation of the oral mucosa produces the feeling of dryness (subjective xerostomia), which need not be accompanied by an objective dryness of the mucosa, since the threshold for this feeling shows great individual variation. Xerostomia is not a single disease with a single cause, as was often thought at the beginning of the century (Chappell 1896, Hamilton 1896), but a symptom whose understanding demands knowledge of the physiology of production, transport, and consumption of the saliva.

Pathophysiology of Xerostomia

The following causes of a negative salivary balance are possible, based on the mechanisms of production of saliva (see Chapter 4) and the factors that determine the consumption of saliva.

- Decreased peripheral stimulus or disturbances of afferent stimulus, which causes secretion of saliva.
- Central disorders.
- Disorders of salivary gland innervation.

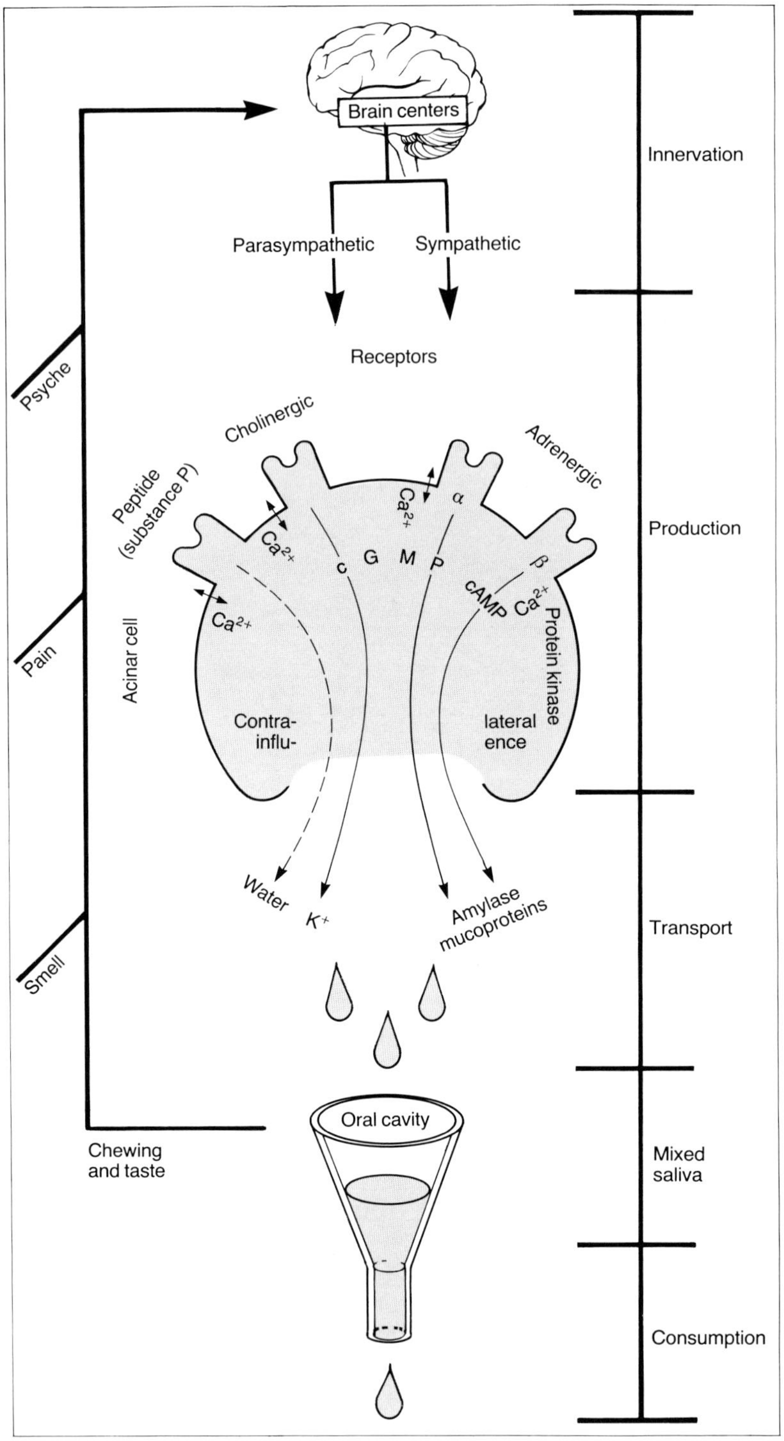

Figure 7.**1** Diagram of the physiology of saliva (Chilla). The quantity of saliva in the mouth is determined by the balance between production and consumption. Disturbances of reflex production and processing (left side of the diagram), disturbances of salivary gland innervation, of salivary production in the acini, of salivary transport, and of increased consumption of saliva (right side of the diagram) can lead to a negative balance of saliva and thus dryness of the mouth.

- Disorders of production in the gland itself:
  a) Absence of the basic materials for the production of saliva.
  b) Absence of acini for the production of saliva.
- Restriction of transport of saliva.
- Increased consumption of saliva.

Decreased Peripheral Stimulus or Disorders of the Afferent Stimulus

The extent to which the summation of peripheral visual, acoustic, thermal, and other stimuli, the spontaneous activity of the salivary nuclei, or the combination of both mechanisms is responsible for the resting secretion of saliva is not accurately known. A limitation of the salivary gland capacity with a decrease in peripheral stimuli and a reduction of central impulses could be the explanation of the dryness of the mouth often found in old people, if no other cause can be found.

Central Disorders

The well-known dryness of the mouth that occurs in stress is a central phenomenon. Previously, xerostomia was mainly ascribed to central disorders (Chappell 1896, Hamilton 1896). Many of the early patients described were post-menopausal women. It is likely that some of the patients described at that time had the as then unknown Sjögren's syndrome (Hadden 1888–1889, Hutchinson 1889).

Xerostomia due to central nervous disorders is a very uncommon disease. It was described by Rauch (1959), and forms a part of the adiposity, oligomenorrhea, and recurrent parotid swelling (AOP) syndrome, a pituitary disorder due to degenerative and hereditary changes in the diencephalon. Xerostomia due to head injury is also very rare (Nickol 1969).

Disorders of Salivary Gland Innervation

The most common cause of xerostomia is a disorder of salivary gland innervation leading to a decrease of salivary secretion. The most common form is an iatrogenic xerostomia induced by drugs, the most important being the antihypertensive agents and the psychotropic drugs, in particular the antidepressive agents (see Chapter 4).

Disorders of Salivary Production

Abnormal salivary production in the gland itself is also a very common cause of dryness of the mouth.

a) Insufficient materials for the production of saliva. The metabolism of the salivary glands depends on general metabolism. Thus, if a patient is deprived of water, the available salivary volume decreases. Heat exposure and dehydration in diabetes mellitus or insipidus are also examples of reduced salivary production due to shortage of water. A chronic deficiency of protein also affects the composition of saliva: for example, it becomes deficient in immunoglobulins for defence against infection (McMurray et al 1977).

b) Lack of acini. Abnormal salivary production due to lack of parenchyma is much more difficult to treat. Marked xerostomia only occurs when the minor salivary glands fail, in addition ot the major glands.

Surgical experience, for example total parotidectomy and unilateral radical neck dissection, shows that loss of one submandibular gland and one parotid gland does not lead to xerostomia. However, it is known that the rare disease of aplasia of the salivary glands leads to dryness of the mouth (Mason & Chisholm 1975, Rauch 1959), although it is not known with certainty whether the minor salivary glands are also involved with this disease.

Radiation xerostomia is important if the salivary glands lie in the field irradiated for the treatment of a tumor. The dose that can lead to irreversible damage of the salivary glands is often overestimated. A dose of 600 rad, which is often used to suppress the salivary secretion while a salivary fistula heals, causes only temporary suppression of gland function. Much higher doses, such as those used for the treatment of tumors, are needed to damage the parenchyma irreversibly (Haubrich 1981). These doses may also affect the oral mucosa directly so that radiation stomatitis is not due solely to the absence of saliva.

Sjögren's syndrome is accompanied by a characteristic xerophthalmia and xerostomia. Its cause is probably an autoimmune chronic sialadenitis of the salivary and lacrimal glands (page 146).

Clinically, the most impressive symptom is the bilateral swelling of the parotid gland accompanied by rheumatoid symptoms, such as arthritis. The atrophy of the parenchyma due to inflammation, particularly of the minor salivary glands, explains the xerostomia.

Limitation of Salivary Transport

Disorders of salivary transport alone are seldom the cause of xerostomia. Salivary calculi almost always affect one of the major glands only. In chronic sialadenitis, stenosis of the ducts is an additional cause of absence of saliva in addition to destruction of parenchyma.

Increased Consumption of Saliva

Chronic mouth breathing and the stimulus of a foreign body (for example new dentures) increase the consumption of saliva, leading to an unpleasant feeling of dryness of the mouth. This does not have the detrimental effects of decreased salivary production on the oral mucosa and the teeth.

Clinical Aspects of Xerostomia

Lack of saliva has considerable effects on the organs within the mouth. The *oral mucosa* becomes dry and red due to inflammation and is often covered by a tenacious film of mucus that

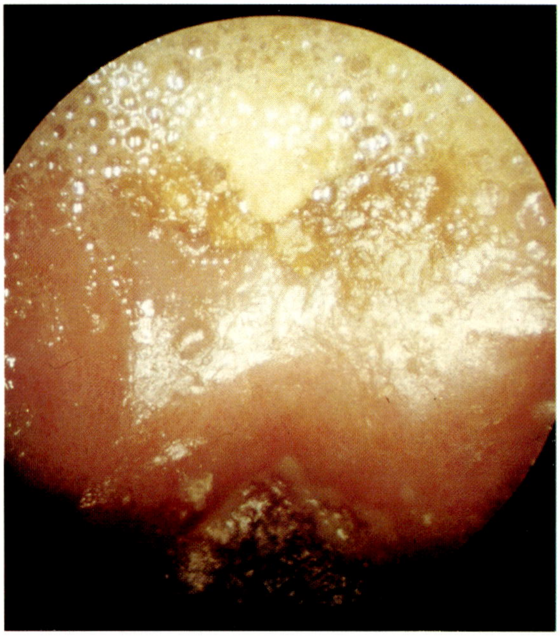

Figure 7.**2** Irradiation xerostomia showing the mucosa of the hard palate, which is red and covered with a tenacious layer of mucus. The patient was submitted to postoperative radiotherapy for carcinoma of the posterior wall of the oropharynx.

can only be scraped off with difficulty (Fig. 7.**2**). The tongue is red and inflamed, its epithelium atrophic, and its surface cracked. The patients complain of *burning of the tongue and abnormal taste.* The *lips* are dry, cracked, and covered with crusts (xerocheilia). The teeth are lost due to progressive caries and periodontal disease. *Chewing and swallowing* become difficult due to damage to the oral mucosa and to the teeth. *Speaking* may also be difficult.

Diagnosis of Xerostomia

If a patient complains of dryness of the mouth, an attempt should be made to measure this symptom, particularly if the typical results of xerostomia cannot be found in the mouth, that is neither the characteristic lesions of the mucosa or teeth or any obvious salivary gland disease. The salivary secretion should be investigated at rest and after stimulation: the term "xerostomia" should only be used, if the flow rate of the total saliva is less than 0.2 ml/15 min, whereas the term "hyposalivation" should be used for values between 0.2 and 0.9 ml/15 min (Bertram 1967). The values given by Rauch (1959) for the parotid and submandibular secretions may be seen in Table 7.**1**.

Since the secretions of all salivary glands are reduced in xerostomia, it is usual to investigate the secretion of only one or two glands, because it is easier to standardize the conditions of collection. Our experience with sialometry of the salivary glands and the appropriate values have already been described in Chapter 5. We do not usually use intraoral application of citrate, supplemented by stimulation with pilocarpine, because of the unpleasant side effects, such as sweating and nausea. We usually use direct methods of investigation, such as sialography, cytology, scanning, and biopsy. Limitation of salivary secretion is only rarely due to an abnormal secretory reflex, so that the citrate test mainly investigates the function of the gland.

If reduced salivary production is not demonstrated by this method, and if the oral mucosa is normal, the dryness of the mouth is due either to increased consumption of saliva or to psychosomatic factors. If the patient has an abnormal oral mucosa in the presence of normal salivary secretion, diseases such as avitaminosis and anemia, either macrocytic or microcytic, should be excluded.

Treatment of Xerostomia

Treatment of the cause of xerostomia is seldom possible. Treatment of metabolic disorders, such as dehydration, will restore salivary secretion to normal. Antidepressive or antihypertensive agents usually cannot be abandoned, but can be modified. The cause of chronic mouth breathing leading to increased consumption of saliva can often be relieved.

However, if the cause of xerostomia is temporary or permanent loss of parenchyma, symptomatic treatment alone is possible. There are three basic methods.

a) Intensive treatment of the oral mucosa and the teeth to prevent the most serious consequences of dry mouth. This requires thorough removal of deposits from the oral mucosa and teeth several times a day.

b) Replacement of the absent saliva. Previously, solutions containing glycerine were often used, but now solutions are prepared that imitate the natural saliva in composition and in particular viscosity. The number of these is increasing constantly (Nakamoto 1979, Shannon et al 1977). We usually use the synthetic saliva (Glandosane) originally described by Matzker and Schreiber (1972).

c) Stimulation of secretion from the remaining parenchyma. Previously, this was done by the use of pilocarpine drops, but now anetholetrithione (Mucinol) is usually used, although this stimulates secretion elsewhere, particularly the gallbladder, leading to corresponding side effects. Indeed, the efficacy of anetholetrithione on xerostomia, particularly in radiation-induced xerostomia (Breunsbach & Dvŏrák 1974) is disputed (Hassenstein et al 1978). It is also not yet clear if radioprotective substances developed in animal experiments (Pratt et al 1980) can have a protective effect on the salivary parenchyma in man.

The many patients, particularly the elderly, who complain of dryness of the mouth in the absence of objective findings have not yet been discussed. The cause is probably a slight reduction of saliva in the presence of a reduced threshold of sensitivity. This can be treated by mild sialogogues.

Xerostomia can thus have numerous causes. Its understanding requires a basic knowledge of salivary physiology. Xerostomia is not always a symptom of salivary gland disease, so that the diagnostic measures must not be confined to the salivary glands, although it must be admitted that in most cases salivary production is indeed decreased. The feeling of dryness of the mouth is not always accompanied by an objective lack of saliva, so that rational treatment is then not available. If saliva is lacking, management ranges from the treatment of the cause (for example, a change of antidepressive drug) to symptomatic procedures, such as the use of synthetic saliva preparations.

Sialorrhea

Drooling is physiologic in childhood at the time of the eruption of the teeth, but it becomes abnormal if it persists beyond this phase of development. This may happen in various neurologic disorders, for example, Parkinson's disease and myasthenia gravis, but particularly in spastic children. In these children drooling may be so severe that the clothes must be changed several times a day or the child must wear a towel round the neck. One cause of drooling in a spastic child is certainly a disordered swallowing reflex (Arnold & Gross 1977, Ekedahl et al 1974, Friedman & Kaplan 1979). Whether saliva is overproduced in addition due to central hyperstimulation (Diamant & Kumlien 1974) is disputed (Arnold & Gross 1977, Friedman & Kaplan 1979, Smith & Goode 1970).

Similar problems also often occur after resection of a tumor of the mouth or pharynx or esophagus, causing difficulty in swallowing. Irradiation used to treat the tumor often limits the production of saliva so that the problem of drooling does not arise, or the patient may even have xerostomia. Drooling in spastic children is not only a nursing problem, but it also hinders rehabilitation, particularly speech therapy and social reintegration. Since longterm treatment with parasympatholytic agents is not possible, physiotherapy must be initiated in early childhood, which is very costly (Bosley 1965, 1966, Mueller 1975). Radiotherapy in small doses is often only temporarily successful, and, furthermore, carries the danger of radiation-induced carcinoma. Surgical methods of treatment of drooling have been described (Selley 1979).

Procedures that may be used alone or in combination include removal of the major salivary glands, rerouting or ligation of the parotid duct, and parasympathetic denervation (Table 7.**2**). The procedure most often used for the treatment of drooling in spastic children is that described by Wilkie (1970), consisting of the removal of both submandibular glands and rerouting of both parotid ducts into the tonsillar fossa (and removal of enlarged tonsils if necessary). This is an extensive procedure, but it was successful in 106 of 123 children (Wilkie & Brody 1977). The disadvantages of this operation are the time it takes and such complications as cyst formation, parotitis, swelling of the cheek (Glass et al 1978, Michel et al 1977, Wilkie & Brody 1977), stenosis of the parotid duct, and disordered reflexes in the hypopharynx and esophageal inlet (Ekedahl et al 1974), possibly leading to aspiration of saliva (Goode & Smith 1970).

Parasympathetic denervation of the major salivary glands leads to an immediate reduction of salivary secretion. Thus, the immediate results of tympanic neurectomy, combined with unilateral or bilateral division of the chorda tympani, are usually better than the long-term results (Arnold & Gross 1977, Michel et al 1977, Mullins et al 1979). However, since a permanent reduction of salivary secretion is needed, parasympathetic denervation for this disease has the same drawbacks as autonomic denervation of vessels and glands. These include the growth of collaterals, the high regenerative capacity of the autonomic nervous system, and the hypersensitivity of denervated organs to neurogenic transmitters (Chapter 4). However, because these operations are not extensive and promise good results in 50% of cases, they are preferred to more extensive methods. One disadvantage of bilateral division of the chorda tympani is loss of the sense of taste from the anterior part of the tongue. It can be obviated by preservation of one chorda tympani combined with removal of one submandibular gland (Diamant & Kumlien 1974, Friedman & Kaplan 1979, Michel et al 1977).

Table 7.2 Operative Treatment of Drooling

No. Subjects	Method	Successes	Period of Follow-up	Reference
14	Bilateral removal of the submandibular gland and bilateral ligation of the parotid duct	12	2 month – 4½ years	Dundas & Peterson 1979
123	Bilateral removal of submandibular gland and bilateral rerouting of the parotid duct	106	1½–13 years	Wilkie & Brodie 1977
14	Bilateral removal of the submandibular gland, 6 by rerouting (Wilkie's method), 6 with bilateral duct ligation, and 2 with unilateral rerouting	5 6 6 2	20–34 months	Glass et al 1978
2	Bilateral tympanic neurectomy and unilateral resection of the chorda tympani	2	6 month – 1½ years	Friedman & Kaplan 1979
4	Bilateral TN and unilateral Ch-R	4	4–9 months	Friedman et al 1974
30*	Bilateral TN and bilateral CH-R	30	2 months	Arnold & Gross 1977
31*	Bilateral TN and bilateral Ch-R	19	24–45 months	Mullins et al 1979
12	Unilateral removal of the submandibular gland and contralateral Ch-R	8	2 years	Diamant & Kumlien 1974
20	Bilateral TN with occasionally bilateral Ch-R	15	Brief (10 successes after 14 months)	Michel et al 1977
5	Bilateral TN & Ch-R	4	2–4 years	Goode & Smith 1970
17	Bilateral Ch-R	7 7 5	Good Partial Failures	Toremalm & Bjerre 1976

* These series consisted of virtually the same patients.
TN = tympanic neurectomy, Ch-R = chorda tympani resection.

References

Arnold, H. G., C. W. Gross: Transtympanic neurectomy: a solution to drooling problems. Dev. Med. Child Neurol. 19 (1977) 509

Bertram, U.: Xerostomia. Acta Odont. Scand., Suppl. 49 (1967) 1

Bosley, E.: Development of sucking and swallowing. Cerebr. Palsy J. 26 (1965) 14

Bosley, E.: Teaching the cerebral palsied to chew. Cerebr. Palsy J. 27 (1966) 8

Breunsbach, J., K. Dvőrák: Erste Erfahrungen mit dem Präparat SL 25 bei der Behandlung der strahleninduzierten Mundtrokkenheit. Strahlentherapie 148 (1974) 298

Chappell, W. F.: Report of three cases of xerostomia or dry mouth. N. Y. med. J. 63 (1896) 277

Chilla, R., M. Opaitz, C. Arglebe: Flußrate, Amylase- und Proteingehalt des Parotisspeichels bei Sialadenose. Z. Laryng. Rhinol. 57 (1978) 274

Diamant, H., A. Kumlien: A treatment for drooling in children with cerebral palsy. J. Laryngol. Otol. 88 (1974) 61

Dundas, D. F., R. A. Peterson: Surgical treatment of drooling by bilateral parotid duct ligation and submandibular gland resection. Plast. Reconstr. Surg. 64 (1979) 47

Ekedahl, C., I. Månsson, N. Sandberg: Swallowing dysfunction in the brain-damaged with drooling. Acta Otolaryngol. 78 (1974) 141

Friedman, W. H., B. Kaplan: Tympanic neurectomy, correction of drooling in cerebral palsy. N. Y. St. J. Med. 75 (1979) 2919

Friedman, W. H., R. S. Swerdlow, J. M. Pornarico: Tympanic neurectomy: a review and an additional indication for this procedure. Laryngoscope 84 (1974) 568

Glass, L. W., G. L. Novel, T. R. Vecchione: Treatment of uncontrolled drooling by bilateral excision of submaxillary glands and parotid duct ligations. Plast. Reconstr. Surg. 62 (1978) 523

Goode, R. L., R. A. Smith: The surgical management of sialorrhea. Laryngoscope 80 (1970) 1078

Hadden, W. B.: Xerostomia (dry mouth). Brain 11 (1888–1889) 484

Hamilton, T. K.: Case of Xerostomia. Zit. nach: Int. Centralbl. Laryngol. Rhinol. 12 (1896) 272

Hassenstein, E., R. Müller, H. Reinhard: Die Wirkung von SL 25 auf die radiogene Xerostomie bei der Strahlentherapie von Tumoren im Hals- und Gesichtsbereich. Strahlentherapie 154 (1978) 554

Haubrich, J.: Etiology and pathogenesis of the inflammatory diseases of the cephalic salivary glands. Adv. Oto-rhino-laryngol. 26 (1981) 39

Hutchinson, J.: A second report on "xerostomia" or "dry mouth", with an additional case. Trans. Clin. Soc. London 22 (1889) 25

Mason, D. K., D. M. Chisholm: Salivary Glands in Health and Disease. Saunders, London 1975

Matzker, J., J. Schreiber: Synthetischer Speichel zur Therapie der Hyposialien, insbesondere bei der radiogenen Sialadenitis. Z. Laryngol. Rhinol. 51 (1972) 422

McMurray, D. N., H. Rey, L. J. Casazza, R. R. Watson: Effect of moderate malnutrition on concentrations of immunoglobulins and enzymes in tears and saliva of young Colombian children. Amer. J. Clin. Nutr. 30 (1977) 1944

Michel, R. G., K. A. Johnson, C. N. Patterson: Parasympathetic nerve section for control of sialorrhea. Arch. Otolaryngol. 103 (1977) 94–97

Mueller, H. A.: Facilitating feeding and pre-speech. In Person, P. H., C. E. Williams: Physical Therapy Services in Development Disabilities. Thomas, Springfield 1975

Mullins, W. M., C. W. Gross, J. M. Moore: Long-term follow-up of tympanic neurectomy for sialorrhea. Laryngoscope 89 (1979) 1219

Nakamoto, R. Y.: Use of saliva in postradiation xerostomia. J. Prosthet. Dent. 42 (1979) 539

Nickol, H.-J.: Xerostomie als Unfallfolge. Arch. Otorhinolaryngol. 194 (1969) 621

Pratt, N. E., M. Sodicoff, J. Liss, M. Davis, M. Sinesi: Radioprotection of the rat parotid gland by WR-2721: morphology at 60 days post-irradiation. Int. J. Radiat. Oncol. Biol. Phys. 6 (1980) 431

Rauch, S.: Die Speicheldrüsen des Menschen. Thieme, Stuttgart 1959

Seifert, G.: Die Sekretionsstörungen (Dyschylien) der Speicheldrüsen. In Cohrs, P., W. Giese, H. Meessen: Ergebnisse der allgemeinen Pathologie und pathologischen Anatomie. Bd. 44. Springer, Berlin 1964 (S. 103)

Selley, W. G.: Remedy for excessive salivation. Brit. Med. J. I (1979) 1355

Shannon, I. L., B. R. Mc Crary, E. N. Starcke: A saliva substitute for use by xerostomic patients undergoing radiotherapy to the head and neck. Oral Surg. 44 (1977) 656

Smith, R. A., R. L. Goode: Sialorrhea. N. Engl. J. Med. 283 (1970) 917

Toremalm, N. G., I. Bjerre: Surgical elimination of drooling. Laryngoscope 86 (1976) 104

Wilkie, T. F.: The surgical treatment of drooling. Plast. Reconstr. Surg. 45 (1970) 549

Wilkie, T. F., G. S. Brody: The surgical treatment of drooling. A ten-year review. Plast. Reconstr. Surg. 59 (1977) 791

8. Sialadenosis

Clinical Findings

The term "sialadenosis" coined by Rauch (1959) embraces a clinically and pathologically well-defined disease characterized by disorders of secretion of all salivary glands, but particularly of the parotid. The disorder may be defined (Seifert 1964) as a noninflammatory salivary disease due to metabolic and secretory disorders of the gland parenchyma accompanied by a recurrent painful bilateral swelling of the glands, in particular the parotid. The disease often gives the patient a hamsterlike appearence, which is often the only reason that the patient seeks advice (Fig. 8.**1**).

The swelling is almost always independent of eating. There is no particular sex predominance, and the peak age incidence lies between the fourth and seventh decade. Disease persisting over 20 years is far from unusual.

The principle of classification of the sialadenoses rests on the results of investigations of numerous patients who have one of the following diseases.

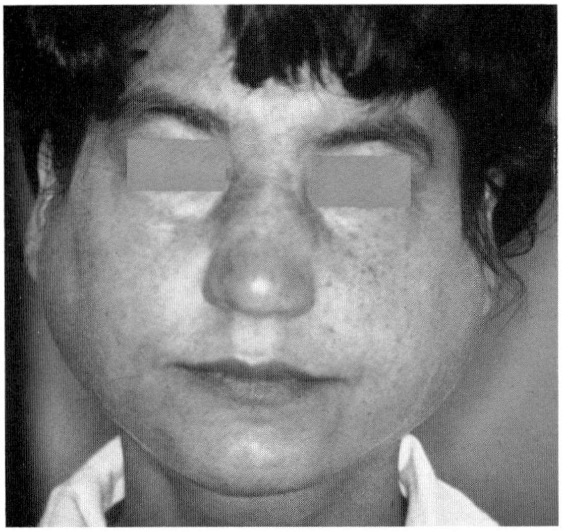

Figure 8.**1** Sialadenosis in a 39-year-old woman with endocrine dysfunction. The typical appearances of a boggy swelling of the parotid on both sides, and the hamsterlike appearance of the patient are well seen.

Sialadenosis in Endocrine Disorders

Gland enlargement due to sialadenosis has been described in virtually all endocrine disorders. The principal one is diabetes mellitus in which there is a disorder of carbohydrate and fat metabolism. Sialadenosis is more common in elderly than in juvenile diabetics.

In many cases, the sialadenosis may manifest itself before the diabetes mellitus.

Disorders of the diencephalon-pituitary system, such as the syndrome of adiposity, oligomenorrhea, and parotid swelling (Rauch 1956), acromegaly, and diabetes insipidus may be accompanied by sialadenosis. Furthermore, sialadenosis may occur in thyroid disorders, particularly hypothyroidism, and dysfunction of the gonads, especially during pregnancy and lactation. Recurrent parotid swellings are observed during phases of hormonal changes, such as puberty and the menopause, and in disorders of the adrenal glands.

Dystrophic-Metabolic Sialadenosis

Salivary swellings in this instance are associated with deficiency of vitamins and proteins in times of famine or in the chronic undernutrition of alcoholics and cirrhotics. Chronic lack of protein in many parts of the world, often associated with vitamin deficiency, is now the causative factor of sialadenosis in kwashiorkor, mang, beriberi, and pellagra.

Neurogenic Sialadenosis

Dysfunction of the autonomic nervous system is assumed to be the cause of neurogenic sialadenosis (Donath & Seifert 1975, Donath 1976, 1979). Rauch (1959) distinguishes a central form due to psychologic causes, antihypertensive agents, such as clonidine, and possibly psychotropic drugs, from a peripheral form due to antihypertensive drugs of the guanethidine group. Parotid gland swelling in anorexia nervosa may fall in both the neurogenic and in the dystrophic-metabolic groups.

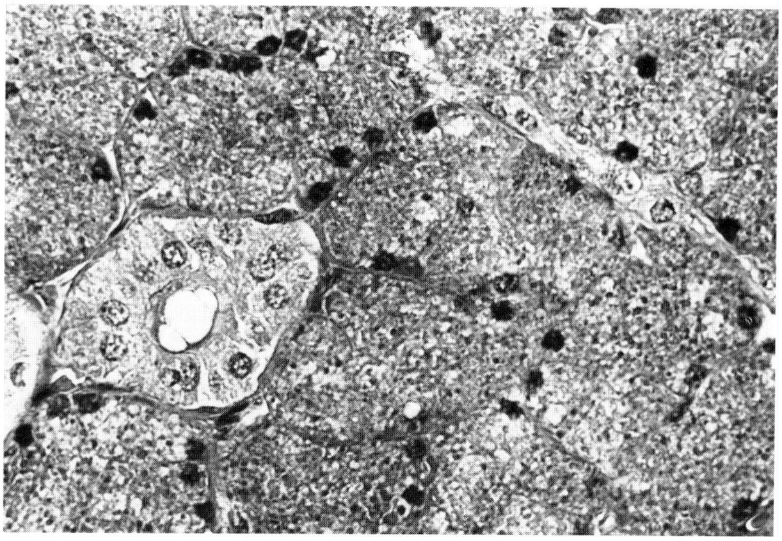

Figure 8.**2** Sialadenosis (granular form) showing marked swelling of the acinar cytoplasm and basal position of the nuclei. On the left of the picture is a striated duct. H & E, 400×.

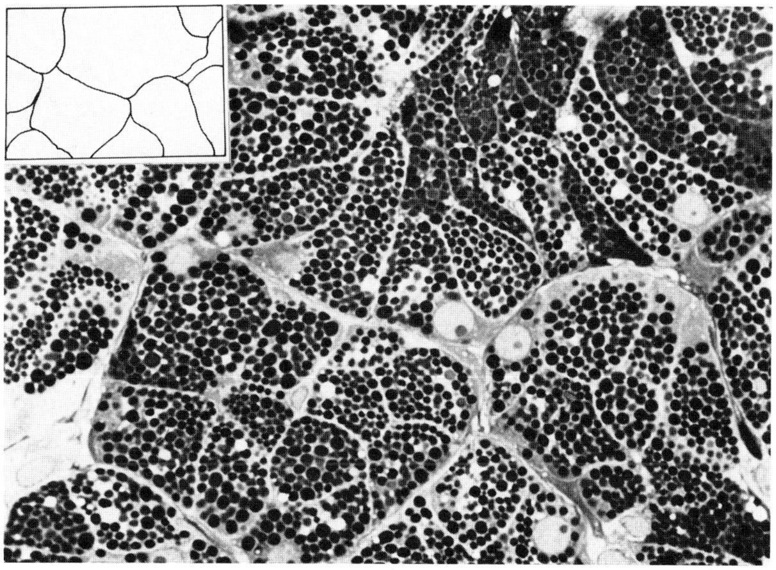

Figure 8.**3** Granular form of sialadenosis showing dense concentration of secretory granules in the cytoplasm. The inset shows a diagram of the acinar borders. Semithin sections stained with toluidine blue. 870×. (Seifert & Donath 1976.)

Pathology

Histopathology shows that the parotid swelling is due to acinar enlargement (Seifert 1964, 1967, 1971, 1981, Donath 1976, 1979, Seifert & Donath 1975). The diameter of the acini increases to twice or three times that of normal (50–70 μm, with a maximum up to 100 μm) compared with the normal acinus of 30–40 μm (Fig. 8.**2**). The nuclei of the individual acinar cells are displaced toward the basal part of the cell and possess a clear nucleolus. Periodic acid–Schiff (PAS)-positive enzyme granules can be demonstrated in the cytoplasm of the swollen cell. Light microscopy of stained sections shows three forms of sialadenosis: the *granular form* (Fig. 8.**3**) is characterized by a dense filling of the cytoplasm with granules, a *honeycomb pattern* (Fig. 8.**4a, b**) demonstrates a vacuolated cytoplasm, and a *mixed form* demonstrates granulated and vacuolated acinar cells. Electron microscopy shows that these differences are not due to the quantity of granules, but that they are determined solely by the optic density of the secretory particles (Fig. 8.**5**). Furthermore, there is almost no correlation between the morphologic appearances and any specific clinical type of sialadenosis. Individual fat cells can be demonstrated in the interstitium of the lobules, but an inflammatory infiltrate is absent. The duct system is slightly compressed by the swollen acini so that the finer peripheral ducts are not demonstrated by sialography. Unlike the parotid gland, the submandibular gland shows a low-grade swelling of the acini, especially of the

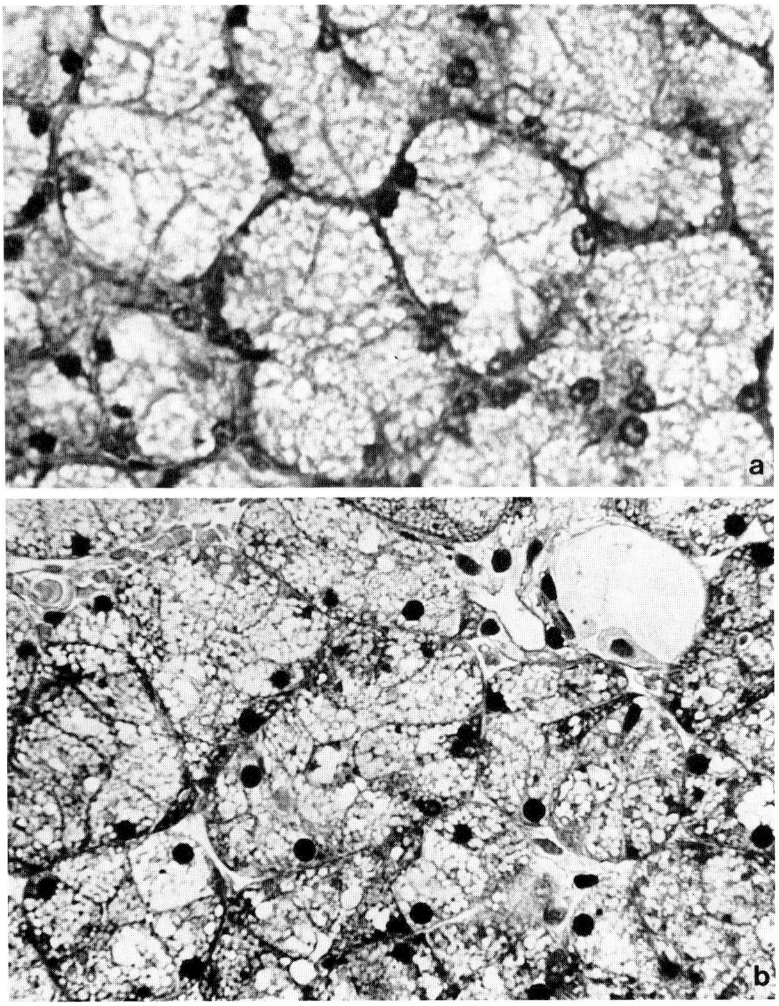

Figure 8.**4** Vacuolated form of sialadenosis: **a** Marked acinar swelling with vacuolar clear areas in the cytoplasm. H & E, 400×. **b** Secretory vacuoles in the cytoplasm. Semithin section. Toluidine blue, 400×.

serous type. The sublingual and minor salivary glands show no gross changes.

Aspiration cytology (Droese 1980) shows extremely large acini and a marked vulnerability of the cytoplasm. Cytologic values for the diameter of the acinus are on average 11 μm higher than in the histologic preparation. Acinar diameters greater than 65 μm should be accepted as cytologic criteria for the presence of sialadenosis.

Electron microscopy (Donath & Seifert 1975) shows lesions of the acinar cells, the myoepithelial cells, and the autonomic nervous system. The cytoplasm of the swollen *acinar cells* includes membrane-limited secretory granules with a diameter of 1–3 μm from the base to the apex (Fig. 8.**5**). The mature granules are smaller and optically dense, whereas the immature granules are larger and optically clear. The coarse endoplasmic reticulum consists of a few parallel-arranged membrane pairs lying basally. The Golgi apparatus is reduced. Condensed vacuoles are scarcely present. Occasionally, paranuclear fat vacuoles can be demonstrated. The *myoepithelial cells* are conspicuous due to degenerative changes. These include nuclear pyknosis, fat vacuoles, and homogeneous condensation zones of the cytoplasm. At some points, progression to myoepithelial cell necrosis may be observed. The main lesions of the *autonomic nervous system* occur on the postganglionic sympathetic neurones. The characteristics include a loss of neurosecretory granules, destruction of the mitochondria, hydropic swelling of the axoplasm, and a terminal axolysis. The initial pattern of damage occurs on the terminal axons of the effector cells, the acinar cells, and the myoepithelial cells. In later stages, lesions of the varicosities of the preterminal axons and on the myelinated nerves in the form of myelin sheaths and osmiophilic granules may also be recorded. The endothelial cells of the capillaries also show atrophic changes.

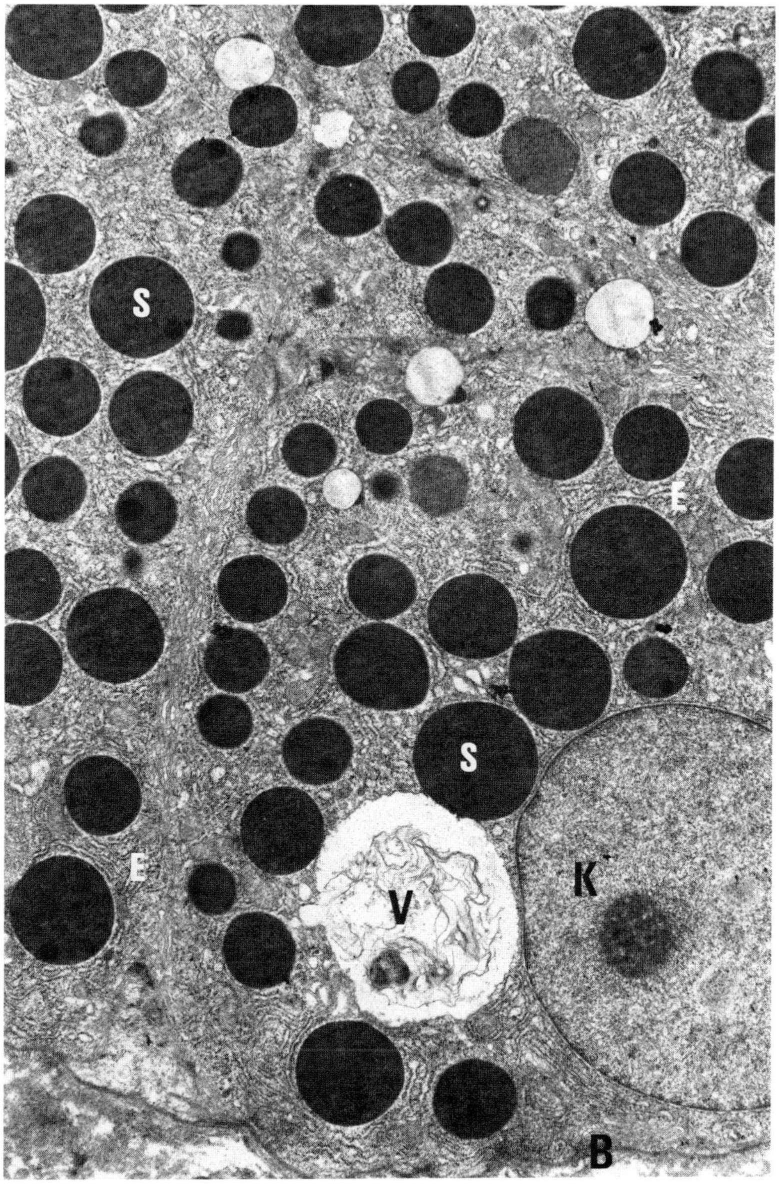

Figure 8.**5** Ultrastucture of the acinar cells in granular sialadenosis showing rich optically dark secretory granules (S) in the cytoplasm with endoplasmic reticulum (e) between them. V = vacuoles in the cytoplasm with myelin-like filamentary structures, K = cell nucleus, B = basal membrane. 7250×. (Seifert & Donath 1976.)

The *triad* of acinar swelling due to concentration of secretory granules, atrophic changes of the myoepithelial cells, and degeneration of the autonomic nervous system characterizes human sialadenosis. Since successive biopsies of human tissue are not available, animal experiments are required to explain the pathogenesis of this disease (Donath 1976). The results of such investigations have led to the conclusion that the main causative factor is a primary neuropathy of the autonomic nervous system that leads to disordered secretion in the acinar cell. Comparison with the regular secretory cycle (Chapter 4) shows that the type of secretory disorder is a disturbance of formation of secretion with two hallmarks: a lengthening of the storage phase of the secretory granules and an arrest of protein synthesis. Both processes produce swelling of the acinar cell (Fig. 8.**6**). Parotid lesions similar to human sialadenosis occur in deprivation of food, destruction of the sympathetic nervous system or overdoses with beta-adrenergic substances.

The clinical findings also support the hypothesis that a *primary neuropathy* of the nervous system is responsible for the sialadenoses. These include bilateral inflammatory recurrent parotid swelling and polyneuropathy in all diseases that coexist with sialadenosis, such as diabetes mellitus, alcoholism, chronic liver disease, disorders of protein metabolism, and nervous diseases. Sialadenoses may also accompany disorders of protein

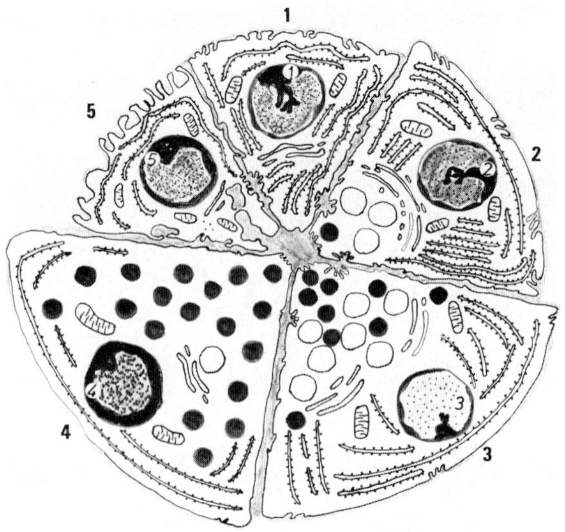

Figure 8.**6** Diagram of the secretory cycle of the parotid gland under adrenergic stimulation: 1 = beginning of synthesis with formation of endoplasmic reticulum, 2–3 = formation and maturation of secretory granules, 4 = prolonged storage phase of secretory granules with increase of the acinar diameter and arrested protein synthesis, 5 = end of secretion after adrenergic stimulation. (Seifert & Donath 1976.)

metabolism and polyneuropathies in patients with tumors having a prolonged course requiring intensive treatment (Günther 1977).

Further evidence that *adrenergic beta-receptors* play a part in the genesis of the sialadenoses is provided by the fact that considerably higher beta receptor concentrations are found after denervation and in the sialadenoses than in healthy salivary tissue (Chilla et al 1981). The parotid gland is

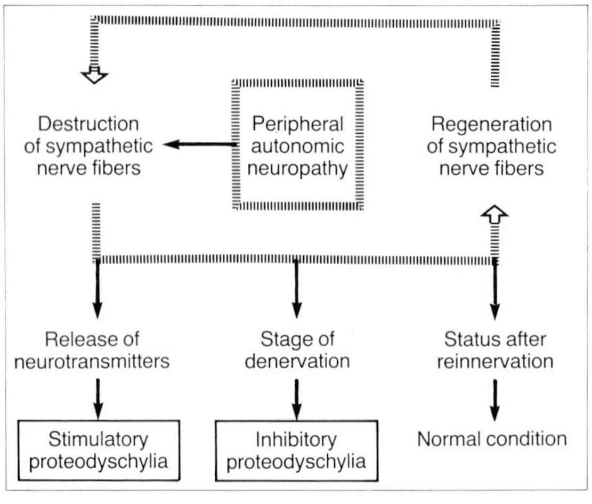

Figure 8.**7** Diagram of neuropathy in sialadenoses with denervation and reinnervation. (Chilla.)

thus oversensitive to the effect of a neurogenic transmitter. During an autonomic neuropathy, alternating denervation and regeneration of autonomic nerve fibers occur, leading to a stimulatory or inhibitory proteodyschylia (Fig. 8.**7**).

The *differential diagnosis* of sialadenosis from other forms of swelling of the cheek, such as sialadenitis, oncocytosis, salivary calculus, cysts, and tumors, requires various diagnostic procedures, including biopsy of the parotid gland (Seifert 1979, Donath 1979, Hornstein 1979, Haubrich 1979).

Etiology

The etiology of sialadenoses has not yet been clearly explained. Any theory about the genesis must take into account the following factors:

- The sialadenoses often occur in hormonal disorders, particularly diabetes mellitus, in nutritional disorders with deficiency of protein and vitamins, in alcoholism, and in various neurologic disorders (Haubrich 1976).
- The swelling of the parenchyma is due to a swelling of the acini, whose diameter is clearly increased. The diagnosis can only be made with certainty by measurement of the acini. Morphometry and aspiration cytology examination are the diagnostic methods of choice. Normal acini have a diameter of about 45 μm, whereas the acini in sialadenosis have a diameter of about 60 μm (Droese 1981).
- The swelling of the acinar cell is due to an increase of its content of zymogen granules. Examination of the acini with the electron microscope shows that these may be divided into a marked protein-containing form (dark form of sialadenosis) or a weak protein-containing form (clear form of sialadenosis) (Donath & Seifert 1975).
- Asthmatics who use sympathomimetics agents in an aerosol for many years can develop sialadenosis (Borsanyi & Blanchard 1967). In animal experiments isoproterenol causes marked swelling of the salivary glands: protein synthesis, protein secretion, and the content of clear zymogen granules in the gland are increased (Selye et al 1961, Johnson & Sreebny 1973, Robinovitch et al 1977).

Some antihypertensive agents, such as guanethidine and related substances, cause salivary gland swellings in man associated with painful secretion of saliva (Bock & Huep 1971, Donath et al 1973). Animal experiments (Donath 1973, Chilla et al 1975) have shown changes in the parotid gland that correspond to the dark form of sialadenosis.

If there were a common cause for the sialadenoses, it would have to explain all the clinical, pathologic, and experimental facts. The accumulation of zymogen granules indicates a disorder of protein secretion. The protein secretion of the salivary gland is mainly regulated by the sympathetic nervous system. Stimulation of beta-adrenergic receptors leads to expulsion exocytosis of secretory granules from the acinar cell (Chilla 1981). If a salivary gland is denervated, it becomes hypersensitive to the neurogenic transmitter (Stefano & Perec 1981). Sympathetic denervation of the parotid gland causes the concentration of the $beta_1$-adrenergic receptors on the acinar cell to increase significantly (Chilla et al 1981). This is probably the cause of the hypersensitivity. The concentration of the $beta_1$-adrenergic receptors also increases in the human parotid gland, if the patient has sialadenosis (Chilla et al 1981). Electron microscopy has shown degenerative changes in the autonomic nerve fibers of the salivary gland of patients with sialadenosis (see before) (Seifert & Donath 1975). The increase of $beta_1$-adrenergic receptors and the demonstration of degenerative changes in the autonomic nerve fibers in sialadenosis leads to the working hypothesis that the sialadenosis results from the sympathetic denervation of the salivary glands. Can such an hypothesis be reconciled with the known facts?

- It is striking that neuropathies are often observed in those diseases in which sialodenosis also occurs frequently, for example, diabetic polyneuropathy, alcoholic neuropathy, and the avitaminoses.
- Sympathetic denervation of a salivary gland must lead to inhibition of protein synthesis. The accumulation of marked protein-containing secretory granules in the dark form of sialadenosis associated with swelling of the acinar cells is consistent with sympathetic denervation.
- The fact that some antihypertensive agents that destroy peripheral sympathetic fibers induce the dark form of sialadenosis in man and experimental animals is also compatible with the hypothesis.

Up to this point, the working hypothesis appears to be reasonably well founded, but the question arises of the genesis of the clear form of sialadenosis caused experimentally by isoproterenol. This sympathomimetic drug activates protein synthesis and secretion, a process directly opposed to sympathetic denervation. A further cause for doubt is the normal protein concentration in the saliva of patients with sialadenoses.

Emmelin and Trendelenburg (1972) especially have investigated the process caused by sympathetic denervation of the salivary gland. After surgical or chemical destruction of sympathetic fibers, their stored norepinephrine is released, leading to degeneration secretion, that is, abnormal protein secretion due to overstimulation. This may be termed "stimulatory proteodyschylia." The pathologic correlate is the clear form of sialadenosis. A denervation phase with inhibited protein secretion follows, and this may be termed an "inhibitory proteodyschylia." The pathologic correlate of this phase is the dark form of sialadenosis.

If denervation is regarded as a dynamic process, the apparent contraindication can be explained. Sympathetic denervation of the acinar cells initially leads to stimulation and then to inhibition of its protein secretion. Because of the high regenerative capacity of the sympathetic nervous system (Murray & Thompson 1957), reinnervation processes often proceed simultaneously. All these events may proceed simultaneously or successively in one gland and induce the different forms of sialadenosis. Simultaneous inhibition and stimulation of protein secretion compensate each other so that the salivary protein concentration remains normal.

Human sialadenosis is thus probably not a disorder of the salivary glands but of the innervation of the glands. Seifert and Donath (1975) regard a peripheral autonomic neuropathy as the basic pathophysiologic principle of sialadenosis that explains the clinical, pathologic, and experimental data, if the term "neuropathy" embraces degeneration secretion, the denervated condition itself, and reinnervation (Fig. 8.**7**).

Diagnosis and Treatment

The history of the patient often shows one of the basic underlying diseases, and the clinical aspects of a bilateral boggy indolent, varying swelling of the parotid gland confirm the suspicion of the diagnosis of sialadenosis. Sialography shows a typical picture, at least in the late stages of the disease. The sialographic findings are caused by the acinar swelling, compressing the proximal ducts. Scanning of the salivary gland with $^{99m}TcO_4$, which is thought to be stored in the intercalated and striated ducts of the parotid gland, often shows concentration of the radioisotope in salivary tissue. However, both increased retention and decreased activity of the diseased gland may be found during the course of the disease.

The surest diagnostic method of verification of sialadenosis is histologic examination of a parotid biopsy. Aspiration cytology (Droese 1980) is also valuable.

Compared with the comprehensive explanation of the etiologic, pathologic, and morphologic aspects of sialadenosis, treatment is as yet unsatisfactory. Endocrine and neurogenic sialadenoses are particularly resistant to treatment. It is striking that even under optimal control of diabetes mellitus the gland swelling due to sialadenosis remains largely unaltered.

Sialadenosis due to antihypertensive agents regresses after withdrawal of the drug. However, in some patients who take guanacline, the symptoms may persist after the drug has been withdrawn, possibly due to irreversible damage to the autonomic nerve fibers by the guanethidine derivative. The effect of isoproterenol on the parotid can be blocked in animal experiments (Arnold & Schaetzle 1973), but treatment of sialadenosis by beta-receptor blockers has not produced appreciable improvement. The exclusive beta-sympatholysis by propranolol leads to functional impairment of the parotid gland due to inhibition of neurohormonally regulated protein secretion.

If the swelling of the gland due to sialadenosis causes an unacceptable cosmetic defect, a subtotal parotidectomy may be considered, but should be the last resort.

References

Arold, R., W. Schätzle: Die "Experimentelle Sialose" und ihre Beeinflussung durch β-Receptoren-Blocker. Arch. klin. exp. Ohr-, Nas.- u. Kehlk.-Heilk. 203 (1973) 274

Bock, K. D., W. W. Huep: Irreversibler Parotisschmerz nach Verabreichung von Guanaclin. Dtsch. med. Wschr. 96 (1971) 1649

Borsanyi, S. J., C. L. Blanchard: Asymptomatic parotid swelling and isoproterenol. Laryngoscope 72 (1967) 1777

Chilla, R.: Sialadenosis of the salivary glands of the head. Adv. Oto-Rhino-Laryng. 26 (1981) 1

Chilla, R., M. Opaitz, C. Arglebe: Flußrate, Amylase- und Proteingehalt des Parotisspeichels bei Sialadenose. Z. Laryng. Rhinol. 57 (1978) 274

Chilla, R., R. Arnold, K.-H. Flucke, C. Arglebe: The effect of clonidine treatment on the salivary glands of the rat. Results of biochemical and histological investigations. Arch. Oto-Rhino-Laryng. 209 (1957) 47

Chilla, R., V. Witzemann, M. Opaitz, C. Arglebe: Possible involvement of parotid beta-adrenergic receptors in the etiology of sialadenosis. Arch. Oto-Rhino-Laryng. 230 (1981) 113

Donath, K.: Ultrastrukturelle Acinusveränderungen der Rattenparotis unter der Einwirkung von Antihypertensiva (Guanacline). Arch. Oto-Rhino-Laryng. 206 (1973) 77

Donath, K.: Die Sialadenose der Parotis. – Ultrastrukturelle, klinische und experimentelle Befunde zur Sekretionspathologie. Fischer, Stuttgart 1976

Donath, K.: Wangenschwellung bei Sialadenose. HNO (Berl.) 27 (1979) 113

Donath, K., G. Seifert: Ultrastructural studies of the parotid gland in sialadenosis. Virchows Arch. Path. Anat. 365 (1975) 119

Donath, K., G. Seifert, W. Pirsig: Parotis-Sialadenose nach Langzeittherapie mit Antihypertensiva (Guanacline). Virchows Arch. Path. Anat. 360 (1973) 33

Droese, M.: Punktionszytologie der Speicheldrüsenerkrankungen. Habil.-Schrift, Göttingen 1980

Droese, M.: Cytological diagnosis of sialadenosis, sialadenitis and parotid cysts by fine-needle aspiration biopsy. Adv. Oto-Rhino-Laryng. 26 (1981) 49

Emmelin, N., U. Trendelenburg: Degeneration activity after parasympathetic or sympathetic denervation. Rev. Physiol. 66 (1972) 147

Günther, W.-L.: Über das Vorkommen der Sialadenose im Obduktionsmaterial. Pathohistologische Untersuchungen. Diss., Hamburg 1977

Haubrich, J.: Differentialdiagnose der Wangenschwellungen (ausschließlich der Speicheldrüsentumoren) aus der Sicht des HNO-Arztes. HNO (Berl.) 27 (1979) 138

Hornstein, O. P.: Differentialdiagnose dermatogener Wangenschwellungen. HNO (Berl.) 27 (1979) 129

Johnson, D. A., L. M. Sreebny: Effect of isoprotenerol on synthesis and secretion in the rat parotid gland. Lab. Invest. 28 (1973) 263

Murray, J. G., J. M. Thompson: Occurence and function of collateral sprouting in sympathic nervous system of the cat. J. Physiol. 135 (1957) 133

Rauch, S.: Zur Differentialdiagnose chronisch-rezidivierender Speicheldrüsenschwellungen. Pract. oto-rhino-laryng. 18 (1956) 272

Rauch, S.: Die Speicheldrüsen des Menschen. Thieme, Stuttgart 1959

Robinovitch, M. R., P. J. Keller, D. A. Johnson, J. M. Iversen, D. L. Kauffman: Changes in rat parotid salivary protein induced by chronic isoproterenol administration. J. dent. Res. 56 (1977) 290

Seifert, G.: Die Sekretionsstörungen (Dyschylien) der Speicheldrüsen. Ergebn. allg. Path. path. Anat. 44 (1964) 103

Seifert, G.: Experimental sialadenosis by isoproterenol and other agents: Histochemistry and electron microscopy. In Schneyer, L. H., Ch. A. Schneyer: Secretory Mechanisms of Salivary Glands. Academic Presse, New York 1967 (p. 191)

Seifert, G.: Klinische Pathologie der Sialadenitis und Sialadenose. HNO (Berl.) 19 (1971) 1

Seifert, G.: Wangenschwellungen bei Speicheldrüsenentzündungen. Pathologisch-anatomische Differentialdiagnose der Sialadenitis. HNO (Berl.) 27 (1979) 119

Seifert, G.: Chronische Mundtrockenheit. Ursachen, Pathologie. Dtsch. Z. Mund-Kiefer-Gesichts-Chir. 5 (1981) 3

Seifert, G., K. Donath: Die Sialadenose der Parotis. Dtsch. med. Wschr. 100 (1975) 1545

Selye, H., R. Veilleux, M. Cantin: Excessive stimulation of salivary gland growth by isoprotenerol. Science 133 (1961) 44

Stefano, F. J. E., C. J. Perec: Denervation supersensitivity in salivary glands. Trends in Pharmacol. Science 2 (1981) 107

9. Sialolithiasis

Clinical Findings and Treatment

Reference to Rauch's extensive treatise on calculus formation in the salivary glands leads to the conclusion that little progress has been made since 1959. The cause of calculus formation is still largely unexplained. Much knowledge has been gained in the intervening period by new techniques, such as scanning electron microscopy (Taniguchi et al 1979), x-ray microanalysis (Taniguchi et al 1979), radiocrystalography (Fichelson et al 1978), infrared spectroscopy (Skurk et al 1972), and atomic absorption spectrometry (Skurk et al 1973) about the composition and structure of salivary calculi. However, it remains unexplained why such calculi form. Unlike calculi in the urinary tract and the gallbladder, methods for dissolving the calculi and for dietetic treatment are not available.

Salivary calculi occur mainly in the large ducts of the salivary glands, and more rarely in the parenchyma, although they have usually developed there in the intraglandular duct system. Salivary calculi are mainly observed in adults (Rauch 1959). Scott (1978) showed that microdeposits of organic material in the intraglandular duct system of the submandibular gland become more numerous with increasing age and that these could play a part in lithogenesis. Salivary calculi are unusual in children (Buchta 1980, Reuther and Hausamen 1976). Usually calculi affect only one gland, and they often recur. Simultaneous involvement of several glands is unusual (Perolta et al 1978). Men are affected twice as commonly as women (Rauch 1959).

Salivary calculi may be present for some time before they block the duct and cause symptoms. In such cases, recurrent swelling of the parenchyma may occur during periods of stimulation of secretion, usually during meal times. The swelling is often extremely painful, but the pain caused by a calculus in the duct system itself is less marked, so that the expression "salivary gland colic" is not entirely accurate. The enlarged gland is tender. If the calculus is not ejected spontaneously, secondary infection almost inevitably occurs in the favorable environment of stagnant secretions. The duct system dilates and the acinar cells atrophy, leading to a *chronic obstructive sialadenitis* (page 137).

The incidence of sialolithiasis varies in the different glands. The following figures were given by Rauch (1959), based on a literature review of 1200 cases:

- Submandibular gland, 83%
- Parotid gland, 10%
- Sublingual gland, 7%

Lithiasis of the minor salivary glands is probably more common than assumed by Rauch (1959). Jensen et al (1979) recorded 47 cases and gave references to other series. The glands of the upper lip and the buccal mucosa were most commonly affected. The symptoms of these salivary calculi are often trivial, so that small calculi may be overlooked.

Sialolithiasis of the Submandibular and Sublingual Glands

There are two reasons why the submandibular gland is much the most frequently affected by sialolithiasis. Firstly, the submandibular saliva is rich in mucus and is thus more viscous than the parotid saliva. Secondly, the submandibular duct ascends when the body is upright, it bends at the posterior edge of the floor of the mouth, and its course is sinuous. These facts all favor stasis of secretion, leading to calculus formation. The sites of predilection within the duct, according to Rauch (1959), are as follows:

- At the ostium, 30%
- In the middle third of the duct, 20%
- At the bend in the duct, 35%
- Peripheral to the bend, 15%.

Calculi peripheral to the bend and some of those in the region of the bend itself lie within the gland (Fig. 9.**1**). The ratio of extra- to intraglandular calculi is 7 : 3.

Rauch (1959) considered that the proportion of sublingual calculi (7%) in his review was artificial-

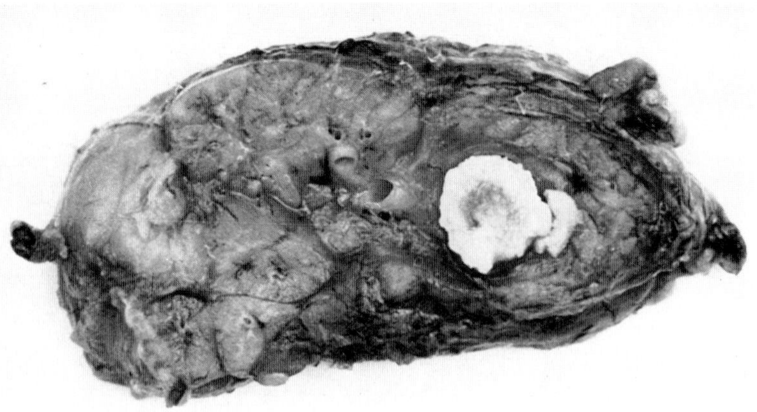

Figure 9.**1** Cut surface of a surgically removed submandibular gland showing an intraglandular salivary calculus of the size of a lentil in a dilated duct.

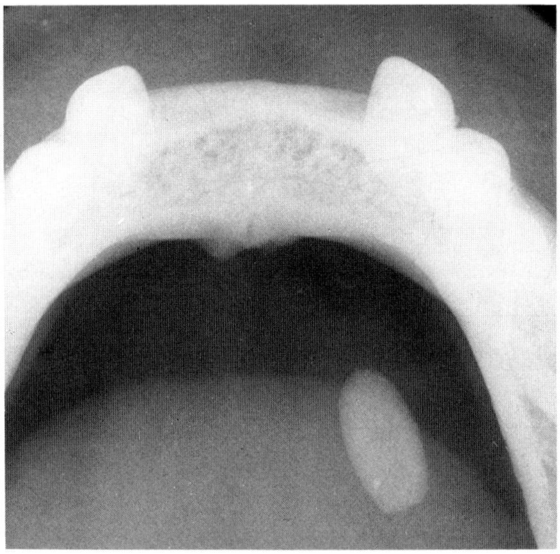

Figure 9.**2** Salivary calculus in the submandibular gland. Radiograph of the floor of the mouth.

ly high. In our experience sublingual calculi are about as frequent as those in the minor salivary glands. Sublingual calculi lie in the floor of the mouth and lead to swelling of the sublingual gland by obstruction of the duct, and this presents as a conspicuous swelling of the floor of the mouth. The swelling may be very painful, if it becomes secondarily infected, and an abscess of the floor of the mouth may develop. Since the sublingual gland has several ducts, some of which open into the submandibular duct, a sublingual calculus may obstruct the latter duct and imitate a submandibular calculus.

Calculi of the submandibular gland are diagnosed by clinical appearances and radiology. If the calculus lies close to the ostium or in the middle third of the duct, it can be palpated in the floor of the mouth. In these cases, radiology usually demonstrates the calculus clearly (Fig. 9.**2**). Radiology is more effective than palpation for calculi at the bend of the duct, whereas both methods are often of no value for intraglandular calculi. The clinical picture of sialolithiasis together with a fluctuating tender, firm swelling of the gland all suggest a salivary calculus. Sialography of the submandibular gland has not yet established itself in the diagnosis of calculi, since dilation of the duct often causes some difficulty.

Treatment

This is almost always surgical. Ejection of the calculus can only seldom be achieved by stimulation of secretion, for example, by sucking lemon slices or with ascorbic acid. This procedure is laborious and causes pain due to the retained secretions. If the calculus is palpable in the floor of the mouth, an attempt may be made to remove it by slitting the submandibular duct. This can usually be carried out under local anesthesia. The slit is made over the calculus, which often slides backward during this manipulation. A prior temporary transmucosal ligature of the duct behind the calculus should prevent this displacement. Finding smaller calculi may be facilitated by dilating the duct. After the calculus is removed, it is sufficient to adapt the mucosal edge. Splinting of the duct by plastic catheters is not necessary, since a fistula in the floor of the mouth causes no symptoms, and stenosis is never observed.

If the calculus lies in the bend of the duct or in the parenchyma of the gland itself, there is little point in making extensive attempts at removal through the mouth, which usually fails in any case. In these instances, it is preferable to remove the submandibular gland in the usual manner.

Division of the chorda tympani nerve has also been recommended for the treatment of sialolithiasis (Zahn & Cooney 1974). The secre-

Figure 9.**3** Salivary calculus in the parotid duct causing chronic recurrent parotitis: **a** Stone in the intraglandular segment of the parotid duct found during parotidectomy. **b** Extremely dilated duct after removal of the stone. **c** Stone after removal.

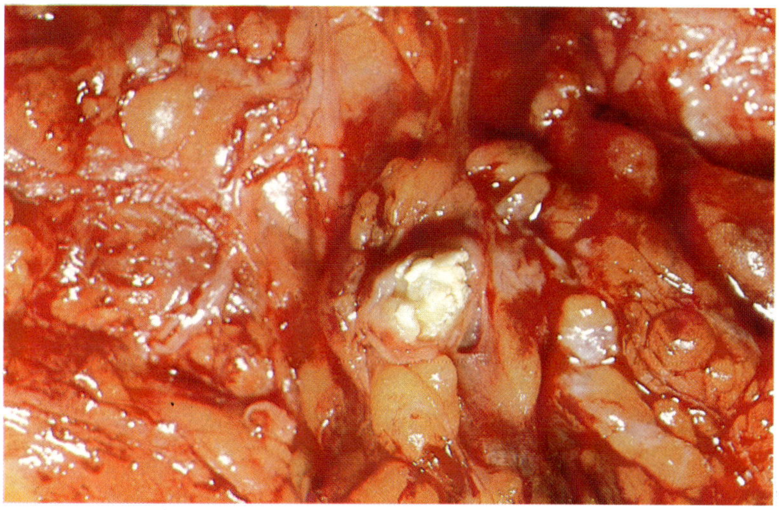

a

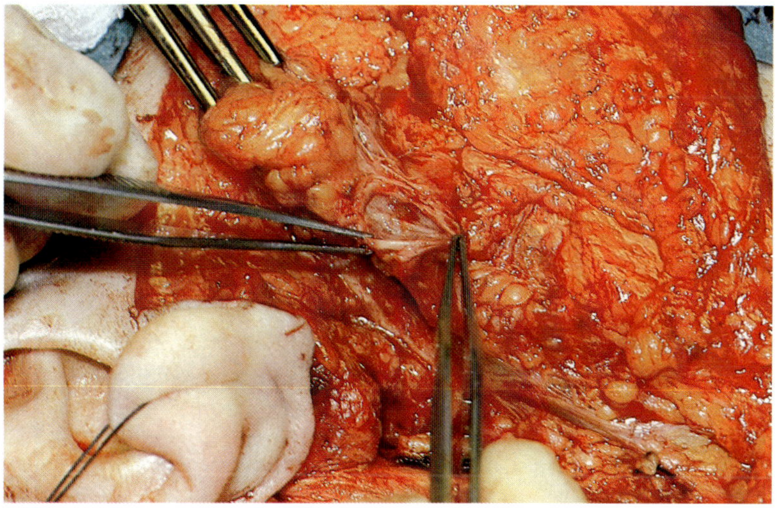

b

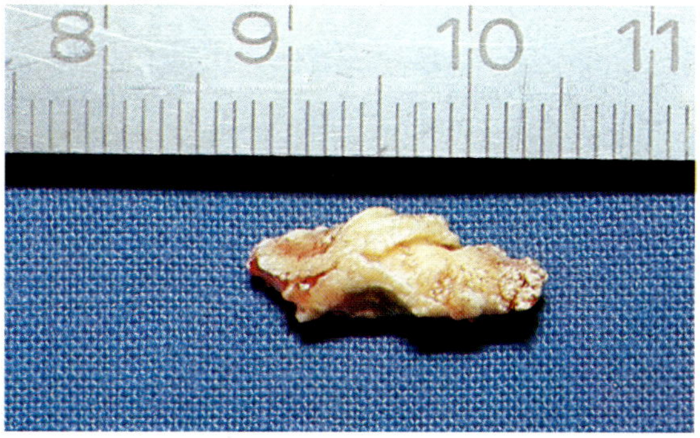

c

tion of the submandibular gland is permanently reduced to a minimum by this parasympathetic denervation (Chilla et al 1979 and 1982). Stagnation of secretion is then no longer possible, the symptoms due to the calculus regress and the gland atrophies. Other surgical methods are to be preferred, however, because division of the chorda tympani is always accompanied by partial loss of the sense of taste, and the calculus remains in the duct system as a possible cause of infection.

Sialolithiasis of the Parotid Gland

Calculi are seldom found in the parotid gland. Doubtless, this is due in part to diagnostic difficulties, especially of radiology. Calculi lying close to the ostium can be palpated and the others can only be demonstrated by radiology. According to Rauch (1959), most parotid calculi, like all other salivary calculi, lie almost exclusively within the duct. The ratio of intra- to extraglandular calculi is about 1 : 35. We regard this estimate as being too high, because intraglandular calculi are difficult to diagnose and are often only discovered accidently at parotidectomy carried out for chronic recurrent parotitis (Fig. 9.**3a–c**). Accord-

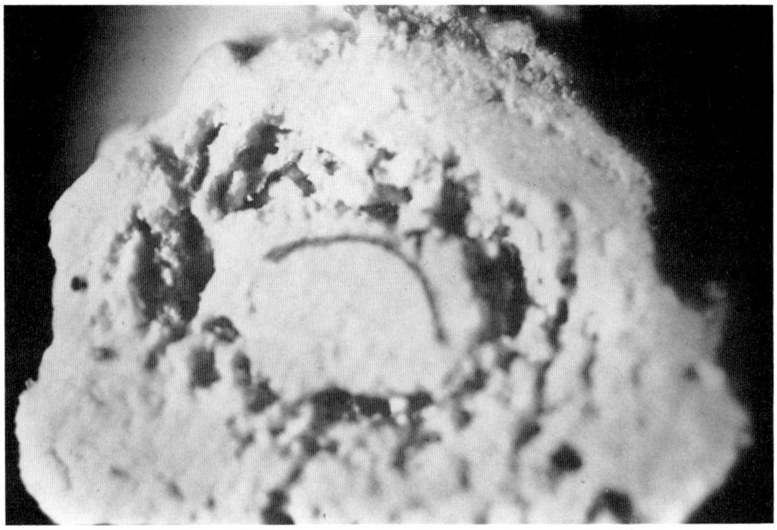

Figure 9.**4** Section through a lamellar submandibular stone.

ing to Suleiman et al (1979), sialolithiasis is the most common cause of unilateral recurrent parotid swelling. Of 109 patients with this symptom, a calculus could be clearly demonstrated in 36 and was the probable cause in another 59.

Parotid calculi are much less often palpable than submandibular calculi. *Radiology* is therefore much more important. A lateral plain view is usually valueless. If an anteroposterior view is combined with an intrabuccal technique using dental films, the success rate increases to 70% (Suleiman & Hobsley 1980). A calculus appears on sialography as a filling defect, although the latter is much more often caused by collections of mucus in the duct system.

The radiologic differential diagnosis of parotid stones includes phleboliths and calcification, which can occur in hemangiomas. Clinically, sialolithiasis of the parotid gland should be distinguished from chronic inflammation, particularly from chronic recurrent parotitis, which is not due to calculus formation.

Treatment

The treatment of parotid calculi may consist of encouragement of spontaneous discharge of small stones. The same methods to stimulate secretion are tried as for the submandibular duct. Successful extraction of palpable calculi may be achieved by an intraoral slit of the parotid duct by an incision around the papilla and then extended posteriorly along the duct. The duct should be splinted over a catheter to prevent stenosis. In other cases, a parotidectomy may be necessary.

Composition, Shape, and Structure of Salivary Calculi

Salivary calculi vary widely in their size and shape, from the size of a grain of semolina to a weight of several grams, for example, 42 g reported by Maskow (1976). According to Rauch (1959), the weight of most salivary calculi lies between 0.1 and 0.3 g. Most calculi are round or oval in shape (Fig. 9.**4**). The surface may be nodular and have angular or pointed projections. Small salivary calculi, especially those of the parotid gland, are more often fissured like coral and cause pain when they are being passed because of their edges, whereas large round calculi are more likely to cause pain by retention of secretions. The color of the calculi ranges from white or yellow to brown.

Salivary calculi consist of organic and inorganic material whose proportions to each other vary widely (Anneroth et al 1975a, 1975b).

The *organic constituents* have been less well investigated than the inorganic. They include precipitated mucus, that is, glycoproteins and mucopolysaccharides, and cell debris. It is not surprising that lipids have also been demonstrated (Anneroth et al 1977).

The *inorganic components* of salivary calculi (Table 9.**1**) consist mainly of calcium phosphate (calcium to phosphate in a ratio of about 2 : 1) (Skurk et al 1972) and calcium carbonate showing the apatite structure. More recent investigations using infrared spectroscopic comparisons between synthetic calcium components and salivary calculi (Skurk et al 1972) confirm the assumption of Blatt et al (1958) that carbonate apatite

Table 9.**1** Inorganic Components of a Submandibular Stone (Skurk et al) Expressed as Dry Weight, or Ash*

	Number	Mean	Range (mean ± 2 SD)
Ash (%)	26	67.0	44.4 –89.6
Ca (%)	20	23.4 33.0*	11.0 –35.8 24.3 –43.1*
Mg (%)	25	0.18 0.26*	0.06– 0.50 0.11– 0.63*
P (%)	22	13.1 17.9*	6.90–19.3 13.9 –21.9*
Mn (ppm)	20	7.2	1.6 –12.4
Fe (ppm)	26	40.0	16.9 –94.7
Cu (ppm)	26	24.1	8.5 –68.3
Zu (ppm)	25	28.8	2.8 –29.8

$[Ca_{10}(PO_4)_6(CO_3)]$ is present and not hydroxylapatite $[Ca_{10}(PO_4)_6(OH)_2]$ (Berthold et al 1970, Harrill et al 1959). Tricalciumphosphate $(Ca_3(PO_4)_2)$ is less common; calcium oxylate dihydrate $(CaC_2O_4 \cdot 2H_2O)$ and dibasic calcium phosphate dihydrate $(CaHPO_4 \cdot 2H_2O)$ may also occassionally be demonstrated (Sakae et al 1981, Yamamoto et al 1983, 1984). This is probably not an artificial complex, as is often assumed (Anneroth et al 1975b). In addition, several trace elements, such as magnesium, iron, copper, zinc, and manganese, may be demonstrated by atomic absorption spectroscopy (Skurk et al 1973). Their content never exceeds 0.5% of the inorganic substances (Skurk et al 1973).

The content of organic and inorganic constituents varies within a calculus. Alternating organic and inorganic layers arranged in lamellae around a well-mineralized spherical nucleus is typical (Fig. 9.**4**). The external covering consists mainly of organic material (Blatt 1964, Taniguchi et al 1979). The structure of a salivary calculus resembles that of the urinary tract rather than a gallstone (Taniguchi et al 1979). However, organic substances such as lipids (Anneroth et al 1977) may be demonstrated in the heavily mineralized zone of salivary calculi (Anneroth et al 1977). Not all salivary calculi have this lamellar construction. Sometimes a typical nucleus is absent, and in other calculi the surface is not homogeneous (Anneroth et al 1975a).

Other aspects of the construction of salivary calculi have been provided by enzyme histochemical studies (Isacsson & Hammarström 1983). A zone of organic material can be demonstrated on the surface of the calculus. This zone includes collagenous fibers and metaplastic squamous epithelium and possesses intense acid phosphatase and lactate dehydrogenase activity. Bordering this is a structureless intermediate zone around the mineralized center of the calculus, with moderate acid phosphatase and succinate dehydrogenase activity, and at some points also alkaline phosphatase and lactate dehydrogenase. The investigators conclude that the calcification process is not passive but is carried out actively by enzymes.

Pathogenesis of Sialolithiasis

It is not yet certain whether a salivary calculus develops from an organic or an inorganic precipitate. In 1959, Rauch thought that it was primarily the minerals that were precipitated and that the organic substances were then laid down around them. Previously, the opinion had been that the opposite was true, and today this is again the general opinion, based on more recent information. According to Harrill et al (1959), the first step is formation of a gel of organic substances in the saliva. Inorganic material is then laid down in the network of the gel. Scott (1978) demonstrated microdeposits of organic material in 48 healthy submandibular glands. These probably consisted of glycoproteins, and their structure resembled the organic part of macroscopic salivary calculi and represented an early stage of lithogenesis. Jensen et al (1979) reported similar findings after investigation of 47 salivary calculi arising in the minor glands. Of these, 11 were heavily mineralized, 23 partially, and 13 not at all. The latter consisted of an organic matrix only, which was identical in both heavily or lightly mineralized stones.

Mineralization of the organic matrix is encouraged by the following factors (Leung & Draus 1962):

- Increasing pH, which favor the precipitation of calcium phosphate compounds in saliva.
- As the mucin concentration in saliva increases, its binding capacity for calcium increases, since calcium in the saliva is partially bound to salivary protein and is thus held in solution. This calcium may be involved in the mineralization of the organic matrix.
- A change in the ionic milieu of the saliva, as has been described in electrolyte sialadenitis (page 137) by Seifert (1964) and Seifert & Donath (1976).

All these factors are also adduced to support the argument of the primary inorganic genesis of salivary stones. A decisive factor is probably the fact that the solubility product of the different calcium phosphate compounds is exceeded, especially in the submandibular gland saliva. This supersaturated solution only remains stable because of the formation of complex pyro- and polyphosphates (McCann 1968) and because a series of calcium reactive proteins is present in saliva (Arglebe 1981). These have a high affinity for calcium and can prevent the precipitation of calcium phosphate in saliva. These proteins include glycoprotein and statherine, a tyrosine-rich protein. This system, which holds the calcium phosphate compounds in saliva in solution, is very sensitive. An increasing pH of the saliva, usually due to a decrease of the bicarbonate concentration, leads to precipitation of calcium salts. As described previously, these are then laid down in a matrix that is already present, consisting of cell debris (Fichelson et al 1959). Alternatively, calcium phosphate crystals (for example apatite compounds) may be surrounded by organic material (Blatt 1964). Further disturbance is possible due to local inflammation, for example. Foreign bodies are also said to act as a nucleus for crystallization, and other mechanical causes include stagnation of secretion and the accompanying formation of sediment (Rauch 1959). Under experimental conditions, calcium phosphate aggregates in the acinar lumen may act as pathogenic factors for later calculus formation due to stimulation of secretion and simultaneous hypercalcemia (Westhofen et al 1984). Finally, there are local causes that have a decisive role in lithogenesis, since it is virtually always only one gland that is subject to sialolithiasis.

The question of whether it is the organic matrix that comes first or the apatite crystals that forms the nucleus of a salivary stone is probably not very important. A large part of the salivary calcium is bound to protein (see Chapter 4), so that the precipitation of a calcium protein complex could indicate that both proteins and minerals were involved in lithogenesis from the start.

References

Anneroth, G., C.-M. Eneroth, G. Isacsson: Morphology of salivary calculi. The distribution of the inorganic component. J. oral Pathol. 4 (1975a) 257

Anneroth, G., C.-M. Eneroth, G. Isacsson: Crystalline structure of salivary calculi. A microradiographic and microdiffractometric study. J. oral Pathol. 4 (1975b) 266

Anneroth, G., C.-M. Eneroth, G. Isacsson: The relation of lipids to the mineral components in salivary calculi. J. oral Pathol. 6 (1977) 373

Arglebe, C.: Biochemistry of human saliva. In Pfaltz, C. R., R. Chilla: Sialadenosis and Sialadenitis. Karger, Basel 1981

Berthold, H., H.-J. Schneider, J. Tscharnke: Struktur und chemischer Aufbau der Speichelsteine. Dtsch. zahnärztl. Z. 25 (1970) 743

Blatt, I. M.: Studies in sialolithiasis. Pathogenesis, diagnosis and treatment. South. Med. J. 57 (1964) 723

Blatt, I. M., R. M. Denning, J. H. Zumberge, J. H. Maxwell: Studies in sialolithiasis. 1. The structure and mineralogical composition of salivary gland calculi. Ann. Otol. 67 (1958) 595

Buchta, R. M.: Submandibular salivary gland calculus. Clin. pediat. 19 (1980) 562

Chilla, R., M. Brüner, C. Arglebe: Function of submaxillary gland following iatrogenic damage to chorda tympani nerve. Acta Otolaryngol. 87 (1979) 152

Chilla, R., J. Nicklatsch, C. Arglebe: Late sequelae of iatrogenic damage to chorda tympani nerve. Acta Otolaryngol. 94 (1982) 461

Fichelson, S., C. P. Tran, T. Frédière, P. Laudenbach: Etude radiocristallographique de 46 calculs salivaires. Hypothèses physiopathogéniques. Rev. Stomat. 79 (1978) 75

Harrill, J. A., J. S. King, W. H. Boyce: Structure and composition of salivary calculi. Laryngoscope 69 (1959) 481

Isacsson, G., L. Hammarström: En enzyme histochemical study of human salivary duct calculi. J. oral Pathol. 12 (1983) 217

Jensen, J. L., F. V. Howell, G. M. Rick, R. W. Correll: Minor salivary gland calculi. A clinicopathologic study of forty-seven new cases. Oral Surg. 47 (1979) 44

Leung, S. W., F. J. Draus: The calcium binding characteristics of a salivary gland mucoid. Arch. oral Biol. 7 (1962) 327

Maskow, H.: Ungewöhnlicher Sialolith der Glandula submandibularis. Z. Laryng. Rhinol. 55 (1976) 237

McCann, H. G.: Inorganic components of salivary secretions. In: Art and Science of Dental Caries Research. Academic Press, New York 1968

Perotta, R. J., J. R. Williams, R. W. Selfe: Simultaneous bilateral parotid and submandibular gland calculi. Arch. Otolaryng. 104 (1978) 469

Rauch, S.: Die Speicheldrüsen des Menschen. Thieme, Stuttgart 1959

Reuther, J., J. E. Hausamen: Sialolithiasis der Gl. submandibularis im Kindesalter. Klin. Pädiat. 188 (1976) 285

Sakae, T., H. Yamamoto, G. Hirai: Mode of occurrence of brushite and whitlockite in a sialolith. J. dent. Res. 60 (1981) 842

Scott, J.: The prevalence of consolidated salivary deposits in the small ducts of human submandibular glands. J. oral Pathol. 7 (1978) 28

Seifert, G.: Die Sekretionsstörungen (Dyschylien) der Speicheldrüsen. Ergeb. allg. Path. path. Anat. 44 (1964) 103

Seifert, G., K. Donath: Die Morphologie der Speicheldrüsenerkrankungen. Arch. Oto-Rhino-Laryng. 213 (1976) 111

Skurk, A., A. Hesse, A. Schmidt, K. Fendel: Infrarotspektroskopische Untersuchungen von Speichelsteinen. Z. Laryng. Rhinol. 51 (1972) 446

Skurk, A., K. Winnefeld, J.-J. Tiedt, A. Schmidt. K. Fendel: Spurenelemente in Speichelsteinen. Die Bestimmung von Ca, Mg, Cu, Zn, Mn und P. Z. Laryng. Rhinol. 52 (1973) 822

Suleiman, S. I., M. Hobsley: Radiological appearances of parotid duct calculi. Brit. J. Surg. 67 (1980) 879

Suleiman, S. I., J. P. S. Thomson, M. Hobsley: Recurrent unilateral swelling of the parotid gland. Gut 2 (1979) 1102

Taniguchi, T., S. Yamamoto, S. Yamada, M. Ohyama: Scanning electron microscopic X-ray microanalytical studies of salivary calculi. Otol. Fukuoka 25, Suppl. 5 (1979) 757

Westhofen, M., H. Schäfer, G. Seifert: Calcium redistribution, calcification and stone formation in the parotid gland during experimental stimulation and hypercalcaemia. Cytochemical and X-ray microanalytical investigations. Virchows Arch. (Path. Anat.) 402 (1984) 425

Yamamoto, H., T. Sakae, M. Takagi, S. Otake, G. Hirai: Wedellite in submandibular gland calculus. J. dent. Res. 62 (1983) 16

Yamamoto, H., T. Sakae, M. Takagi, S. Otake: Scanning electron microscopic and X-ray microdiffractometric studies on sialolith-crystals in human submandibular glands. Acta Path. Jpn. 34 (1984) 47

Zahn, H., T. C. Cooney: Chorda tympani neurectomy – a new approach to submandibular salivary obstruction. Brit. J. Surg. 61 (1974) 391

10. Salivary Gland Cysts

Definition and Classification

Cysts of the salivary glands are non-neoplastic, localized lesions of the duct system. Three types may be distinguished:

- Dysgenetic cysts (see Chapter 6)
- Secondary acquired cysts lined by epithelium (duct cysts, lymphoepithelial cysts, and retention mucoceles).
- Pseudocysts without an epithelial lining (extravasation mucocele).

The non-neoplastic cysts and pseudocysts form about 6% of lesions of the salivary glands (Table 10.**1**). Seventy-five percent of these are constituted by mucoceles of the minor salivary glands, followed in decreasing order of frequency by parotid duct cysts (about 10%), lymphoepithelial cysts (about 6%), and ranula (about 5%). Congenital sialectasia and dysgenetic cystic parotid are very rare.

The non-neoplastic cysts must be distinguished from cystic changes in the ducts occurring in certain forms of chronic sialadenitis, such as chronic sialectatic parotitis and chronic myoepithelial parotitis in Sjögren's syndrome, and from cystic tumors (cystadenolymphoma, cystic mucoepidermoid tumor, cystic duct adenoma, cystic adenocarcinoma, and cystic pleomorphic adenoma).

Mucoceles

Mucoceles are spherical, nontender, circumscribed mucosal swellings of varying size that contain mucus. Two forms may be distinguished: extravasation and retention.

Extravasation Mucoceles

More than 80% of mucoceles are of this type; an alternative term is mucous granuloma (Hamperl 1932, Seifert 1964, Seifert et al 1980, 1981). The macroscopic appearances are those of a spherical cyst with a diameter of 1–1.5 cm, which bulges the surface and which is mobile over the surrounding tissue. Almost 80% lie in the lower lip, another 15% in the cheek or the floor of the mouth, and the remaining 5% in the palate, tongue, and upper lip. The peak incidence is in the second decade. Extravasation mucoceles become increasingly uncommon after the age of 50 years; 60% arise in men.

Histology demonstrates three phases of development of an extravasation mucocele. In the *initial*

Table 10.**1** Classification of Salivary Gland Cysts in the Salivary Gland Register of the Pathological Institute of the University of Hamburg. This Register Contains 7336 Specimens of Salivary Lesions

Cyst Type	Main Site	Number	Per cent
Mucoceles	Minor salivary glands	371	77
Extravasation mucoceles	Lower lip	312	65
Retention mucoceles	Lip, cheek, palate, floor of mouth	59	12
Duct cyst	Parotid	51	10.5
Lymphoepithelial cyst	Parotid, floor of mouth	29	6
Ranula	Sublinguinal	25	5
Congenital sialectasis	Parotid	5	1
Dysgenetic cystic parotid	Parotid	2	0.5
Total		483	

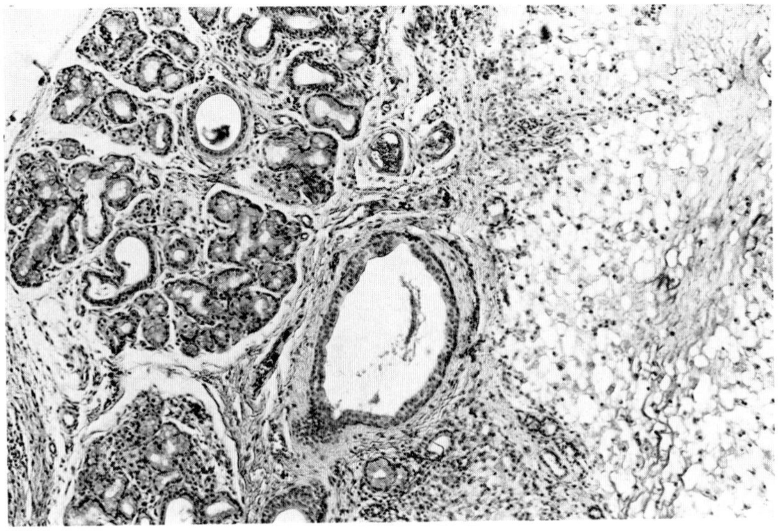

Figure 10.**1** Extravasation mucocele of the lower lip showing the early phase with periductal extravasation of mucus (right), dilated duct and intact glandular tissue (left). Astra blue, 63×.

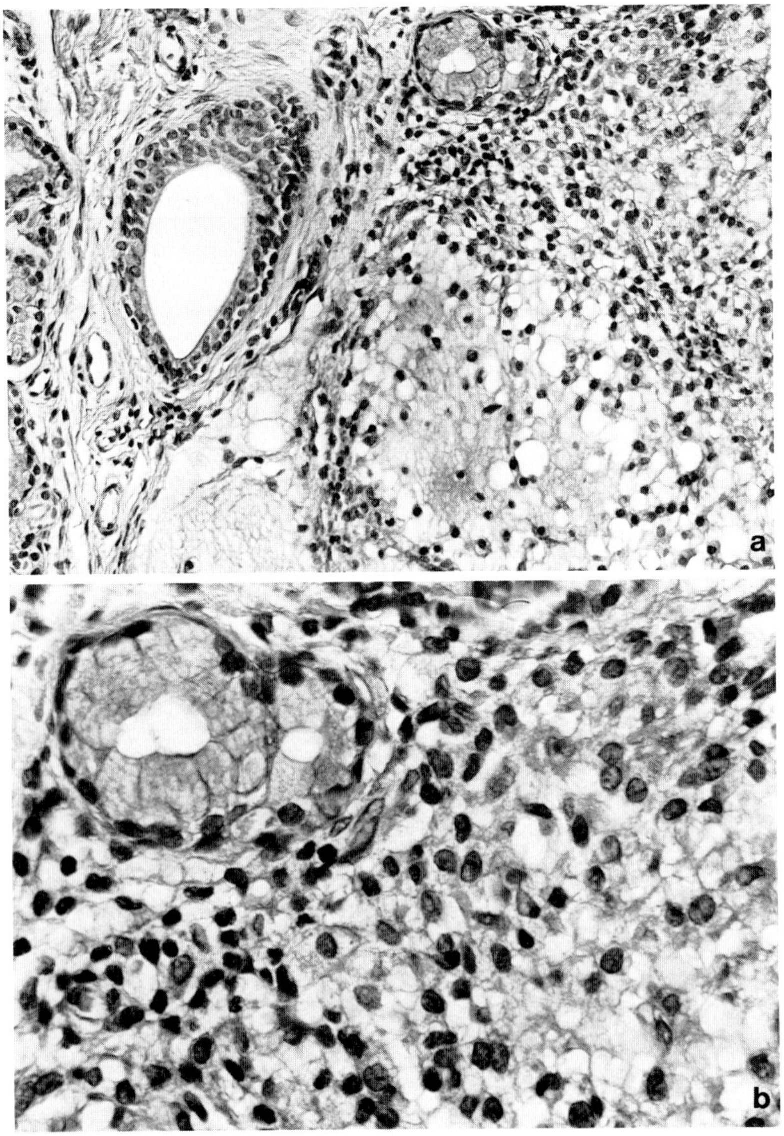

Figure 10.**2** Extravasation mucocele of the lower lip showing periductal and mucous masses with infiltration by histiocytes, foam cells, and occasional leukocytes. Astra blue. **a** 160×, **b** 400×.

Figure 10.**3** Resorption phase in an extravasation mucocele showing infiltration by macrophages and multinucleated foreign body giant cells. **a** Astra blue, 160×, **b** PAS, 400×.

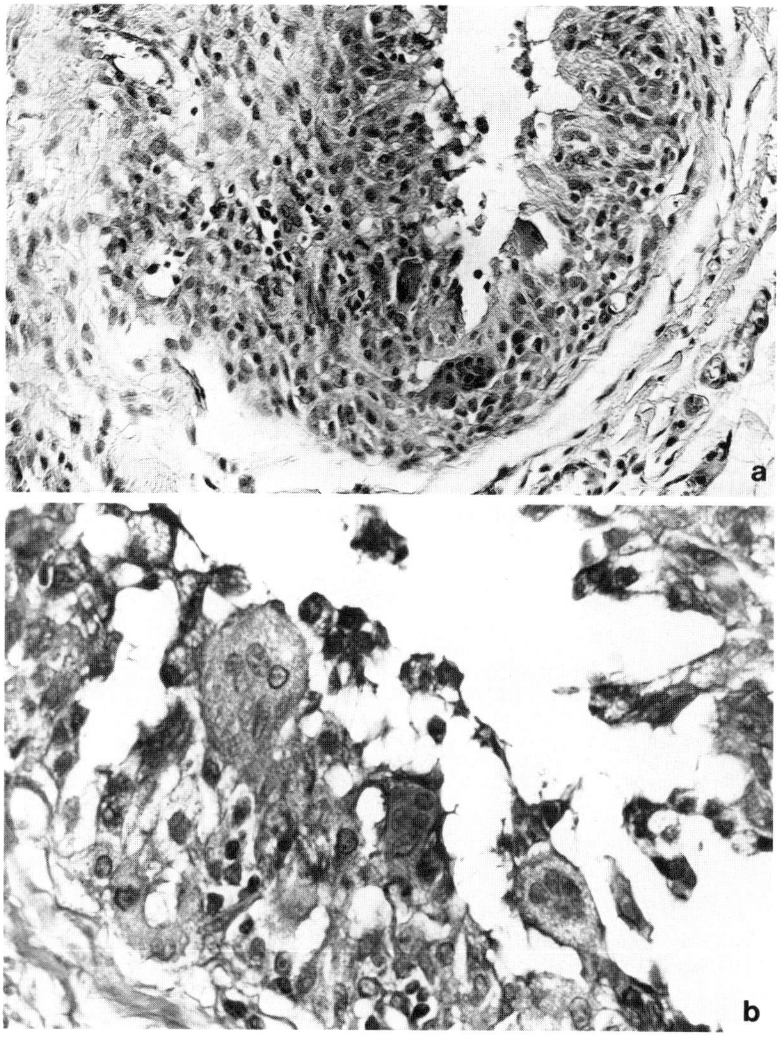

stage (Figs. 10.**1**, 10.**2a, b**), mucus penetrates the interstitium from the duct system and parenchyma. The deposits of mucus are initially not well circumscribed and contain neutral and acid mucopolysaccharides. A few leukocytes and histiocytes lie around the extravasated material. A mucous granuloma develops in the *resorption phase* (Fig. 10.**3a, b**). This contains histiocytes, macrophages, and foam cells in whose cytoplasm resorbed masses of mucus can be demonstrated. In addition, multinucleated foreign body giant cells with intracytoplasmic mucus particles may be demonstrated. Electron microscopy shows that the macrophages and giant cells contain mucous vacuoles and occasionally crystalline secretion products. In the *end phase* (Figs. 10.**4a, b,** 10.**5**) a mucus-filled pseudocyst develops from the mucous granuloma. A connective tissue capsule with an endothelioid lining develops around the mucous mass, which does not itself have an epithelial covering.

Extravasation mucoceles may be produced *experimentally* by ligation or division of the duct (Harrison & Garrett 1972, 1975, Bhaskar et al 1976).

Two factors are important in **pathogenesis:** the amount of extravasated mucus combined with the intensity of the secretory stimulus, and the speed with which the mucus is phagocytosed by the granulation tissue.

The preferred site is the lower lip in young people: this indicates that *recurrent microtrauma* due to biting plays an important role in the causation of extravasation mucoceles. This is also true of mucous granulomas that develop in the region of a denture.

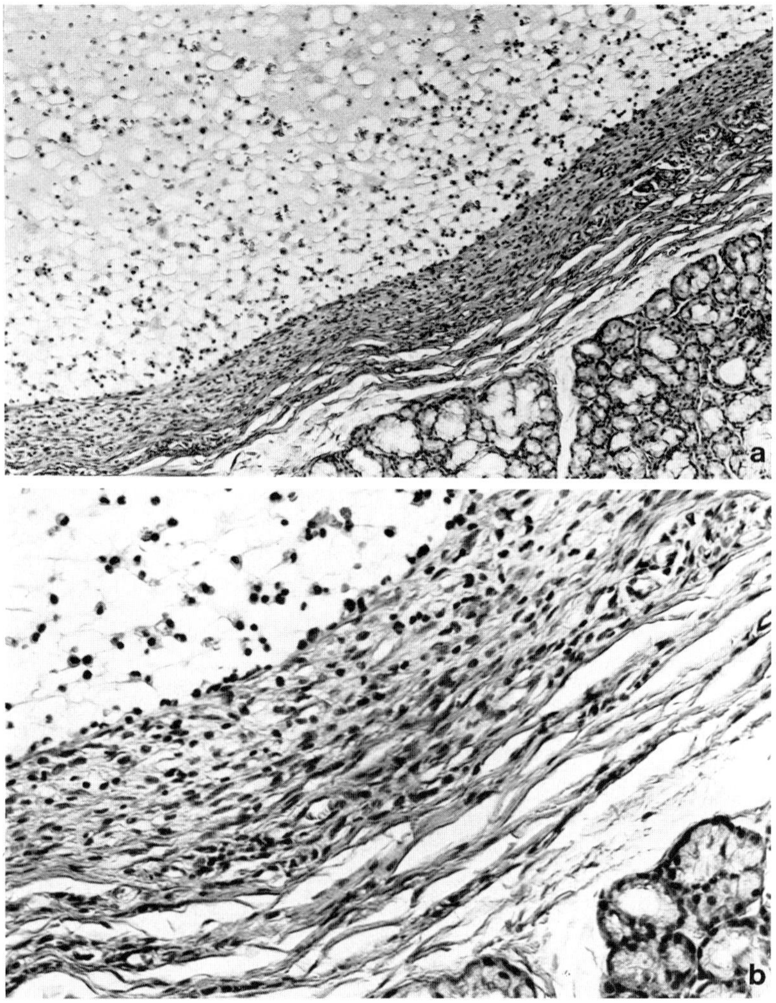

Figure 10.**4** End phase of an extravasation mucocele showing a mass of mucus bordered by a pseudocyst with no epithelial lining. Mucous acini retained outside the pseudocyst. H & E. **a** 63×, **b** 160×.

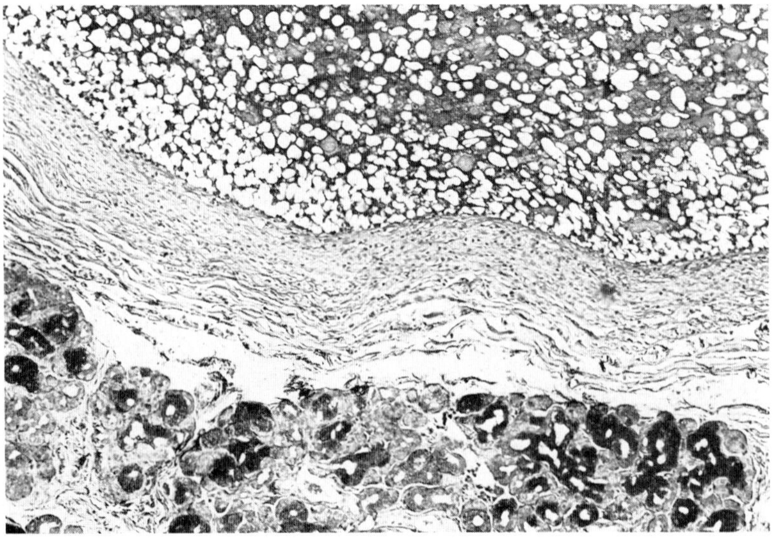

Figure 10.**5** Extravasation mucocele showing mucous-filled pseudocyst with connective tissue wall and intact gland lobules in the surrounding tissue. PAS, 63×.

Retention Mucocele (Mucous Retention Cyst)

These are considerably less common than extravasation mucoceles, but are more common in the older age groups, with a peak incidence in the eighth decade. They are distributed evenly among the minor glands (20% each in the lower lip and cheek, 15% each in the upper lip, palate, floor of the mouth, and tongue).

The **histologic characteristics** of a retention mucocele are a triad of an epithelial lining, a retained mucous mass, and a connective tissue capsule (Fig. 10.**6**). The structure of the epithelium of the cyst wall resembles the various segments of the duct system. The various types that can be distinguished include flat, cuboidal epithelium resembling that of the intercalated duct, an oncocyte cyst wall resembling that of the striated duct, and epithelial units arranged in multiple rows similar to the excretory ducts of the interlobular type (Figs. 10.**7**–10.**9**). Occasionally, squamous metaplasia or papillary prominences may be seen that resemble the structure of a monomorphic cystadenoma. The mucous secretion is finely flocculated and may also contain spheroliths or microliths that fill the lumen of the cyst. The wall of the mucous retention cyst shows little evidence of the inflammation that is characteristic of an extravasation mucocele. In rare cases, mucus may be extravasated due to tearing of a retention cyst to produce a mixed form.

Partial obstruction of the duct due to microliths, inspissated secretion, or bends in the duct system plays the main role in the **pathogenesis** of retention mucoceles (Harrison 1975). Furthermore, it has been suggested that this lesion may be an early manifestation of a monomorphic cystadenoma (Southam 1974). This hypothesis is supported by the fact that the age and sex distribution of retention mucoceles is similar to that of duct adenomas (Seifert & Schulz 1979). Furthermore, areas with oncocytic-cystic differentiation often occur in this tumor.

Salivary Duct Cysts

Duct cysts occur mainly in the parotid gland and constitute about 10% of all non-neoplastic cysts of the salivary glands (Seifert & Waller 1982, Pieterse & Seymour 1981, Richardson et al 1978, Shaheen et al 1975). The peak age incidence is in the seventh decade and 77% occur in men. The cyst is usually unilocular and varies in size from a lentil to the size of a plum, with an average diameter of 2–3 cm.

The **histologic appearances** of the duct cyst resemble those of the retention mucocele of the minor salivary glands: the lesion is lined by a duct epithelium of varying differentiation and contains mucous secretion. The duct epithelium may be flat, but it may also be arranged in several rows or may be differentiated into oncocytes (Fig. 10.**10a, b**). Squamous metaplasia occurs occasionally. Secretory deposits (Fig. 10.**11**) of spheroliths and crystalline particles can develop within the mass of mucus (Takeda & Ishikawa 1983). The cyst wall contains loose connective tissue without a pronounced inflammatory reaction. Small local mucus granulomas may form due to extravasation of mucus from the cyst into the interstitium. Secretions are retained in the neighboring gland tissue due to increasing size of the cyst: in the

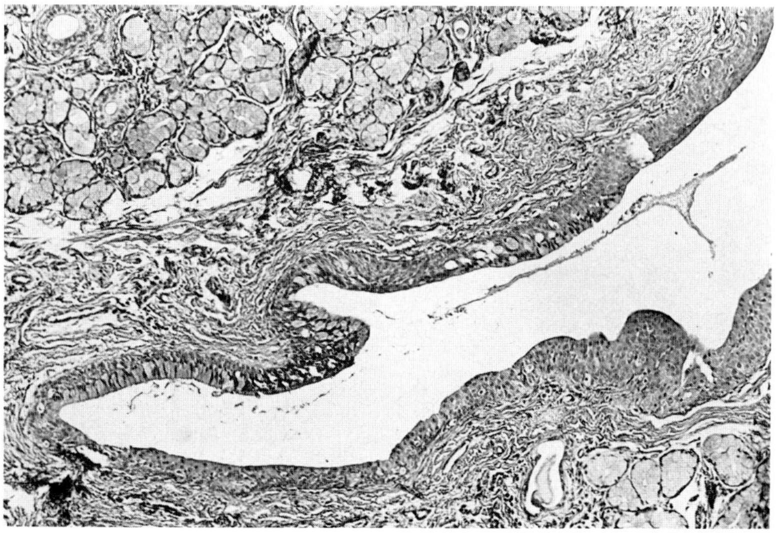

Figure 10.**6** Retention mucocele of the glands of the cheek. The mucous cyst is lined by multilayered duct epithelium, showing squamous metaplasia on the right. Astra blue, 60×.

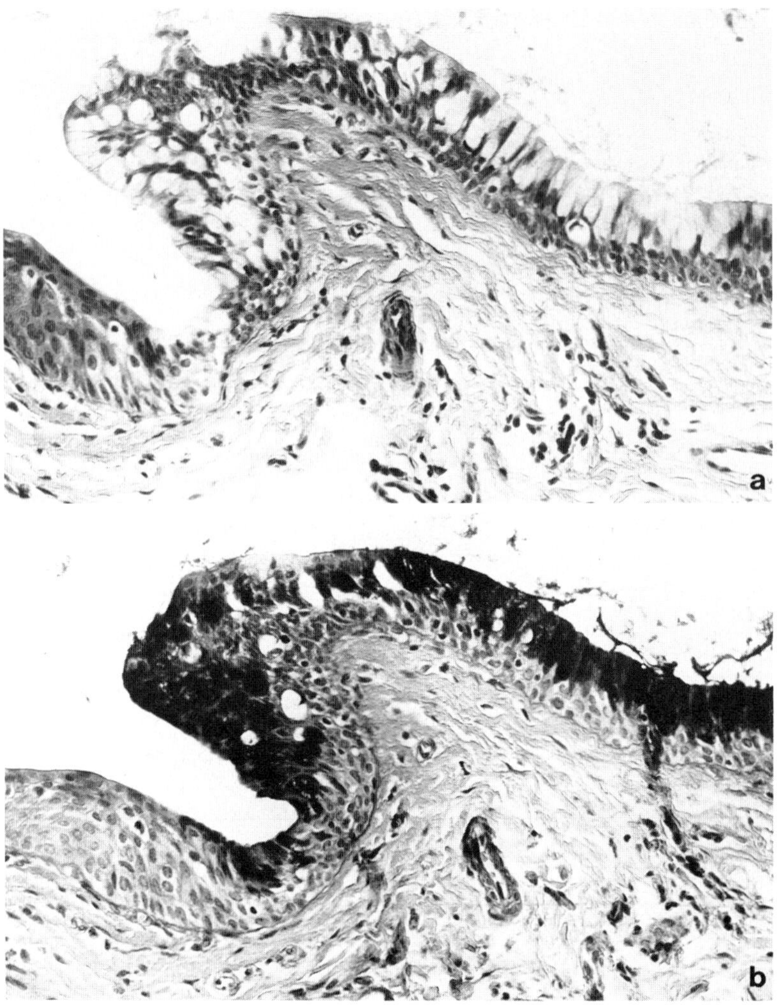

Figure 10.**7** Retention mucocele showing multilayered duct epithelium with mucous secretion and squamous metaplasia. The cyst wall is on the left side. **a** H & E, 160×, **b** PAS, 160×.

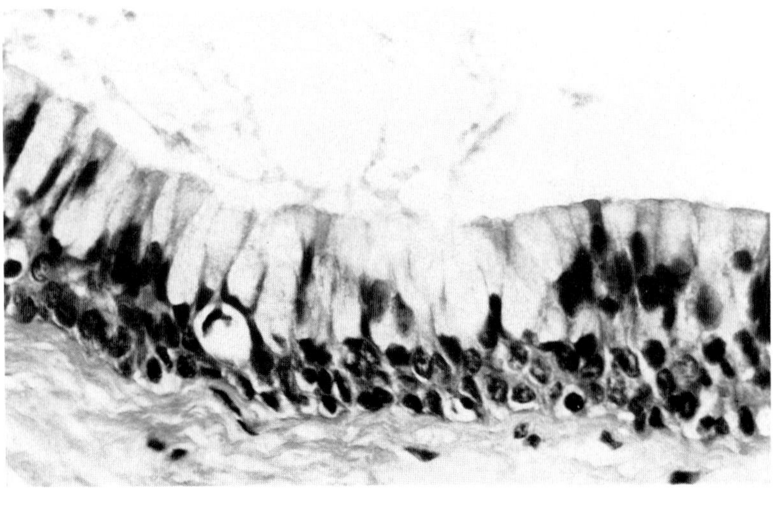

Figure 10.**8** Retention mucocele: multilayered columnar epithelium with formation of mucus in the luminal layers and basal dark reserve cells. H & E, 400×.

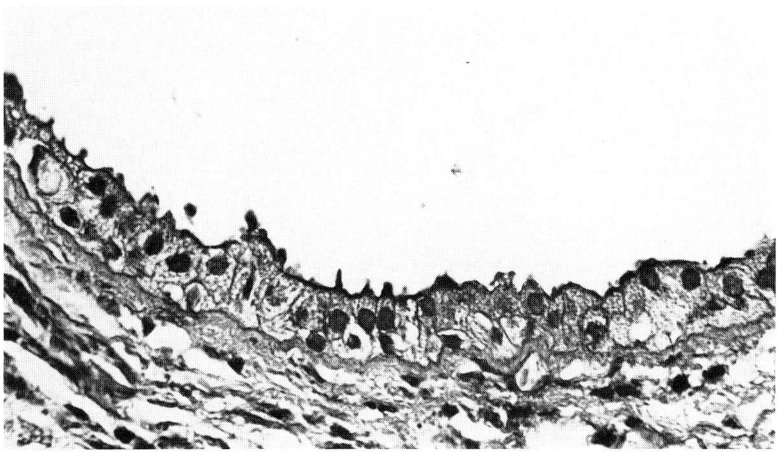

Figure 10.**9** Retention mucocele lined by a flat multilayered duct epithelium. PAS, 400×.

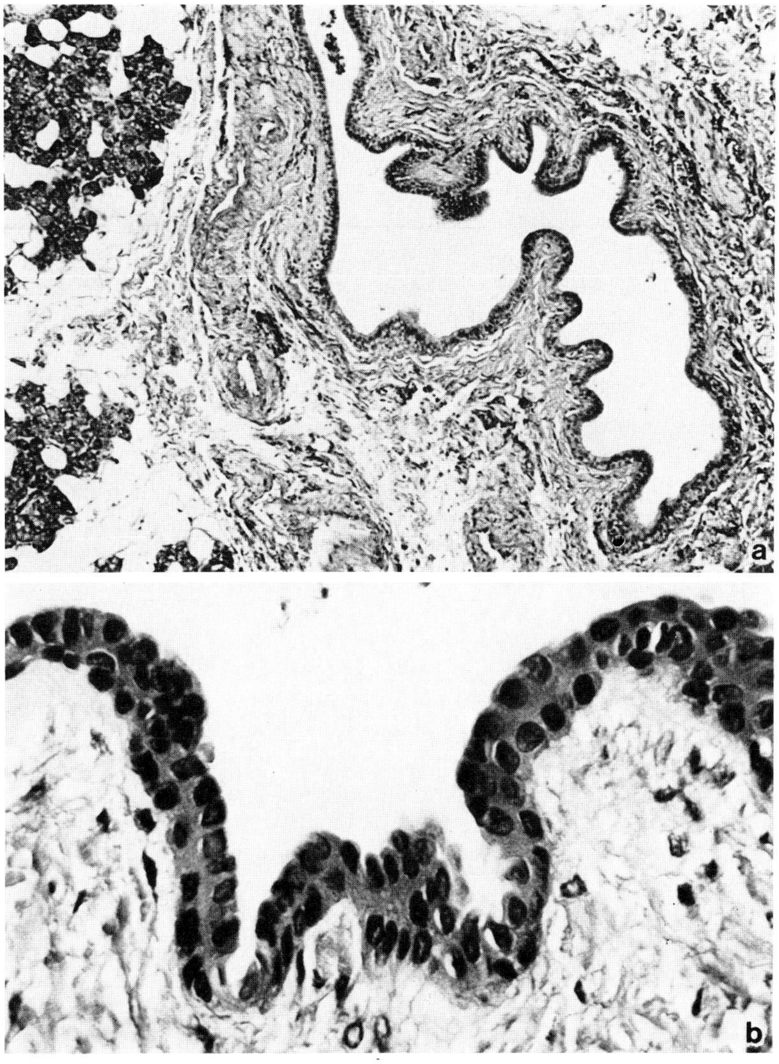

Figure 10.**10** Duct cyst of the parotid gland: **a** Complete epithelial lining of the cyst lumen, bounded by gland tissue (left) and by loose connective tissue. H & E, 45×. **b** Section of the cyst wall showing double-layered duct epithelium. H & E, 280×.

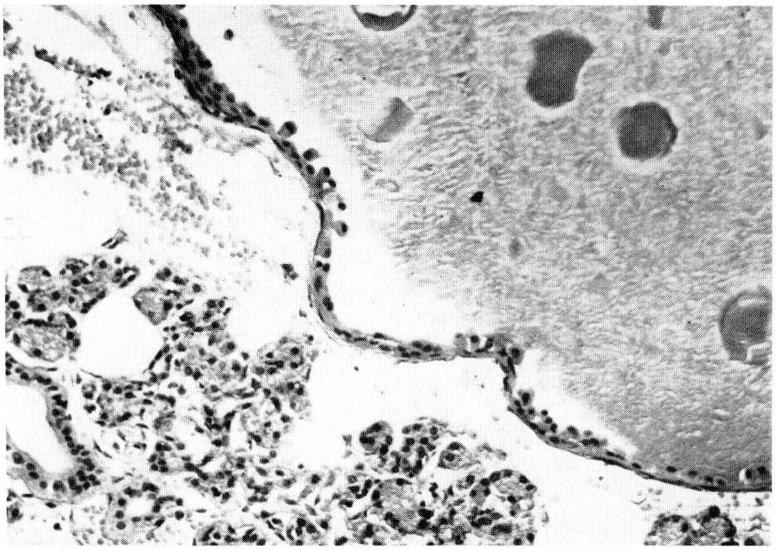

Figure 10.**11** Parotid duct cyst: clumped precipitates of secretion and flattening of the cyst epithelium. H & E, 160×. (Seifert & Waller 1982.)

course of time, this leads to a focal obstructive parotitis in 80% of patients.

The **pathogenesis** of the duct cyst may be compared closely with that of the mucous retention cyst. The predilection for the older age groups is evidence against a dysgenetic cause and indicates rather that cystic dilation of the ducts occurs due to local retention of secretions or bends in the duct system. The dilation increases in size in the course of time.

Lymphoepithelial Cysts

Lymphoepithelial cysts occur mainly in the parotid gland, but also in the floor of the mouth. The size of the average cyst is 1 cm, which is less than that of a duct cyst. One third of the cases are multilocular in structure (Seifert & Waller 1982).

Histology. The histologic examination shows the cyst to be bounded by a flattened multilayered epithelium that is always surrounded by a lymphoid stroma with lymphoid follicles (Fig. 10.**12**). Occasional goblet cells and sebaceous glands may also be found within the multilayered epithelium. Sometimes, the cyst is bounded externally by a multilayered squamous epithelium with clear keratinization on the surface (Fig. 10.**13a, b**). The cyst contains a serous fluid with inclusions of desquamated epithelium, lymphocytes, and foam cells. However, mucous secretion is not present, as it is in the duct cyst. The lymphoid stroma may demonstrate atrophic changes with hyalinization.

The cellular composition of lymphocytes, plasma cells and histiocytes resembles that of a lymph node. Granulomas with multinucleated foreign body giant cells are sometimes found lying close to squamous epithelial units with keratinization. Very occasionally, cholesterol granulomas may be found. A focal obstructive parotitis may be found in the periphery of a lymphoepithelial cyst, but less often and of lesser intensity than in duct cysts.

Pathogenesis. The descriptive term "lymphoepithelial cyst" coined by Bernier and Bhaskar (1958) refers to the cystic lymphoepithelial structure, but leaves the question of histogenesis open (Bhaskar 1966). Chronic inflammation leading to a local epithelial proliferation in the surrounding lymphoid stroma has been suggested as a cause for the cysts in the oral cavity. Lymph follicles with parenchymatous inclusions are relatively frequent in the parotid gland, and these are probably the basis for the development of lymphoepithelial cysts (Fujibayashi & Itoh 1981).

The synonymous term *brachiogenic parotid cyst* (Bhaskar & Bernier 1958), should only be used if the cyst clearly lies in the lateral part of the neck in the branchial region (Ungerecht 1981). This point is also made by Stoll (1980), who distinguishes the branchial fistula (a branchial arch derivative) from the branchial cyst, which is a lymph node with a parenchymatous inclusion. The epithelial proliferation in the initial phase is the result of an inflammatory process. In the later phase, the growth of the cyst is encouraged by breakdown and metabolic products in the cyst lumen. The lymphoepithelial cysts belong to the group of lymphoepithelial salivary gland lesions (Seifert 1980), including the benign lymphoepithelial lesion, chronic myoepithelial

Figure 10.**12** Lymphoepithelial cyst of the parotid showing the cyst bounded by multilayered flat epithelium and lymphoid stroma with lymphoid follicles (left) and parotid tissue (right). H & E, 63×.

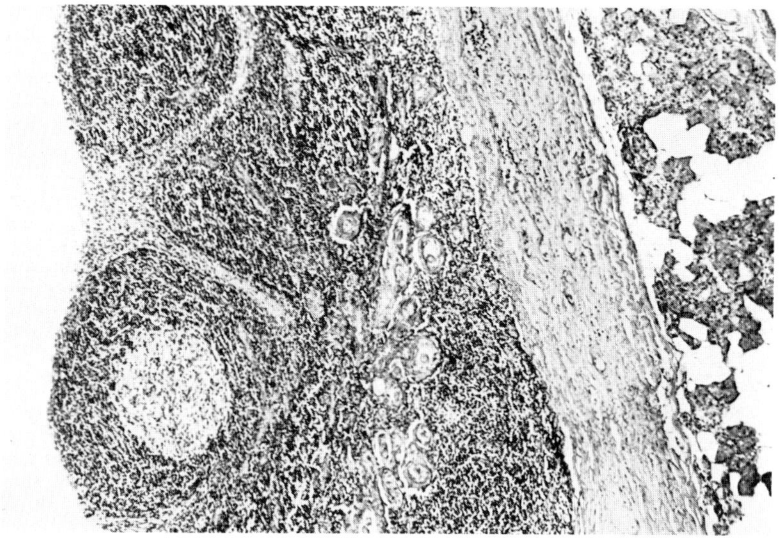

Figure 10.**13** Lymphoepithelial cyst of the parotid: **a** Border of multilayered squamous epithelium and lymphoid stroma. **b** Lining of keratinized squamous epithelium. H & E, 160×.

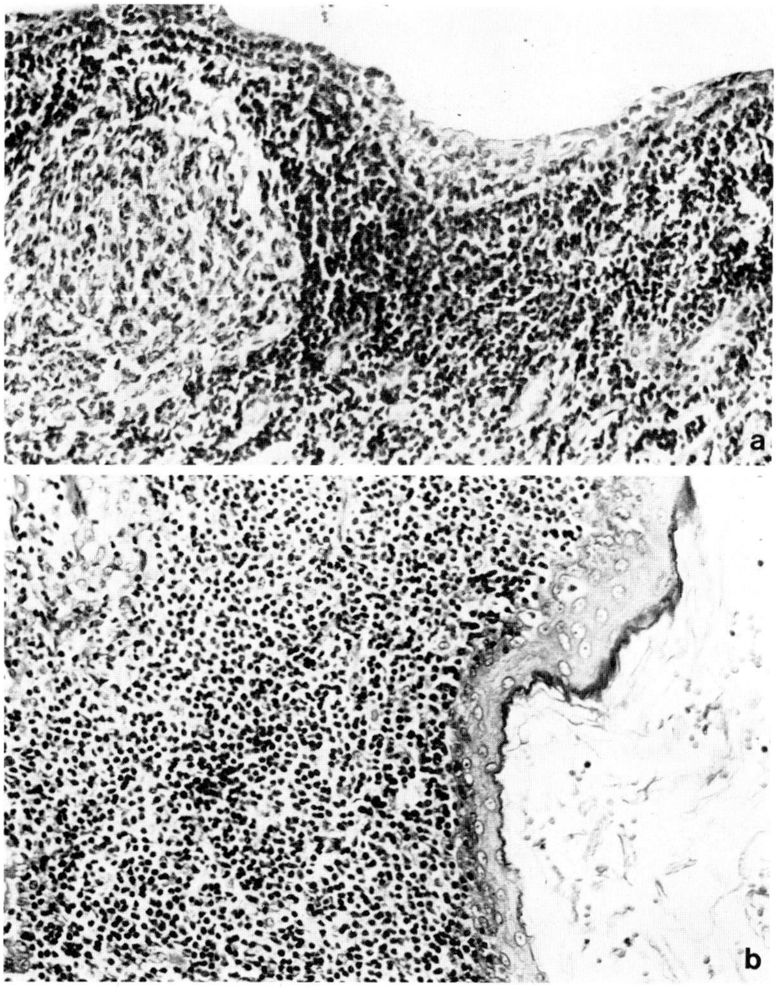

sialadenitis (Sjögren's syndrome) and the metaplastic type of cystadenoma lymphomatosum of the parotid (Seifert et al 1980).

Treatment

The treatment of choice is the complete removal of the cyst, observing the principles of surgery of the facial nerve. Incision or incomplete removal leads to recurrence, a fistula, or progressive chronic inflammation.

Treatment is discussed further in Chapters 13 and 22.

References

Bernier, J. L., S. N. Bhaskar: Lymphoepithelial lesions in salivary glands: classification and histogenesis based on 186 cases. Cancer 11 (1958) 1156

Bhaskar, S. N.: Lymphoepithelial cysts of the oral cavity. Report of twenty-four cases. Oral Surg. 21 (1966) 120

Bhaskar, S. N., J. L. Bernier: Histogenesis of branchial cysts. A report of 468 cases. Amer. J. Path. 35 (1958) 407

Bhaskar, S. N., T. E. Bolden, J. P. Weinmann: Pathogenesis of mucoceles. J. Dent. Res. 35 (1956) 863

Fujibayashi, T., H. Itoh: Lymphoepithelial (so-called branchial) cyst within the parotid gland. Report of a case and review of the literature. Int. J. Oral Surg. 10 (1981) 283

Hamperl, H.: Über "Schleimgranulome" und "glanduläre Erosionen" in den Speicheldrüsen und der Magenschleimhaut. Beitr. path. Anat. 88 (1932) 193

Harrison, J. D.: Salivary mucoceles. Oral Surg. 39 (1975) 268

Harrison, J. D., J. R. Garrett: Mucocele formation in cats by glandular duct ligation. Arch. oral Biol. 17 (1972) 1403

Harrison, J. D., J. R. Garrett: Experimental salivary mucoceles in cat. A histochemical study. J. oral Pathol. 4 (1975) 297

Pieterse, A. S., A. E. Seymour: Parotid cysts. An analysis of 16 cases and suggested classification. Pathology 13 (1981) 225

Richardson, G. S., A. A. Clairmont, E. R. Erickson: Cystic lesions of the parotid gland. Plast. Reconstr. Surg. 61 (1978) 364

Seifert, G.: Die Sekretionsstörungen (Dyschylien) der Speicheldrüsen. Ergebn. allg. Path. path. Anat. 44 (1964) 103

Seifert, G.:- Lymphoid lesions of the oral cavity. Pathol. Res. Pract. 167 (1980) 179

Seifert, G., C.-P. Schulz: Das monomorphe Speichelgangadenom. Klassifikation und Analyse von 79 Fällen. Virchows Arch. Path. Anat. 383 (1979) 77

Seifert, G., D. Waller: Klassifikation der Parotiszysten. Differentialdiagnose der Speichelgangzysten und lymphoepithelialen Zysten. Z. Laryng. Rhinol. 61 (1982) 78

Seifert, G., H. G. Bull, K. Donath: Histologic classification of the cystadenolymphoma of the parotid gland. Analysis of 275 cases. Virchows Arch. Path. Anat. 388 (1980) 13

Seifert, G., K. Donath, Ch. v. Gumberz: Mucozelen der Speicheldrüsen. Extravasations-Mucozelen (Schleimgranulome) und Retentions-Mucozelen (Schleim-Retentionscysten). HNO (Berl.) 29 (1981) 179

Shaheen, N. A., G. T. Harboyan, R. I. Nassif: Cysts of the parotid gland: review and report of two unusual cases. J. Laryngol. Otol. 89 (1975) 435

Southam, J. C.: Retention mucoceles of the oral mucosa. J. oral Pathol. 3 (1974) 197

Stoll, W.: Laterale Halszysten und laterale Halsfisteln: zwei verschiedene Krankheitsbilder. Z. Laryng. Rhinol. 59 (1980) 385

Takeda, Y., G. Ishikawa: Crystalloids in salivary duct cysts of the human parotid gland. Scanning electron microscopical study with electron probe X-ray microanalysis. Virchows Arch. Path. Anat. 399 (1983) 41

Ungerecht, K.: Parotiszyste mit branchiogenem Anteil als Relikt der 1. Kiemenfurche und Äquivalent einer Hals-Ohrfistel. Z. Laryng. Rhinol. 60 (1981) 225

11. Miscellaneous Noninflammatory Epithelial Lesions

Oncocytosis

Diffuse oncocytosis of the parotid gland, unlike the oncocytic tumors such as cystadenolymphoma and oncocytoma, is a very rare non-neoplastic parotid lesion due to oncocytic metaplasia of the ductal and acinar epithelium (Becker et al 1982, Thackray & Lucas 1974, Vigliani & Genetta 1982). Only two cases were found in 7336 salivary gland specimens in the Salivary Gland Register between 1965 and 1981.

Histology. The histologic examination (Figs. 11.**1**–11.**3**) shows a complete oncocytic metaplasia of the gland lobules affecting both the acini and the ducts. The oncocytic cells possess a swollen granular acidophilic cytoplasm. Fat cells are sometimes found in the interstitium. The oncocytes of the ducts can only be differentiated from oncocytic acinar cells by their position and not by their structure. A periductal infiltrate of lymphocytes and plasma cells is occasionally seen.

The common **electron microscopic** characteristic of all oncocytes is the richness of mitochondria. The mitochondria are usually swollen, show crystalization, and contain osmiophilic granules. The ductal oncocytes possess occasional tonofilaments, and the myoepithelial oncocytes, peripheral myofilaments. The autonomic nervous

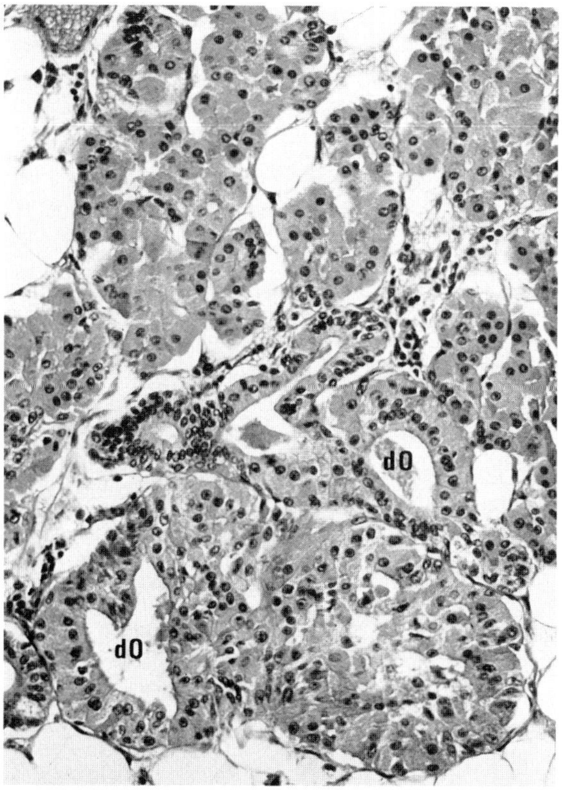

Figure 11.**1** Diffuse oncocytosis of the parotid gland showing acinar oncocytes (above), duct oncocytes (dO), and individual fat cells in the interstitium. H & E, 160×. (Becker et al 1982.)

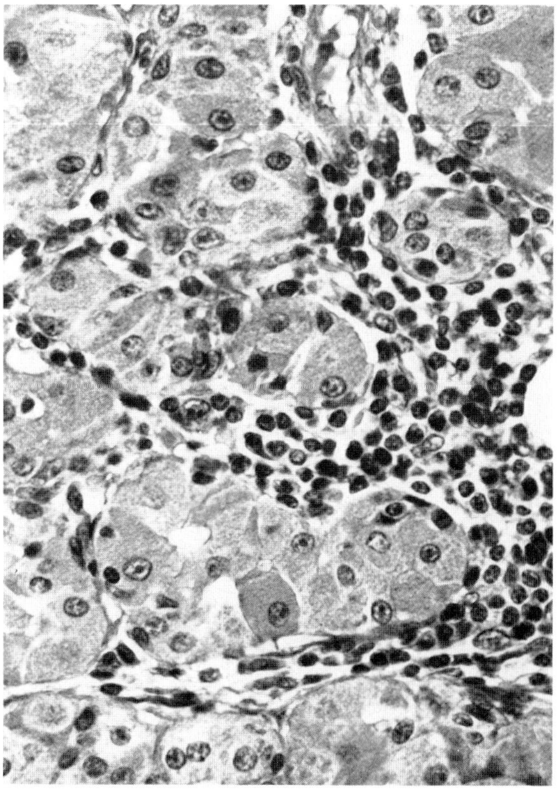

Figure 11.**2** Diffuse oncocytosis of the parotid gland showing an infiltrate of lymphocytes and plasma cells between the oncocytic cell units. H & E, 400×. (Becker et al 1982.)

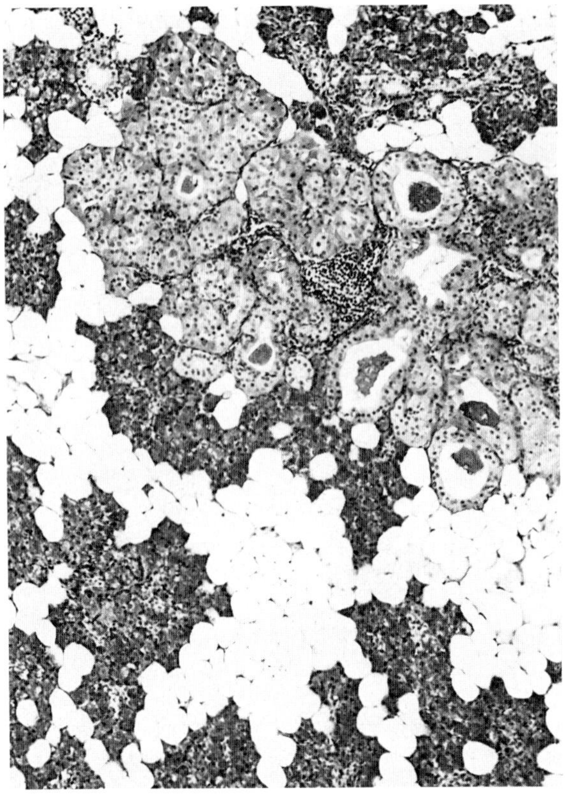

Figure 11.**3** Diffuse oncocytosis of the parotid gland showing remnants of acini with enzyme granules (dark area) and fatty tissue in the region of oncocytic cell units. H & E, 63×. (Becker et al 1982.)

system shows loss of neurosecretory granules in the terminal axones and dissolution of neurotubules and mitochondria.

The diffuse oncocytosis is an intracellular metabolic disorder with mitochondriopathy. The occurrence in the older age groups is ascribed to an age-dependent metabolic defect (Becker et al 1982). Oncocytosis is almost always unilateral, unlike sialadenosis, which is bilateral.

Multifocal oncocytic adenomatous hyperplasia (Shwartz & Feldman 1969), unlike diffuse oncocytosis, is a partly micronodular and partly macronodular adenomatous hyperplasia arising by oncocytic buds from the ductal epithelium. Remnants of the original salivary tissue with acini and fatty tissue are usually present between the oncocytic foci. The macronodular foci are up to 1 cm in size and have a solid trabecular structure. There is an occasional interstitial infiltration of lymphocytes and plasma cells. Since focal oncocytic hyperplasia can be demonstrated in the region of a typical oncocytoma, it is assumed that the oncocytic adenomatous hyperplasia is a focal neoplastic transformation from which the oncocytoma can arise by confluent growth and later formation of a capsule. Oncocytomas have an average size of 3–4 cm, and the peak age incidence 1–2 decades later than that of focal oncocytic hyperplasia. The differential diagnostic characteristics of diffuse oncocytosis, focal oncocytic hyperplasia, and oncocytoma are summarized in Table 7.**1**.

Table 11.**1** Differential Diagnosis of Diffuse Oncocytosis, Oncocytic Adenoma, Adenomatous Hyperplasia, and Oncocytoma of the Parotid Gland (Becker et al)

Characteristic	Diffuse Oncocytosis	Oncocytic Hyperplasia	Oncocytoma
Frequency	Extremely rare: 0.01% of all salivary diseases	Extremely rare: 0.1% of all salivary diseases	Very rare: 0.5% of all salivary diseases
Maximum age incidence	Seventh decade	Sixth decade	Seventh and eight decades
Macroscopy	Diffuse without capsule	Multifocal without a capsule	Usually solitary with a capsule
Size of nodes	—	Micronodular, 0.1 cm Macronodular, 1.0 cm	3–4 cm
Microscopy	Lobular, occasional intersital fatty tissue	Lobular, inclusion of gland remnants	Lobar, without inclusion of gland remnants
Arrangement	Acinar	Ductular	Ductular, microcystic solid, trabecular
Cell structure	Acidophil-granular	Acidophil-granular, focal clear cells	Acidophil-granular, rarely focal clear cells
Septae	—	—	Focal
Tissue of origin	Acini, duct system	Duct system	Duct system
Malignant transformation	—	—	Rare

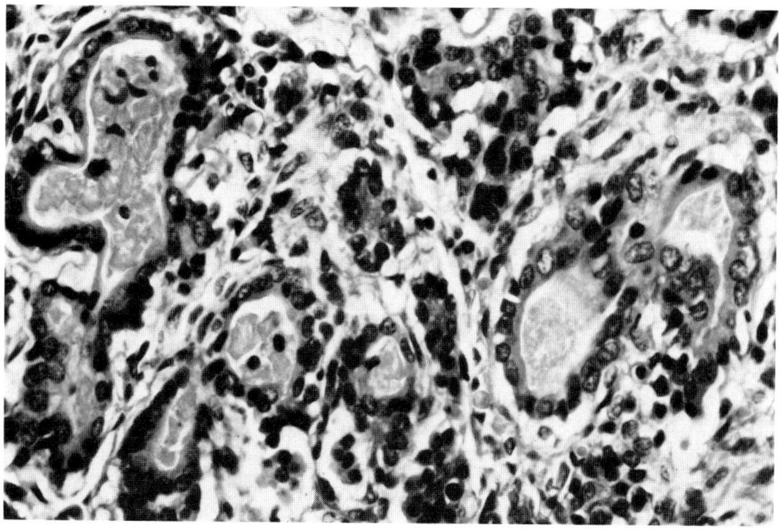

Figure 11.4 Cystic fibrosis of the parotid gland: duct ectasia and viscous inspissation of secretion with interstitial fibrosis. H & E, 400×.

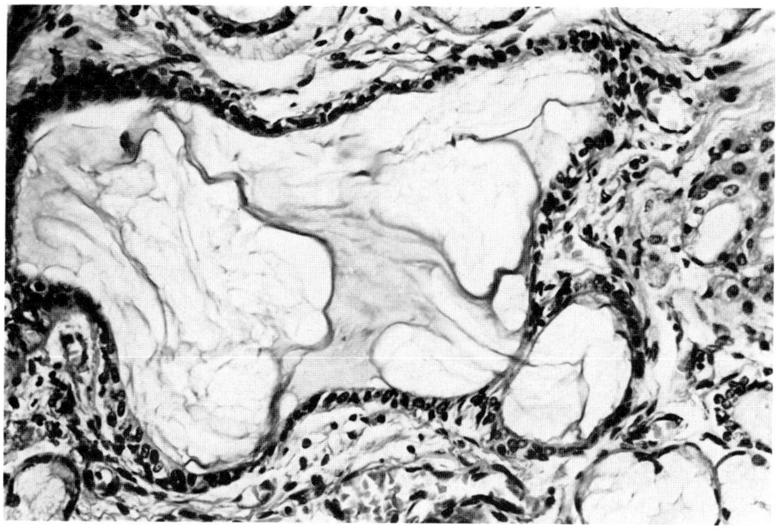

Figure 11.5 Cystic fibrosis of the sublingual gland showing dilated ducts with viscous masses of secretion. H & E, 250×.

Cystic Fibrosis

The characteristics of cystic fibrosis (mucoviscidosis) include changes in the composition of saliva (Muenzel 1976, Chilla et al 1977, Meyer et al 1980), and histologic and ultrastructural changes in the acini and duct system (Blomfield et al 1976, Seifert 1966, Seifert & Donath 1976). Dilations or cysts of the lumen of the acinus are caused by formation of viscous masses of mucus; duct ectasia also occurs due to inspissation of mucus in the ducts (Figs. 11.**4**, 11.**5**). Mucous particles arranged in layers like an onion ring are found in the sublingual gland particularly. The lumpy microliths (Figs. 11.**6**, 11.**7**) consist of mucoprotein-calcium complexes. Electron microscopy demonstrates conversion of amorphous calcium phosphate particles into star-shaped hydroxylapatite crystals, not only in the cytoplasm of the acinus, but also in the acinar and duct lumen. The calcium content, particularly of the submandibular secretion, is increased. The protein profile of the parotid saliva shows the most marked changes, and new protein groups are recorded (Meyer et al 1980).

Atrophy

Atrophy of the glandular tissue, particularly of the secreting serous acini, occurs with increasing age (Drummond & Chisholm 1984). It also occurs in all diseases associated with tissue destruction and limitation of function of the organ, such as

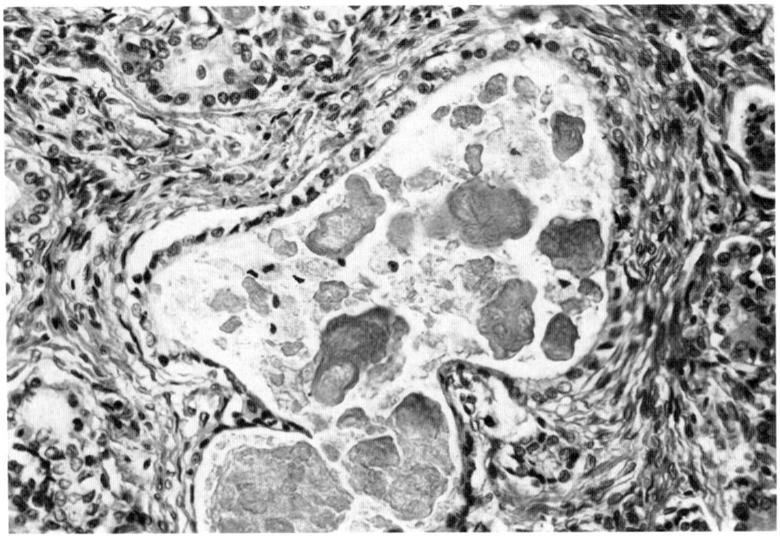

Figure 11.**6** Cystic fibrosis of the parotid gland showing microliths in the duct. H & E, 250×.

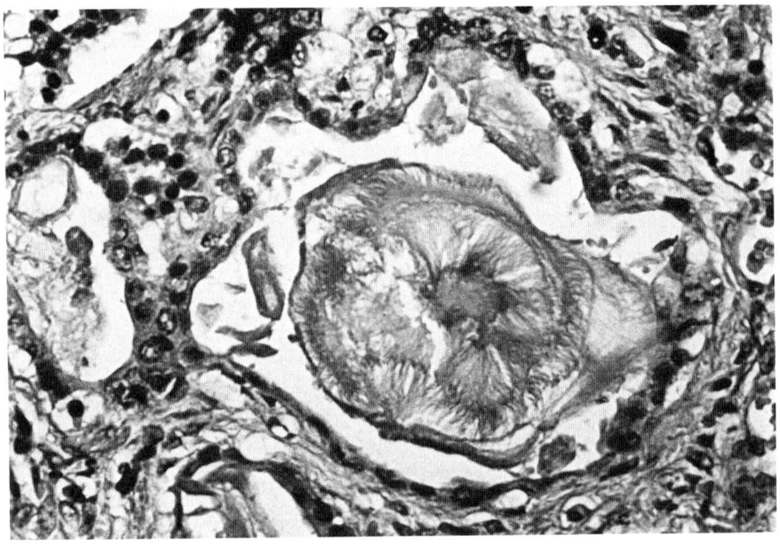

Figure 11.**7** Cystic fibrosis of the submandibular gland: microliths in a dilated duct with radial layers. H & E, 400×.

hunger, tumor cachexia, and chronic infections. The space is filled in by fat tissue. Marked parenchymal atrophy can also occur after chronic radiation treatment. The gland parenchyma within the intraglandular lymph nodes also shows increasing atrophy in the older age groups. Initially, the acini disappear and later also the ducts enclosed in lymphoid tissue (Seifert & Geiler 1956).

Lipomatous parotid atrophy is an unusual form (Seifert 1959). Macroscopically, the gland consists almost exclusively of fatty tissue. Histologic examination shows atrophic remnants of acini and slender segments of the duct system in the middle of fatty tissue arranged in lobules. Inflammatory infiltrate or fibrosis do not occur. The occurence of lipomatous pancreatic atrophy in infants and young children, together with experimental findings, indicates that the cause may be a previous virus infection, particularly by the coxsackievirus B. The parenchyma destroyed by the virus is replaced by fatty tissue.

Necrotizing Sialometaplasia (Salivary Gland Infarct)

More than 50 cases have now been recorded since the original description by Abrams et al (1973) of ischemic lesions in the minor salivary glands of the palate. This lesion is found in 0.03% of all oral biopsies (Mesa et al 1984). Donath (1979a, b) coined the term "salivary gland infarct" because the lesion resembles that in other organs, such as the prostate gland. Most cases are localized to the palate (Santis et al 1982, Grouls 1982, Krueger &

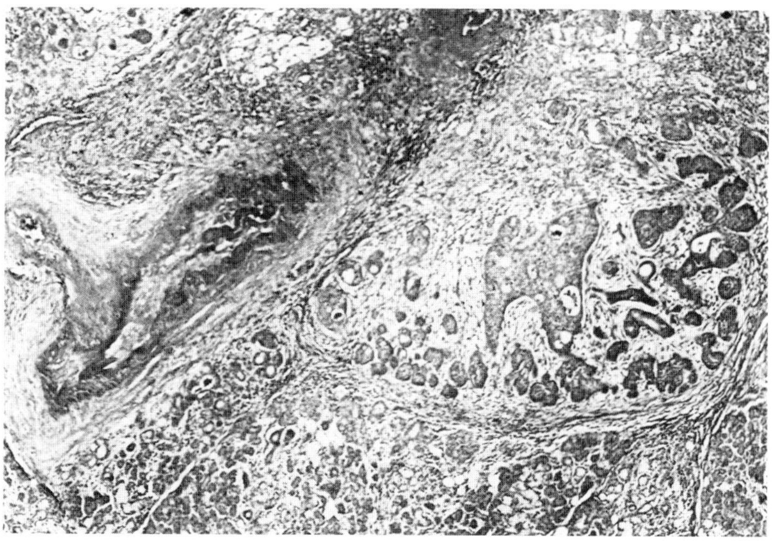

Figure 11.**8** Necrotizing sialometaplasia of the submandibular gland: lobular arrangement of salivary gland infarcts (right) and obliterative thrombosis of a small artery (left) in the postoperative period. H & E, 63×.

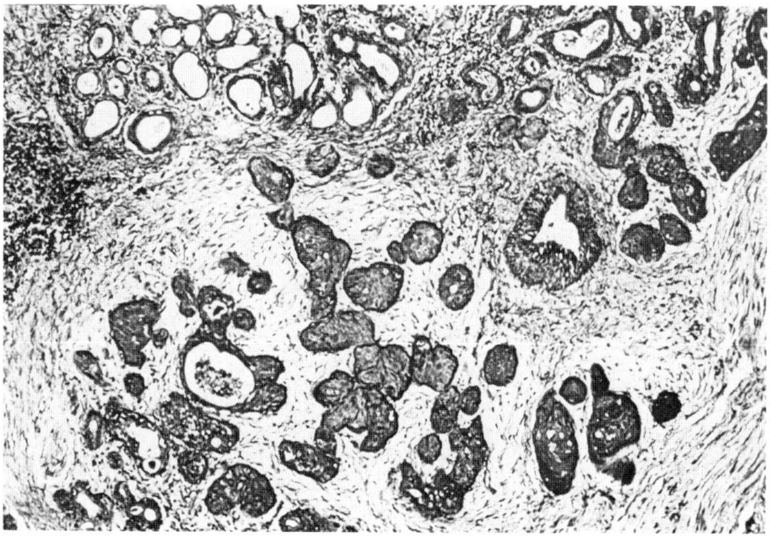

Figure 11.**9** Necrotizing sialometaplasia of the palatal glands: lobular arrangement of squamous cell metaplasia, remnants of palatal glands with dilated ducts (top). Masson-Goldner, 63×.

Dietrich 1982). Necrotizing sialometaplasia has been described more rarely in other salivary glands, including the submandibular gland and the minor glands of the lower lip and the gingiva (Forney et al 1977, Gad et al 1980, Beer & Neuwirth 1983). Thirty-two cases were found in the material of the Salivary Gland Register from 1965 to 1981, including several in the major glands (Donath 1979a).

Histology. Necrotizing sialometaplasia shows a lobular arrangement, a finding interpreted by Thackray and Lucas (1974) as lobular gland regeneration. In the center lies the regular dichotomous branching duct system with squamous cell metaplasia (Figs. 11.**8**–11.**10**). Necrotic acini, inflammatory resorptive cell infiltrate, or fatty tissue are found peripherally. These are usually surrounded by intact glandular tissue. Goblet cells may occur within the squamous cell metaplasia, a finding that can lead to confusion with a mucoepidermoid tumor (Fig. 11.**11**). Further vascular changes have been described in interlobular connective tissue around the salivary gland infarct (Fig. 11.**8**), including stenosis, thrombosis, or obliteration of vessels, particularly after operations.

The **cause** of necrotizing sialometaplasia is assumed to be vascular. Similar lesions can be produced experimentally by vascular ligation especially of the arteries (Donath 1979b, Standish & Shafer 1957). The squamous cell metaplasia in the center of the lesion represents a relatively ischemic zone, and the outer layer of necrosis is a zone of absolute ischemia. The relative ischemia

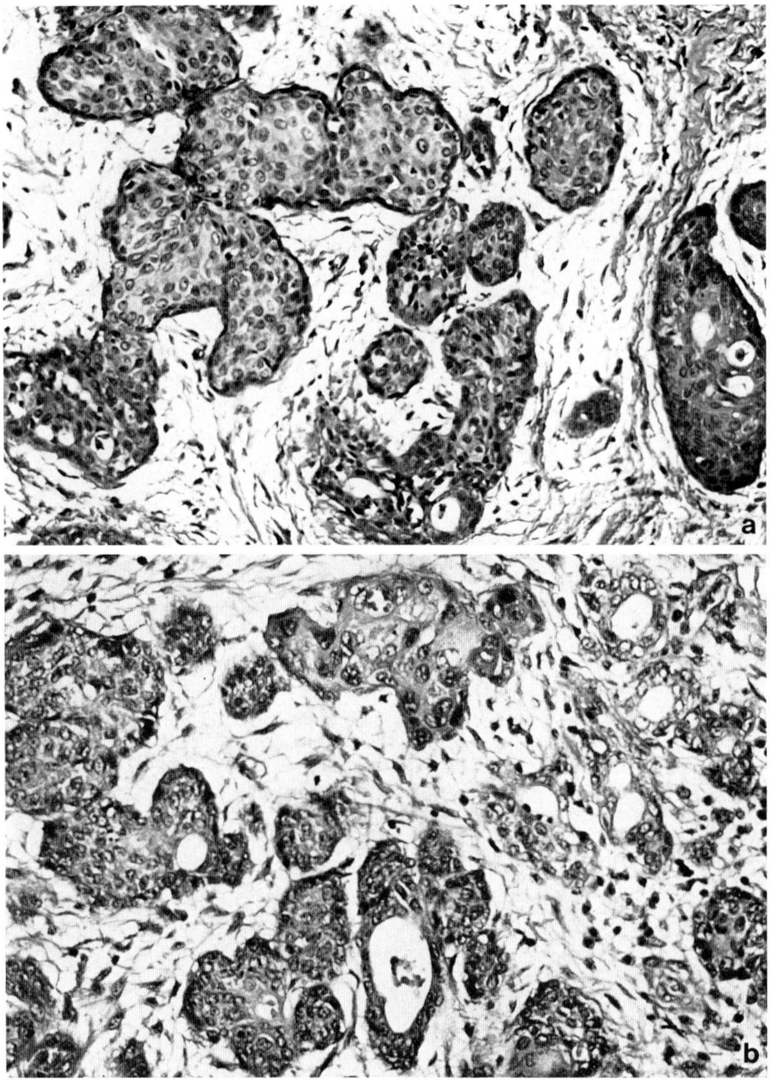

Figure 11.**10** Necrotizing sialometaplasia (see Fig. 11.**9**): **a** Dichotomously branched duct system with squamous cell metaplasia. **b** Remnants of duct lumen and inflammatory infiltrate with gland regeneration (right). Masson-Goldner, 160×.

damages the highly differentiated ductal epithelium, which is followed by replacement with squamous epithelium and by a regenerative hyperplasia of the undifferentiated basal reserve cells. Similar mechanisms are also proposed for squamous cell metaplasia in other tissues, such as that of the prostate, bronchi, and the uterine cervix. Another piece of evidence in favor of a vascular cause is the fact that necrotizing sialometaplasia was found affecting the parotid, submandibular, and minor salivary glands of patients who had a biopsy or a tumor operation a few weeks previously. Such operations are always associated with local vascular changes.

The **differential diagnosis** of necrotizing sialometaplasia includes squamous cell carcinoma and a mucoepidermoid tumor.

Other Epithelial Metaplasias

Sebaceous Gland Metaplasia.

This lesion is most commonly found in children and adolescents. It may be explained by the fact that the epithelium of the ducts is a derivative of the oral ectoderm and thus possesses the potential for forming sebaceous glands like the epithelium of the epidermis (Seifert 1966). Sebaceous gland foci occur particularly in the terminal duct system (Fig. 11.**12**). The presence of sebaceous glands in normal salivary glands explains the development of salivary tumors with similar patterns of differentiation (sebaceous gland adenoma, sebaceous gland carcinoma).

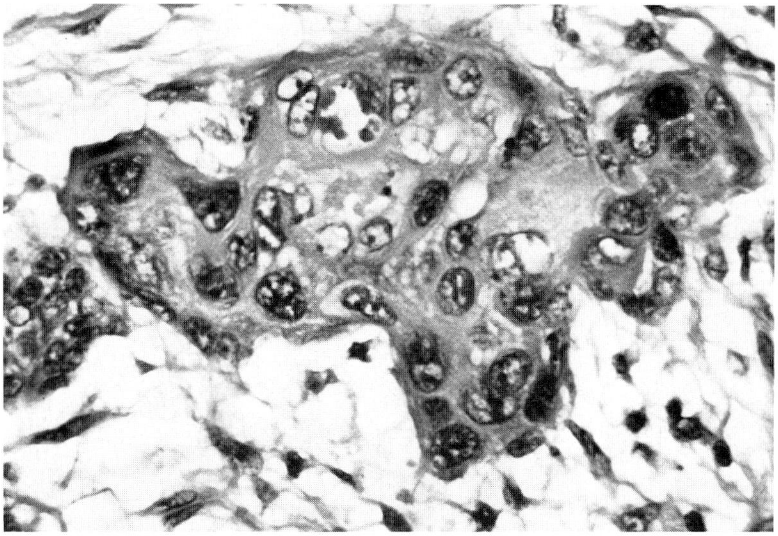

Figure 11.**11** Necrotizing sialometaplasia (see Fig. 11.**9**): detail of epithelial metaplasia with bizarre nuclear forms that could be confused with squamous cell carcinoma. H & E, 400×.

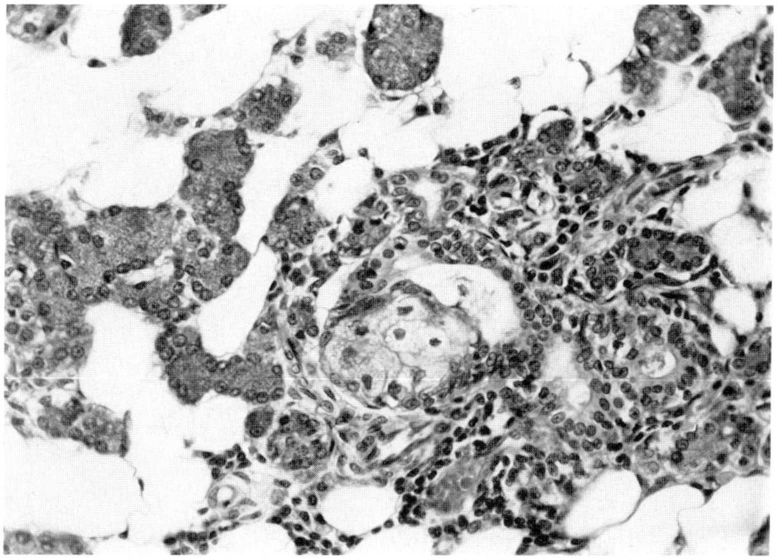

Figure 11.**12** Sebaceous metaplasia in a terminal duct of the parotid gland. H & E, 160×.

Goblet Cell Metaplasia

Goblet cell metaplasia (Fig. 11.**13**) frequently affects the duct system of the child's parotid gland, and the frequency of goblet cell metaplasia thereafter decreases with increasing age. Goblet cell metaplasia may occur in radiation sialadenitis, necrotizing metaplasia, and cystadenolymphoma, and it is especially characteristic of mucoepidermoid tumors.

Squamous Cell Metaplasia

This lesion is mainly found in chronic inflammation and deficiency disorders, such as avitaminoses, in addition to vascular disorders, especially necrotizing sialometaplasia. Squamous cell metaplasia is also a typical finding in sialolithiasis. The ductal epithelium is usually replaced by squamous epithelium in the presence of encrusted microliths (Fig. 11.**14**).

Oncocytic Metaplasia

Oncocytic metaplasia (Hamperl 1962) is observed more frequently with increasing age, so that it can be found in 80% of all glands by the age of 70 years (Hamperl 1931a, 1931b). Oncocytic metaplasia (Figs. 11.**15**, 11.**16**) affects the duct system of the sublingual gland particularly, whereas the parotid gland demonstrates this type of metaplasia much less often. Oncocytes are defined as swollen acidophilic cells with small chromatin-dense cell nuclei and granular cytoplasm. Electron microscopy shows that the granules represent a dense permeation of the cytoplasm by

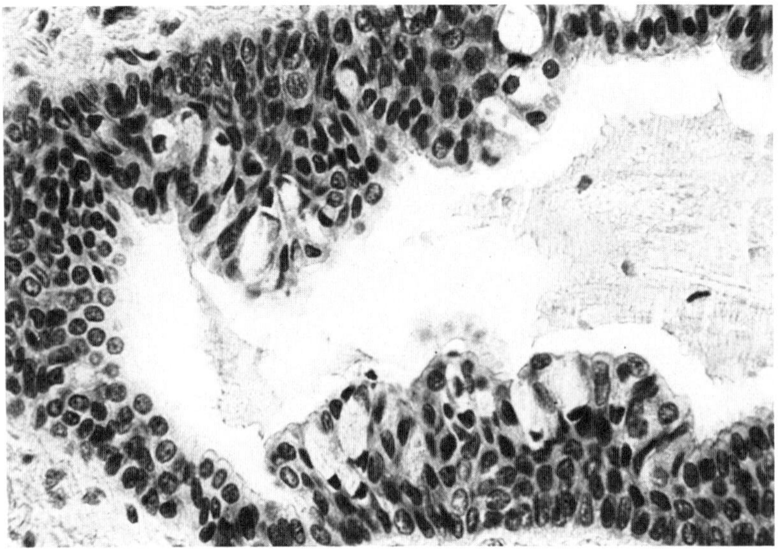

Figure 11.**13** Goblet cell metaplasia in an excretory duct of the parotid gland. H & E, 160×.

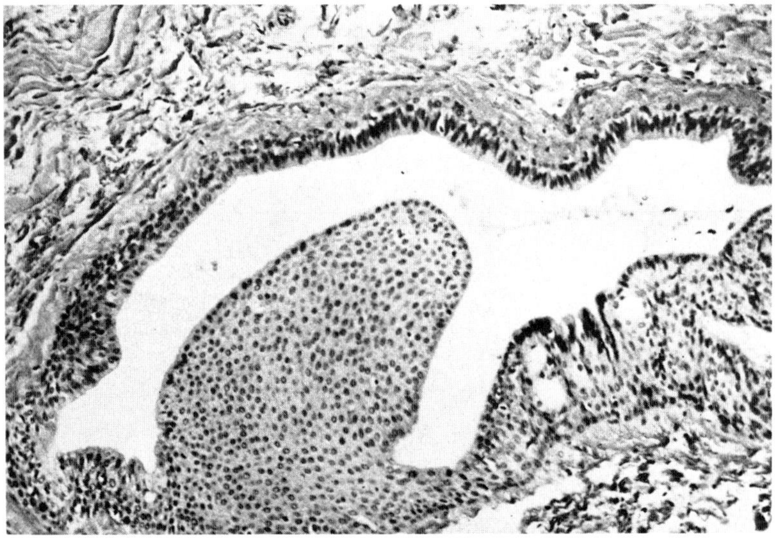

Figure 11.**14** Squamous cell metaplasia in an excretory duct of the palatal glands. H & E, 160×.

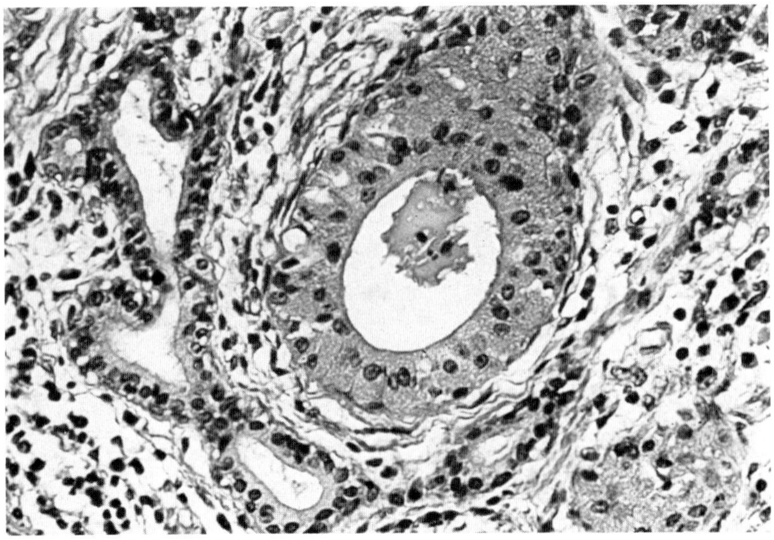

Figure 11.**15** Oncocytic metaplasia in the parotid ducts. H & E, 160×.

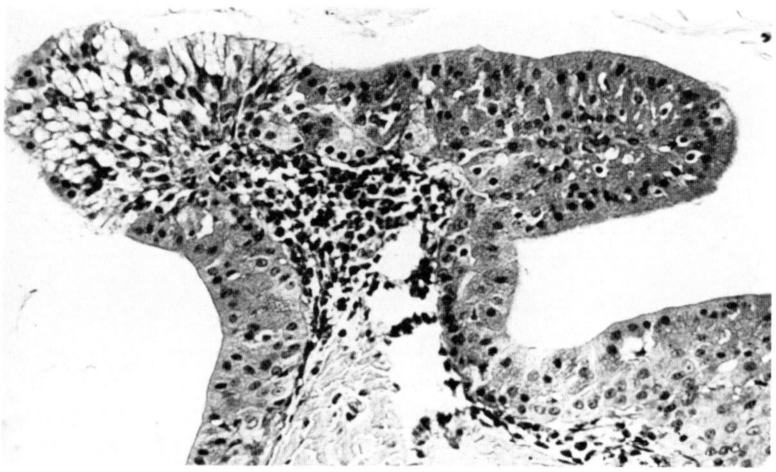

Figure 11.**16** Oncocytic metaplasia (right and top) and focal goblet cell metaplasia in a minor gland duct of the lower lip. H & E, 160×.

mitochondria. Histochemistry shows that the oncocytes are characterized by a high activity of oxidative and hydrolytic enzymes (cytochrome oxidase, succinodehydrogenase, diphosphopyridine nucleotide and triphosphopyridine nucleotide diaphorase). Obviously, oncocytic metaplasia represents a change of cell metabolism, which is accompanied by a mitochondriopathy.

Oncocytosis is discussed on page 101, and oncocytic tumors on page 213.

References

Abrams, A. M., R. J. Melrose, F. V. Howell: Necrotizing sialometaplasia: A disease simulating malignancy. Cancer 32 (1973) 130

Becker, K., K. Donath, G. Seifert: Die diffuse Onkozytose der Parotis. Definition und Differentialdiagnose. Z. Laryng. Rhinol. 61 (1982) 691

Beer, G. M., A. Neuwirth: Nekrotisierende Sialometaplasie (Speicheldrüseninfarkt) der Glandula submandibularis. Laryng. Rhinol. Otol. 62 (1983) 468

Blomfield, J., A. R. Rush, H. M. Allars, J. M. Brown: Parotid gland function in children with cystic fibrosis and child control subjects. Pediat. Res. 10 (1976) 574

Chilla, R., K. M. Doering, H. Lubahn, C. Arglebe: Über das Auftreten "schneller Isoamylasen" im Mukoviszidosespeichel. Arch. Oto-Rhino-Laryng. 214 (1977) 367

Donath, K.: Pathohistologie des Parotisinfarktes (Necrotizing sialometaplasia). Z. Laryng. Rhinol. 58 (1979a) 70

Donath, K.: Eine experimentelle Studie zur Ätiopathogenese der nekrotisierenden Sialometaplasie. Arch. Oto-Rhino-Laryng. 223 (1979b) 191

Drummond, J. R., D. M. Chisholm: A qualitative and quantitative study of the ageing human labial salivary glands. Arch. oral Biol. 29 (1984) 151

Forney, S. K., J. M. Foley, W. E. Sugg jr., G. W. Oatis jr.: Necrotizing sialometaplasia of the mandible. Oral Surg. 43 (1977) 720

Gad, A., H. Willén, R. Willén, S. Thorstensson, L. Ekman: Necotizing sialometaplasia of the lip simulating squamous cell carcinoma. Histopathology 4 (1980) 111

Grouls, V.: Nekrotisierende Sialometaplasie (Speicheldrüseninfarkt). Pathologe 3 (1982) 339

Hamperl, H.: Beiträge zur normalen und pathologischen Histologie der Speicheldrüsen. Z. mikroskop.-anat. Forschg. 27 (1931a) 1

Hamperl, H.: Onkozyten und Geschwülste der Speicheldrüsen. Virchows Arch. Path. Anat. 282 (1931b) 724

Hamperl, H.: Das Onkozytom der Speicheldrüsen. Z. Krebsf. 64 (1962) 427

Krüger, R., H. G. Dietrich: Der Speicheldrüseninfarkt (Necrotizing sialometaplasia). Differentialdiagnose und Pathogenese. Pathologe 3 (1982) 342

Mesa, M. L., R. S. Gertler, L. C. Schneider: Necrotizing sialometaplasia: Frequency of histologic misdiagnosis. Oral Surg. 57 (1984) 71

Meyer, P., R. R. Kleber, K. W Mittenzwey: Zur Sialochemie des Parotis- und Submandibularisspeichels bei Mukoviszidose. Z. Laryng. Rhinol. 59 (1980) 274

Münzel, M.: Die Biochemie der menschlichen Speicheldrüsensekrete. Arch. Oto-Rhino-Laryng. 213 (1976) 209

Santis, H. R., S. P. Kabani, A. Rederiques, J. M. Driscoll: Necrotizing sialometaplasia: An early, nonulcerative presentation. Oral Surg. 53 (1982) 387

Schwartz, J. S., M. Feldman: Diffuse multinodular oncocytoma ("oncocytosis") of the parotid gland. Cancer 23 (1969) 636

Seifert, G.: Lipomatöse cystische Pankreasfibrose und lipomatöse Pankreasatrophie. Beitr. path. Anat. 121 (1959) 64

Seifert, G.: Mundhöhle, Mundspeicheldrüsen, Tonsillen und Rachen. In Doerr, W., E. Uehlinger: Spezielle pathologische Anatomie, Bd. 1. Springer, Berlin 1966 (S. 1)

Seifert, G., K. Donath: Die Morphologie der Speicheldrüsenerkrankungen. Arch. Oto-Rhino-Laryng. 213 (1976) 111

Seifert, G., G. Geiler: Zur Pathologie der kindlichen Kopfspeicheldrüsen. Beitr. path. Anat. 116 (1956) 1

Standish, S. M., W. G. Shafer: Serial histologic effects of rat submaxillary and sublingual salivary gland duct and blood vessel ligation. J. Dent. Res. 36 (1957) 886

Thackray, A. L., R. B. Lucas: Tumors of the major salivary glands. Atlas of Tumor Pathology, 2. ser. fasc. 10. Armed Forces Institute of Pathology, Washington 1974

Vigliani, R., C. Genetta: Diffuse hyperplastic oncocytosis of the parotid gland. Case report with histochemical observations. Virchows Arch. Path. Anat. 397 (1982) 235

12. Sialadenitis

Classification

A classification of inflammation of the salivary glands must cover several facets. The first is the tissue that is subject to inflammation: infection may be divided into sialangitis affecting the ductal system and sialadenitis affecting the parenchyma. The second is the gland that is affected (the parotid, the submandibular, the sublingual, or the minor glands). The third is the course of the disease (acute, chronic, or recurring). The fourth is the pathogenesis (ascending inflammation or hematogenous causes), and the fifth is the numerous etiologic agents, such as infection, disorders of secretion, lesions of the duct, immunologic factors. Furthermore, it must be decided whether the patient has an isolated, local inflammation or whether the inflammation of the salivary glands is merely one manifestation of a generalized disorder, such as chronic infection, tumor cachexia, diabetes mellitus, renal insufficiency, or other systemic disorders.

Data about the *frequency of inflammation of the salivary glands* are difficult to assess, since they usually relate to a selected population. This is particularly true of acute inflammation. In contrast, chronic inflammation is easier to assess, because tissues are almost always removed both for diagnostic and therapeutic purposes, allowing the disease to be classified by histopathology (Table 12.**1**).

Table 12.**1** Frequency of Chronic Salivary Gland Inflammation

Type of Sialadenitis	N	%
Chronic reccurrent parotitis	429	21.0
Chronic sialadentitis of the submandibular gland (Küttner tumor)	686	33.5
Chronic sialadenitis of the sublinguinal gland	37	2.0
Chronic sialadenitis of the minor glands (all forms)	201	10.0
Chronic myoepithelial parotitis	152	7.5
Chronic epithelioid cell parotitis	46	2.5
Salivary gland tuberculosis	2	–
Radiation sialadenitis	27	1.5
Obstructive electrolyte sialadenitis	438	21.5
Rare forms	11	0.5
Total	2029	100.0

Effective treatment is based on knowledge of the etiology, of which part of which gland is affected, of the course of the disease (acute, subacute, chronic, etc.) and on the clinical findings. The following remarks are therefore based on an etiologic classification (Table 12.**2**), but, any etiologic classification must take into account the fact that inflammatory processes often have a multifactorial basis. The complexity of the course of the inflammation can only be explained by the interplay of several etiologic factors.

Etiology

Several general (just mentioned) and local factors play a part in the genesis of salivary gland inflammation.

The *generalized factors* include reduction of the *resistance* and the *immunologic defense mecha-*

Table 12.**2** Etiologic Classification of Sialadenitis (Seifert)

- Bacterial sialadenitis
  - Acute purulent parotitis
  - Chronic recurrent parotitis
- Viral sialadenitis
  - Epidemic parotitis
  - Cytomegalovirus
  - Other forms, e. g., coxsackievirus, ECHO virus, parainfluenza virus, types 1–3
- Radiation sialadenitis
- Obstructive electrolyte sialadenitis
- Chronic sclerosing sialadenitis (Küttner tumor) of the submandibular gland
- Immune sialadenitis
  - Myoepithelial sialadenitis (Sjögren's syndrome)
  - Epithelioid cell sialadenitis (Heerfordt's syndrome)

nisms. This explains the frequency of inflammation of the salivary glands in a wide range of serious, usually chronic, generalized diseases, such as malignant cachexia, uremia, diabetes mellitus, chronic intoxication, undernourished states, chronic infective diseases, and the postoperative state. *Age and sex* are additional generalized factors.

Local predisposing factors include abnormalities of the *salivary secretion and of the duct system.* Saliva of normal amount and composition coupled with a functioning secretory immune system provides a natural protection against inflammation. A sufficient flow of saliva and a normal ductal system prevent penetration of toxins into the duct system or inspissation of secretion. A reduction of the flow of saliva, a change in its electrolyte concentration, or retention of secretion in the duct system predispose to the development of infection. The ductal factors include congenital anomalies, such as sialectasis, diverticuli, and stenoses, and acquired lesions, such as strictures, secondary duct ectasia, and obstructions. The length and branching of the ductal system is also important in the varying frequency with which inflammation affects the individual salivary glands.

Complementary etiologic noxae in addition to general and local factors must be invoked to explain the polymorphous picture of sialadenitis. *Acute forms of sialadenitis* are usually caused by *bacteria or viruses,* whereas *secretory disorders and immunopathologic reactions* play an increasingly important role in *chronic inflammation.* It is easy to demonstrate bacterial or viral infection in acute inflammation by the isolation of streptococci or staphylococci in the saliva, by the isolation of viruses, and by positive serologic complement-binding reactions. In contrast, organisms can seldom be isolated in chronic inflammation, and antibacterial therapy is almost always valueless. From this, it can be concluded that chronic inflammatory processes are mainly due to secretory disorders and immunologic mechanisms.

Secretory disorders change the amount and chemical composition of the saliva, including that of protein, mucins, and electrolytes (Münzel 1976, Arglebe 1981). The pathologic basis is viscous inspissation of secretions, spheroliths, and microliths, with appropriate histochemical parameters. The altered properties of the secretion are accompanied by changes in the glandular tissue, such as epithelial metaplasia and ductal obstruction, proliferation, and dilation. The chronic forms of sialadenitis accompanied by secretory disorders are encompassed by the term *electrolyte sialadenitis* (Seifert 1964, Seifert & Donath 1977). Experimental models include iodide sialadenitis (Seifert & Junge-Hülsing 1965) and calciphylactic sialadenitis (Immenkamp & Seifert 1969).

Immune mechanisms lead to lesions of the duct system, especially in chronic inflammation, producing *immune sialadenitis* (Seifert 1979, Donath & Seifert 1981, Caselitz & Seifert 1982). The clinical findings are changes of salivary and blood chemistry, such as immune complexes, antibodies and autoantibodies, rheumatoid factors, and hypergammaglobulinemia. Histopathologic examination shows a change in composition of the immunoglobulin-forming plasma cells, the development of lymphoid follicles, and antibodies against ductal epithelium, and myoepithelial cell islands. Immunopathologic and secretory phenomena can potentiate each other, as may occur in chronic sclerosing sialadenitis (Küttner tumor) of the submandibular gland (Seifert & Donath 1977).

The main lesion of *radiation sialadenitis* is irradiation-induced damage to the parenchyma and the resulting secondary disturbance of secretion. There is a direct relationship between the dose of radiation and the extent of damage to the gland.

Pathogenesis

In any inflammation of the salivary glands, the pathogenic agent must be identified in addition to the etiologic factors. The organism may reach the glandular tissue via the ductal system, by the bloodstream, or more readily by lymphatic spread. Inflammation spreading via the ducts must be distinguished from hematologic or lymphatic spread.

Acute bacterial inflammation is usually due to organisms ascending the duct system from the mouth. In the later stages, the inflammation may invade the parenchyma of the gland after overcoming the duct barrier. In chronic inflammation, also the duct system is the most important pathway of spread of the inflammation. Both secretory disorders and immunologic lesions affect the duct especially and lead to increasing destruction of the lobular system, even in the absence of any pathogenic organism, causing a further decrease in the secretory capacity of the gland tissue.

The bloodstream plays a role in generalized septic diseases, virus infections, and immunopathies. Bacteria may be carried by the vascular system to the salivary gland and infect the gland by pericanalicular or periacinar capillary spread. The viremia causes excretion of viruses in the saliva, and also leads to a virus sialadenitis. Immune complexes, antibodies, and autoantibodies reach the salivary glands via the bloodstream, and in addition to local immune factors maintain the chronic inflammatory process.

Lymphatic pathogenesis is much rarer. It should be considered if intra- or periglandular lymph node diseases affect the gland: lymphatic diseases may also extend from neighboring tissue.

References

Arglebe, C.: Biochemistry of human saliva: Sialadenosis and sialadenitis. In: Pfaltz, C. R., R. Chilla, Advances in ORL, Vol. 26. Karger, Basel 1981

Caselitz, J., G. Seifert: Das lokale Abwehr- und Immunsystem der Speicheldrüsen unter physiologischen und pathologischen Bedingungen. Dtsch. Z. Mund-Kiefer-Gesichts-Chir. 6 (1982) 93

Donath, K., G. Seifert: Immunologische und immunpathologische Reaktionen der Speicheldrüsen. Allergologie 4 (1981) 110

Immenkamp, M., G. Seifert: Zur Pathogenese der experimentellen Speicheldrüsen-Calciphylaxie. Virchows Arch. Abt. A 347 (1969) 211

Münzel, M.: Die Biochemie der menschlichen Speicheldrüsensekrete. Arch. Oto-Rhino-Laryng. 213 (1976) 209

Seifert, G.: Die Sekretionsstörungen (Dyschylien) der Speicheldrüsen. Ergebn. allg. Path. path. Anat. 44 (1964) 103

Seifert, G.: Mundhöhle, Mundspeicheldrüsen, Tonsillen und Rachen. In Doerr, W., E. Uehlinger: Spezielle pathologische Anatomie, Bd. 1. Springer, Berlin 1966 (S. 1)

Seifert, G.: Wangenschwellungen bei Speicheldrüsenentzündungen. Pathologisch-anatomische Differentialdiagnose der Sialadenitis. HNO (Berl.) 27 (1979) 119

Seifert, G.: Chronische Mundtrockenheit. Ursache, Pathologie. Dtsch. Z. Mund-Kiefer-Gesichts-Chir. 5 (1981) 3

Seifert, G., K. Donath: Die Morphologie der Speicheldrüsenerkrankungen. Arch. Oto-Rhino-Laryng. 213 (1976) 111

Seifert, G., K. Donath: Zur Pathogenese des Küttner-Tumors der Submandibularis. Analyse von 349 Fällen mit chronischer Sialadenitis der Submandibularis. HNO (Berl.) 25 (1977) 81

Seifert, G., G. Junge-Hülsing: Untersuchungen zur Jodid-Sialadenitis und Jod-131-Aktivität der Speicheldrüsen. Frankf. Z. Path. 74 (1965) 485

Bacterial Sialadenitis

Acute Purulent Sialadenitis (Parotitis)

Acute ascending infections usually affect the parotid gland; they affect the submandibular glands less commonly. The most common organisms are group A streptococci and Staphylococcus aureus. Reduced or absent saliva appears to be the most important pathogenic factor, whereas changes in the composition of the saliva have a subordinate role. It is worthy of note that parotitis almost never occurs in patients with extensive tumors of the mouth, which are heavily infected. In contrast, a serious parotitis occurs in coma of various causes and in intestinal diseases accompanied by reduction or failure of the flow of saliva. It is obvious that the normal flow of saliva provides mechanical or anti-infective defenses.

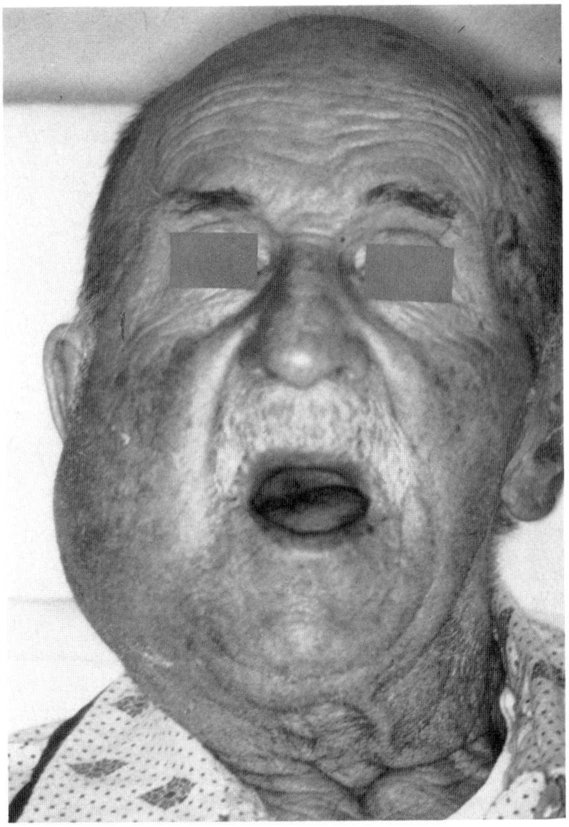

Figure 12.**1** Acute purulent parotitis with parotid abscess.

The **clinical picture** is characterized by tender, often fluctuant, circumscribed, or diffuse swelling of the parotid gland (Fig. 12.**1**). The ear lobes may be displaced laterally, and turbid secretion drains from the duct. Occasionally, a fistula forms as a result of an abscess, and purulent secretion drains from it. The abscess may track via the pterygomaxillary fissure into the pterygopalatine fossa or via Santorini's fissure into the external auditory meatus. The facial nerve is largely resistant to the inflammatory process. A facial paralysis almost always indicates a lesion other than acute parotitis.

Macroscopically (Fig. 12.**2**), the parotid is very swollen with increased vascularity and liquifaction of tissue to form abscesses.

Histologic examination shows that the process begins as an acute sialangitis (Fig. 12.**3**), characterized by swelling and desquamation of the ductal epithelium, an increased accumulation of mucus in the duct lumen, with inclusions of bacteria and periductal inflammatory edema. Later in the disease, the leukocytic infiltrate affects the periductal tissue, with destruction of duct epithelium (Figs. 12.**4**–12.**6**). This inflammatory

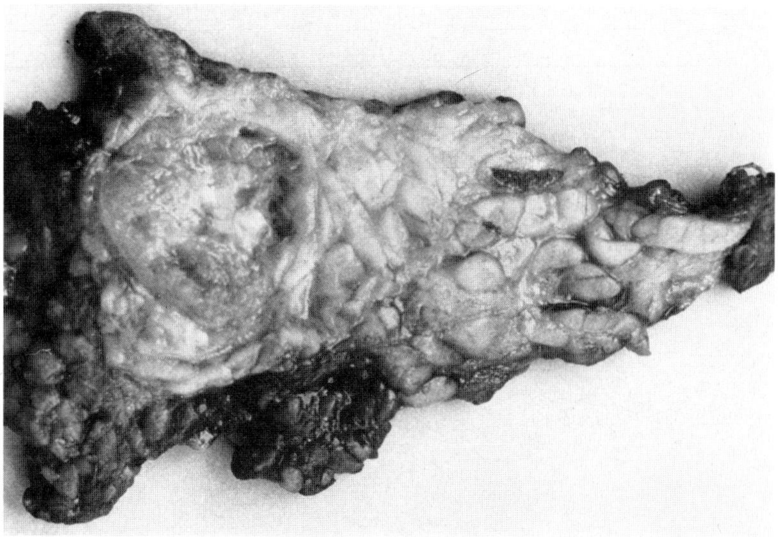

Figure 12.**2** Acute purulent parotitis showing abscesses on the cut surface.

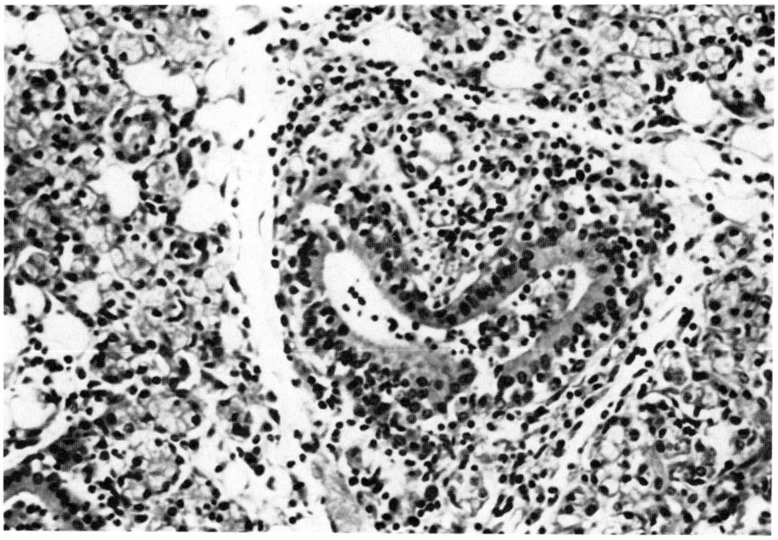

Figure 12.**3** Acute purulent parotitis showing a collection of leukocytes in the duct (sialangitis) and periductal inflammatory edema. H & E, 160×.

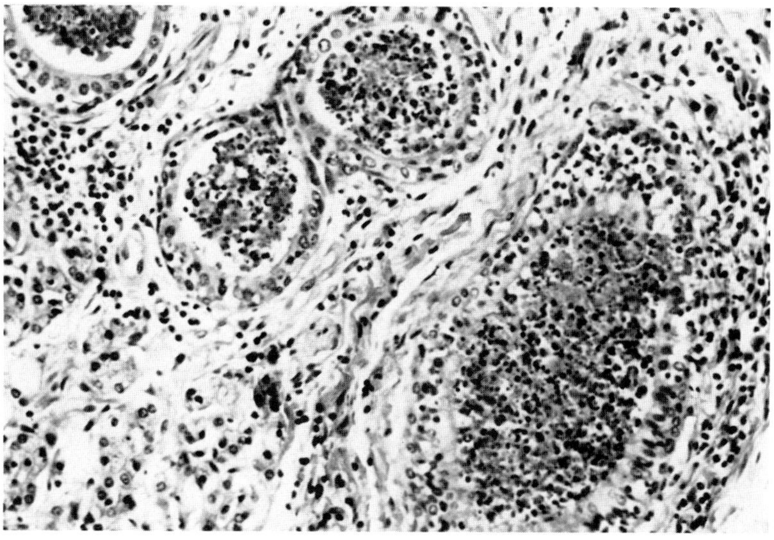

Figure 12.**4** Acute purulent parotitis showing a collection of pus in the dilated duct, and periductal inflammatory infiltrate. H & E, 160×.

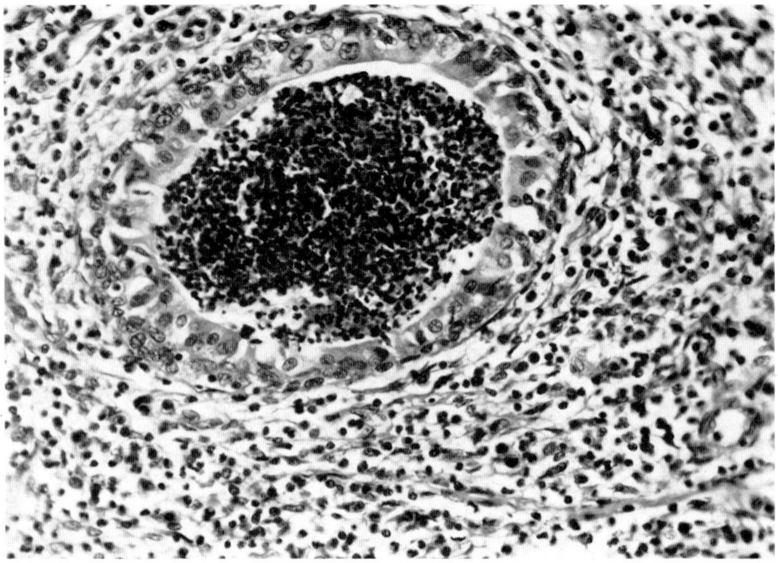

Figure 12.**5** Severe purulent sialangitis and perisialangitis of the parotid gland. H & E, 160×.

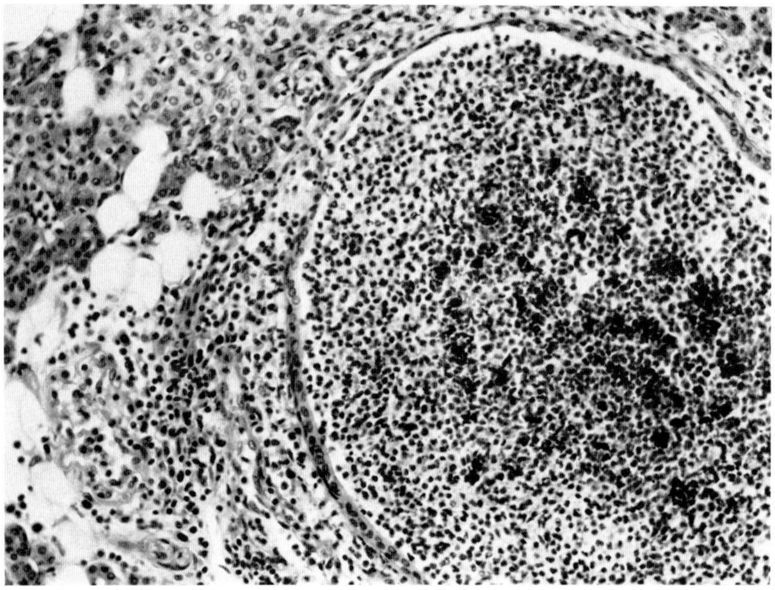

Figure 12.**6** Parotid abscess in a patient with diabetes mellitus showing collections of pus and bacteria in the dilated duct, and dissolution of the duct epithelium. H & E, 160×.

process is accompanied by a loss of acini and formation of microabscesses. In patients with reduced general resistance, particularly those with postoperative parotitis, the abscesses may increase in number and size, penetrate the periglandular tissue, and form a fistula. Septicemia may develop if the organisms penetrate the bloodstream.

The differential diagnosis includes arthritis of the temporomandibular joint, unerupted molars, and dental abscess.

Since the **diagnosis** of acute parotitis is easily made in most cases, further diagnostic procedures, such as biochemical analysis of the saliva, are unneccessary and usually of no practical value.

The **treatment** of choice is the appropriate antibiotic determined by culture and sensitivity tests. Antibiotics should be administered parenterally: adminstration by the salivary ducts is not necessary. If an abscess forms, it must be drained by incisions parallel to the fibers of the facial nerve to avoid damage to the nerve.

Seemann (1969) conducted 200 postmortem examinations and found a purulent sialangitis on 18 occasions and a severe parotid abscess on eight occasions in patients with severe cachetic diseases, such as hepatic or diabetic coma and enterocolitis. The peak age incidence was in the sixth and seventh decades.

Acute Postoperative Parotitis

This is an unusual form of circumscribed purulent parotitis. It presents after major abdominal operations particularly, but also after other major prodecures. According to Thörner (1963), the cause is staphylococcal infection accompanied by hyposalivation and dehydration. Vascular toxic factors and proteolytic enzymes activated by tissue kinases in the parenchyma of the gland are also important. The incidence of postoperative parotitis is quoted as being between 0.09 and 0.88% (Mathis 1954, Bach & Buttenberg 1958).

The fact that postoperative parotitis can occur even during intensive antibiotic therapy indicates that the cause is not a straightforward bacterial inflammation. The similarity of the clinical picture and pathologic course of postoperative parotitis to acute pancreatitis is striking.

There is a close functional relationship between the pancreas and the parotid, so that lesions of the autonomic nervous system and toxic and allergic lesions may be included within the scope of the disease. Hypoxic tissue damage due to increased capillary permeability leads, in turn, to involvement of the secretory parenchyma and thus to the extravasation of parotid secretion into the surrounding tissue. If trypsinogen is then converted by activators to trypsin, an autodigestive enzymatic process develops that is often complicated by secondary infection.

The submandibular gland, unlike the parotid gland, is only rarely affected, possibly because of its high content of mucinous secretion with particularly active protective agents.

Postoperative parotitis has declined in frequency in recent years, but its **treatment** still presents difficulties. Radiotherapy and stellate ganglion blokade are recommended at the earliest sign of the disease. It is said that stellate ganglion blokade interrupts the abnormal autonomic impulses. This also applies to infiltration of the parotid gland with procaine (Karst 1955, Köster 1961). Drainage through generous incisions is necessary, if the gland fluctuates. The trypsin inactivator aprotinin has proved useful in inhibiting the autodigestive process (Forell 1961).

Chronic Recurrent Parotitis

Two types of chronic recurrent parotitis must be distinguished, one affecting children and the other adults.

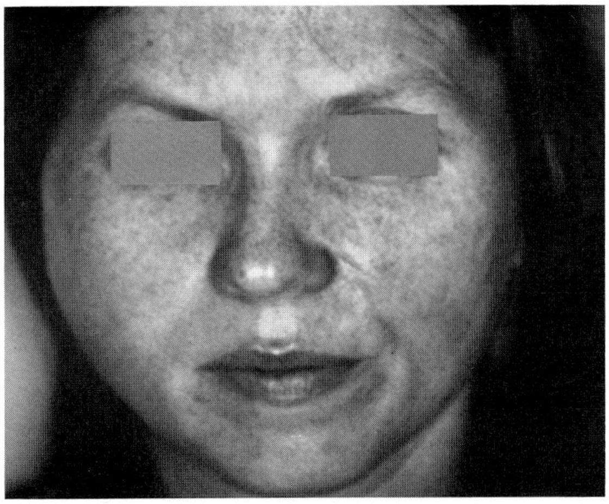

Figure 12.**7** Chronic recurrent parotitis in a 34-year-old woman.

Clinical Picture. The disease is characterized by recurrent tender swelling of one or both glands (Fig. 12.**7**). The swelling may persist for days or weeks, and the interval between episodes of inflammation varies from weeks to months or years. In symptom-free intervals, the glands may be clinically unremarkable or slightly indurated. Usually, salivation is present, and the sodium content of the saliva is increased. As the inflammatory episodes increase, the salivation becomes more and more prominent, thus favoring the progress of the inflammatory process.

Chronic recurrent parotitis in children is distinguished from that in adults only by its prognosis. Chronic recurrent parotitis in children very often resolves spontaneously at puberty. Treatment must thus be as conservative as possible for as long as possible.

Treatment is usually easy, based on the typical history and findings on palpation. Sialogram usually shows impressive and typical findings: diffuse spherical ectasia and stenosis. In many cases, a large dilation of the duct predominates (Diamant & Forsberg 1959, Becker et al 1960). The duct ectasia may be regarded as the end stage of the results of the inflammatory process spreading throughout the gland. The duct ectasia causes an appearance like a string of pearls on the sialogram due to alternating dilation and narrowing of the duct system. The most certain diagnostic method is a biopsy, but this is usually superfluous because of the typical clinical findings.

Macroscopically, the glandular tissue is indurated and shows coarsening of the lobular structure. The regional intra- or periglandular lymph nodes may be enlarged.

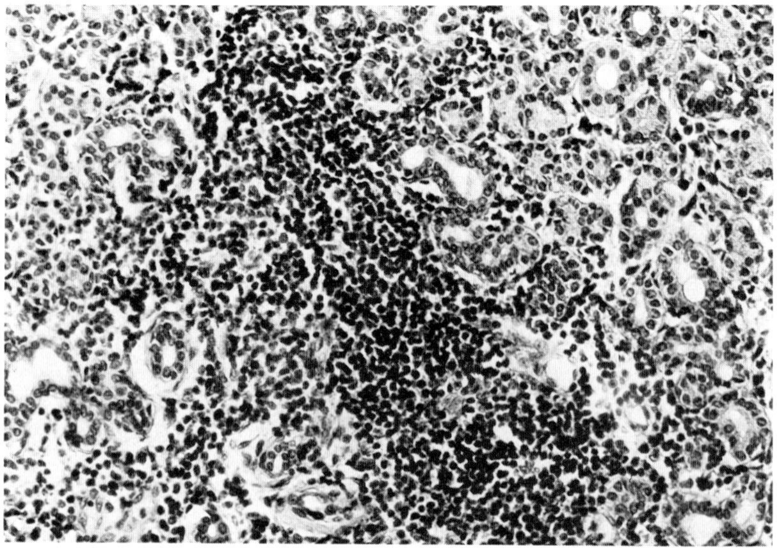

Figure 12.**8** Chronic recurrent parotitis showing focal interstitial lymphocytic infiltration. H & E, 160×.

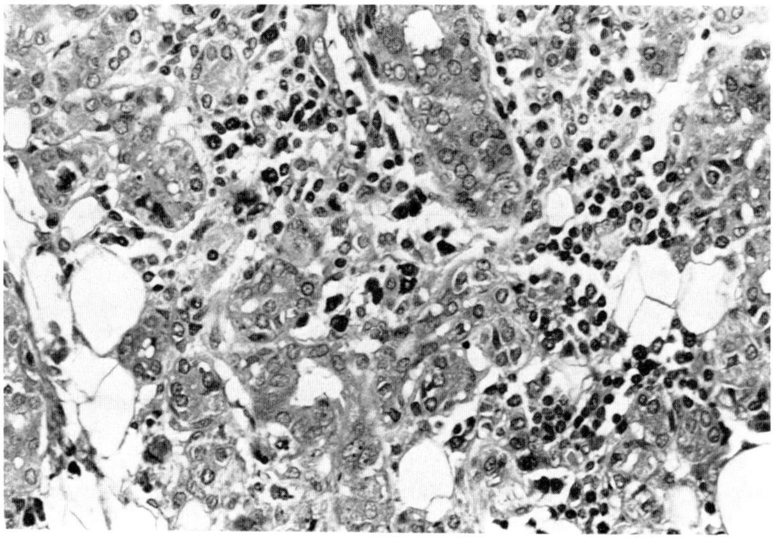

Figure 12.**9** Demonstration of IgA-forming plasma cells in the interstitium in chronic parotitis. Immunoperoxidase, 400×.

Histologic examination (Figs. 12.**8**–12.**10**) demonstrates a varying expression of the inflammatory process, depending on the length of history of the disease and the presence of infection at the time the tissue is harvested (Donath & Gundlach 1979, Steinbach & Strohm 1952). The *early stages* are characterized mainly by ductal lesions, including a modest dilation of the lumen of the intercalated and striated ducts and interlobular ducts. The duct lumen contains inspissated mucous secretion and desquamated duct epithelium, but only rarely inflammatory cells. The periductal connective tissue is expanded by edema and suffused by occasional lymphocytes. The acini are swollen and the acinar cells filled with secretory granules. In the *later stages,* the periductal inflammatory reaction increases, recognizable by marked connective tissue fibrosis and cellular infiltration with lymphocytes, histiocytes, and mast cells. The duct lumen is wider in the proximal part and is accompanied by degenerative changes of the duct epithelium.

In the *advanced stages* (Figs. 12.**11a, b,** 12.**12a, b**), the lobular structure is more and more destroyed, although the severity of the lesions in the individual lobules varies considerably. The volume of secreting gland parenchymal tissue is progressively reduced and replaced by proliferation of interstitial fatty and connective tissues. Duct proliferations develop from the terminal ducts and they may be so well developed on individual lobules that the atrophic lobule consists solely of ductal proliferations and connective and fatty tissues. The duct system shows particularly marked changes. Increased mitoses are found in

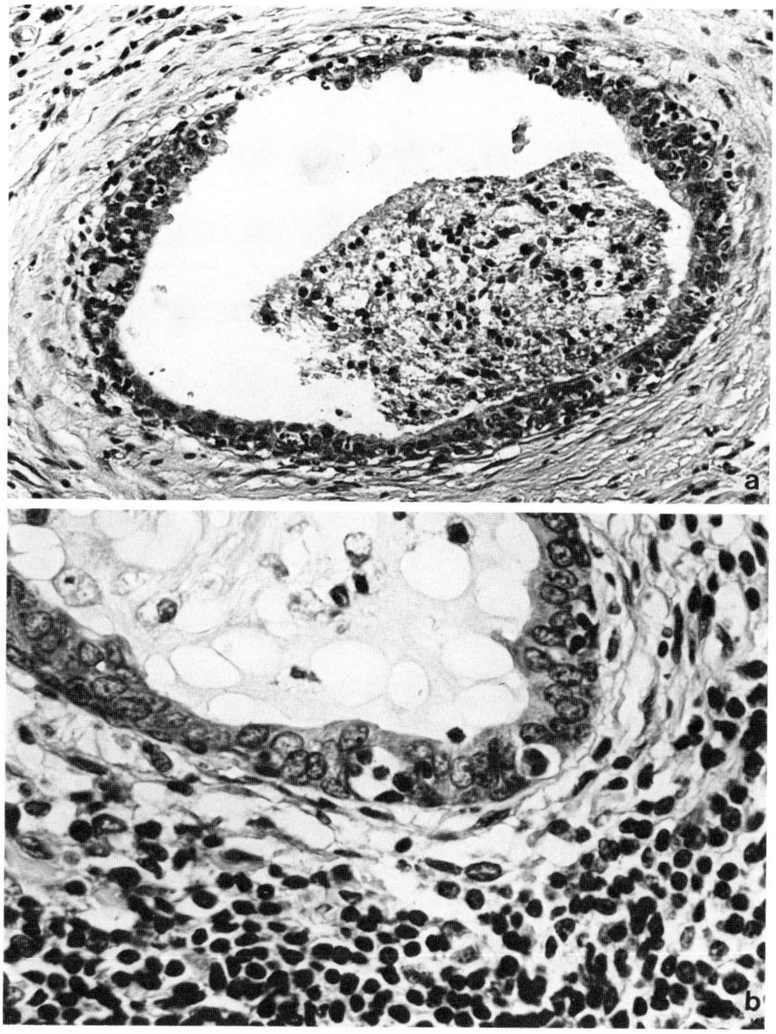

Figure 12.**10** Chronic recurrent parotitis. **a** Circumscribed ductal dilation with mucous secretion and desquamated epithelium. **b** Multilayered ductal epithelium with basal epithelial regeneration and periductal lymphocytic infiltration. H & E. **a** 160×, **b** 400×.

the terminal ducts, and the epithelium of the striated ducts is replaced by undifferentiated duct cells and myoepithelial cells. Epithelial metaplasia and dysplastic epithelial regeneration complement these changes.

Chronic sialectatic parotitis shows a particularly characteristic picture (Figs. 12.**13**–12.**16**). The spherical duct ectasia is encircled by dense lymphocytic infiltrate and newly formed lymphoid follicles. The duct epithelium shows metaplasia and is heavily infiltrated by lymphocytes. The periductal lymph follicles demonstrate degenerative changes with hyaline transformation. Occasional islands of myoepithelial cells underline the significance of immunologic factors in the late stage of the inflammation. A richly inspissated secretion blending with larger flakes of secretion and microliths are found in the duct lumen.

The duct ectasia, parenchymal atrophy, and retention of secretions in the duct lumen found in chronic recurrent parotitis resembles the findings after experimental ligature of the duct (Donath et al 1973). This is evidence that abnormal formation and transport of secretion play an important role in the pathogenesis of chronic recurrent parotitis and demonstrates that there are parallels to obstructive electrolyte siadalenitis. The marked lymphocytic periductal inflammatory reaction in the later stages, the occasional islands of myoepithelial cells, and the occasional associated ductal lesions indicate that immunologic reactions complement the inflammatory process. The pathogenesis of the disease is thus multifactorial.

The electron microscopic findings in chronic recurrent parotitis in children are of interest with respect to the multifactorial pathogenesis of the disease (Takeda 1982). Tubuloreticular structures with a diameter of 15–25 nm were observed in the perinuclear cytoplasm of endothelial cells of the

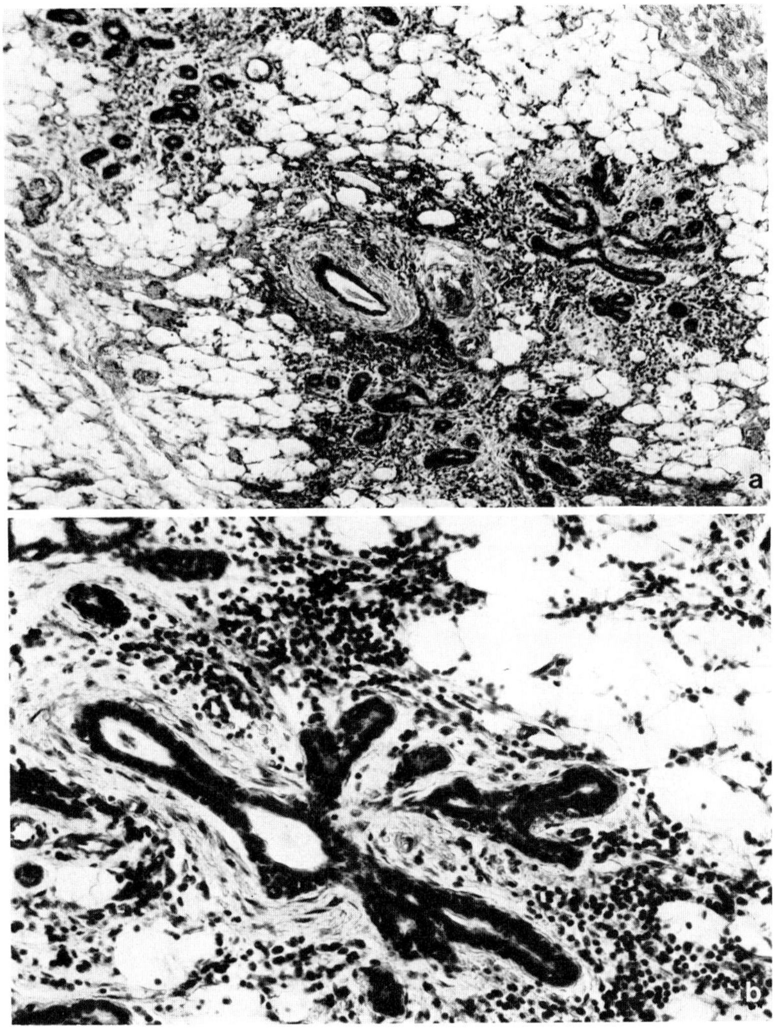

Figure 12.**11** Late phase of a chronic recurrent parotitis showing destruction of the lobular architecture, disappearance of the acini, and ductular proliferation. H & E. **a** 63×, **b** 160×.

parotid gland. These microtubular structures obviously arise from the endoplasmic reticulum and could represent incomplete expression of a virus infection.

The range of **therapeutic procedures** extends from conservative methods via partial surgery to total parotidectomy. Appropriate antibiotics should always be the first line of attack, and they are often successful, particularly in the early stage of the disease. However, recurrent episodes of inflammation can only be controlled by a reduction of secreting parenchyma; therefore appropriate measures, such as radiation therapy, must be taken (Glasenapp et al 1970). A superficial dose of 600 rad produced a favorable effect (Glasenapp et al 1970), although scanning demonstrated no reduction of salivary tissue after exposure to irradiation. In most cases the benefit of irradiation is short lived.

Several *surgical procedures* are available, with the common goal of elimination of the pathogenic role of the ductal system. These procedures include ligature of the parotid duct or occlusion of the duct system with amino acid solution. *Ligature of the parotid duct* has been recommended by many investigators (Diamant 1958, Diamant & Enfors 1965, Sazama 1969, Morgan 1973, Garvar & Kringstein 1974, Steinbach 1976, Münzel & Meister 1977). These methods carry the danger of damming up the saliva, leading to slipping of the ligature if functioning salivary tissue remains. Some investigators therefore recommended complementary radiation therapy in doses of 5–12 Gy (Diamant 1974, Münzel & Meister 1977). Animal experiments have shown that it is feasible to eliminate the secretion of saliva by the injection of amino acid solution into the duct system of the parotid as an alternative to ligature of the duct (Rettinger et al 1981 and 1983, Schröder et al

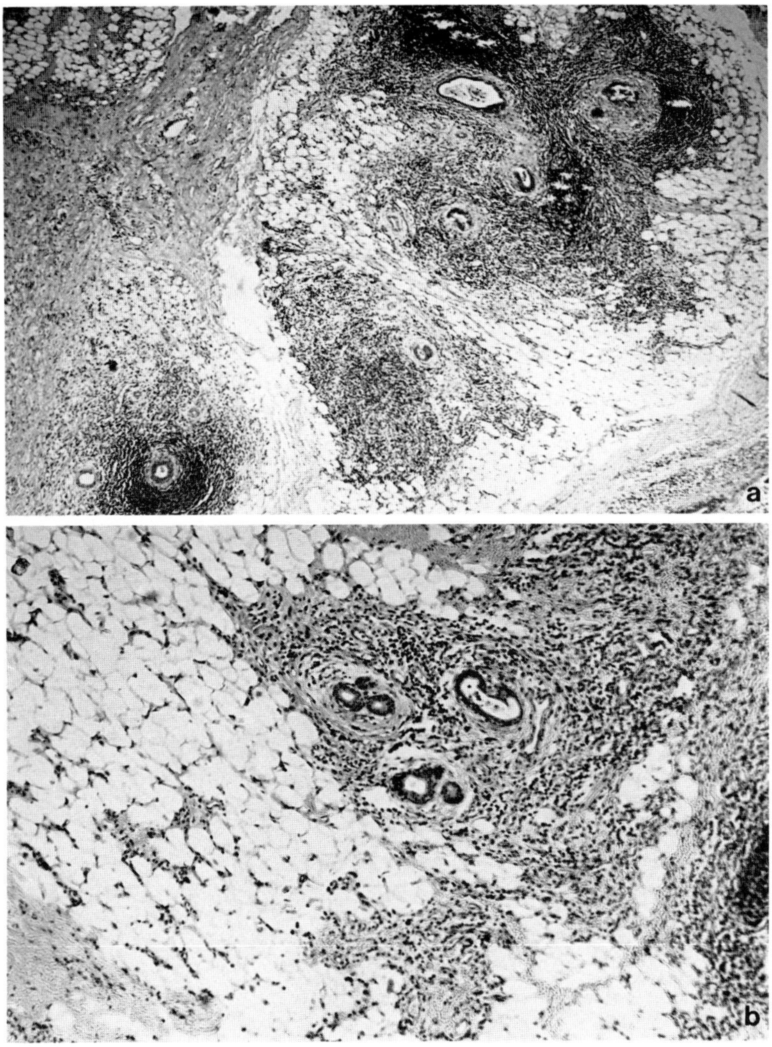

Figure 12.**12** End stage of a chronic recurrent parotitis showing shrunken gland remnants with irregular arrangement of duct structures and replacement of the glandular tissue by connective tissue, fatty tissue, and inflammatory infiltrate. H & E. **a** 25×, **b** 63×.

1982). The researchers maintain that this procedure is as easy to perform as sialography. Filling of the duct can be repeated if atrophy of the gland is incomplete. The occlusion method requires further experimental investigation because of the possible late damage: long-term clinical observations are also necessary to define the place of this method.

Opinions differ about the value of denervation of the parotid by stripping of the tympanic plexus, combined on occasion with division of the chorda tympani (Chilla 1981). The principle of the procedure was described as early as 1914 by the French surgeon Leriche. He divided the auriculotemporal nerve in a patient with multiple salivary fistulas, thus blocking the parasympathetic innervation. The technical difficulties of the extratemporal procedure have been solved by transtympanic neurectomy in which the tympanic branch of the vagus nerve and the chorda tympani are divided. This procedure rests on the following anatomic principles: the parasympathetic fibers of the XIth cranial nerve leave the inferior salivatory nucleus as Jacobson's nerve, follow the glossopharyngeal nerve, and then pass between the jugular bulb and the carotid canal to enter the middle ear. Initially, the nerve runs vertically on the medial wall of the middle ear and often gives off a branch in the hypotympanon. The further course of the nerve is via the superficial petrosal nerve where the preganglionic segment ends in the otic ganglion. The postganglionic fibers reach the parotid gland via the auriculotemporal nerve. Supplementary division of the chorda tympani is based on several clinical reports that have shown that the secretory capacity of the parotid gland is reduced by 30–50% by division of this nerve.

Our experiences have not encouraged us to attempt to popularize this procedure, because we were not convinced that this operation modified

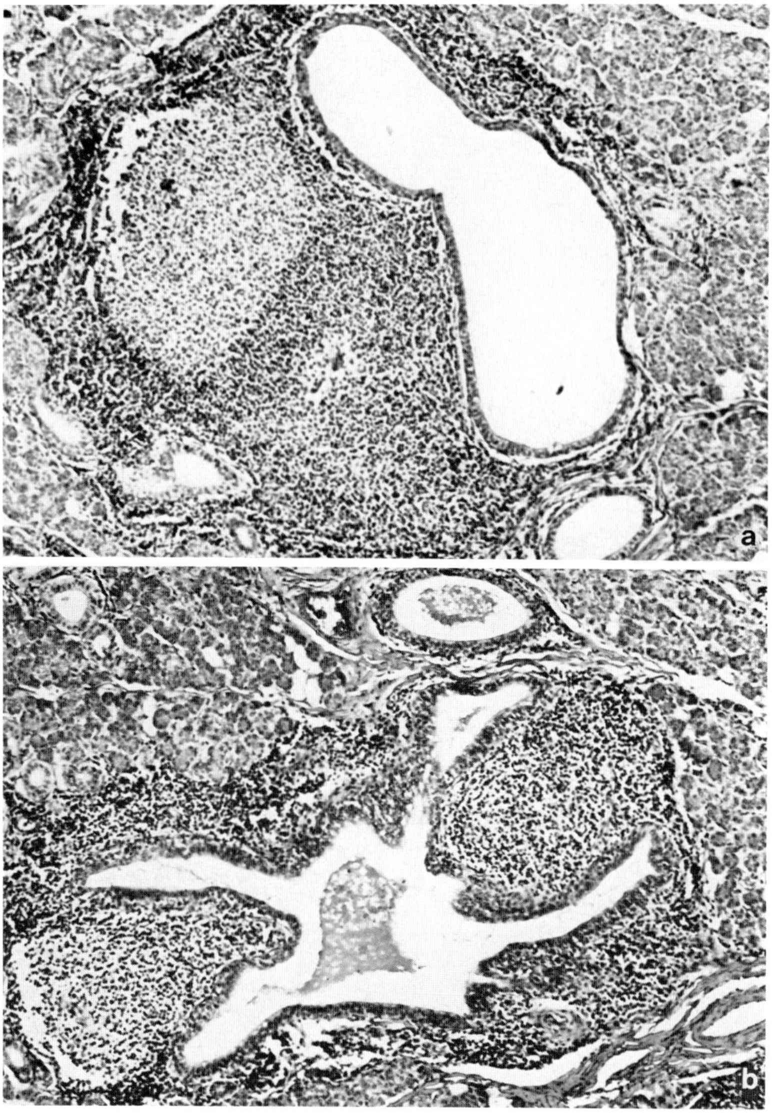

Figure 12.**13** Chronic sialectatic parotitis: **a** Ectatic duct with periductal lymphocytic infiltration and inclusion of an active lymphoid follicle. **b** Dilated salivary duct with fingerlike projections surrounded by lymphoid follicles. H & E. **a** and **b** 63×.

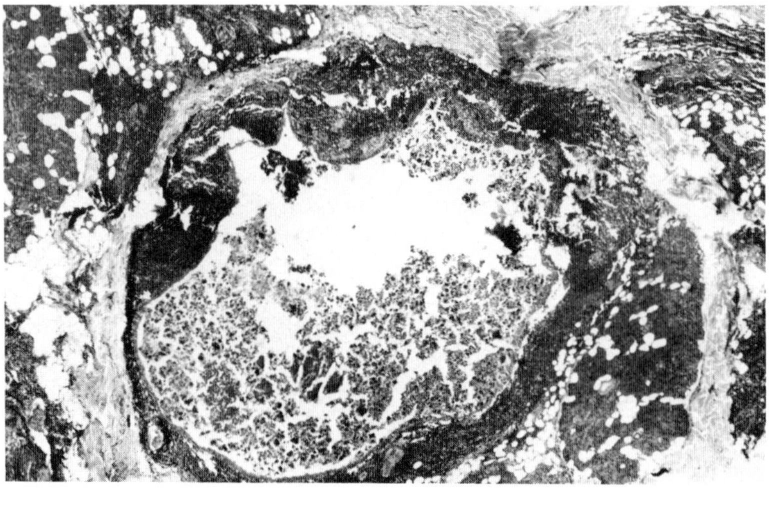

Figure 12.**14** Chronic sialectatic parotitis showing spherical sialectasis with purulent content. H & E, 25×.

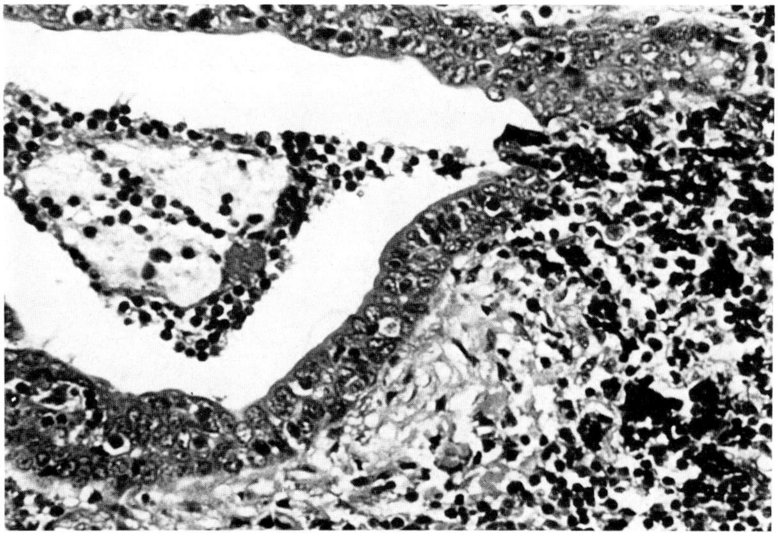

Figure 12.**15** Chronic sialectatic parotitis showing metaplastic duct epithelium, secretion, and desquamated cells in the duct lumen, periductal sclerosis, and inflammatory infiltrate. H & E, 400×.

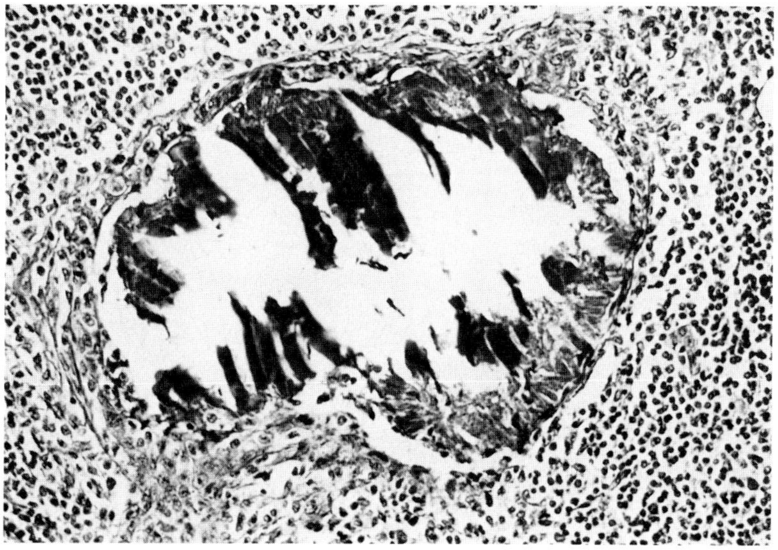

Figure 12.**16** Chronic sialectatic parotitis showing calcified flakes of secretion with occlusion of a duct, duct epithelial metaplasia, and periductal inflammatory infiltrate. PAS, 160×.

the course of chronic recurrent parotitis. Münzel and Meister (1977) also expressed reservations about the efficacy of parasympathetic denervation of the parotid gland, but Allam (1975) reported encouraging results.

If all other measures fail, the only recourse is a total parotidectomy. The operation is very demanding in this disease, since the fibers of the facial nerve adhere closely to the chronically inflammed salivary tissue (Chilla et al 1982). The success rate of parotidectomy could possibly be improved by combination with other procedures, such as ductal occlusion, although complete elimination of active secretory gland tissue is the basic determinant of the success of this procedure.

Tuberculosis of the Salivary Glands

Tuberculosis almost always affects the intra- and periglandular lymph nodes in the parotid gland, whereas invasion of the parenchyma itself is only rarely seen. Preoperative diagnosis in the absence of calcification of the nodes on radiography is very difficult, if not impossible, in most cases. It is often impossible to distinguish this disease from a true neoplasm, so that operation should be recommended in every case, if dissemination from a lung focus is not present. The extent of the procedure ranges from removal of an individual lymph node to total parotidectomy. The place of antituberculous treatment must then be discussed. Surgery prevents extension of the disease to the surrounding tissue, and often the development of a very obstinate fistula. The disease affects the

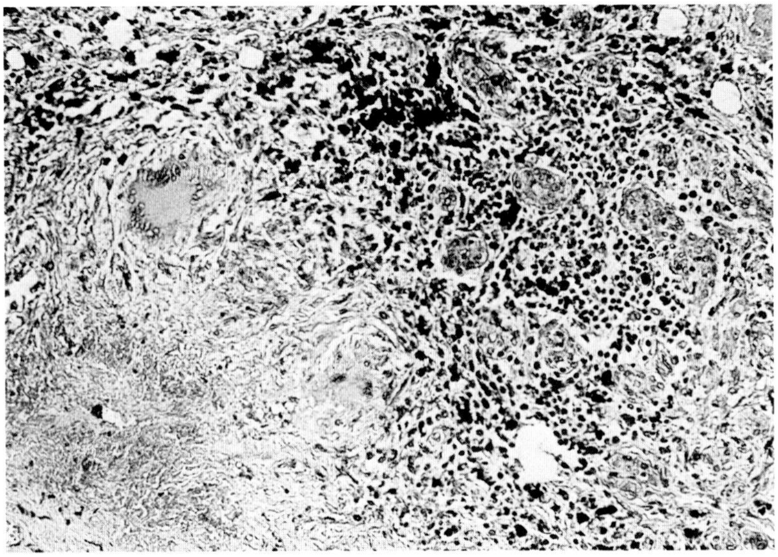

Figure 12.**17** Tuberculosis of the parotid gland showing a tuberculous granuloma with Langhans' giant cell (left) surrounded by IgA-forming plasma cells and lymphocytes. Immunoperoxidase, 160×.

parotid gland in 75% of cases and the submandibular gland in 25% (Becker 1963).

Tuberculosis of salivary tissue must be distinguished from those infections arising from intra- or periglandular lymph nodes and that then invade the salivary tissue secondarily. Parenchymatous tuberculosis is seldom seen in the parotid or submandibular glands, but then follows primary tuberculosis with a lymphatic or hematogenous spread. In the productive form (Fig. 12.**17**), granulomas of varying sizes are found within the lobules, consisting of epithelioid cells, lymphocytes, and Langhans'-type giant cells. The even rarer caseating form is accompanied by large necrotic areas, advanced destruction of parenchyma, and the formation of fistulas. Productive parenchymatous tuberculosis must be distinguished from sarcoid, with its epithelioid cell sialadenitis. *Intra- or periglandular lymph node tuberculosis* ist much more common than parenchymatous tuberculosis. The Salivary Gland Register (1965–1981) contains only two cases of parenchymatous tuberculosis of the parotid gland, but 46 of intra- or periglandular lymph node tuberculosis. 26 affecting the parotid and 20 the submandibular gland. The infection usually has a lymphatic origin and its course may be productive or exudative-caseating. If the tuberculosis remains confined to the lymph nodes, the lymphadenopathy may compress the duct system, leading to a focal obstructive nonspecific sialadenitis.The mixed picture of parenchymatous and lymph node tuberculosis arises, if the lymph node capsule ruptures.

Tuberculous sialadenitis of the minor salivary glands is occasionally observed in the course of oral mucosal tuberculosis or lupus vulgaris and affects the glands of the lip and palate especially.

Other Bacterial Inflammations

Other specific diseases of the salivary glands are rare. Syphilis and gonorrhea may cause inflammation of the parotid gland characterized by bilateral involvement and an almost entirely painless swelling. The diagnosis rests on serologic investigations.

In the older literature, actinomycosis was mentioned, but it, too, is now very rare. It mainly affects the minor salivary glands and may spread in two ways: an ascending infection via the ducts or by penetration of the inflammatory process into the parenchyma of the gland. The latter route appears to be the more frequent. The clinical picture consists of the well-known boardlike infiltration of the soft tissues of the cheek, characterized by lack of pain, but by discoloration of the skin and fistulas (Schuchardt 1959, Seifert 1971).

The **histopathologic picture** in syphilis and other specific disorders with cellular immune reactions is characterized by the formation of specific granulomas whose histologic appearance cannot be distinguished from that in other organs. The extreme rarity of these diseases is amply demonstrated by the fact that not a single case of syphilis, actinomycosis, or other specific infections of the salivary glands was observed in the 8000 cases in the salivary gland register seen between 1965 and 1982. The older literature contains individual reports of syphilis affecting the parotid gland especially, or actinomycosis of the submandibular gland (Seifert 1966, Haubrich 1976).

Of 58 patients operated on for chronic parotitis at the Goettingen ENT clinic, only one patient had syphilis (Chilla et al 1982).

References

Allam, A. F.: Transtympanic neurectomy in chronic recurrent parotid sialoadenitis. J. Laryng. 90 (1975) 405

Bach, H., G. Buttenberg: Zur postoperativen Parotitis. Münch. med. Wschr. 100 (1958) 532

Becker, W.: Erkrankungen der Speicheldrüsen einschließlich Tumoren, jedoch ausschließlich Fazialischirurgie. In Berendes, J., R. Link, F. Zöllner: Hals-Nasen-Ohren-Heilkunde, Bd. II/1. Thieme, Stuttgart 1963

Becker, W., J. Matzker, J. Ruckes: Zur Morphologie der „diffusen, kugelförmigen Gangektasien" in der Glandula Parotis. Z. Laryng. Rhinol. 39 (1960) 479

Chilla, R.: Vegetative Hirnnervenstrukturen. Arch. Oto-Rhino-Laryngol. 231 (1981) 353

Chilla, R., H.-O. Meyfarth, C. Arglebe: Über die operative Behandlung der chronischen Ohrspeicheldrüsenentzündung. Arch. Oto-Rhino-Laryngol. 234 (1982) 53

Diamant, H.: Ligation of the parotid duct in chronic recurrent parotitis. Acta Otolaryngol. (Stockh.) 49 (1958) 375

Diamant, H., B. Enfors: Treatment of chronic recurrent parotitis. Laryngoscope 75 (1965) 153

Diamant, H., A. Forsberg: La sialographie: méthode d'investigation de la glande parotide. Rev. Laryng. (Bordeaux) 80 (1959) 957

Donath, K., K. K. H. Gundlach: Ein Beitrag zur Ätiologie und Pathogenese der chronisch-rezidivierenden Parotitis. Dtsch. zahnärztl. Z. 34 (1979) 45

Donath, K., H.-U. Hirsch-Hoffmann, G. Seifert: Zur Pathogenese der Parotisatrophie nach experimenteller Gangunterbindung. Ultrastrukturelle Befunde am Drüsenparenchym der Rattenparotis. Virchows Arch. Abt. A 359 (1973) 31

Forell, M. M.: Aktivierung und Inaktivierung pathologischer Fermente des Pankreas und ihre klinische Bedeutung. Dtsch. med. Wschr. 86 (1961) 981

Glasenapp, G. B., L. Kessler, W. Schmidt, H. J. Otto: Zur Behandlung der chronisch-rezidivierenden Parotitis mit Röntgenbestrahlung unter szintigraphischer Kontrolle. Z. Laryng. Rhinol. 48 (1970) 520

Garvar, L. R., G. J. Kringstein: Recurrent parotitis in childhood. J. Oral. Surg. 32 (1974) 373

Haubrich, J.: Klinik der nichttumorbedingten Erkrankungen der Speicheldrüsen. Arch. Oto-Rhino-Laryng. 213 (1976) 1

Karst, W.: Über die Behandlung der postoperativen Parotitis. Chirurg 26 (1955) 319

Köster, H.: Die Behandlung der postoperativen Parotitis mit Novocaininfiltrationen des Ganglion stellatum. Med. Klin. 56 (1961) 1319

Leriche, R.: Behandlung der permanenten Parotisfistel durch die Entnervung der Speicheldrüse. Zbl. Chir. 41 (1914) 754

Mathis, H.: Die Erkrankungen der Speicheldrüsen. Hanser, München 1954

Morgan, W. R.: Parotid duct ligation and tympanic neurectomy. Arch. Otolaryng. 98 (1973) 179

Münzel, M., P. Meister: Zur Ligatur des Stenonschen Ganges bei der chronisch-rezidivierenden Parotitis. Z. Laryng. Rhinol. 56 (1977) 902

Rettinger, G., M. Stolte, C. Bäumler: Ausschaltung von Speicheldrüsen durch temporäre Okklusion des Gangsystems mit einer Aminosäurenlösung. Tierexperimentelle Studie zu einem neuen Therapieverfahren. HNO (Berl.) 29 (1981) 294

Sazama, L.: Considérations sur la pathogénice et le traitement de la parotidite recidivante de l'enfant. Rev. Stomatol. 69 (1969) 309

Schröder, M., R. Chilla, C. Arglebe, M. Droese: Occlusion of Stenon's duct by prolamine: a possible treatment of chronic parotitis? Preliminary experience from animal experiments. ORL 44 (1982) 1

Schuchardt, K.: Spezifische Infektionen im Gesichts-Kieferbereich. In: Die Zahn-, Mund- u. Kieferheilkunde. Wiss. Handbuch für die zahnärztliche Praxis, Bd. III/2. Urban & Schwarzenberg, München 1959

Seemann, N.: Pathohistologische Untersuchungen zur Häufigkeit der Sialolithiasis und Sialadenitis der Parotis. HNO 17 (1969) 3

Seifert, G.: Mundhöhle, Mundspeicheldrüsen, Tonsillen und Rachen. In Doerr, W., E. Uehlinger: Spezielle pathologische Anatomie, Bd. 1. Springer, Berlin 1966 (S. 1)

Seifert, G.: Klinische Pathologie der Sialadenitis und Sialadenose. HNO 19 (1971) 1

Steinbach, E.: Zur chirurgischen Behandlung der chronisch-rezidivierenden Parotitis. Arch. Oto-Rhino-Laryng. 213 (1976) 389

Steinbach, E., M. Strohm: Zur Pathogenese der chronisch-rezidivierenden sialektatischen Parotitis. Z. Laryng. Rhinol. 61 (1982) 66

Takeda, Y.: Tubuloreticular structures in chronic recurrent parotitis in childhood. Japn. J. oral Biol. 24 (1982) 1027

Thörner, H. J.: Die postoperative Parotitis. Neue Behandlungswege mit dem Ferment-Inaktivator Trasylol. Chirurg 43 (1963) 195

Virus Sialadenitis

Virus diseases of the salivary glands are due to a viral infection of the gland tissue (Seifert 1984).

Viruses and the Salivary Glands

Viruses may affect the salivary tissue in five different ways (Table 12.**3**).

Primary viral absorption via the saliva appears to be exceedingly unlikely, both from clinical obser-

Table 12.**3** Viruses and the Salivary Glands

Primary viral infection via the saliva
Secondary excretion of virus in the saliva
Viral transmission in viremia without infection of the salivary glands
Viruses in the saliva that act as a source of infection
Poliomyelitis
Hepatitis
Rabies
Rubella
Viral influenza
Viral sialadenitis
Viruses with sialadenotropism
Epidemic parotitis
Cytomegalovirus
Concomitant viral sialadenitis
Coxsackievirus infection
Infectious mononucleosis
Measles
Whooping cough
Encephalomyocarditis virus infection
ECHO virus infection
Latent viruses in the salivary glands
Cytomegalovirus
Epstein-Barr virus
Oncogenic viruses
Virus-induced salivary tumors
Polyoma virus
Adeno virus
Simian virus 40
Virusassociated salivary tumors
Epstein-Barr virus

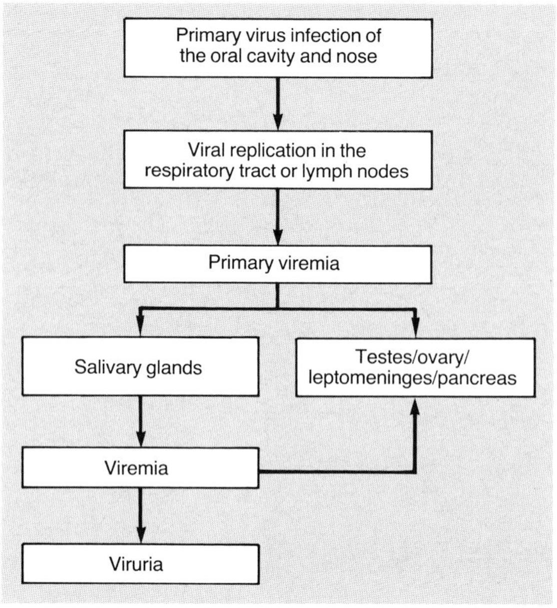

Figure 12.**18** Diagram of mumps infection

vations and experimental findings. The immune system of the salivary glands protects the glands from invasion, if the salivary secretion is normal: secretory immunoglobulin A (IgA) in particular neutralizes viruses (Caselitz & Seifert 1982).

Secondary excretion of viruses in the saliva has been demonstrated for numerous viruses, including both the typical sialotropic virus infections (epidemic parotitis, cytomegalovirus) and other viral diseases without sialadenotropism. The virus reaches the salivary glands via the bloodstream and is excreted in the saliva after simple viral passage without producing sialadenitis. The excreted saliva then constitutes a source of infection. Examples of virus passage through the saliva are poliomyelitis, hepatitis, rabies, rubella, and virus influenza (Berger 1959, 1960, Seifert 1966).

Viral sialadenitis is caused by the viremia of a sialadenotropic virus leading to a virus induced inflammatory reaction by a local cytopathogenic effect. Typical forms of viral sialadenitis include epidemic parotitis (mumps) and the cytomegalovirus. Several other viral infections, such as infective mononucleosis, encephalomyocarditis, measles, whooping cough, lymphocytic choriomeningitis, and diseases caused by coxsackievirus and ECHO viruses, may be accompanied by viral sialadenitis. Usually, the lesions can only be demonstrated in experimental animals but have also occasionally been recorded clinically (Seifert 1966, Brill & Gilfillan 1977, Cullen & Baublis 1980, Mor et al 1982).

It is assumed that there is a viral latency in the salivary glands for cytomegalovirus and Epstein-Barr virus (Niederman et al 1976, Morgan et al 1979, Wolf et al 1981, Wilmes & Wolf 1981). Viral latency is defined as a condition in which there are no acute or persistent symptoms of a viral infection and an infective virus cannot be demonstrated, but virus-dependent factors, such as virus DNA and viral-specific antigens or antibodies, can be demonstrated. It has so far not been clearly defined which tissues or cells in the salivary glands constitute the virus reservoir and which factors form the virus latency. The significance of a latent virus is that it may be reactivated leading to viremia, if the immunologic environment changes. The parotid gland may form a reservoir for the site of replication for the Epstein-Barr virus (Wolf et al 1981). The Epstein-Barr virus genome has been demonstrated by nucleic acid hybridization in situ and by kinetic analysis. Whether the virus is a transitory phenomenon or whether it has a place in the cause of undifferentiated parotid carcinoma remains undecided (see pages 267 and 273).

Several *oncogenic viruses* can cause virus-induced or virus-associated salivary gland tumors (see page 276).

Epidemic Parotitis (Mumps)

Epidemic parotitis is caused by a paramyxovirus, the mumps virus. The term "epidemic parotitis" is unfortunate: it is true that in most cases the parotid gland is involved, but mumps may also affect other organs, such as the pancreas, the gonads, and the central nervous system, without affecting the parotid glands.

The mumps virus is transmitted by droplet infection in saliva. The *mode of infection* (Fig. 12.**18**) is characterized by a primary viral infection of the oral and nasal cavity accompanied by a multiplication of the virus in the upper respiratory tract and the regional lymph nodes. The resulting viremia leads to a hematogenous infection of the salivary glands, and sometimes of other glands, such as the testes or ovary, the leptomeninges, and the pancreas. Renewed viremia and viruria may occur late in the disease. The saliva remains infective for up to 6 weeks, even in clinically silent infection. Mumps is most prevalent between the ages of 2 and 14 years. Newborn children are usually protected in the first few months of life by maternal antibodies transmitted across the placenta. Protection in this way is very common, since the infection rate with the mumps virus is very high, attaining 90% by the age of 14 years in Germany.

About 50% of all mumps infections are clinically silent. In the other cases, various prodromal features, such as pain in the head and neck and mild fever, appear after an incubation period of about 18 days. Inflammatory swelling of one parotid gland is followed within hours or days by swelling of the other gland in 75% of cases. The characteristic boggy tender swelling is often accompanied by edema, causing swelling of the eyelids and narrowing of the external auditory meatus. Trismus often occurs also. The parotitis dominates the clinical picture for 1 to 2 weeks and is accompanied by slight to moderate fever. The other salivary glands may also be inflamed at this time, and then inflammation of other organs, such as the pancreas, the gonads, the breast, and the central nervous system, often follows. However, these diseases may often precede the parotitis, which may indeed be absent altogether. The infection endows the patient with lifelong immunity.

Mumps carries two dangerous complications: After puberty mumps is accompanied in 10–30% of cases by *orchitis*, leading almost always to sterility if both testes are affected. In contrast, the ovary is seldom infected.

Infection of the *central nervous system* is much more common than previously thought, although it is often clinically silent. The infection is usually a serous meningoencephalitis whose symptoms are usually slight, but can on occasion be intense. Cranial nerve paralyses may occur, particularly of the VIIIth nerve leading to persistent deafness. Fortunately, usually only one nerve is affected.

The clinical **diagnosis** may be confirmed by the complement-binding reaction. An increase of antibody titer by at least fourfold compared with initial values is required to substantiate the diagnosis. Initial *leukopenia* is often found, and the serum amylase is often increased. Differentiation of isoamylases shows that this increase is due to salivary isoamylase and is usually found in acute inflammation of the salivary glands (Fig. 12.**19**). An additional increase of pancreatic isoamylase indicates involvement of the pancreas (Škrha et al 1979).

The **histologic appearances** are those of an interstitial salivary inflammation affecting mainly the parotid gland (Figs. 12.**20**–12.**22**) and the submandibular and sublingual glands to a lesser extent. The interstitial infiltrate consists of lymphocytes and plasma cells permeating the periductal and periacinar interstitial tissue (Boström 1968, Henson et al 1971). This inflammatory infiltrate is accompanied by a dissolution of the serous acini and vacuolation of the ductal epithelium (Figs. 12.**23**, 12.**24**). The ducts contain increased mucous secretion. Several stages may be distinguished in the dissolution of the acinar cells. Initially there is swelling and vacuolation of the cytoplasm and later loss of the enzyme granules and pyknosis of nuclei. Comparison with animal experiments on mumps infection (Johnson & Goodpasture 1936) shows that the mumps virus has a cytopathogenic effect on the cell organelles of the acinar cell. These effects include dissolution of the endoplasmic reticulum and of the secretory granules and the formation of virus particles visible on light microscopy as small inclusion bodies. Similar interstitial inflammatory processes with lymphocytic and plasma cell infiltration can occur transitorily in the pancreas, testes, heart muscle, and other organs, such as leptomeninges and brain.

Figure 12.**19** Hyperamylasemia in acute parotitis with elevation of the salivary amylase (S). The pancreatic amylase (P) is unchanged. Normal findings are shown on the left and the findings in acute parotitis on the right.

Treatment of epidemic parotitis is restricted to symptomatic measures, such as the treatment of pain and reduction of fever. Gamma globulin may be used to protect from orchitis if the infection occurs during puberty. Administration of gamma globulin prevents infection of the second testis in unilateral orchitis. The use of corticosteroids in orchitis and central nervous system infections has been tried. Immunization in childhood is recommended because of the undesirable complications that the mumps virus may cause.

Cytomegalovirus

The *cytomegalovirus* is a DNA virus of the herpes group (Smith 1959, Hanshaw 1968). The polygo-

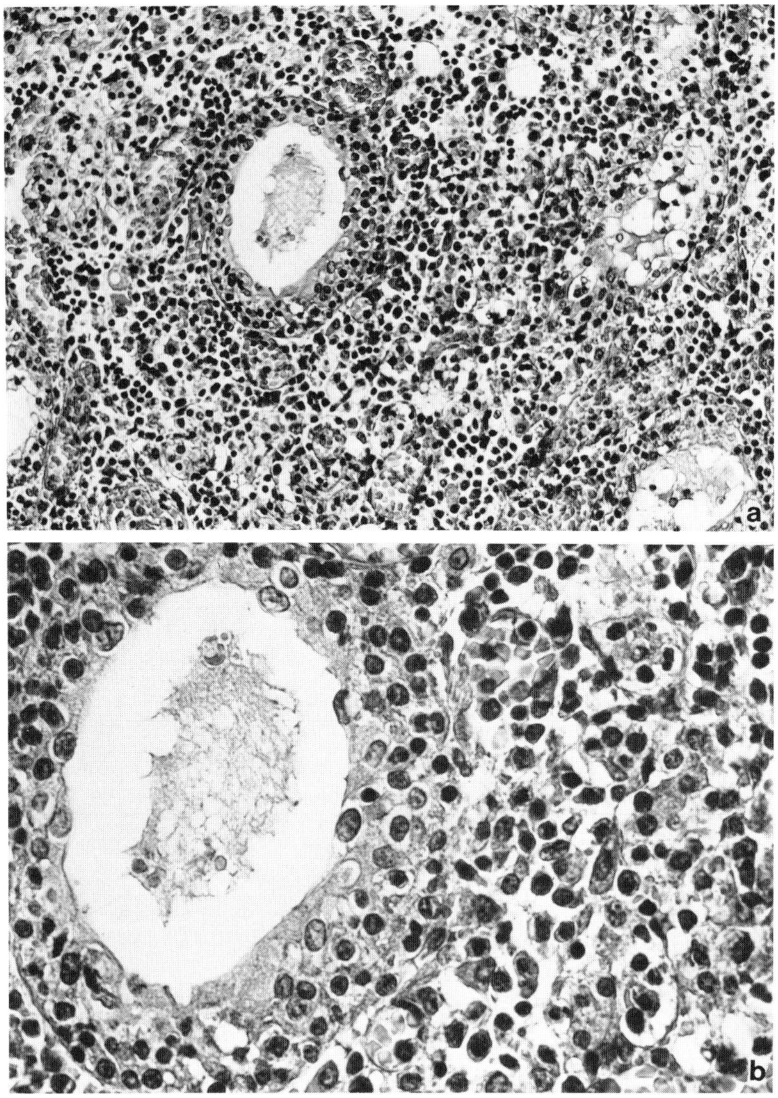

Figure 12.**20** Epidemic parotitis showing dense lymphocytic and plasma cell infiltration of the gland tissue. A duct is shown in the center of the figure. H & E. **a** 160×, **b** 400×.

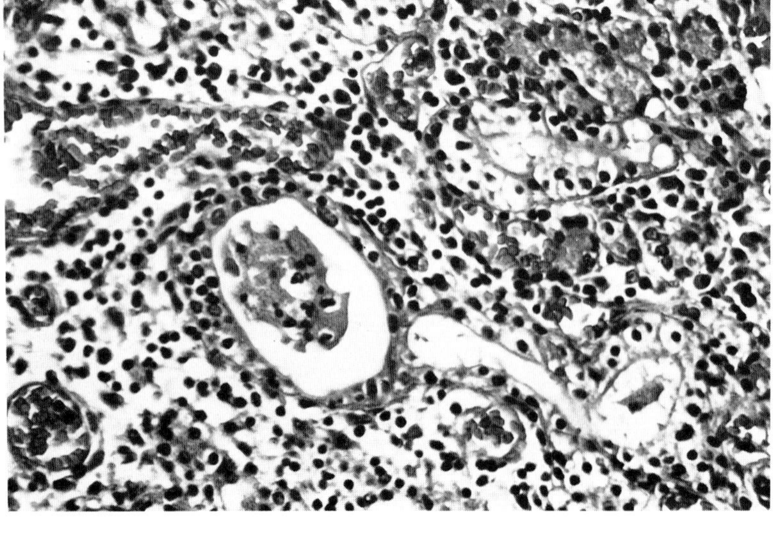

Figure 12.**21** Epidemic parotitis showing clumps of secretion and desquamated epithelium in the duct, and a periductal cell infiltrate. H & E, 250×.

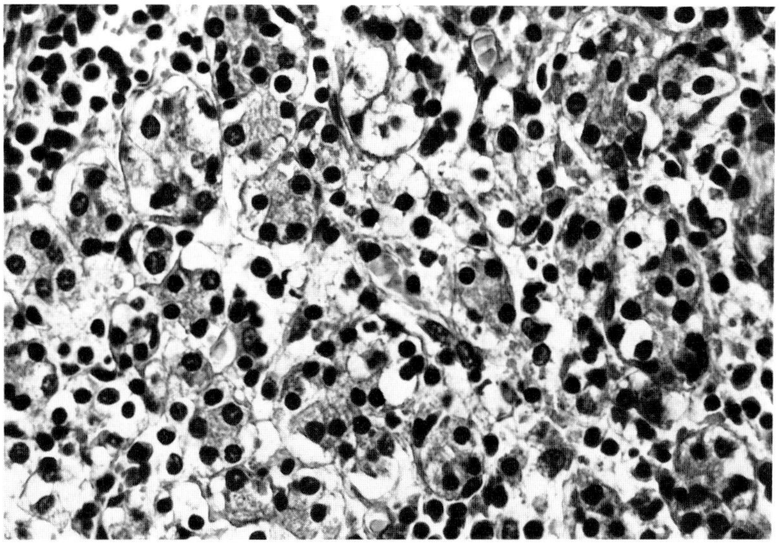

Figure 12.**22** Epidemic parotitis showing marked swelling of the acini, and interstitial edema with abundant plasma cells. H & E, 400×.

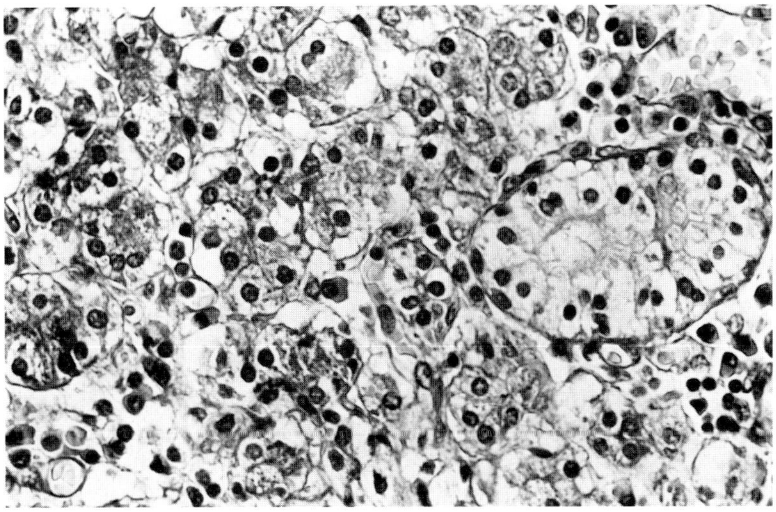

Figure 12.**23** Epidemic parotitis: vacuolar transformation of the ductal and acinar epithelium and disappearance of zymogen granules. PAS reaction, 400×.

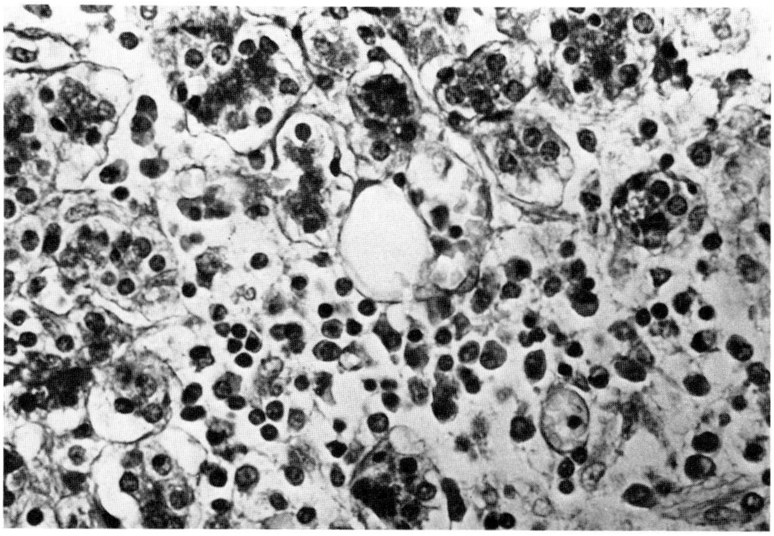

Figure 12.**24** Epidemic parotitis: extensive acinar necrosis and interstitial edema with abundant collections of plasma cells. H & E, 400×.

nal virus particles are 100–140 nm in size and consist of a virus nucleoid 60 nm in size surrounded by a capsid 20–30 nm in size with 162 capsomeres. The virus particles are enclosed by an external membrane and after extrusion into the cytoplasm are also enclosed by a nucleocapsid envelope. The cytopathogenic effect of the cytomegalovirus is characterized by formation of giant cells, including inclusion bodies in the cell nuclei and also inclusions in the cytoplasm (Seifert & Oehme 1957, Seifert 1973). The demonstration of cytomegalic cells is pathognomonic of cytomegalovirus disease.

The **clinical course** of cytomegalovirus infection depends on the patient's age (Krech et al 1971, Luthardt 1976). Prenatal congenital cytomegalovirus is transmitted across the placenta from the infected mother (Benirschke et al 1974). Transmission by infected cervical secretion (Wenckebach & Curry 1976) or mother's milk plays and important role in perinatal or early postnatal infection. Infection during adolescence and adulthood may be caused by infected urine or saliva and also by blood tranfusion, organ transplants, or chronic dialysis. *Prenatal cytomegalovirus disease* leads either to a localized clinically silent form or to a severe generalized form, depending on the severity of the infection and the immune status of the host (Table 12.**4**).

Generalized cytomegalovirus disease is characterized by lesions of the brain, the eyes, the internal organs, and the skeleton. The histologic diagnosis (Figs. 12.**25**–12.**27**) rests on the demonstration of typical giant cells and lymphocytic inflammation of numerous organs. The giant cells in the salivary glands arise from duct epithelium. They may also be demonstrated in the saliva after they have been desquamated into the duct lumen. The giant cells are 30 μm in size and contain a 15 μm cell nucleus displaced to the base of the cell, which contains a 10 μm nuclear inclusion body with a clear areola. The nuclear inclusion body is composed of granular nuclear chromatin and DNA virus particles. Granular cytoplasmic inclusions with a size of 1.5–3.0 μm consisting partly of virus particles and partly of cytoplasmic secretion products are found in the cytoplasm at the luminal cell pole.

Prenatal cytomegalovirus disease is 20 times more common than perinatal cytomegalovirus disease.

Adult cytomegalovirus disease (Table 12.**4**) is of considerable current importance. The infection may cause an illness resembling mononucleosis with episodes of fever, lymphadenopathy, thrombopenia, and leukopenia. Other forms include cytomegalovirus hepatitis (Henson et al 1974, myocarditis, or polyradiculitis (Guillain-Barré syndrome), an atypical bronchopneumonia, gastric or intestinal ulceration, and an exanthema.

Cytomegalovirus is being increasingly recorded in the adult (Nash 1982, Parham 1981, Press et all 1980, Strayer et al 1981), as a secondary phenomenon in patients with malignant tumors, such as carcinoma, lymphoma, and leukemia, after immunosuppression, blood transfusion, in the postperfusion syndrome, and after transplantations of the kidney, heart, liver, lungs, and the

Table 12.**4** Types of Cytomegalovirus

Prenatal Cytomegalovirus	Adult Cytomegalovirus
Generalized form	Cytomegalus mononucleosis
Cerebral lesions	Episodes of fever
Microcephalus	Lymphadenopathy
Internal hydrocephalus	Thrombocytopenia and leukopenia
Micro- and polygyria	Hepatitis
Intracranial calcification	Myocarditis
Encephalitis and ependymitis	Polyradiculitis
Eye lesions	Guillain-Barré syndrome
Chorioretinitis	Atypical bronchopneumonia
Microphthalmia	Gastric and intestinal ulceration
Optic atrophy	Exanthema
Visceral lesions	
Hemolytic disease of the newborn	
Hepatosplenomegaly	
Hepatitis, bile duct atresia	
Interstitial pneumonia	
Bone lesions	
Localized occult form	

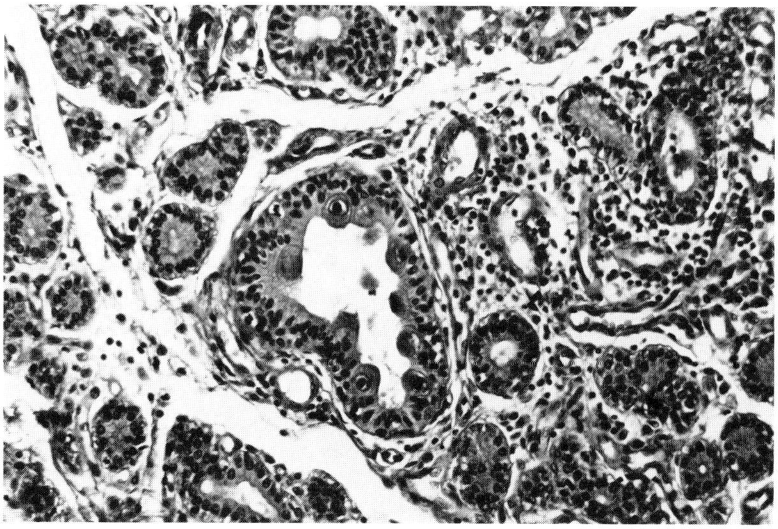

Figure 12.**25** Cytomegalo-virus of the parotid gland showing multiple giant cells with inclusion bodies in the region of the duct system and interstitial lymphocytic infiltration. H & E, 63×.

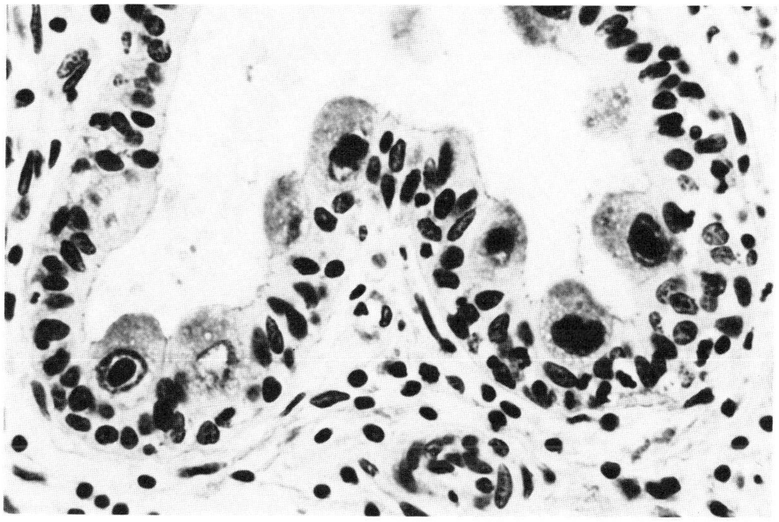

Figure 12.**26** Cytomegalo-virus infection of the parotid gland showing a duct with multiple mononuclear giant cells. Masson-Goldner, 400×.

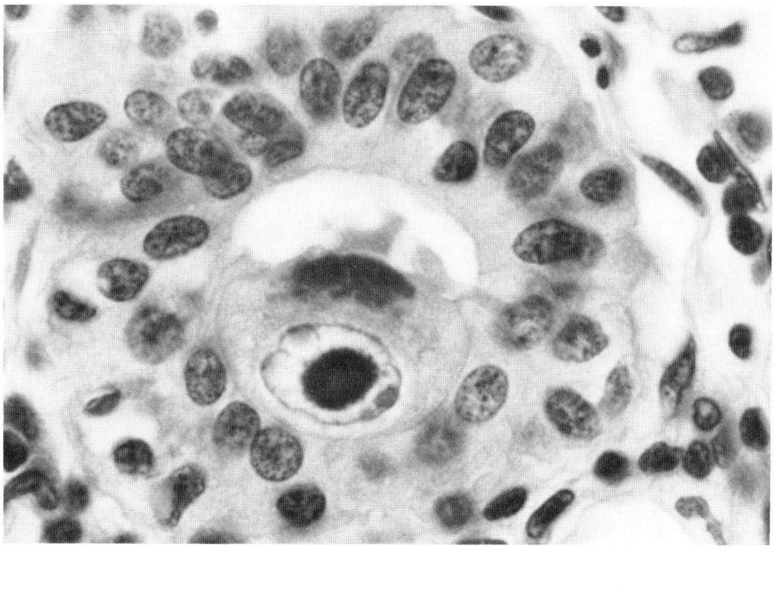

Figure 12.**27** Cytomegalo-virus of the parotid gland: owl eye cell with nuclear inclusion bodies, a clear areola with small particles on the nuclear membrane, and inclusion particles in the cytoplasm on the luminal cell pole. H & E, 600×.

bone marrow. In addition concomitant infection with other organisms, such as Pneumocystis carinii, toxoplasmosis, Klebsiella, Candida, aspergillosis, and Epstein-Barr virus, are observed (Table 12.**5**).

The **diagnosis** of cytomegalovirus rests on the demonstration of an increase of IgM antibody titer against cytomegalovirus to at least 1 : 64 (Heni et al 1976, Ziegelmaier et al 1979), the enzyme linked immunosorbent assay test (ELISA), an increase of complement binding reaction, a positive immunofluorescence test, the demonstration of virus in urine, saliva, or blood, and the demonstration of giant cells with typical cell nuclei and cytoplasmic inclusion bodies by cytologic or histologic examinations (Fig. 12.**28**).

Table 12.**5** Diseases Associated with Cytomegalovirus infection

Malignant tumors
Carcinoma
Lymphoma
Leukemia
Immunosuppressive therapy
Blood transfusion
Post perfusion syndrome
Organ transplantation
Kidneys
Heart
Liver
Lungs
Bone marrow
Double infection
Pneumocystis carinii
Toxoplasmosis
Klebsiella
Monilia
Aspergilosis
Epstein-Barr virus

The *pathogenic factors* of cytomegalovirus infection include productive infection by cells with immune function and the resulting prolonged cellular immunosuppression (Hamilton 1982, Papadimitrioú et al 1982). The productive infection affects leukocytes, lymphocytes, and macrophages. After the infection, the lymphocyte reactivity against bacterial antigens and mitogens is considerably reduced (Ten Napel & The 1980). This leads to an increased sensitivity to other infections, particularly in adults. Experimental cytomegalovirus interstitial pneumonia (Brody et al 1978) causes changes in the cell membrane, particularly disorders of cellular polarity, with an increase of intracellular pinocytic transport.

A *viral latency* may occur after the primary infection (Fig. 12.**29**). Numerous cell systems have been discussed as the possible reservoir for the latent virus, including the splenic B lymphocyte (Olding et al 1975), peritoneal macrophages (Brautigam et al 1979), cells of the salivary glands (Jordan 1978), and stromal cells of the ovaries or the testicular coat (Brautigam & Oldstone 1980). Certain *risk factors*, such as immune deficiency, pregnancy, malignant tumors, immunosuppressive agents, operations (mainly transplants), or chronic dialysis, may cause *reactivation*.

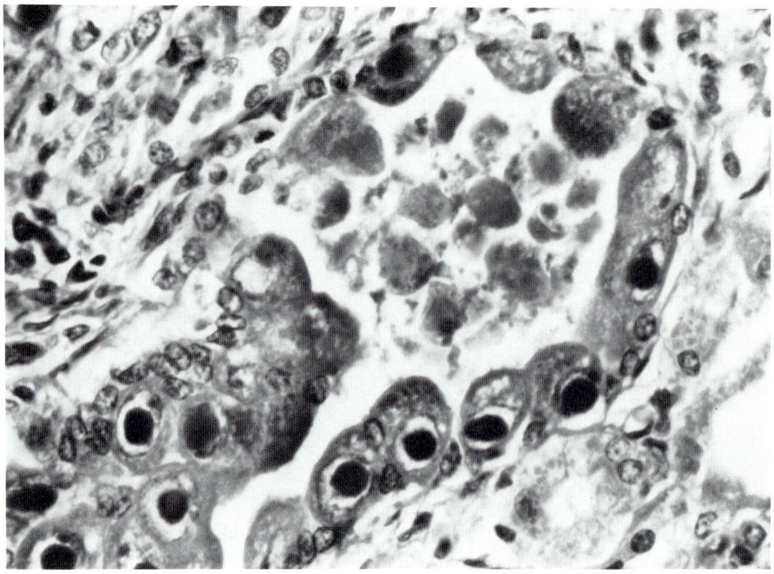

Figure 12.**28** Cytomegalo-virus of the kidneys: numerous giant cells around a renal tubule. H & E, 400×.

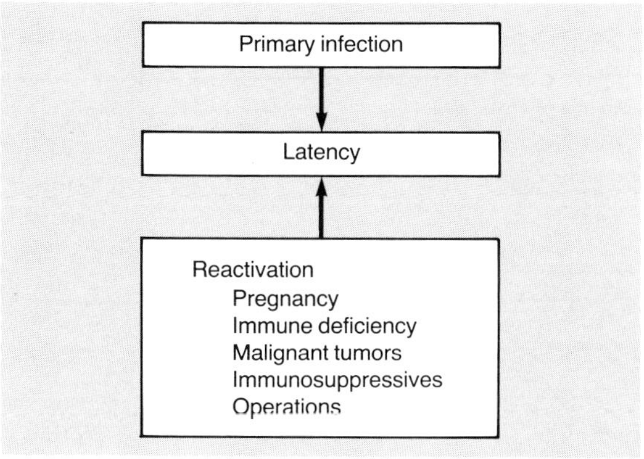

Figure 12.**29** Latent phase of cytomegalo-virus.

Coxsackievirus Sialadenitis and Other Viral Infections

The clinical and pathologic aspects of infection by the coxsackievirus A resemble epidemic parotitis. The virus is excreted by the pharyngeal mucosa and the intestine and is spread by contact. The following triad is said to occur: parotitis, gingivitis, and herpangina (Howlett et al 1957). The disease often begins with pharyngitis, rapidly followed by a soft swelling of the parotid gland similar to that seen in mumps. The differential diagnosis from other infective salivary disorders rests on epidemiology and determination of serologic titers.

Other viruses such as the influenza virus may in exceptional cases produce a disease similar to mumps (Brill & Gilfillan 1977), particularly in patients with reduced defense mechanisms (Cullen & Baublis 1980).

Sialadenitis may also occur during the course of infectious mononucleosis, with extensive interstitial infiltrates consisting of monocytes and lymphocytes (Seifert & Geiler 1956).

The *morphologic findings* in coxsackievirus infection are largely identical to those of epidemic parotitis, that is, an interstitial lymphocytic sialadenitis accompanied by acinar cell necrosis. This may lead in the long term to lipomatous parotid atrophy (see page 104). Multinuclear giant cells with oxyphilic nuclear and cytoplasmic inclusion bodies have occassionally been described in measles and whooping cough (Broz 1955).

References

Andersen, H. K., E. S. Spencer: Cytomegalovirus infection among renal allograft recipients. Acta med. Scand. 186 (1969) 7
Benirschke, K., G. R. Mendoza, P. L. Bazeley: Placental and fetal manifestations of cytomegalovirus infection. Virchows Arch. B. Cell Path. 16 (1974) 121
Berger, U.: Neue Viruskrankheiten der Speicheldrüsen. Dtsch. zahnärztl. Z. 14 (1959) 932
Berger, U.: Viren als Erreger von Speicheldrüsenaffektionen. Fortschr. Kiefer- u. Gesichts-Chir. 6 (1960) 307
Boström, K.: Patho-anatomical findings in a case of mumps. With pancreatitis, myocarditis, orchitis, epididymitis and seminal vesiculitis. Virchows Arch. Abt. A 344 (1968) 111
Brautigam, A. R., M. B. A. Oldstone: Replication of murine cytomegalovirus in reproductive tissues. Amer. J. Pathol. 98 (1980) 213
Brautigam, A. R., F. J. Dutko, L. B. Olding, M. B. A. Oldstone: Pathogenesis of murine cytomegalovirus infection: the macrophage as a permissive cell for cytomegalovirus infection, replication and latency. J. gen. Virol. 44 (1979) 349
Brill, S. J., R. F. Gilfillan: Acute parotitis associated with influenza. Type A: Twelve cases. New Engl. J. Med. 296 (1977) 1391
Brody, A. R., Ph. C. Kelleher, J. E. Craighead: A mechanism of exsudation through intact alveolar epithelial cells in the lungs of cytomegalovirus-infected mice. Lab. Invest. 39 (1978) 281
Broz, O.: Zur Frage der Ätiologie der Riesenzellpneumonie bei Kindern. Zbl. allg. Path. path. Anat. 93 (1955) 370
Caselitz, J., G. Seifert: Das lokale Abwehr- und Immunsystem der Speicheldrüsen unter physiologischen und pathologischen Bedingungen. Dtsch. Z. Mund-Kiefer-Gesichts-Chir. 6 (1982) 93
Cullen, S. J., J. V. Baublis: Parainfluenza type 3 parotitis in two immunodeficient children. J. Pediatr. 96 (1980) 437
Hamilton, J. D.: Cytomegalovirus and Immunity. In Melnick, J. L.: Monographs in Virology, Vol. 12. Karger, Basel 1982
Hanshaw, J. B.: Cytomegaloviruses. In Gard, S., C. Hallauer, K. F. Meyer: Virology Monographs, Vol. 3. Springer, Wien 1968 (p. 1)
Heni, N., P. Glogner, H. Schmitz: Klinik und Diagnostik der akuten Cytomegalie-Infektion bei primär gesunden Erwachsenen. Klin. Wschr. 54 (1976) 1117
Henson, D. E., Ph. M. Grimley, A. J. Strano: Postnatal cytomegalovirus hepatitis. An autopsy and liver biopsy study. Human Path. 5 (1974) 93
Henson, D., St. Siegel, A. J. Strano, A. Primack, D. A. Fucillo: Mumps virus sialadenitis. An autopsy report. Arch. Path. 92 (1971) 469
Howlett, J., F. Somlo, F. Kalz: A new syndrome of parotitis with herpangina caused by coxsackievirus. Canad. med. Ass. J. 77 (1957) 5
Johnson, C. D., E. W. Goodpasture: Histopathology of experimental mumps in the monkey macasus rhesus. Amer. J. Pathol. 12 (1936) 495
Jordan, M. C.: Interstitial pneumonia and subclinical infection after intranasal inoculation of murine cytomegalovirus. Infect. Immunity 21 (1978) 275
Krech, U. H., M. Jung, F. Jung: Cytomegalovirus infections in man. Karger, Basel 1971
Mor, S., S. Pitlik, S. Dux, J. B. Rosenfeld: Parotitis and pancreatitis complicating infectious mononucleosis. Isr. J. Med. Sci. 18 (1982) 709
Morgan, D. G., J. C. Niederman, G. Miller, H. W. Smith, J. M. Dowalby: Site of Epstein-Barr virus replication in the oropharynx. Lancet 1979/II, 1154
Nash, G.: Pathologic features of the lung in the immunocompromised host. Human Pathol. 13 (1982) 841
Niederman, J. C., G. Miller, H. A. Pearson, J. S. Pagano, J. M. Dowalby: Infectious mononucleosis. Epstein-Barr virus shedding in saliva and the oropharynx. New Engl. J. Med. 294 (1976) 1355
Olding, L. B., F. C. Jensen, M. B. A. Oldstone: Pathogenesis of cytomegalovirus infection. I. Activation of bone marrow-derived lymphocytes by in vitro allogenic reaction. J. exp. Med. 141 (1975) 561
Papadimitriou, J. M., G. R. Shellam, J. E. Allan: The effect of the beige mutation on infection with murine cytomegalovirus. Histopathologic studies. Amer. J. Pathol. 108 (1982) 299
Parham, D. M.: Post-transplantation pancreatitis associated with cytomegalovirus (report of a case). Human Pathol. 12 (1981) 663
Press, M. F., R. H. Riddell, J. Ringus: Cytomegalovirus inclusion disease. Its occurrence in the myenteric plexus of a renal transplant patient. Arch. Pathol. Lab. Med. 104 (1980) 580
Seifert, G.: Mundhöhle, Mundspeicheldrüsen, Tonsillen und Rachen. In Doerr, W., E. Uehlinger: Spezielle pathologische Anatomie, Bd. I. Springer, Berlin 1966 (S. 1)
Seifert, G.: Pathologische Anatomie der Cytomegalie. Klin. Wschr. 51 (1973) 533

Seifert, G.: Virale Erkrankungen der Speicheldrüsen. Dtsch. Z. Mund-Kiefer-Gesichts-Chir. 8 (1984) 187
Seifert, G., G. Geiler: Zur Pathologie der kindlichen Kopfspeicheldrüsen. Beitr. path. Anat. 116 (1956) 1
Seifert, G., J. Oehme: Mumps. In Gsell, O., W. Mohr: Infektionskrankheiten, Bd. I/1. Springer, Berlin 1967 (S. 419)
Škrha, J., J. Štěpán, E. Sixtová: Amylase isoenzymes in mumps. Eur. J. Pediatr. 132 (1979) 99
Smith, M. G.: The salivary gland viruses of man and animals (cytomegalic inclusions disease). Progr. med. Virol. 2 (1959) 171
Strayer, D. S., G. B. Phillips, K. H. Barker, Th. Winokur, K. de Schryver-Kecskemeti: Gastric cytomegalovirus infection in bone marrow transplant patients: An indication of generalized disease. Cancer (Philad.) 48 (1981) 1478
Ten Napel, Chr. H. H., T. H. The: Acute cytomegalovirus infection and the host immune response. II. Relationship of suppressed in vitro lymphocyte reactivity to bacterial recall antigens and mitogens with the development of cytomegalovirus-induced lymphocyte reactivity. Clin. exp. Immunol. 39 (1980) 272
Wells jr., S. A., A. S. Rabson, R. A. Mahngren, A. S. Ketcham: In vitro neoplastic transformation of newborn hamster salivary gland tissue by oncogenic DNA viruses. Cancer (Philad.) 19 (1966) 1411
Wenckebach, G. F. C., B. Curry: Cytomegalovirus infection of the female genital tract. Histologic findings in three cases and review of the literature. Arch. Path. Lab. Med. 100 (1976) 609
Wilmes, E., H. Wolf: Der Nachweis von Epstein-Barr-Virus-Genom in der Ohrspeicheldrüse. Z. Laryng. Rhinol. 60 (1981) 7
Wolf, H., G. J. Bayliss, E. Wilmes: Biological properties in Epstein-Barr virus. In Grundmann, E.: Cancer Campaign, Vol. 5. Fischer, Stuttgart 1981 (p. 101)
Ziegelmaier, R., F. Behrens, G. Enders: ELISA: Nachweis von IgG- und IgM-Antikörpern bei Cytomegalie- und Rötelninfektionen. Laboratoriumsbl. 29 (1979) 149

Radiation Sialadenitis

This form of sialadenitis becomes more and more important with the ever-increasing use of radiotherapy. The extent of lost function of the gland depends on the quality and quantity of the radiotherapy and the period of time over which the irradiation is applied, that is, on the dose and its fractionation. The response also depends on whether the gland itself is the primary target of the radiotherapy or whether it lies on the edge of an irradiated field. Development of Sjögren's syndrome also depends on the rate of salivary flow before irradiation therapy (Eneroth et al 1972, Mira et al 1981, Mossman et al 1981 and 1982). If the parotid gland lies immediately within the radiation field, the flow rate of saliva is suppressed to 50% and the protein secretion is reduced to 40% after a few weeks of treatment. This condition persists for the next 3 to 4 weeks. The glycoproteins are more severely affected than amylase. Chromatography gives the impression that radiation damage affects not so much protein synthesis as the protein itself (Mossman et al 1981). The parotid gland is much more sensitive to radiation than the submandibular gland (Shannon et al 1978). The severity of Sjögren's syndrome therefore depends considerably on whether the parotid gland is included in the field: it contributes to 33% of the entire salivary secretion.

In most cases, the secretion of the salivary gland decreases to one tenth by the end of a complete tumor dose. The patient has a distressing dryness of the treatment itself (Mossman et al 1982). It is not yet clear whether these longstanding changes of salivary gland function result from lesions of the ducts and acinic system or whether they are due to damage to other components. Eneroth et al (1972) measured salivary flow rate and found a return of function of the salivary glands 8 months after the end of irradiation.

Statistics show a 50% complication rate, including reduction of salivary flow and disturbances of protein secretion 5 years after irradiation to a dose of 70 Gy. However, our investigations have shown that a permanent Sjögren's sydnrome may be induced by a dose as low as 40–65 Gy.

The following factors contribute to the pathogenesis of radiation-induced Sjögren's syndrome: reduction of salivary flow with increasing viscosity of the saliva, reduction of the enzyme activity, disruption of protein secretion, and reduction of the blood supply to the gland. This favors bacterial infection. The oral mucosa is often infected with Candida albicans during irradiation.

The response of the salivary glands to irradiation may be classified in three stages (Hülse 1971):

1. An early reaction with temporary reduction of salivary flow.
2. A period of dryness after irradiation to a dose of 15 Gy per field.
3. Long-term damage accompanied by a severe loss of secretory gland parenchyma.

Although the salivary tissue is capable of an astonishing degree of functional recovery, the salivary glands nonetheless have permanent injury in most cases.

The sensitivity to irradiation of the individual salivary gland depends on the construction and differentiation of the gland tissue. The highly differentiated serous gland acini show a more severe pattern of damage than the relatively resistant mucous glands. In addition, there is a direct correlation between the dose of irradiation and the severity of the damage.

Irradiation injury initially affects the serous acini in particular. The **histologic characteristics** are swelling, vacuoles, and degranulation of the acinar cells, leading later to acinar cell necrosis. An acute serous-cellular inflammatory reaction with swelling of the ductal epithelium develops in the duct system (Figs. 12.**30**–12.**33**). The blood vessels also demonstrate edema of the wall with swelling of the endothelial cells (Seifert & Geier

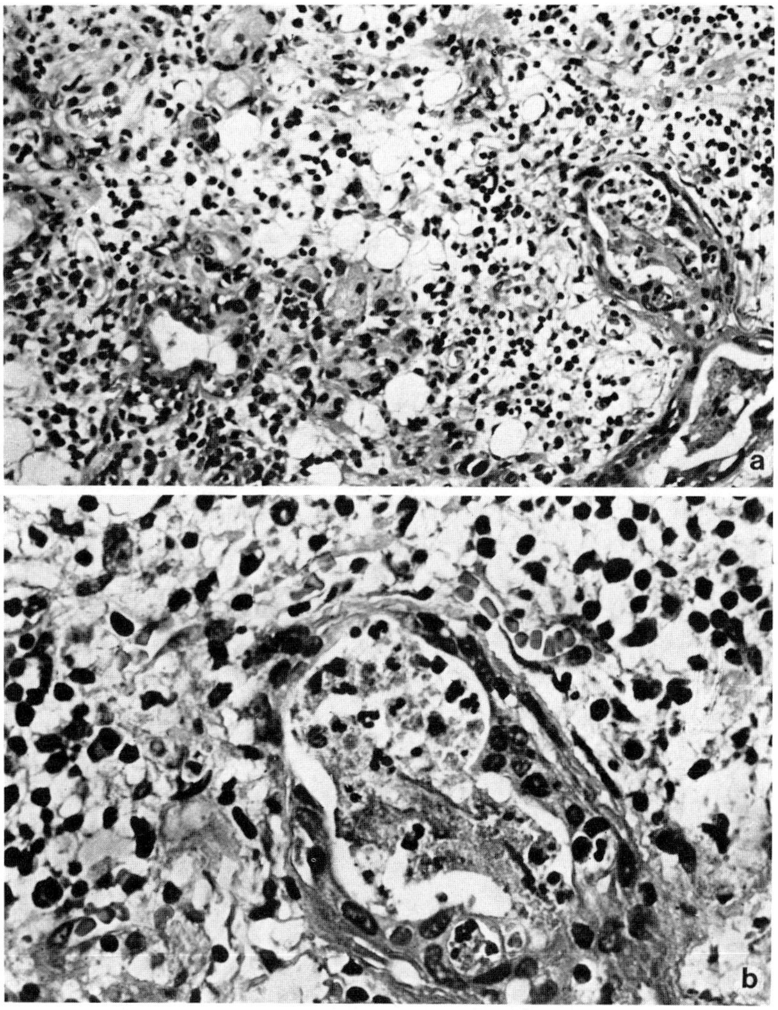

Figure 12.**30** Radiation sialadenitis of the parotid gland: **a** Dissolution of gland acini and interstitial inflammatory edema. **b** Segment of a dilated duct with secretion and cell debris in the duct, epithelial metaplasia, and periductal inflammation. H & E. **a** 160×, **b** 400×.

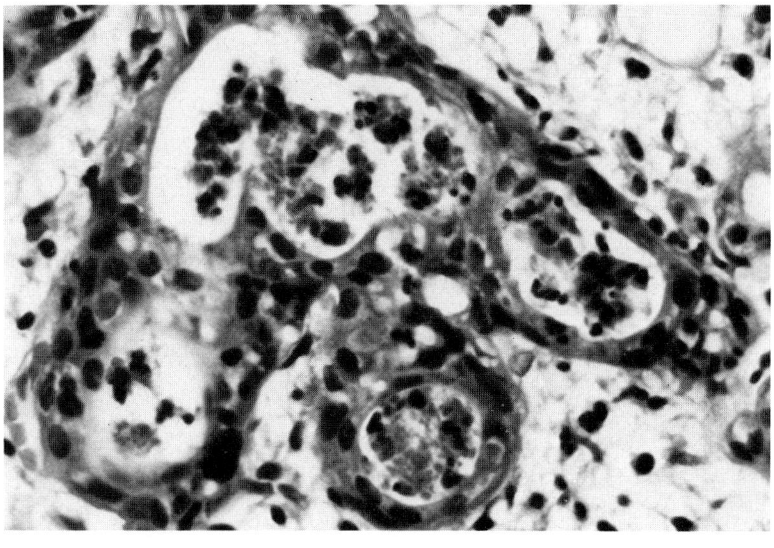

Figure 12.**31** Radiation sialadenitis of the submandibular gland: swelling and necrosis of the ductal epithelium and inflammatory infiltrate in the duct lumen. H & E, 400×.

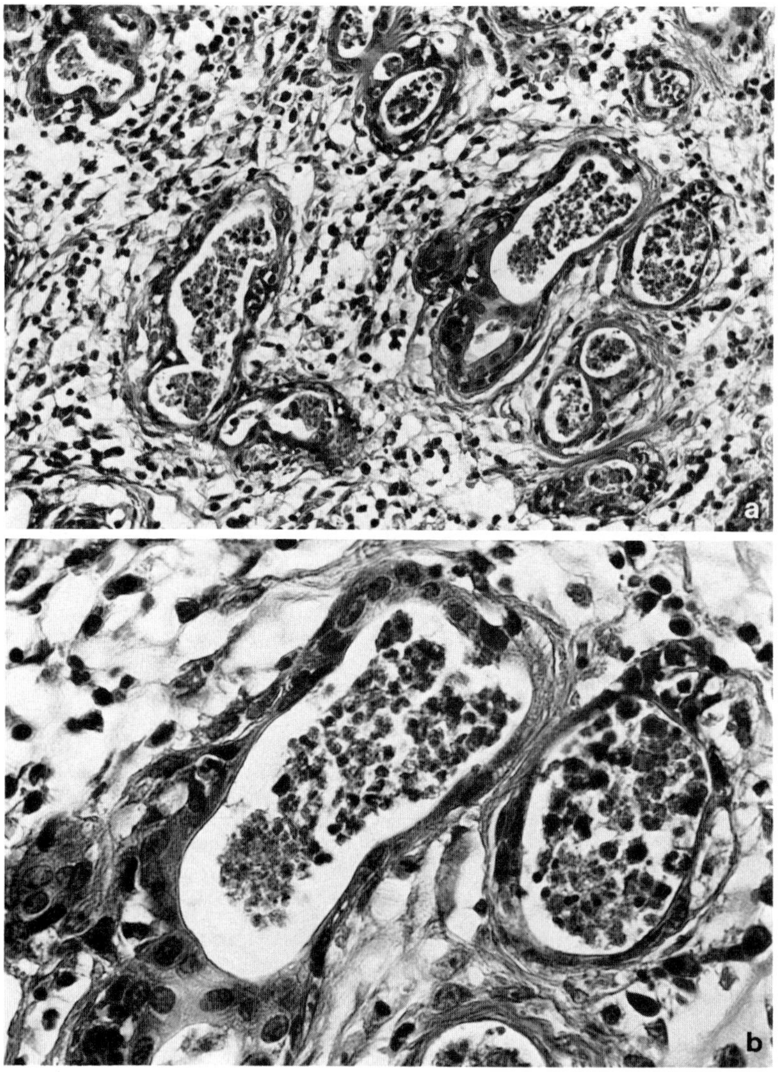

Figure 12.**32** Radiation sialadenitis of the submandibular gland showing widespread destruction of the acini, massive inflammatory infiltrate in the duct lumen and the interstitium. H & E. **a** 160×, **b** 400×.

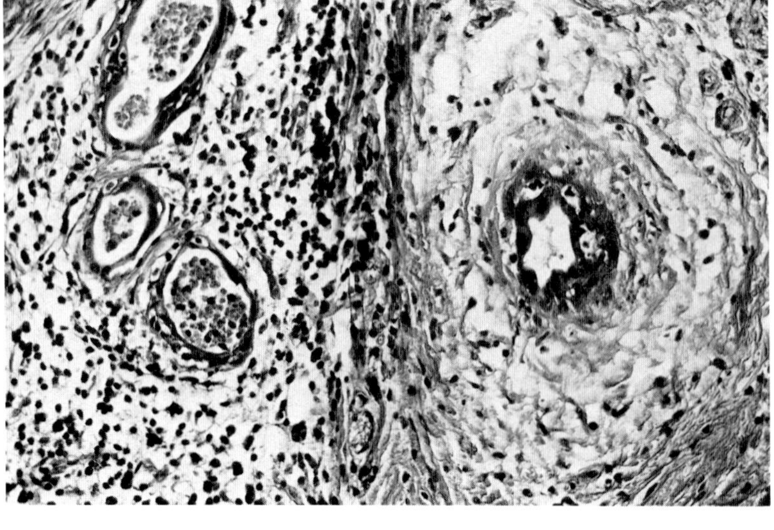

Figure 12.**33** Radiation sialadenitis of the submandibular gland showing necrosis of the ductal epithelium in the right half of the field, and periductal edema. PAS, 160×.

Figure 12.**34** Radiation sialadenitis of the submandibular gland: **a** Inflammation of the duct system and interstitium. **b** Focal goblet cell metaplasia. H & E. **a** 160×, **b** 400×.

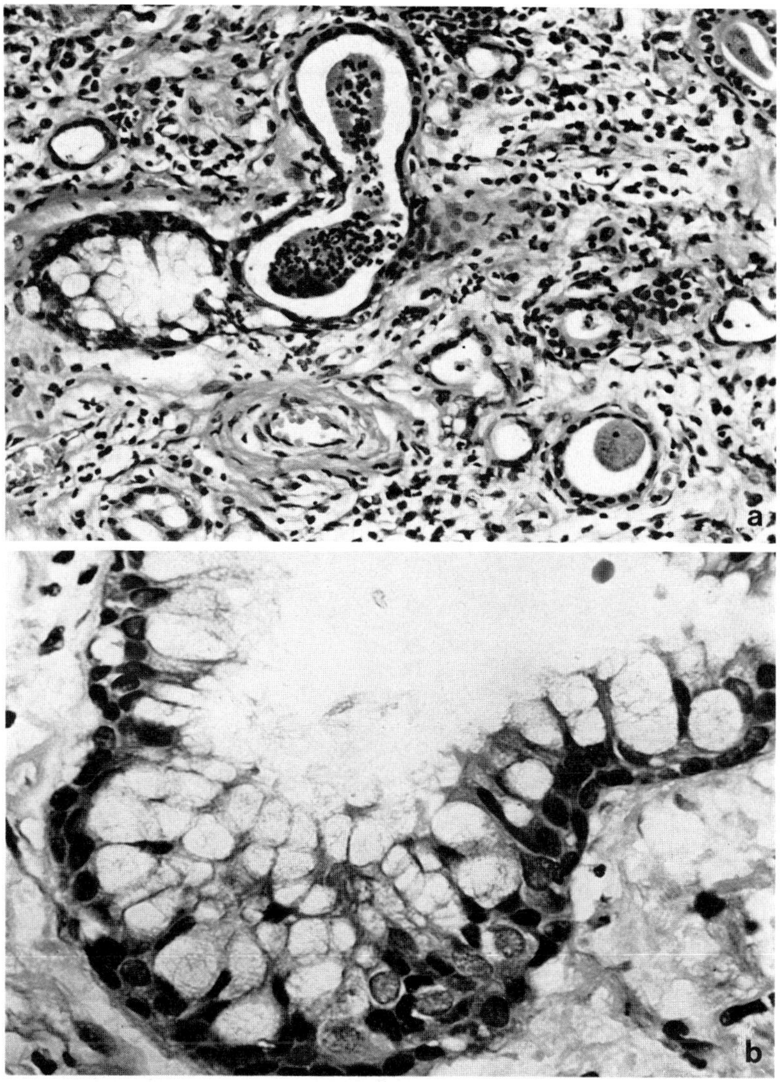

1971, Glücksman & Cherry 1971, Harwood et al 1973, Kashima et al 1965, Fajardo & Berthrong 1981).

The *chronic forms* of radiation sialadenitis are typified by parenchymatous atrophy, interstitial fibrosis, marked changes in the ductal system with duct ectasia, epithelial metaplasia, and ductular proliferation (Figs. 12.**34**–2.**36**). The ductal system also demonstrates dysplastic epithelial degeneration and goblet cell metaplasia.

The *ultrastructural changes* have mainly been shown by animal experiments (Stern et al 1976, Sholley et al 1981, Chomette et al 1981). The endoplasmic membrane and the secretory granules of the serous acini show dissolution. In the later course of the disease, membrane-bounded vacuoles, cytolysozymes and focal degeneration of cytoplasm are seen. Crystalloids are precipitated in the cytolysosomes. Lesions of the mitochondria, such as vacuolization, crystallization, and destruction of the basal cytoplasmic infoldings occur in the striated ducts. This process is accompanied by a loss of enzymes and an electrolyte imbalance in the saliva (Anderson et al 1981). The autonomic nervous system shows lesions similar to those of sialadenosis, such as swelling of the axons, dissolution of the neurofilaments and neurosecretory granules, and loss of the synaptic vesicles.

Recent animal experiments throw new light on the **pathogenesis** of radiation-induced salivary gland lesions (Abok et al 1984). The serous granulated cells are particularly radiosensitive, whereas the mucous cells and the duct epithelium are more radioresistant. This is explained by the

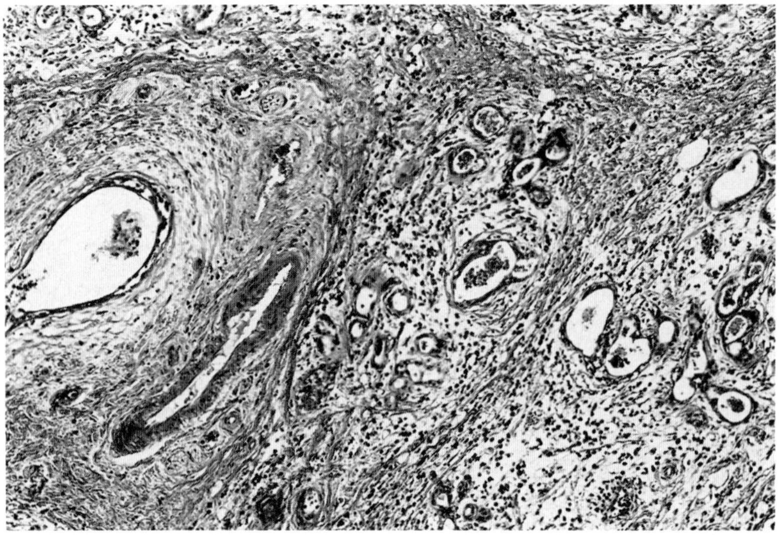

Figure 12.**35** Radiation sialadenitis of the submandibular gland: glandular destruction with inflammatory interstitial fibrosis and atrophy of the parenchyma. H & E, 63×.

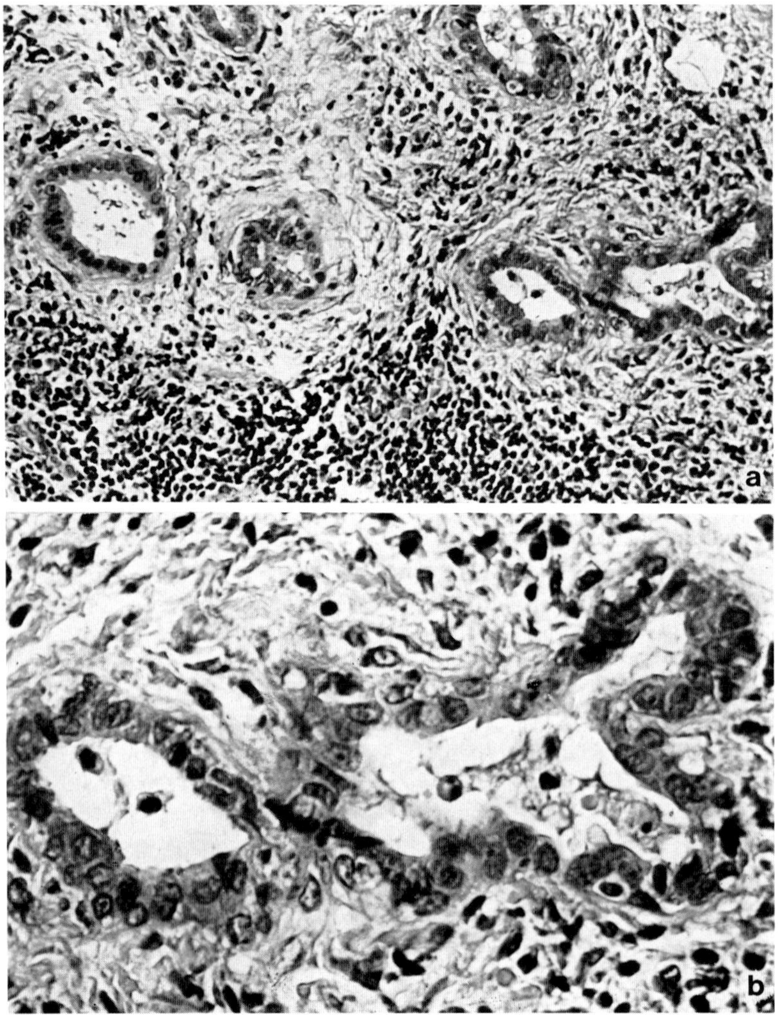

Figure 12.**36** Radiation sialadenitis of the submandibular gland: inflammatory interstitial fibrosis with atrophy of the acini and epithelial proliferations in the irregular ducts. H & E. **a** 160×, **b** 400×.

fact that the secretory granules contain heavy metals, such as zinc, manganese, and iron, and the granule membrane is integrated by the effect of the radiation, allowing the heavy metal to catalyze a lipid oxidation.

The **treatment** of *irradiation-induced sialadenitis* is difficult. The main thrust of treatment is to compensate for the absent saliva and the resulting dryness of the mouth. Beer with a low alcohol content, lozenges to moisten the mucosa, and pilocarpine drops (Hülse 1971), and 1% pilocarpine solution are recommended (Breuninger 1983). A synthetic saliva (Matzker & Schreiber 1972) has been developed, which many patients find to be successful. The preparation is injected into the mouth before a meal so that the swallowing of food is considerably facilitated.

References

Abok, K., U. Brunk, B. Jung, J. Ericsson: Morphologic and histochemical studies on the differing radiosensitivity of ductular and acinar cells of the rat submandibular glands. Virchows Arch. (Cell Pathol.) 45 (1984) 443

Anderson, M. W., K. T. Izutu, J. C. Rice: Parotid gland pathophysiology after mixed gamma and neutron irradiation of cancer patients. Oral Surg. 52 (1981) 495

Breuninger, H.: Medikamentöse Therapie der Hals-Nasen-Ohren-Krankheiten, 4. Aufl., Thieme, Stuttgart 1983

Chomette, G., M. Auriol, J. M. Vialannt, J. Ch. Bertrand, Ch. Chenal: Effect of irradiation on the submandibular gland of the rat. An enzyme histochemical and ultrastructural study. Virchows Arch. (Pathol. Anat.) 391(1981) 291

Eneroth, C. M., C. O. Henrikson, P. A. Jakobsson: Effects of fractionated radiotherapy on salivary gland function. Cancer 30 (1972) 1147

Fajardo, L. F., M. Berthrong: Radiation injury in surgical pathology. Part. III. Salivary glands, pancreas and skin. Amer. J. Surg. Path. 5 (1981) 279

Glücksman, A., C. P. Cherry: Effects of irradiation in salivary glands. In Berdjis, C. C.: Pathology of Irradiation. Williams and Wilkins, Baltimore, 1971 (p. 290)

Harwood, T. R., C. J. Staley, H. Yokoo: Histopathology of irradiated and obstructed submandibular salivary glands. Arch. Pathol. 96 (1973) 189

Hülse, R.: Symptomatik und Therapie von Strahlenreaktionen im Kopf-Hals-Bereich. Z. Laryng. Rhinol. 50 (1971) 133

Kashima, H. K., W. R. Kirkham, J. R. Andrews: Postirradiation sialadenitis. Amer. J. Roentgen. Rad. Ther. Nucl. Med. 94 (1965) 271

Matzker, J., J. Schreiber: Synthetischer Speichel zur Therapie der Hyposialien, insbesondere bei der radiogenen Sialadenitis. Z. Laryng. Rhinol. 51 (1972) 422

Mira, J. G., W. B. Wescott, E. N. Starcke, I. L. Shannon: Some factors influencing salivary function when treating with radiotherapy. Int. J. Radiat. Oncol. Biol. Phys. 7 (1981) 535

Mossman, K., A. R. Shatzman, J. D. Chencharick: Effects of radiotherapy on human parotid saliva. Radiat. Res. 88 (1981) 403

Mossman, K., A. R. Shatzman, J. D. Chencharick: Long-term effects of radiotherapy on taste and salivary function in man. Int. J. Radiat. Oncol. Biol. Phys. 8 (1982) 991

Seifert, G., W. Geier: Zur Pathologie der Strahlen-Sialadenitis. Z. Laryng. Rhinol. 50 (1971) 376

Shannon, I. L., J. N. Trodahl, E. N. Starcke: Radiosensitivity of the human parotid gland. Proc. Soc. exp. Biol. Med., 157 (1978) 50

Sholley, M. M., N. E. Pratt, M. Sodicoff: Cytoplasmic crystalloids in irradiated rat parotid glands. J. oral Pathol. 10 (1981) 192

Stern, M. H., J. E. Turner, L. S. Jett, H. Mincer, J. P. McGinnis: Electron microscopic changes in rat parotid and submandibular glands subsequent to total body irradiation with fast neutrons. Oral Surg. 42 (1976) 620

Electrolyte Sialadenitis

Electrolyte sialadenitis affects the submandibular gland in 90% of cases and the parotid gland in only 10%. Initially, the electrolyte content of the saliva is disturbed, causing increased viscosity of the saliva and retention of mucus in the terminal ducts. Sialolithiasis is the end stage of this dyschylia (Seifert 1964). In most cases, dyschylic secretory disorders have no clinical expression (see Chapter 9).

Histology of the early stages of electrolyte sialadenitis is characterized by viscous masses of secretion in the duct and modest duct ectasia (Seifert & Donath 1976). These are followed by precipitation of secretion as spheroliths that contain an organic matrix of mucoprotein complexes (Figs. 12.**37**–12.**40**). Radial or lamellar microliths form by further appositional growth on these spheroliths. Histology of the parotid gland shows intraductal spheroliths or microliths in 25% of patients with metabolic disorders, such as diabetes mellitus or cirrhosis of the liver (Semann 1969). These intraductal inspissations of secretion are almost always associated with duct ectasia and periductal inflammatory lesions. In the *later stages,* the obstructive lesions of the duct increases in severity. These lesions include duct ectasia, squamous cell metaplasia, and ductular proliferation (Figs. 12.**41,** 12.**42**). The secretory parenchyma undergoes increasing atrophy and shows increasing periductal fibrosis in the interstitial tissue and a cellular infiltrate consisting mainly of lymphocytes, histiocytes, and plasma cells. In the late stages, the lesions resemble those of atrophy due to ligation of the duct (Donath et al 1973).

The altered composition of the saliva plays a decisive role in the **pathogenesis** of this condition. This is encompassed by the term "dyschylia" (Seifert 1964). The start of the process is characterized by dyschylic disorders of secretion and its end by sialolithiasis (see Chapter 9). Obstructive factors are shared by chronic recurrent parotitis (Donath & Gundlach 1979) and chronic sialadenitis of the submandibular gland (Seifert & Donath 1977). Focal ductal obstruction by salivary gland cysts and lymph node diseases or tumors are the cause of circumscribed obstructive inflammatory processes with dyschylic disorders of secretion (see Chapter 10). In the minor glands there is a relationship between the occurrence of retention cysts and microliths (Jensen et al 1979).

Microliths occur mainly in the older age groups in the glands of the lip and cheek. The center of the microlith consists of an organic, relatively homogeneous, matrix that encloses inspissated

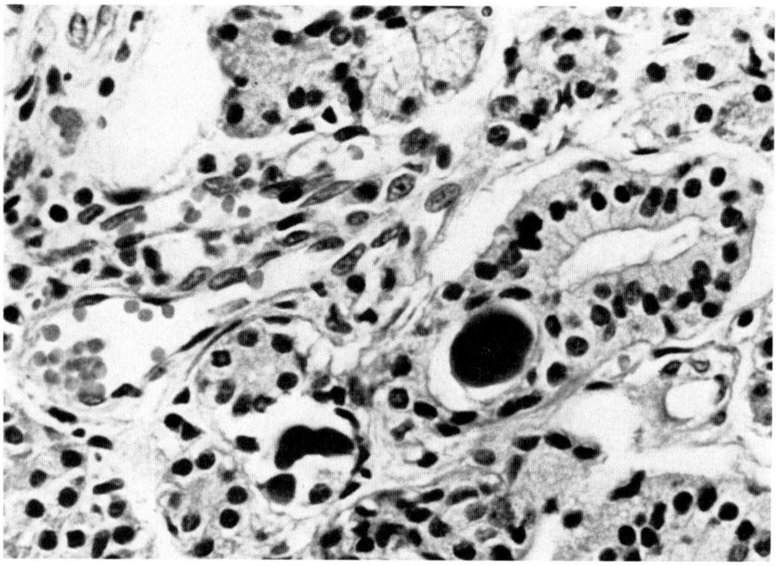

Figure 12.**37** Electrolyte sialadenitis of the parotid gland: speroliths in the terminal duct system. PAS, 400×.

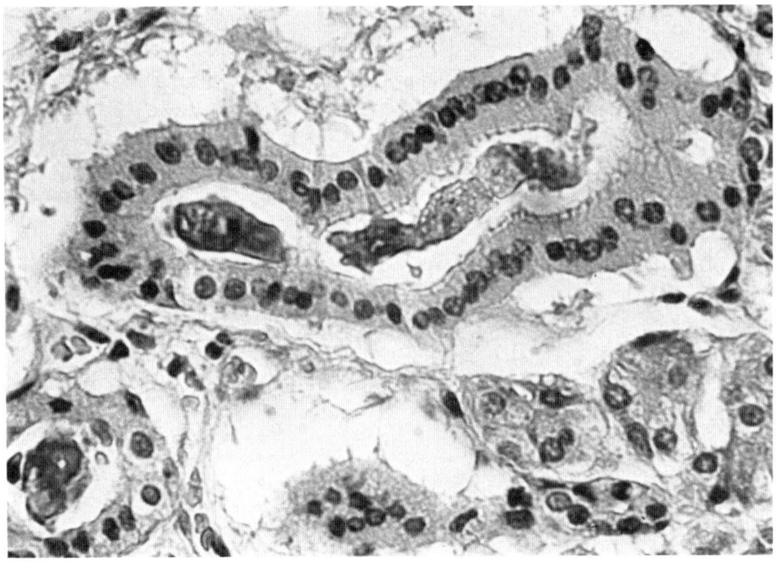

Figure 12.**38** Electrolyte sialadenitis of the submandibular gland: clumps of secretion and speroliths in the terminal duct system. H & E, 400×.

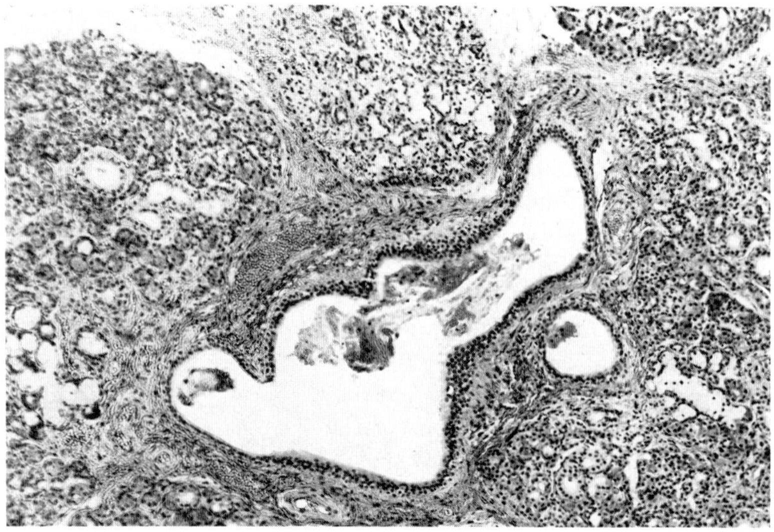

Figure 12.**39** Electrolyte sialadenitis of the submandibular gland: sialectasis with viscous clumps of secretion and periductal inflammatory fibrosis. H & E, 63×.

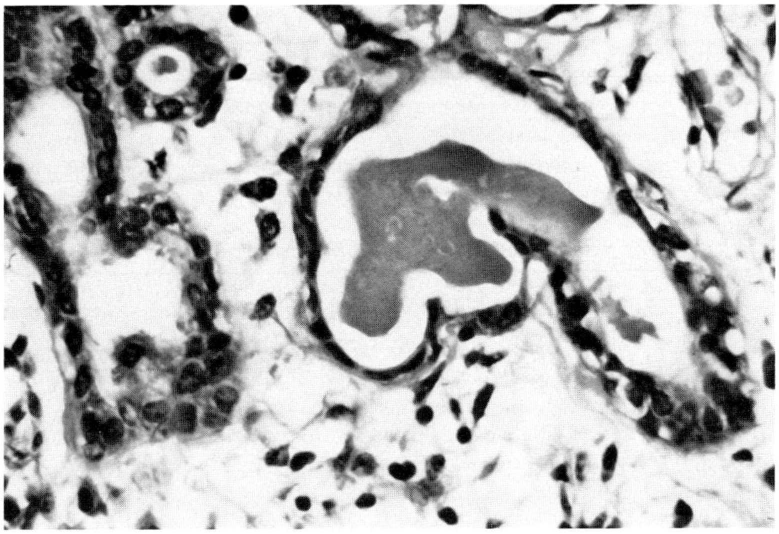

Figure 12.**40** Electrolyte sialadenitis of the submandibular gland: ectasia of peripheral ducts with clumps of secretion in the lumen and swelling of the ductal epithelium. H & E, 400×.

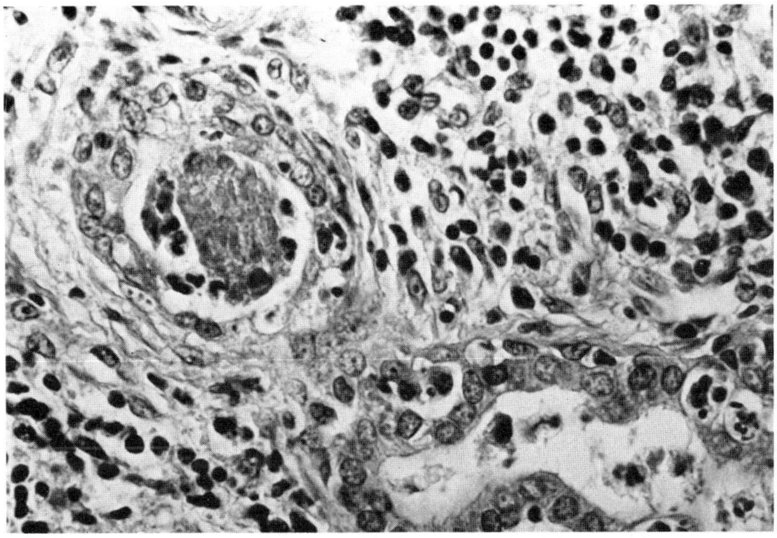

Figure 12.**41** Electrolyte sialadenitis of the submandibular gland: viscous masses of secretion in small salivary ducts, metaplasia of the duct epithelium, and interstitial inflammation. H & E, 400×.

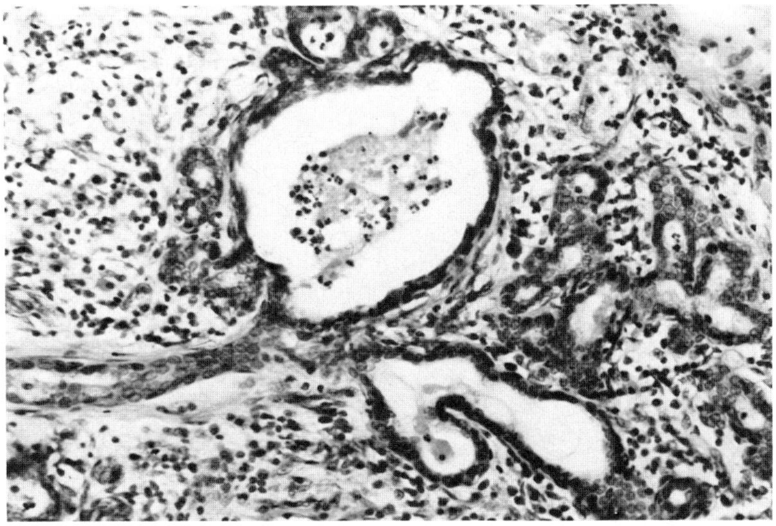

Figure 12.**42** Electrolyte sialadenitis of the submandibular gland: irregular duct ectasia, ductular proliferations, and interstitial inflammatory fibrosis. H & E, 160×.

mucous masses. The degree of mineralization of this matrix varies. The ductal system demonstrates squamous metaplasia, ductal ectasia, and proliferation; the interstitial tissue, as in the major glands, shows chronic inflammation with parenchymatous atrophy (Pullon & Miller 1972, Eversole & Sabes 1971, Holst 1971). Morphologic analysis of the microliths reveals similar findings to that of the major salivary gland calculi of the parotid and submandibular glands (Anneroth et al 1975a, 1975b, Burstein et al 1979). Microradiography demonstrates a crystalline inorganic matrix consisting mainly of hydroxylapatite and magnesium octocalcium phosphate. The configuration and mineralization of salivary calculi varies widely. The greater frequency of obstructive sialadenitis in the submandibular gland is ascribed to the higher mucus and calcium contents of the saliva of the submandibular gland, to the ascending duct system of the gland, and to the relative narrow opening of the ducts, all of which favor stagnation of secretions (Anneroth et al 1975a).

References

Anneroth, G., C.-M. Eneroth, G. Isacsson: Morphology of salivary calculi. The distribution of the inorganic component. J. oral Pathol. 4 (1975a) 257

Anneroth, G., C.-M. Eneroth, G. Isacsson: Crystalline structure of salivary calculi. A microradiographic and microdiffractometric study. J. oral Pathol. 4 (1975b) 266

Burstein, L. S., A. L. Boskey, P. J. Tannenbaum, A. S. Posner, I. D. Mandel: The crystal chemistry of submandibular and parotid salivary gland stones. J. oral Pathol. 8 (1979) 284

Donath, K., K. K. H. Gundlach: Ein Beitrag zur Ätiologie und Pathogenese der chronisch-rezidivierenden Parotitis. Dtsch. zahnärztl. Z. 34 (1979) 45

Donath, K., H.-U. Hirsch-Hoffmann, G. Seifert: Zur Pathogenese der Parotisatrophie nach experimenteller Gangunterbindung. Ultrastrukturelle Befunde am Drüsenparenchym der Rattenparotis. Virchows Arch. Abt. A 359 (1973) 31

Eversole, L. R., W. R. Sabes: Minor salivary duct changes due to obstruction. Arch. Otolaryngol. 94 (1971) 19

Holst, E.: The clinical entity of sialolithiasis of the minor salivary glands. Acta odont. scand. 29 (1971) 75

Jensen, J. L., F. V. Howell, G. M. Rick, R. W. Correll: Minor salivary gland calculi. A clinicopathologic study of forty-seven new cases. Oral. Surg. 47 (1979) 44

Pullon, P. A., A. S. Miller: Sialolithiasis of accessory salivary glands: Review of 55 cases. J. oral Surg. 30 (1972) 832

Semann, N.: Pathohistologische Untersuchungen zur Häufigkeit der Sialolithiasis und Sialadenitis der Parotis. HNO (Berl.) 17 (1969) 636

Seifert, G.: Die Sekretionsstörungen (Dyschylien) der Speicheldrüsen. Ergebn. allg. Path. path. Anat. 44 (1964) 103

Seifert, G., K. Donath: Die Morphologie der Speicheldrüsenerkrankungen. Arch. Oto-Rhino-Laryng. 213(1976) 111

Seifert, G., K. Donath: Zur Pathogenese des Küttner-Tumors der Submandibularis. Analyse von 349 Fällen mit chronischer Sialadenitis der Submandibularis. HNO (Berl.) 25 (1977) 81

Chronic Sclerosing Sialadenitis (Küttner Tumor) of the Submandibular Gland

In 1896, Küttner described a disease that expressed itself by hardness and swelling of the submandibular gland. Clinically, the lesion cannot be distinguished from a true tumor. The diagnosis is made after the gland has been removed: histologic examination then allows the lesion to be distinguished from true tumors.

Four degrees of severity of inflammation may be distinguished by histologic examination (Seifert & Donath 1977).

Stage 1 is marked by a focal chronic inflammation with nests of lymphocytic infiltration around the salivary ducts (Fig. 12.**43**). The ducts are moderately dilated and contain inspissated secretion as

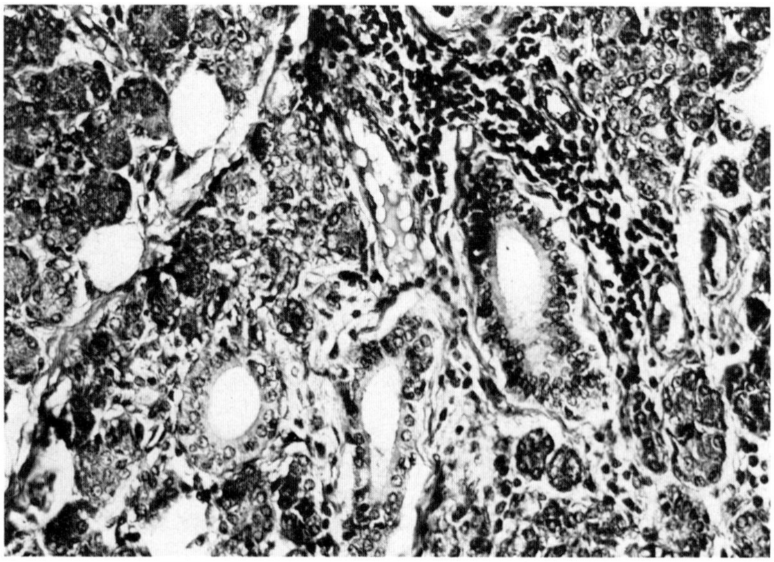

Figure 12.**43** Stage 1 of chronic sclerosing sialadenitis (Küttner tumor): focal periductal lymphocytic infiltrate. H & E, 160×

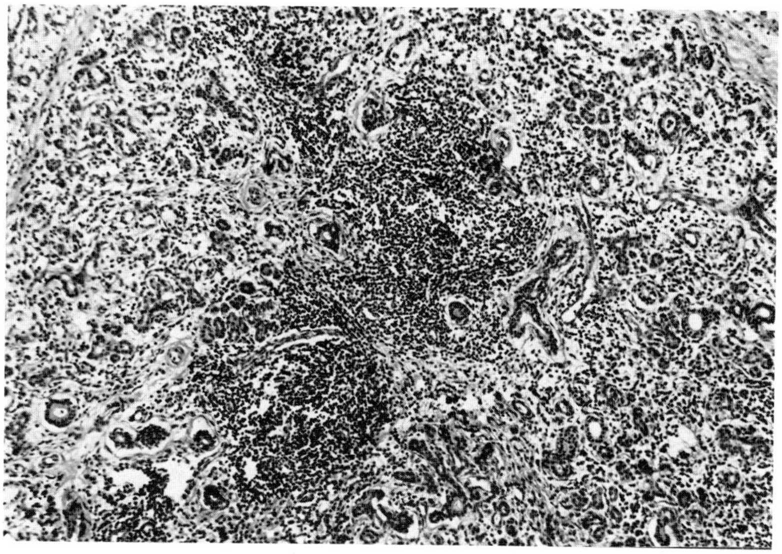

Figure 12.**44** Stage 2 of chronic sclerosing sialadenitis (Küttner tumor): diffuse lymphocytic infiltration. H & E, 63×.

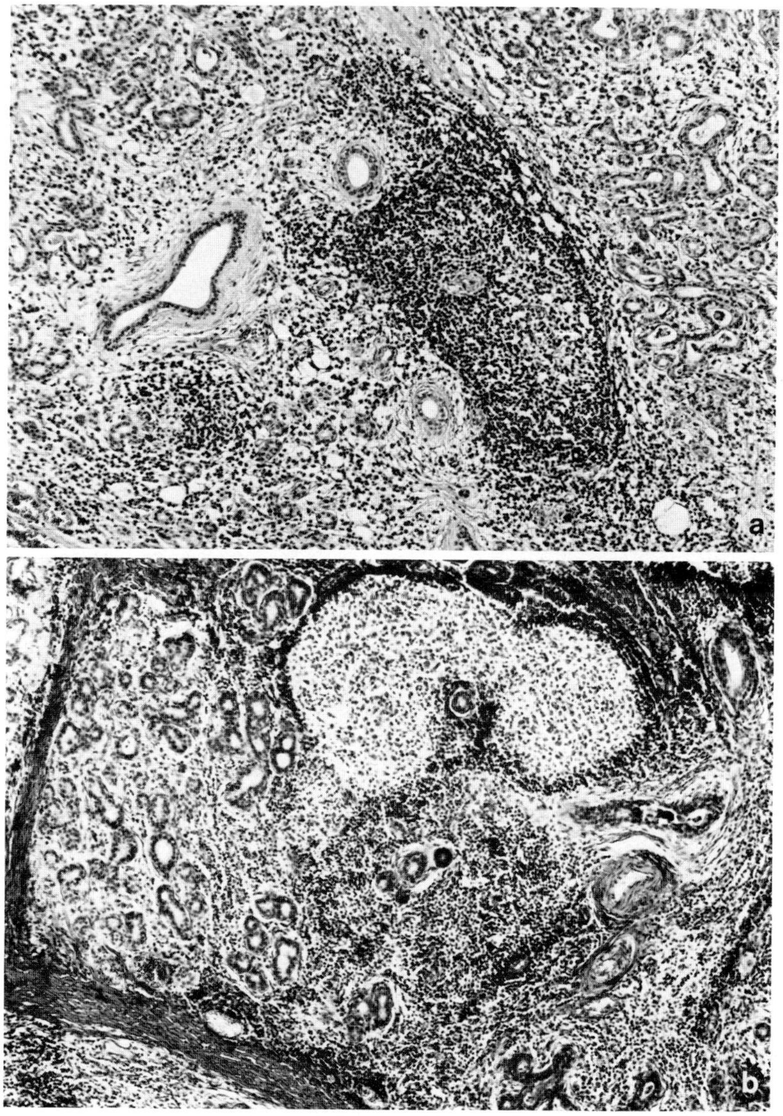

Figure 12.**45** Stage 2 of chronic sclerosing sialadenitis (Küttner tumor): **a** Early periductal formation of lymphoid follicles. **b** Pronounced follicle formation with activated follicular center in the upper part of the figure, and interstitial fibrosis. H & E. **a**, **b** 63×.

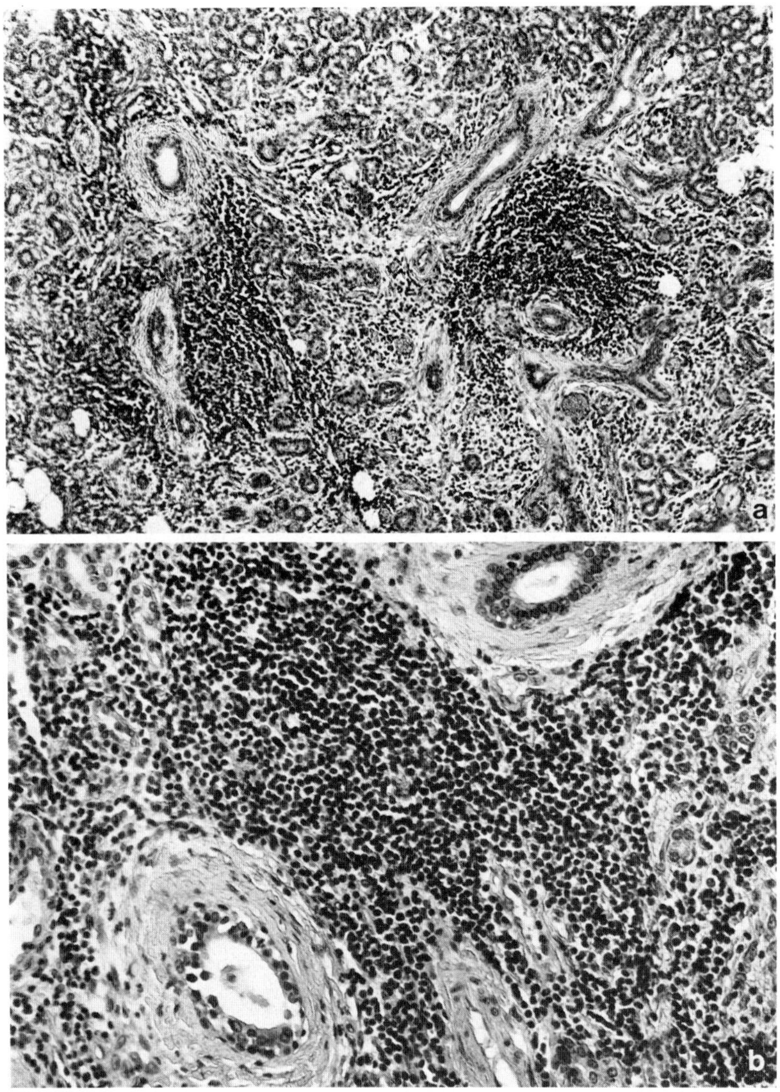

Figure 12.**46** Stage 3 of chronic sclerosing sialadenitis (Küttner tumor): **a** Interstitial sclerosis with reduction of secreting gland parenchyma. **b** Pronounced periductal sclerosis and dense lymphocytic infiltration. H & E. **a** 63×, **b** 160×.

evidence of a disorder of secretion. The structure of the gland is largely retained. Focal lymphocytic sialadenitis of the submandibular gland is relatively frequent in a random series of sections (Waterhouse & Doniach 1966, Chisholm et al 1970).

In *stage 2* (Figs. 12.**44**, 12.**45a, b**), the diffuse lymphocytic infiltration is more marked and is accompanied by a more severe periductal fibrosis. The duct system shows dyschylic inspissation of secretions in addition to focal metaplasia and proliferation of the duct epithelium. Periductal lymph follicles are well developed. The fibrosis affects the center of the lobule and is accompanied by atrophy of the serous acini in particular.

Stage 3 (Figs. 12.**46**–12.**48**) may be defined as a chronic, sclerosing sialadenitis. The advanced sclerotic scar tissue is obviously the histologic correlate of the palpable indurated pseudotumor. At some points, the ducts are surrounded by marked hyalinization. The extent of lymphocytic infiltration and formation of lymph follicles is greater than in stage 2, as is the parenchymatous atrophy. The duct system demonstrates squamous and goblet cell metaplasia in addition to periductal extravasation of secretion with development of extravasation mucoceles (see Chapter 10). Ductular, relatively primitive, duct buds are seen also.

In *stage 4* (end stage), the progressive inflammatory process is so marked that the lobular architecture resembles that of cirrhosis of the liver. Indeed, this stage may be described as salivary gland cirrhosis (Figs. 12.**49**–12.**51**). Gland parenchyma is seldom to be found so that the gland may be described as burnt out.

A marked connective tissue sclerosis and occasional lipomatosis accompany an inflammatory

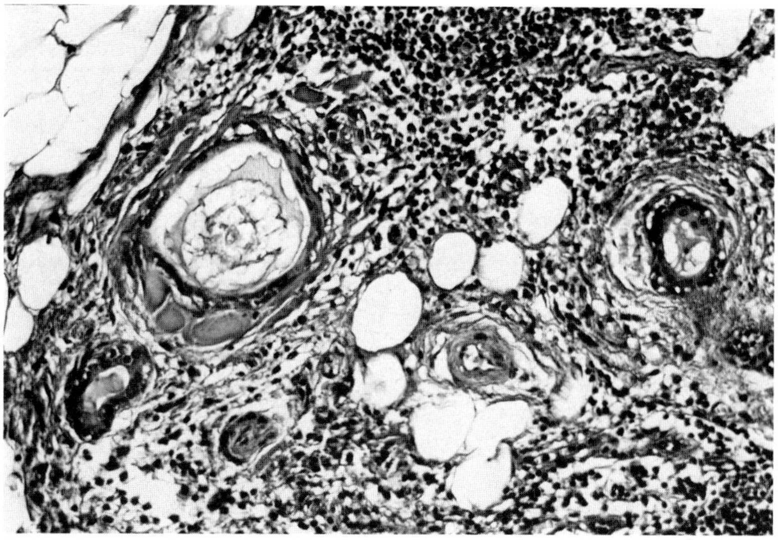

Figure 12.**47** Stage 3 of chronic sclerosing sialadenitis (Küttner tumor): clumps of secretion in the ducts with periductal extrusion of mucus and distinct loss of parenchyma. H & E, 160×.

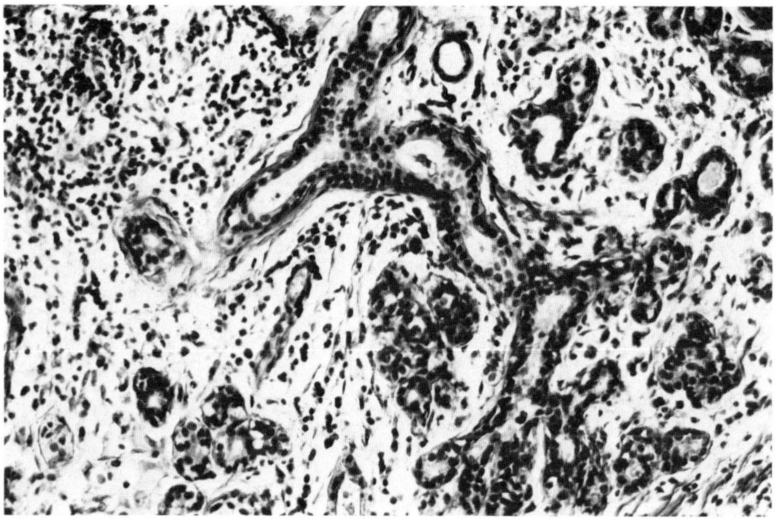

Figure 12.**48** Stage 3 of chronic sclerosing sialadenitis (Küttner tumor): pronounced ductular proliferation and loss of secreting glandular tissue. H & E, 160×.

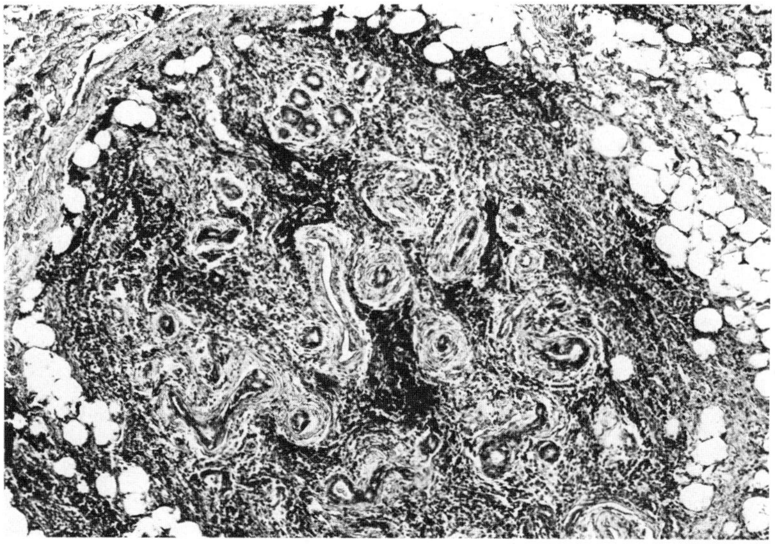

Figure 12.**49** Stage 4 of chronic sclerosing sialadenitis (Küttner tumor): destruction of lobular structure, replacement of parenchyma by sclerotic connective tissue, inclusions of ductular proliferations, and focal lipomatosis. H & E, 63×.

Figure 12.**50** Stage 4 of chronic sclerosing sialadenitis (Küttner tumor): burnt-out gland with cirrhotic transformation and ductular proliferations with epithelial metaplasia. H & E. **a** 63×, **b** 160×.

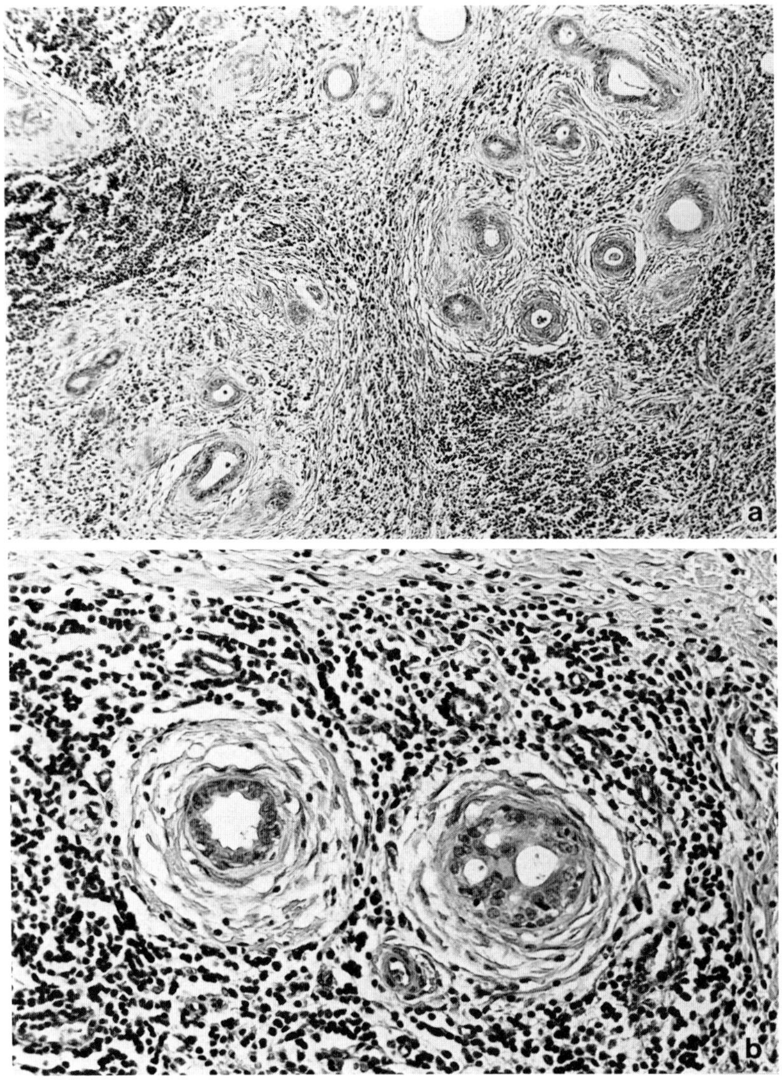

infiltrate and lymphoid follicles. The ductal system is largely destroyed. On occasion, undifferentiated duct sprouts, epithelial metaplasia and dysplasia, and myoepithelial cell islands are found.

The **pathogenesis** is dominated initially by an obstructive electrolyte sialadenitis (Fig. 12.**52**). The later course is marked by abnormal immunologic reactions (Herberhold 1984), accompanied by parenchymatous atrophy, increasing gland sclerosis, and lesions of the ducts (Räsänen et al 1972). The stages are distinguished by the following characteristics (Herberhold 1984): stage 1 by an increase of IgA-containing plasma cells, stage 2 by stimulation of lactoferrin and lysozyme production and increase of IgA and IgG plasma cells, and stage 3 and 4 by destruction of the local nonspecific immune system and degeneration of immunoglobulin-forming plasma cells. The increasing development of lymphoid follicles and the marked infiltration by lymphocytes, associated with the appearance of myoepithelial cell islands mark a transition to an autoimmune sialadenitis. Twenty-five percent of all cases are in stage 1, 20%, in stage 2, 40%, in stage 3, and 15%, in stage 4. About 50% of patients with chronic sclerosing adenitis also manifest sialolithiasis. The peak age incidence is in the fourth and fifth decades.

A review of the data on this lesion leads to the conclusion that it represents a primary obstructive electrolyte sialadenitis caused by a secretory disorder. The disease is progressive, leading to immunologic destruction of the submandibular gland. There are etiologic and pathogenic correlations between progressive obstructive immune sialadenitis of the submandibular gland and the chronic myoepithelial parotitis of Sjögren's syndrome (Seifert 1981).

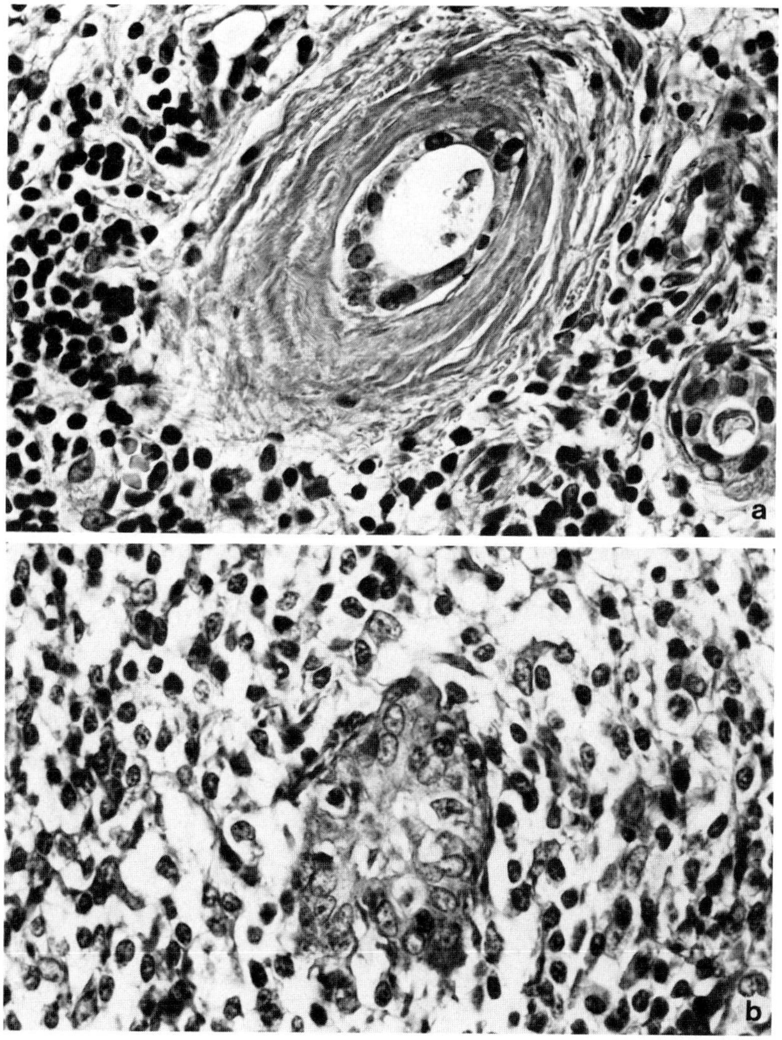

Figure 12.**51** Stage 4 of chronic sclerosing sialadenitis (Küttner tumor): pronounced ductal changes. **a** Concentric periductal sclerosis. **b** Development of a myoepithelial island with surrounding lymphocytic infiltrate. H & E. **a**, **b** 400×.

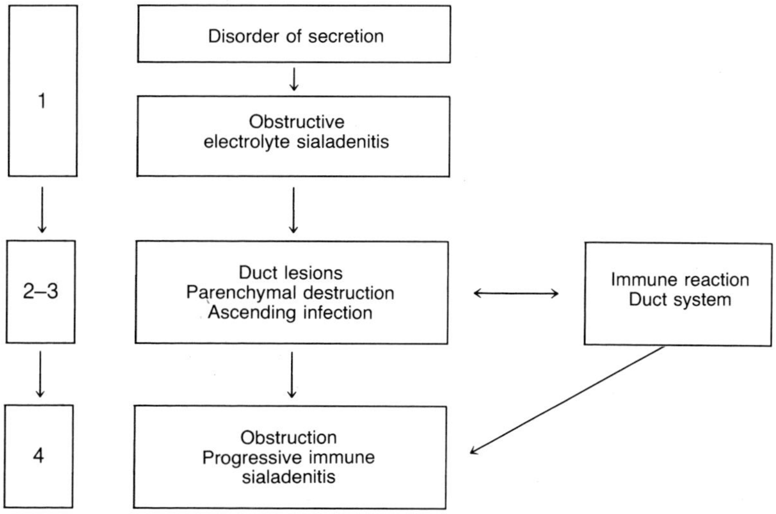

Figure 12.**52** Stages and pathogenic factors of chronic sclerosing sialadenitis (Küttner tumor) of the submandibular gland (Seifert & Donath).

References

Chisholm, D. M., J. P. Waterhouse, D. K. Mason: Lymphocytic sialadenitis in the major and minor salivary glands: A correlation in postmortem subjects. J. Clin. Path. 23 (1970) 690
Herberhold, C.: Immunpathologische Reaktionen im Ablauf der chronischen Sialadenitis der Glandula submandibularis (sog. Küttner-Tumor). Laryng. Rhinol. Otol. 63 (1984)
Räsänen, O., K. Jokien, K. Dammert: Sclerosing inflammation of the submandibular salivary gland (Küttner-Tumor) – A progessive plasmacellular ductitis. Acta oto-laryng. 74 (1972) 297
Seifert, G.: Chronische Mundtrockenheit. Ursachen, Pathologie. Dtsch. Z. Mund-Kiefer-Gesichts-Chir. 5 (1981) 3
Seifert, G., K. Donath: Zur Pathogenese des Küttner-Tumors der Submandibularis. Analyse von 349 Fällen mit chronischer Sialadenitis der Submandibularis. HNO (Berl.) 25 (1977) 81
Waterhouse, J. P., I. Doniach: Post-mortem prevalence of focal lymphocytic adenitis of the submandibular glands. J. Path. Bact. (Edinb.) 91 (1966) 53

Immune Sialadenitis

The term "immune sialadenitis" encompasses an acute or chronic salivary gland inflammation caused by a disorder of the immune system. This range of diseases does not include the bacterial inflammations due to a lowering of the defense mechanism, for example, in the postoperative period. Immune sialadenitis in its strict sense also includes those forms of inflammation due to hyperreactivity of the immune system. This is especially true of acute allergic sialadenitis and autoimmune sialadenitis.

Allergic Sialadenitis

Acute allergic sialadenitis, evoked by the action of various antigen-antibody complexes on the salivary glands, is rare. A fleeting swelling of the salivary glands appears only to disappear after elimination of the allergen. Allergens include foodstuffs and drugs, particularly phenylbutazone (Garfunkel et al 1974, Simpson 1966) and nitrofurantoin (Pellinen & Kalske 1982, Griffin & Penn 1982). The histopathologic findings include dissolution of gland acini, and periductal and perivascular inflammatory infiltration by lymphocytes, leukocytes, and histiocytes. They resemble the experimental findings of *immune complex sialadenitis* (Boss et al 1975, Dishon et al 1973). This disease can be evoked by antibodies against the basal membrane and against consituents of blood plasma. The antibody must be injected into the ductal system of previously sensitized rats. The inflammation may also be induced by introducing the preformed immune complexes into the ductal system in the absence of sensitization and may be prevented by antihistamines (Sela 1975, Ulmansky et al 1972).

Myoepithelial Sialadenitis (Sjögren's Syndrome)

It is assumed that autoimmune mechanisms are the main cause of Sjögren's syndrome, so that the term *autoimmune sialadenitis* is justified (Donath & Seifert 1981, Caselitz & Seifert 1982). Synonymous terms include benign lymphoepithelial lesion (Godwin 1952, Kahn 1979), chronic myoepithelial sialadenitis (Seifert & Geiler 1957, Donath & Seifert 1972, Seifert 1981), and autoimmune sialadenopathy.

In 1933, the Swedish ophthalmologist Sjögren, established that patients with xerophthalmia also demonstrated reduced secretions of the salivary glands in addition to the reduced lacrimal secretion that was the cause of the keratoconjunctivitis. The disease affected older women almost exclusively: their salivary glands, mainly the parotids, were swollen and they often had rheumatoid arthritis. Sjögren concluded that the keratoconjunctivitis sicca was a generalized disease. This syndrome was named after Sjögren and is probably identical with the disease described by Gougerot in 1925. Morgan and Castleman (1953) concluded on the basis of histopathology that the syndrome described by von Mikulicz (1888, 1892) is the same as Sjögren's syndrome. The disease could therefore be described as Gougerot-von Mikulicz-Sjögren syndrome.

Sjögren's syndrome remains to this day a clinical diagnosis that may be made if two or three of the following triad are present (Bloch et al 1965):

1. Keratoconjunctivitis sicca
2. Xerostomia
3. Rheumatoid arthritis or other connective tissue disorders, such as disseminated lupus erythematosus, progressive scleroderma, polymyositis, and panarteritis nodosa.

Specific diseases of the lacrimal and salivary glands, such as tuberculosis or sarcoid, should not be included in Sjögren's syndrome. If the first two components of the triad alone are present, the term *primary Sjögren's syndrome* should be used. If these two are accompanied by rheumatoid arthritis, the term *secondary Sjögren's syndrome* should be used.

Based on this clinical definition of Sjögren's syndrome, chronic epithelial sialadenitis is very common in biopsies of the major and minor salivary glands. A chronic unilateral parotid swelling, on the other hand, often hides a myoepithelial sialadenitis without the clinical symptoms of Sjögren's syndrome and without later involvement of other salivary and lacrimal glands. The same is also true of autoantibodies against cytoplasmic

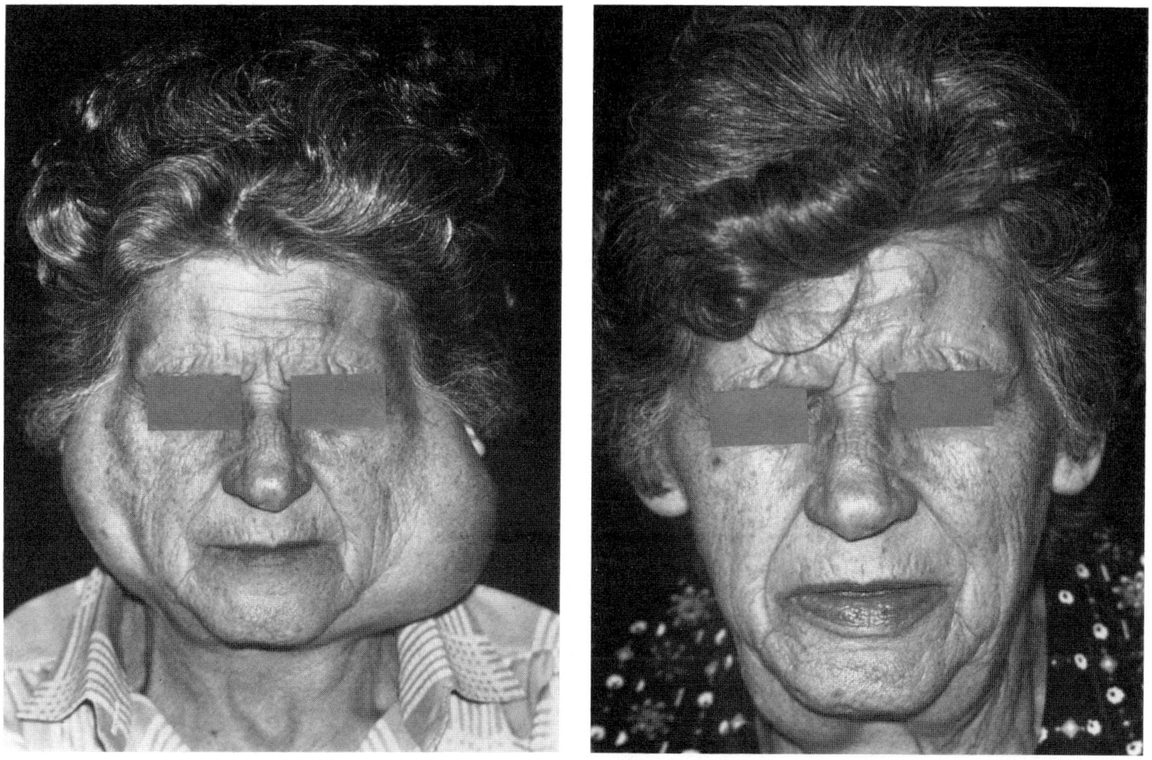

Figure 12.**53** Bilateral parotid swelling in a patient with Sjögren's syndrome. **a** Before operation, **b** after operation. A parotidectomy was carried out for cosmetic reasons.

antigens of the salivary duct epithelium which have been demonstrated in the serum of 75% of patients with Sjögren's syndrome (Bertram & Halberg 1964). However, this type of antigen is also observed in patients without Sjögren's syndrome and in various collagenoses, for example, in 27% of patients with disseminated lupus erythematosus and in 12.5% of patients with Hashimoto's thyroiditis (Bertram 1967).

The term "Sjögren's syndrome" may be further refined by using the term "complete Sjögren's syndrome," if myoepithelial sialadenitis and ductal antibodies can be demonstrated in the serum in addition to the clinical symptoms. Batsakis (1982) distinguishes between a benign lymphoepithelial lesion, which may be a localized salivary gland disease, or may be one manifestation of Sjögren's syndrome.

The **clinical picture** of Sjögren's syndrome is dominated by the reduction of tears and saliva, the resulting keratoconjunctivitis sicca, and objective xerostomia due to hyposalivation or absence of saliva (Chapter 7). The appropriate glands may be swollen due to chronic inflammation. Bilateral swelling of the parotid glands is typical, but other glands, particularly the submandibular gland, may be affected. The disease is most common in women, with a peak age incidence between 50 and 60 years (Figs. 12.**53a, b,** 12.**54**). The salivary gland parenchyma may undergo secondary infection in some cases (Cohen & Bankhurst 1979). This secondary infection can recur and simulate chronic recurrent parotitis (Chilla et al 1982). The resulting tenderness of the parotid swelling is not typical of Sjögren's syndrome.

The reduced salivary production influences the function of the oral mucosa (see Chapter 7). The reduced lacrimal secretion leads to metabolic disturbances of the cornea and the conjunctiva. The activity of other mucosal glands apart from those of the eye and oral cavity may be affected, so that the sicca phenomenon may extend to the upper airway, the esophagus, and the stomach (Bloch et al 1965). Extraglandular manifestations of Sjögren's syndrome with the characteristic lymphocytic infiltrate have been described, for example, in the kidneys and lung (Talal et al 1967, 1971).

The clinical appearances of Sjögren's syndrome vary, depending on the occurrence of rheumatoid arthritis and on disorders that often accompany Sjögren's syndrome, such as macrocytic anemia, recurrent pancreatitis, diabetes mellitus, and Hashimoto's thyroiditis (Whaley et al 1973, Bloch et al 1965).

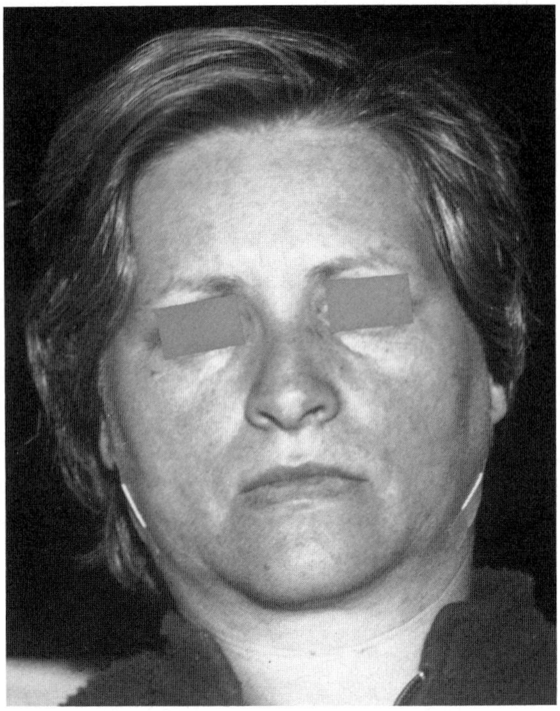

Figure 12.**54** Mainly unilateral parotid swelling in myoepithelial sialadenitis without Sjögren's syndrome.

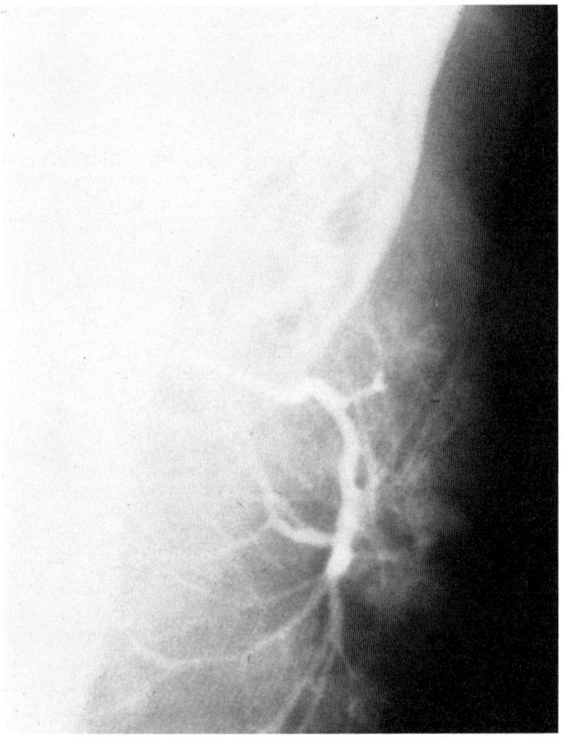

Figure 12.**55** Sialography in Sjögren's syndrome.

The **diagnosis** of Sjögren's syndrome offers no difficulty in the full-blown disease. The diagnosis may be confirmed by a biopsy from the parotid or submandibular glands or from the minor salivary glands, particularly those of the lip. Laboratory findings can be divided into three groups:

1. *Nonspecific signs of inflammation* such as increased erythrocyte sedimentation rate and increased levels of gamma globulins in the serum.
2. Autoantibodies against cytopasmic antigens of the ductal epithelium are the most important of the *disease-specific phenomena*. From a literature review (Moutsopoulos et al 1980), it appears that these are found in 69% of patients with secondary Sjögren's syndrome, but in only 25% of patients with primary Sjögren's syndrome, and in 26% of patients with rheumatoid arthritis but without Sjögren's syndrome.
3. The *nonspecific immune phenomena*, which may be demonstrated in Sjögren's syndrome, include antinuclear factors (in about 50%), antigamma-globulin factors and numerous autoantibodies, for example, against plasma antigens of the salivary follicle cells, the gastric epithelium (Whaley et al 1973) and pancreatic duct epithelium (Ludwig et al 1978).

Involvement of the salivary glands in Sjögren's syndrome leads inevitably to the use of specific methods of investigation, such as analysis of the saliva and sialography. There is no specific sialographic picture of myoepithelial sialadenitis (Haubrich 1976). The sialographic changes resemble those of recurrent parotitis (Fig. 12.**55**). Analysis of the saliva is only possible if material can be obtained, but this is not possible in advanced myoepithelial sialadenitis, either from the individual glands or from the oral cavity. Electrophoresis demonstrates that two proteins specific for Sjögren's syndrome are found if some secretory activity remains (Benedek-Spät et al 1980). Sialochemistry shows that individual constituents of the saliva, such as sodium, chloride, IgA, IgG, lactoferrin, and albumin, are increased in concentration, whereas others, such as phosphate, are reduced (Stuchel et al 1984).

The **histopathologic appearances** consist of a triad of parenchymatous atrophy, interstitial lymphocytic cell infiltration, and myoepithelial cell islands. Depending on the degree of severity, early, middle, and advanced stages of the inflammatory process can be distinguished (Figs. 12.**56**, 12.**57**). The early lesions are a periductal lymphocytic infiltrate and a focal involution of the acini. In the later course of the disease, the lym-

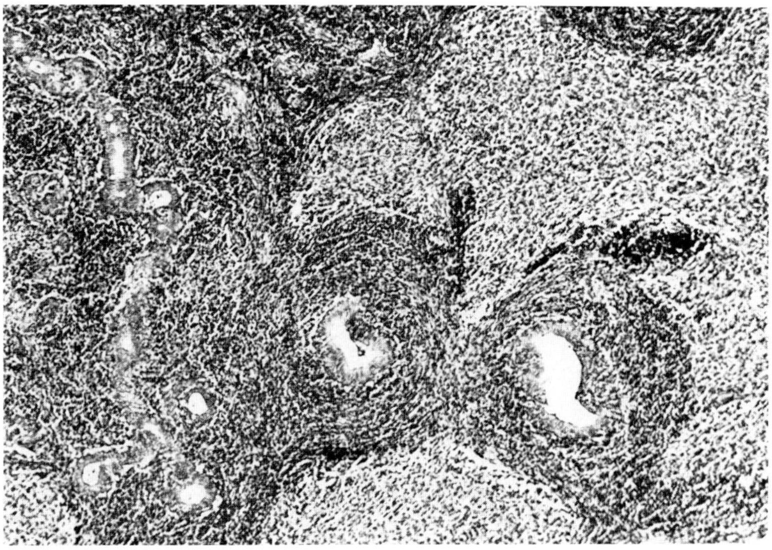

Figure 12.**56** Immune sialadenitis of the parotid gland showing periductal lymphocytic infiltrate, formation of lymph follicles, and loss of parenchyma. H & E, 63×.

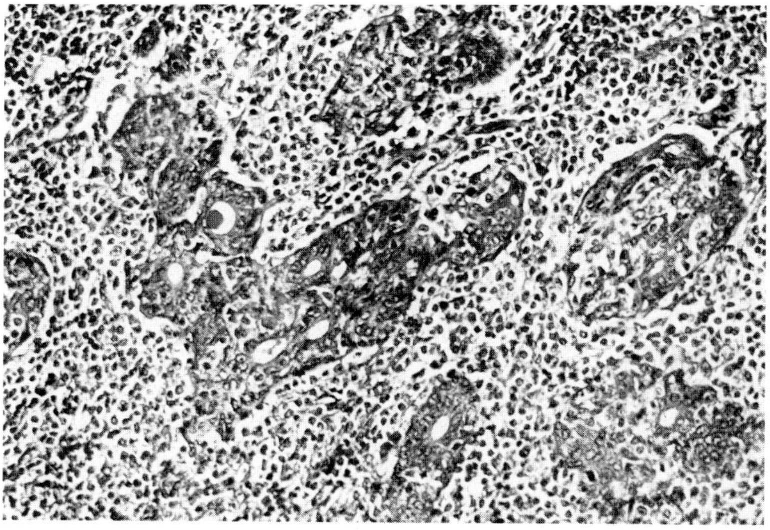

Figure 12.**57** Myoepithelial parotitis in Sjögren's syndrome: multiple epithelial cell islands surrounded by lymphocytic infiltration and complete loss of parenchyma. H & E, 160×.

phocytic infiltration and parenchymatous atrophy increase. The ductal system shows metaplasia of its epithelium and proliferation of myoepithelial cells. The development of the myoepithelial cell islands shows different phases (Fig. 12.**56**). Initially, the cell islets retain a lumen (Fig. 12.**58a, b**), but with increase of the lymphocytic infiltrate, this remnant disappears and the cell islets undergo hyaline transformation (Figs. 12.**59**, 12.**60a, b**). The external basal membrane is thus gradually destroyed (Fig. 12.**61a, b**).

Electron microscopy demonstrates young myoid cells that migrate into the interstitium and that are said to be responsible for the accumulation of membrane material and the later collagenous sclerosis (Chomette et al 1983).

The severity of the focal lesions varies enormously, as shown by sialography. Occasionally, duct ectasia may be found demonstrating retention of secretion, inspissated secretions, and microliths (Fig. 12.**62**). The ductal epithelium shows proliferation, and extensive hyaline transformation may occur on its external surface.

Immunohistochemistry in the later phases demonstrates a marked increase of IgG-containing plasma cells, whereas in chronic sialadenitis without autoimmune phenomena the IgA-containing plasma cells are predominant (Gumberz & Seifert 1980). Within the myoepithelial cell islands, plasma cells are scarce compared with an abundance of lymphocytes. This phenomenon indicates a change of local immune status and an invasion by

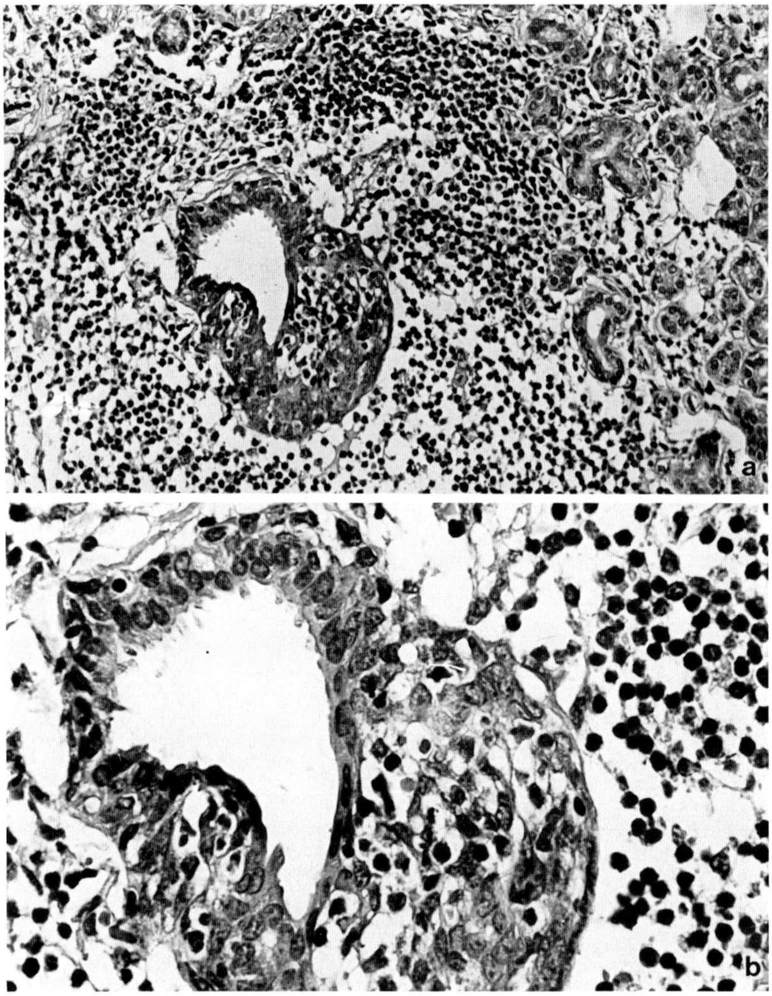

Figure 12.**58** Myoepithelial parotitis: myoepithelial cell islands with residual lumen and focal cell proliferations. H & E. **a** 160×, **b** 400×.

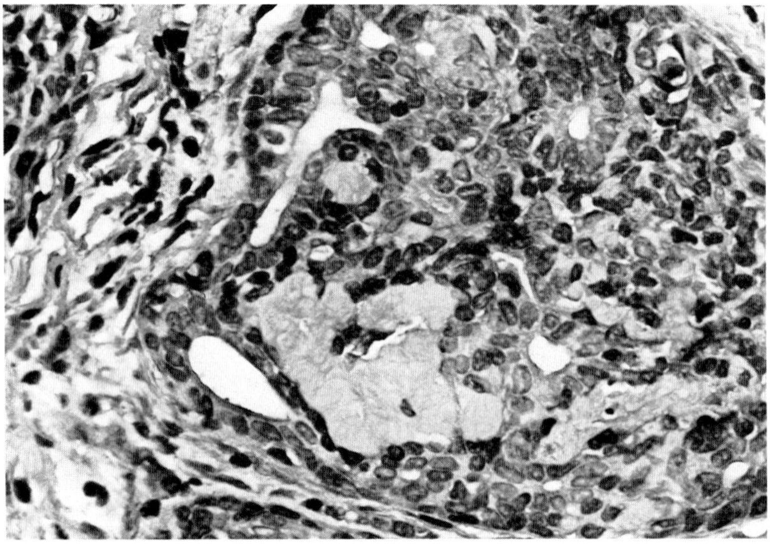

Figure 12.**59** Myoepithelial cell island with residual lumen and early hyalinization. H & E, 400×.

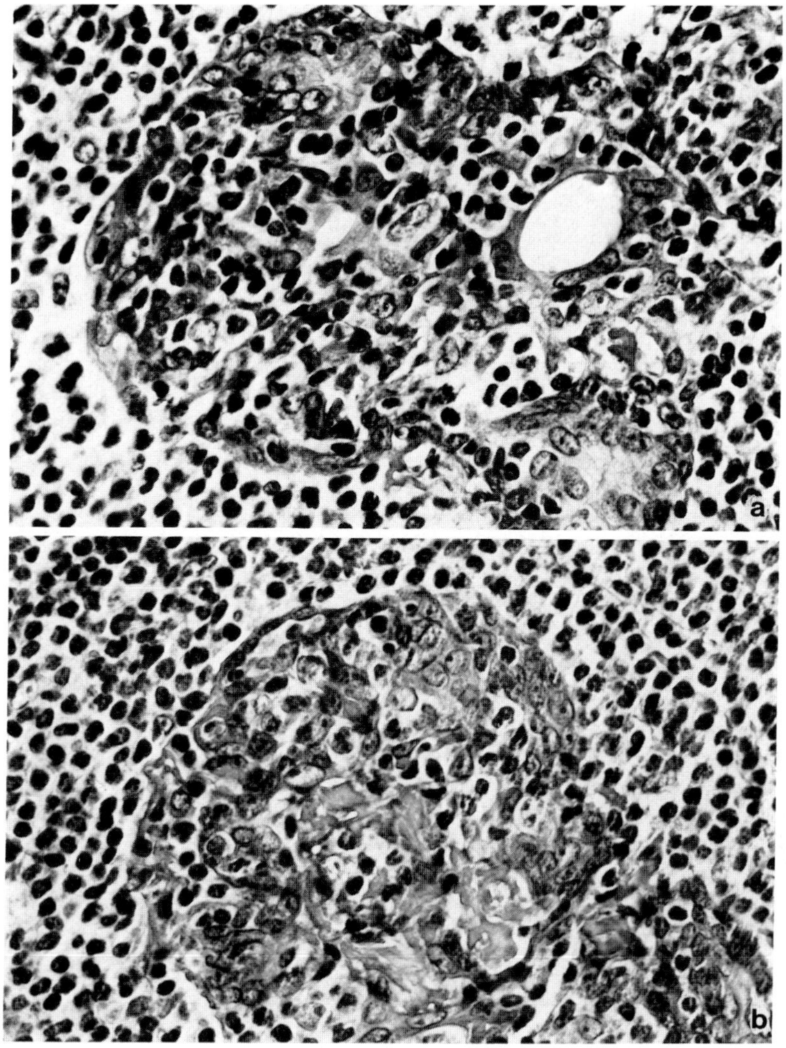

Figure 12.**60** Developmental stage of myoepithelial cell islands: **a** Island with residual lumen and lymphocytic infiltration. **b** Island with complete hyalin transformation. H & E. **a**, **b** 400×.

new plasma cell clones with special IgG formation. Epithelioid cell granulomas also occur occasionally in myoepithelial sialadenitis (Fig. 12.**63a, b**). These often lie in the neighborhood of the myoepithelial cell islands (de Wilde et al 1984). The development of epithelioid cell granulomas probably represents a secondary step and is the expression of an immune defect of the B and T lymphocytes (Seifert et al 1980). The demonstration of *antiductal antibodies* is particularly important (Cummings & Tarpley 1978, Kassan & Gardy 1978), especially in patients with Sjögren's syndrome and rheumatoid arthritis (Ludwig et al 1978). The demonstration of this antibody does not necessarily correlate with the density of the lymphocytic infiltrate. Further antibodies against definite nuclear constituents are also often observed in Sjögren's syndrome. The order of the immunologic system expresses itself not only in a change of the humoral defense, but also in a shift of the T and B cell population. Recent immunocytochemical investigations have shown a T lymphocyte predominance and also a marked individual variation with respect to the distribution of T helper and T suppressor cells (Kilpi et al 1983). The polyclonal lymphocyte infiltration can be accompanied by IgG paraprotein (Basu et al 1983). The increase of IgA-positive cells probably plays a role in the local accumulation of T lymphocytes (Kilpi et al 1983).

The *minor salivary glands,* particularly those of the lip, are inflamed in addition to the major glands (Greenspan et al 1974, Luhn et al 1981, Sapiro & Eisenberg 1978, Tarpley et al 1974, Chomette et al 1981, Konttinen 1981). Histologic examination (Fig. 12.**64**) shows duct ectasia, lymphocytic infiltrate, and marked sclerosis of glands with atrophy of acini and destruction of the lobules. However, myoepithelial cell islands are rarely found in the minor salivary glands (de

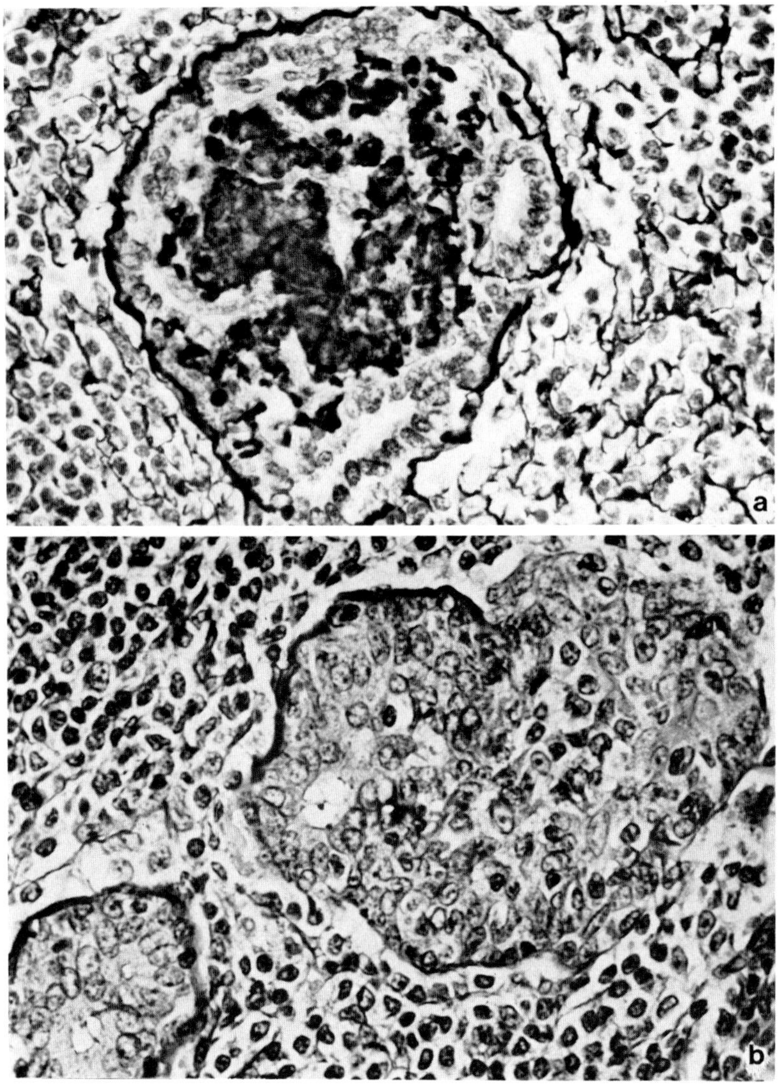

Figure 12.**61** Border of a myoepithelial cell island: **a** Basal membrane on the external surface and hyaline transformation within. Gomori, 400×. **b** Partial dissolution of the PAS positive basal membrane and lymphocytic infiltrate. PAS, 400×.

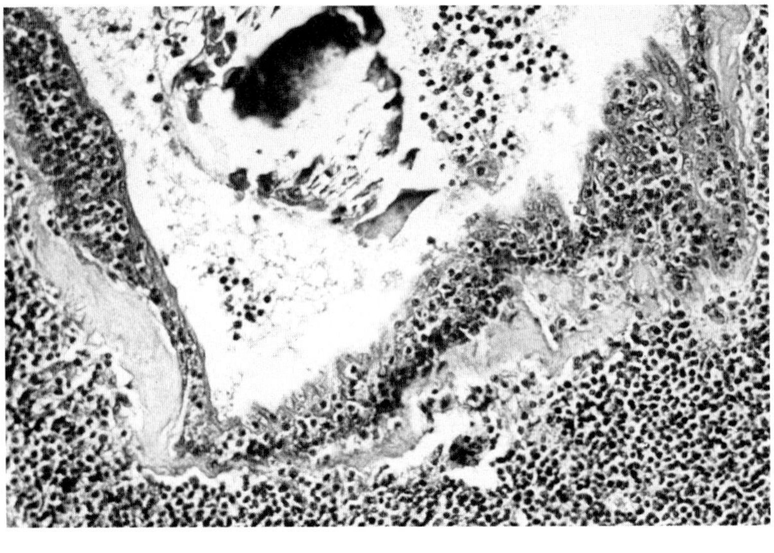

Figure 12.**62** Myoepithelial parotitis: focal duct ectasia with inspissated secretion and formation of microliths, proliferation of the duct epithelium, and periductal sclerosis. H & E, 160×.

Figure 12.**63** Myoepithelial parotitis: **a** Epithelioid cell granuloma lying close to a myoepithelial cell island (**b**). H & E. **a**, **b** 400×.

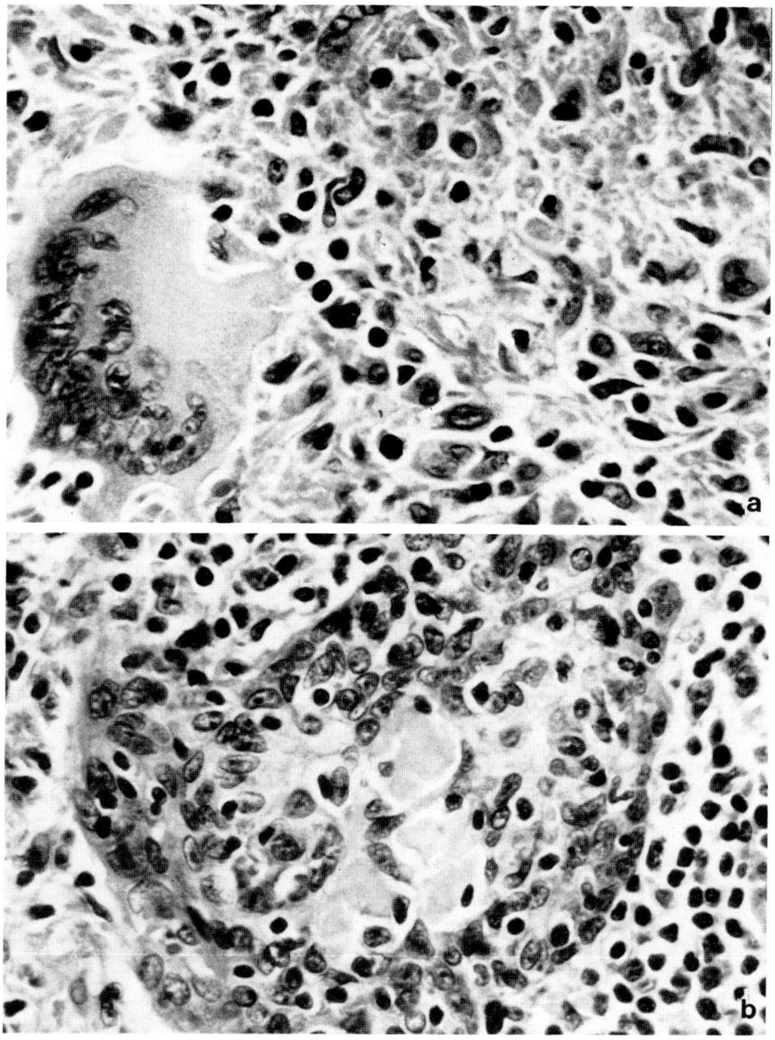

Figure 12.**64** Chronic immune sialadenitis of the palatal glands in Sjögren's syndrome: duct ectasia, and extensive lymphocytic infiltrate and parenchymatous atrophy. H & E, 160×.

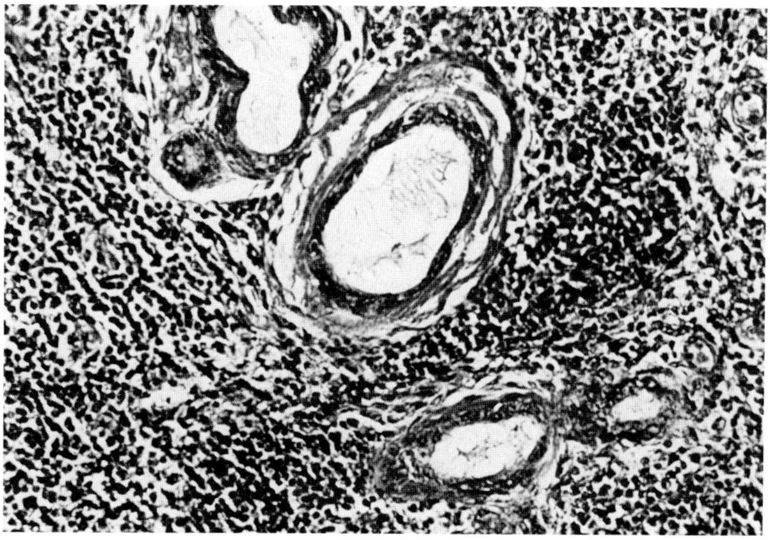

Wilde et al 1984). The severity of the lesions correlates with the findings in the parotid gland. Decreasing enzyme activity, an ultrastructural injury pattern of the cell organelles, and defective salivation parallel the morphologic lesions (Ben-Aryeh et al 1981). The finding that patients with graft-versus-host reaction show similar changes in their salivary glands is interesting and indicates the significance of immunologic reactions in Sjögren's syndrome (Sale et al 1981).

Sjögren's syndrome is now classified with the autoimmune disorders, which include Hashimoto's thyroiditis, rheumatoid arthritis, and disseminated lupus erythematosus. Although the **pathogenic mechanism** leading to the development of Sjögren's syndrome is so far unexplained, a whole range of abnormal immunologic reactions and experimental investigations strongly suggest the presence of an autoimmune disease (Moutsopoulos et al 1980). These include:

1. The demonstration by immunofluorescence of autoantibodies in the serum, usually IgG, against cytoplasmic antigens of the salivary duct epithelium (Bertram & Halberg 1964, Cummings & Tarpley 1978, Kassan & Gardi 1978). Other autoantibodies occur, for example, against salivary follicular cells and gastric epithelium.
2. Genetic anomalies of the immune system have been suggested (Shearn 1971). Thus, two lymphocytic antigens (HLA-B8 and HLA-DW3) occur in patients with Sjögren's syndrome, which may be coded by the histocompatibility complex. These two immune response genes obviously affect the course of the autoimmune reaction.
3. Repeated demonstration of specific B cell populations in the presence of Sjögren's syndrome (Moutsopoulos et al 1978 and 1979).
4. There is much evidence of hyperreactivity of the B cells in Sjögren's syndrome, including polyclonal hypergammaglobulinemia and nonorgan-specific autoantibodies (Alspaugh & Tan 1975, Alspaugh et al 1976), probably due to a defect of T suppressor cells (Kaufman & Boswick 1979). Parallels arise here with disseminated lupus erythematosus (Talal 1976, Fauci et al 1978, Jonsson et al 1982), which itself obviously demonstrates analogies to the autoimmune models in the mouse (Theofilopoulos et al 1979). However, an increase of circulating B cells that secrete spontaneously polyclonal antibodies is not to be found in Sjögren's syndrome (Mountsopoulos et al 1980). Possibly these B cells are sequestered in lymphatic organs in Sjögren's syndrome.
5. Many strains of mice, for example NZB, and NZB × NZW F_1, which demonstrate genetically determined autoimmune diseases, develop histologic changes in the lacrimal and salivary glands that resemble myoepithelial sialadenitis (Kessler 1968). A further model is provided by the experimental autoallergic sialadenitis in the SL/Ni mouse (Takeda & Ishikawa 1983).
6. Patients who develop a graft-versus-host reaction, for example as a result of bone marrow transplantation (Gratwohl et al 1977), develop changes typical of Sjögren's syndrome in their salivary glands (Sale et al 1981).

The spectrum of Sjögren's disease extends from isolated involvement of the lacrimal and salivary glands through interstitial lymphocytic infiltrate of other exocrine glands, with an extraglandular extension of this infiltrate to *malignant lymphatic disorders* (Talal et al 1967, Anderson & Talal 1971). Non-Hodgkin's malignant lymphoma has been described repeatedly in association with Sjögren's syndrome in recent years (Rothman et al 1951, Talal & Bunim 1964, Ferlito & Cattai 1980, Hordijk & Meyer 1981, Heckmayr et al 1976, von Gumberz & Seifert 1980, Schmid et al 1982). Most of these non-Hodgkin's lymphomas were not localized to the salivary glands themselves, although obviously these sites are at increased risk (Azzopardi & Evans 1971). Our material from the years 1965–1975 included 16 patients with primary non-Hodgkin's lymphoma of the salivary glands, and one women had had Sjögren's syndrome for many years.

The risk of the development of a malignant tumor in patients with or without Sjögren's syndrome has been analyzed carefully (Kassan et al 1978).

The relative risk (that is, observed to expected cases) for non-lymphatic malignancy is only increased slightly to 1.2 : 1. For non-Hodgkin's lymphoma, the relative risk increases to 43.8 : 1. Patients with a parotid swelling are particularly at risk (with a relative risk of 66.7 : 1), whereas those without swelling have a relatively lower risk (12.5 : 1). It is interesting that Sjögren's patients with non-Hodgkin's lymphoma show no autoantibodies against salivary duct epithelium (Pritchard et al 1978) and that patients without such an autoantibody show a tendency to marked lymphocytic infiltrate (Anderson et al 1973).

The clinical signs of the development of a malignant lymphoma in a preexisting myoepithelial sialadenitis include a rapidly progressive swelling of the cheek, particularly in older women. Further details of the classification of lymphomas is given on page 321.

The **treatment** of Sjögren's syndrome is unsatisfactory. In the secondary forms, precedence is given to the treatment of the rheumatoid arthritis by drugs, including the antirheumatic preparations, steroids, and immune suppressants. The progressive irreversible failure of the lacrimal and salivary gland parenchyma cannot usually be prevented. Synthetic preparations, mainly on a methylcellulose basis, are now used to mitigate the results of lack of tears and saliva (see Chapter 7).

Myoepithelial sialadenitis is rarely an indication for surgery. Apart from cosmetic indications because of extreme swelling of the salivary glands, there are only two purposes for removal of the glands:

Parotidectomy may be indicated for diagnostic purposes, if the clinical appearances and the results of biopsy do not confirm the presence of a myoepithelial sialadenitis. This is particularly true of a unilateral myoepithelial sialadenitis (Fig. 12.**54**), which can occur without acute inflammatory symptoms and without the clinical appearance of Sjögren's syndrome. The suspicion of a tumor becomes stronger if a salivary gland in a patient with Sjögren's syndrome grows rapidly, particularly because the increased incidence of malignant lymphoma in the salivary glands in this syndrome is well known.

The secondarily infected forms of myoepithelial sialadenitis can present as a resistant recurrent parotitis and can then only be controlled by removal of the inflamed gland.

Epithelioid Cell Sialadenitis (Sarcoidosis of the Salivary Glands, Heerfordt's Syndrome)

The **etiology** of sacoidosis is so far unknown. Since it may be an allergic reaction to an as yet unidentified allergen, epithelioid cell sialadenitis as a manifestation of sarcoidosis of the salivary glands is included under the heading of allergic sialadenitis. Typically, sarcoidosis affects the lymph nodes, particularly those of the hilum of the lung, causing a hilar adenopathy, but many other organs may be affected by this systemic disease. Between 1 and 6% of patients with sarcoidosis have disease of the salivary glands (Mayock et al 1963, Pfeiffer 1963 and 1968). In our series of patients with chronic parotitis, 8.6% had epithelioid cell parotitis. The chronic form is typical: unlike recurrent parotitis, the swelling of the gland is constant and pain is slight or absent. Often, only one parotid gland is diseased. A pronounced xerostomia is unusual, in contrast to that in the usually bilateral myoepithelial parotitis. The parotid swelling in epithelioid cell inflammation usually shows a modest firm consistency and is often multinodular, because of variable involvement of the parenchyma or because of involvement of para- and intraglandular lymph nodes. It is said that the minor salivary glands of the palate and lips are often affected by sarcoidosis in addition to the parotid gland (Cahn et al 1964, Chisholm et al 1971).

The **diagnosis** must be confirmed by biopsy. The *tuberculin test* can be used to distinguish the disease from tuberculosis, since the test is usually negative in sarcoidosis. The positive outcome of the *Kveim test* (a skin test) is largely specific for sarcoidosis, but the necessary antigen is not commercially available so that this test cannot be used as a routine procedure. Increase of the serum calcium level in sarcoidosis correlates with bony involvement. Furthermore, sarcoidosis is accompanied by changes in activity of the serum enzymes, but these are not specific for this disease. The determination of *angiotensinase I* is more useful. This enzyme, which is produced especially in the vascular endothelium of the lungs, acts on angiotensin I to split off angiotensin II, which influences the blood pressure. Its serum level is increased in sarcoidosis (Wurm 1981). Determination of the enzyme does not replace biopsy, but is useful for follow-up during and after treatment.

Analysis of the saliva shows a reduced flow rate, a depressed amylase content with normal protein concentration, and an increase of lysozymes and albumin content of the parotid saliva (Chisholm et al 1971, Beeley & Chisholm 1976, Bhoola et al 1969), but this analysis has very little diagnostic value. These changes are not typical of an epithelioid cell parotitis, since they occur in other chronic salivary inflammations. The sialographic picture in sarcoidosis of the salivary glands is equally nonspecific.

If sarcoidosis arising primarily in the salivary glands is diagnosed, a thorough search for other manifestations must follow, looking especially for lesions of the lungs and eyes. Combined involvement of the eye and parotid gland by sarcoidosis is described as *Heerfordt's syndrome*, named for the Danish ophthalmologist who first described it. In 1909, he reported three cases of uveoparotid fever, affecting the parotid gland and the uvea of the eye, and often complicated by paralysis of the cranial nerves. The first description thus encompassed a further manifestation of sarcoidosis, namely, involvement of neural tissue, particularly the cranial nerves, such as the facial nerve.

Histologic examination shows that recurrent swelling of the parotid is caused by a granulomatous

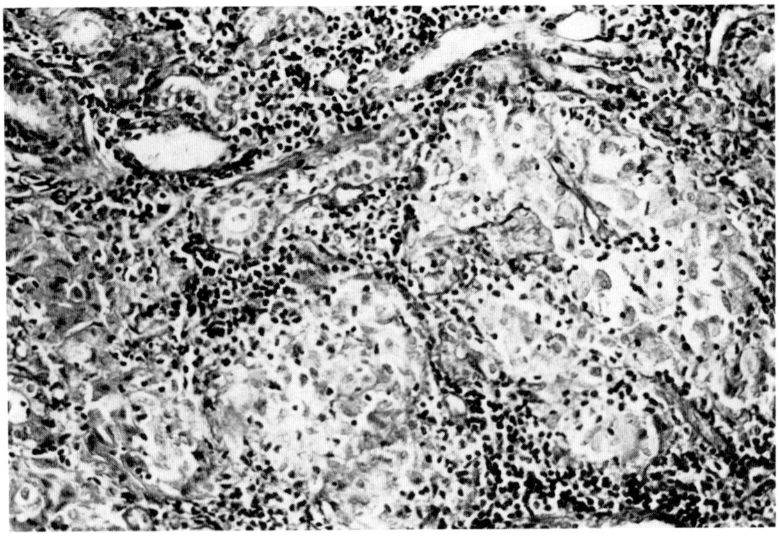

Figure 12.**65** Epithelioid parotitis: permeation of the gland lobule by granulomas consisting of epithelioid cells and occasional lymphocytes. H & E, 160×.

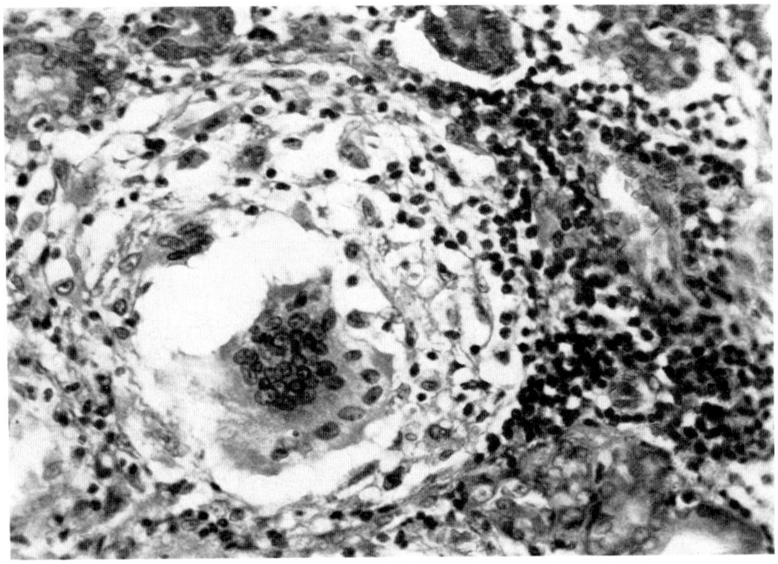

Figure 12.**66** Epithelioid cell parotitis: segment of a granuloma with a multinuclear Langhans' giant cell, epithelioid cells and lymphocytes. H & E, 400×.

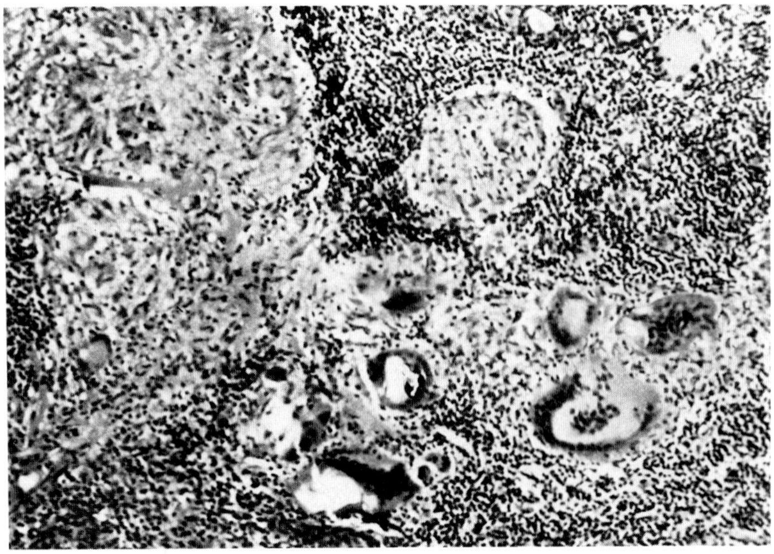

Figure 12.**67** Epithelioid cell parotitis showing granuloma formation with inclusion of numerous giant cells. H & E, 160×.

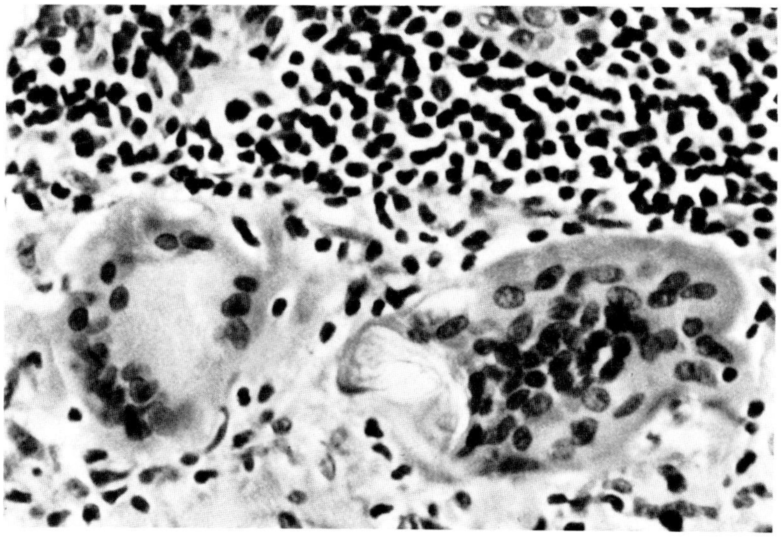

Figure 12.**68** Epithelioid cell parotitis: granuloma formation with multinuclear giant cells and inclusion of foreign body particles. H & E, 400×.

inflammation of the lobules of the gland (Figs. 12.**65**, 12.**66**). The granulomas consist of epithelioid cells, lymphocytes, and multinuclear giant cells of Langhans' type. Caseation does not occur. Smaller granulomas tend to form larger nodes. The lobules are gradually destroyed by chronic progressive inflammation. Foreign-body giant cells arise due to ductal obstruction and inspissation of secretions, and the giant cells may contain birefringent particles (Figs. 12.**67**, 12.**68**). Occasionally, mucous granulomas (mucoceles of extravasation type) are found with remnants of extravasated mucous masses in the interstitium.

The following forms of sarcoidosis may be distinguished, depending on the *site*.

- Epithelioid cell granulomas of the parenchyma of the major salivary glands, particularly the parotid,
- Primary affection of the intra- or periglandular lymph nodes with possible secondary invasion of the parenchyma,
- Supplementary involvement of the minor salivary glands (Tarpley et al 1972, Nesson & Jacoway 1979).

The rare *coincidence of myoepithelial and epithelioid cell parotitis* is particularly interesting (Seifert et al 1980). This finding relatively often accompanies immunopathies, such as gamma dysproteinemia, immunoglobulin defect, and tumors (see Chapter 17). Obviously, there is a reduction of T cell function and a corresponding increase of B cell function, not only in myoepithelial cell parotitis, but also in Heerfordt's syndrome (Cottier 1980, Daniele et al 1981). The development of epithelioid cell granulomas is a secondary phenonemon analogous to the epithelioid cell-rich lymphogranulomatosis (Lennert & Mestdagh 1968).

The **treatment** of sarcoidosis consists of long-term steroids, usually supervised by an internist.

References

Alspaugh, M. A., E. M. Tan: Antibodies to cellular antigens in Sjögren's syndrome. J. clin. Invest. 55 (1975) 1067

Alspaugh, M. A., N. Talal, E. M. Tan: Differentiation and characterization of autoantibodies and their antigens in Sjögren's syndrome. Arthr. Rheum. 19 (1976) 216

Anderson, L. G., N. Talal: The spectrum of benign to malignant lymphoproliferation in Sjögren's syndrome. Clin. exp. Immunol. 9 (1971) 199

Anderson, L. G., T. M. Tarpley, N. Talal, N. A. Cummings, R. O. Wolf, G. L. Schall: Cellular-versus-humoral autoimmune responses of salivary gland in Sjögren's syndrome. Clin. exp. Immunol. 13 (1973) 335

Azzopardi, J. G., D. J. Evans: Malignant lymphoma of parotid associated with Mikulicz disease (benign lymphoepithelial lesion). J. clin. Path. 24 (1971) 744

Basu, M. K., J. D. Price, J. B. Matthews: Benign lymphoepithelial lesion in a patient with Sjögren's disease and IgG paraprotein. J. oral Path. 12 (1983) 515

Batsakis, J. G.: The pathology of head and neck tumors: the lymphoepithelial lesion and Sjögren's syndrome. Head Neck Surg. (N. Y.) 5 (1982) 150

Beeley, J. A., D. M. Chisholm: Sarcoidosis with salivary gland involvement: Biochemical studies on parotid saliva. J. Lab. clin. Med. 88 (1976) 276

Ben-Aryeh, H., A. Spielman, R. Szargel, D. Gutman, J. Scharf, M. Nahir, Y. Scharf: Sialochemistry for diagnosis of Sjögren's syndrome in xerostomic patients. Oral Surg. 52 (1981) 487

Benedek-Spät, E., M. Puskás, J. Rajki: Electrophoretic protein pattern of human parotid saliva in Sjögren's syndrome and sialosis. Acta Otolaryngol. 90 (1980) 275

Bertram, U.: Xerostomia. Acta odont. scand., Suppl. 49 (1967) 1

Bertram, U., P. Halberg: A specific antibody against the epithelium of the salivary ducts in sera from patients with Sjögren's syndrome. Acta allerg. 19 (1964) 458

Bhoola, K. D., M. W. McNicol, S. Oliver, J. Foran: Changes in salivary enzymes in patients with sarcoidosis. New Engl. J. Med. 281 (1969) 877

Bloch, K. J., W. W. Buchanan, M. J. Wohl, J. H. Bunim: Sjögren Syndrome. Medicine 44 (1965) 187

Boss, J. H., J. Sela, M. Ulmansky, T. Dishon, E. Rosenmann:

Experimental immune sialadenitis. A review. Israel J. Dent. Med. 24 (1975) E 15
Cahn, L. R., L. Eisenbud, M. M. Blake, D. Stern: Biopsies of normal appearing palates of patients with known sarcoidosis. Oral Surg. 18 (1964) 342
Caselitz, J., G. Seifert: Das lokale Abwehr- und Immunsystem der Speicheldrüsen unter physiologischen und pathologischen Bedingungen. Dtsch. Z. Mund-Kiefer-Gesichts-Chir. 6 (1982) 93
Chilla, R., H.-O. Meyfarth, C. Arglebe: Über die operative Behandlung der chronischen Ohrspeicheldrüsenentzündung. Arch. Otorhinolaryng. 234 (1982) 53
Chisholm, D. M., A. Lyell, T. S. Haroon, D. K. Mason, J. A. Beeley: Salivary gland function in sarcoidosis. Oral Surg. 31 (1971) 766
Chomette, G., M. Auriol, N. van Cat, H. Szpirglas, P. Tranbaloc, J. M. Vaillant: Biopsie des glandes salivaires labiales dans le syndrome de Gougerot-Sjögren. Étude clinicopathologique, histoenzymologique et ultrastructurale. Virchows Arch. Path. Anat. 392 (1981) 339
Chomette, G., P. Laudenbach, M. Auriol, H. Szpirglas: Les glandes salivaires accessoires dans le syndrome de Sjögren. Étude histologique et ultrastructurale. – Correlations avec les modifications des sialographies dans les glandes principales. Rev. Stomatol. Chir. maxillofac. 84 (1983) 121
Cohen, M., A. D. Bankhurst: Infectious parotitis in Sjögren's syndrome: a case report and review of the literature. J. Rheumat. 6 (1979) 185
Cottier, H.: Pathogenese. Springer, Berlin–New York 1980
Cummings, N. A., T. M. Tarpley: Detection of antisalivary duct antibody from Sjögren's syndrome by an autoradiographic method. J. immunol. Meth. 23 (1978) 161
Daniele, R. D., J. H. Dauber, M. D. Rossman: Immunologic abnormalities in sarcoidosis. Ann. int. Med. 92 (1981) 406
Dishon, T., J. Sela, M. Ulmansky, E. Rosenmann, J. H. Boss: Experimental allergic sialadenitis. VI. Prevention by antihistamine and induction by intraductal instillation of performed immune complexes. Virchows Arch. Abt. A Path. Anat. 359 (1973) 283
Donath, K., G. Seifert: Ultrastruktur und Pathogenese der myoepithelialen Sialadenitis. Virchows Arch. Abt. A Path. Anat. 356 (1972) 315
Donath, K., G. Seifert: Immunologische und immunpathologische Reaktionen der Speicheldrüsen. Allergologie 4 (1981) 110
Fauci, A. S., A. D. Steinberg, B. F. Haynes, G. Whalen: Immunoregulatory aberrations in systemic lupus erythematosus. J. Immunol. 121 (1978) 1473
Ferlito, A., N. Cattai: The so-called "benign lymphoepithelial lesion" Part II. Clinical and pathological considerations with regard to evolution. J. Laryng. Otol. 94 (1980) 1283
Garfunkel, A. A., N. W. Roller, C. Nichols, I. I. Ship: Phenylbutazone-induced sialadenitis. Oral Surg. 38 (1974) 223
Godwin, J. T.: Benign lymphoepithelial lesion of the parotid gland (adenolymphoma, chronic inflammation, lymphoepithelioma, lymphocytic tumor, Mikulicz's disease). Report of 11 cases. Cancer (Philad.) 5 (1952) 1089
Gougerot, H.: Insuffisance progressive et atrophie des glandes salivaires et muqueuses de la bouche, des conjonctives etc. Bull. Soc. frc. dermat. syph. 32 (1925) 376
Gratwohl, A. A., H. M. Moutsopoulos, T. M. Chused, M. Akizuki, R. O. Wolf, J. B. Swett, A. B. Deisseroth: Sjögren-type syndrome after allogeneic bone-marrow transplantation. Ann. int. Med. 87 (1977) 703
Greenspan, J. S., D. E. Daniels, R. A. Sylvester: The histopathology of Sjögren's syndrome in labial salivary gland biopsies. Oral Surg. 37 (1974) 217
Griffin, J. P., R. G. Penn: Nitrofurantoin-induced parotitis. Brit. med. J. 285 (1982) 654
Gumberz, Chr. v., G. Seifert: Immuno-globulin-containing plasma cells in chronic parotitis and malignant lymphomas of the parotid gland. Comparing immunocytochemical observations of frequency and localization. Virchows Arch. Path. Anat. 389 (1980) 79
Haubrich, J.: Klinik der nichttumorbedingten Erkrankungen der Speicheldrüsen. Arch. Oto-Rhino-Laryng. 213 (1976) 1
Heckmayr, M., G. Seifert, K. Donath: Maligne Lymphome und Immun-Sialadenitis. Z. Laryng. Rhinol. 55 (1976) 593
Heerfordt, C. F.: Über ein „Febris uveo-parotidea subchronica" an der Gl. parotis und der Uvea des Auges lokalisiert und häufig mit Paresen cerebrospinaler Nerven kompliziert. Arch. klin. exp. Ophthal. 70 (1909) 254
Hordijk, G. J., C. J. L. M. Meyer: Benign lymphoepithelial lesion and malignancy. Arch. Oto-Rhino-Laryng. 230 (1981) 201
Jonsson, R., D. Bratthall, G. Nyberg: Histologic and sialochemical findings indicating sicca syndrome in patients with systemic lupus erythematosus. Oral Surg. 54 (1982) 635
Kahn, L. B.: Benign lymphoepithelial lesion (Mikulicz's disease) of the salivary gland: An ultrastructural study. Human Pathol. 10 (1979) 99
Kassan, S. S., M. Gardy: Sjögren's syndrome: An update and overview. Amer. J. Med. 64 (1978) 1037
Kassan, S. S., T. L. Thomas, H. M. Moutsopoulos, R. Hoover, R. P. Kimberly, D. R. Budman, J. Costa, J. L. Decker, T. M. Chused: Increased risk of lymphoma in sicca syndrome. Ann. intern. Med. 89 (1978) 888
Kaufman, D. B., E. Boswick: Defective suppressor T-cell activity in systemic lupus erythematodes. Clin. Immunol. Immunopath. 13 (1979) 9
Kessler, H. S.: A laboratory model for Sjögren's syndrome. Amer. J. Path. 52 (1968) 671
Kilpi, A., Y. T. Konttinen, M. Malmström, V. Bergroth, S. Reitamo, T. Helve: Immunocompetent cells in labial salivary glands in secondary Sjögren's syndrom associated with SLE. J. oral Path. 12 (1983) 465
Konttinen, Y.: In situ characterization of the cellular infiltrate in labial and palatine glands in Sjögren's syndrome. Scand. J. Rheumat. 10 (1981) 321
Lennert, K., J. Mestdagh: Lymphogranulomatosen mit konstant hohem Epitheloidzellgehalt. Virchows Arch. Path. Anat. 344 (1968) 1
Ludwig, H., G. Schernthaner, O. Scherak, G. Kolarz: Pankreasgang-Antikörper beim Sjögren-Syndrom und bei chronischer Polyarthritis. Verh. Dtsch. Ges. Rheumatol. 5 (1978) 144
Luhn, J.-P., K. Donath, E. Haneke: Veränderungen der Lippenspeicheldrüsen bei Glossodynie. Pathohistologische und morphometrische Analyse. HNO (Berl.) 29 (1981) 10
Mayock, R. L., P. Bertrand, C. E. Morrison, J. H. Scott: Manifestations of sarcoidosis. Analysis of 145 patients with a review of 9 series selected from the literature. Amer. J. Med. 35 (1963) 67
v. Mikulicz, J.: Verhandlungen des Vereins für wissenschaftliche Heilkunde zu Königsberg in Preußen. Berl. klin. Wschr. 25 (1888) 759
v. Mikulicz, J.: Über eine eigenartige symmetrische Erkrankung der Tränen- und Mundspeicheldrüsen. Beitr. Chir. Festschrift Billroth 2 (1892) 610
Morgan, W. S., B. A. Castleman: A clinicopathologic study of "Mikulicz's disease". Amer. J. Pathol. 29 (1953) 471
Moutsopoulos, H. M., D. L. Mann, A. H. Johnson, T. M. Chused: Genetic differences between primary and secondary sicca syndrome. New Engl. J. Med. 301 (1979) 761
Moutsopoulos, H. M., T. M. Chused, A. H. Johnson, B. Knudsen, D. L. Mann: B Lymphocyte antigens in sicca syndrome. Science 199 (1978) 1441
Moutsopoulos, H. M., T. M. Chused, D. L. Mann, J. H. Klippel, A. S. Fauci, M. M. Frank, T. J. Lawley, M. I. Hamburger: Sjögren's syndrome (sicca syndrome): Current Issues. Ann. intern. Med. 92 (1980) 212
Nesson, V. J., J. R. Jacoway: Biopsy of minor salivary glands in the diagnosis of sarcoidosis. New Engl. J. Med. 301 (1979) 922
Pellinen, T. J., J. Kalske: Nitrofurantoin-induced parotitis. Brit. med. J. 285 (1982) 344
Pfeiffer, K.: Über die Boeck'sche Erkrankung der Kopfspeicheldrüsen, zugleich ein Beitrag zur Analyse des Mikulicz-Syndroms. Radiol. 3 (1963) 165
Pfeiffer, K.: Die Röntgendiagnostik der Speicheldrüsen und ihrer Ausführungsgänge. In: Handbuch der Med. Radiologie, Bd. VI. Springer, Berlin 1968
Pritchard, K. I., A. M. M'seffar, A. Weinstein, A. Katz, D. A. Cordon, M. A. Baker: The prevalence of Sjögren's syndrome in non-Hodgkin's lymphoma. Proc. Amer. Ass. Cancer Res. 19 (1979) 418
Rothman, S., M. Block, F. V. Hauser: Sjögren's syndrome associated with lymphoblastoma and hypersplenism. Arch. Dermat. Syph. 63 (1951) 642
Sale, G. E., H. M. Shulman, M. M. Schubert, K. M. Sullivan, K. J. Kopecky, R. C. Hackman, Th. H. Morton, R. Storb, E. D. Thomas: Oral and ophthalmic pathology of graft versus host diseases in man: predictive value of the lip biopsy. Human Pathol. 12 (1981) 1022
Sapiro, S. M., E. Eisenberg: Sjögren's syndrome (sicca complex). Oral Surg. 45 (1978) 591
Schmid, U., D. Helbron, K. Lennert: Development of malignant lymphoma in myoepithelial sialadenitis (Sjögren's syndrome). Virchows Arch. Path. Anat. 395 (1982) 11
Seifert, G.: Lymphoid lesions of the oral cavity. Path. Res. Pract. 167 (1980) 179

Seifert, G.: Chronische Mundtrockenheit. Ursachen. Pathologie. Dtsch. Z. Mund-Kiefer-Gesichts-Chir. 5 (1981) 3
Seifert, G., G. Geiler: Vergleichende Untersuchungen der Kopfspeichel- und Tränendrüsen zur Pathogenese des Sjögren-Syndroms und der Mikulicz-Krankheit. Virchows Arch. Path. Anat. 330 (1957) 402
Seifert, G., K. Donath, Chr. v. Gumberz: Granulomatöse Reaktionen der Speicheldrüsen. Klassifikation und Pathogenese. Verh. Dtsch. Ges. Path. 64 (1980) 250
Sela, J., J. A. Bab, T. Dishon, E. Rosenmann, J. H. Boss: Experimental allergic sialadenitis. VII. Reactivity of the parotid gland to antigenic challenge in passively immunized rats. J. oral Pathol. 4 (1975) 11
Shearn, M. A.: Sjögren's Syndrome. Saunders, Philadelphia 1971
Simpson, R. W.: Salivary gland enlargement and phenylbutazone. Brit. Med. J. II (1966) 113
Sjögren, H.: Zur Kenntnis der Keratoconjunctivitis sicca. Acta ophthal. 10, Suppl. II (1933) 1
Stuchell, R. N., I. D. Mandel, H. Baurmash: Clinical utilization of sialochemistry in Sjögren's syndrome. J. oral Path. 13 (1984) 303
Takeda, Y., G. Ishikawa: Experimental autoallergic sialadenitis in mice. Histopathological and ultrastructural studies. Virchows Arch. Path. Anat. 400 (1983) 143
Talal, N.: Disordered immunologic regulation and autoimmunity. Transplant. Rev. 31 (1976) 240
Talal, N., J. J. Bunim: The development of malignant lymphoma in the course of Sjögren's syndrome. Amer. J. Med. 36 (1964) 529
Talal, N., L. Sokoloff, W. F. Barth: Extrasalivary lymphoid abnormalities in Sjögren's syndrome (reticulum cell sarcoma, "pseudolymphoma", macroglobulinemia). Amer. J. Med. 43 (1967) 50
Tarpley, Th. M., L. G. Anderson, C. L. White: Minor salivary gland involvement in Sjögren's syndrome. Oral Surg. 37 (1974) 64
Tarpley, Th. M., L. G. Anderson, Ph. Lightbody, J. N. Sheagren: Minor salivary gland involvement in sarcoidosis. Report of 3 cases with positive lip biopsies. Oral Surg. 33 (1972) 755
Theofilopoulos, A. M., R. A. Eisenberg, M. Bourdon, J. S. Crowell, F. J. Dixon: Distribution of lymphocytes identified by surface markers in murine strains with systemic lupus erythematosus-like syndromes. J. exp. Med. 149 (1979) 516
Ulmansky, M., T. Dishon, E. Rosenmann, J. Sela, J. H. Boss: Experimental allergic sialadenitis. IV. Studies on the etiopathogenetic mechanisms of the acute and chronic inflammatory process. Israel J. med. Sci. 8 (1972) 1791
Whaley, K., J. Webb, B. A. McAvoy, G. R. V. Hughes, P. Lee, R. N. M. MacSween, W. W. Buchanan: Sjögren's Syndrome. Quart. J. Med., New Ser. XLII (1973) 513
Wilde, P. C. M. de, P. J. Slootweg, R. J. Hené, J. P. A. Baak, L. Kater: Multinucleate giant cells in sublabial salivary gland tissue in Sjögrens's syndrome. Virchows Arch. (Pathol. Anat.) 403 (1984) 247
Wurm, K.: Sarkoidose-Diagnostik. Dtsch. med. Wschr. 106 (1981) 1356

Sialadenitis of the Minor Salivary Glands

In principle, the same etiologic and pathogenic principles apply to inflammation of the minor salivary glands as to that of the major glands (see page 118ff). Local factors, too, play a role.

Obstructive sialadenitis of the minor salivary glands is a relatively constant finding in the area around a tumor (Fig. 12.**69**). It is also found in localized retention of secretions due to dentures, a poorly seated dental crown, or cystic processes, particularly extravasation mucoceles or mucous retention cysts.

A *radiation sialadenitis* occurs in the irradiated field of tumors of the head and neck and is characterized histologically by loss of serous acini, an interstitial cell infiltrate, and ductal changes.

An inflammatory reaction of the minor salivary glands, particularly those of the lip (page 163), occurs mainly in *immunosialadenitis* in Sjögren's syndrome and less often in Heerfordt's syndrome.

Inflammation is found particularly often in the *labial glands,* and the following specific forms must be distinguished. *Cheilitis glandularis apostematosa* (Seifert 1966) arises in a heterotopic minor salivary gland in the margin of the lower lip exposed to bite injuries causing extravasation of mucus into the interstitium, as in extravasation mucoceles. *Granulomatous cheilitis* (Miescher 1945) affects the upper lip preferentially, producing an appearance like an elephant's trunk. Usually, this is one manifestation of the Melkersson-Rosenthal syndrome (Hornstein & Schuermann 1962, Hornstein & Haneke 1980). Histologic findings (Figs. 12.**70**, 12.**71**) show an epithelioid

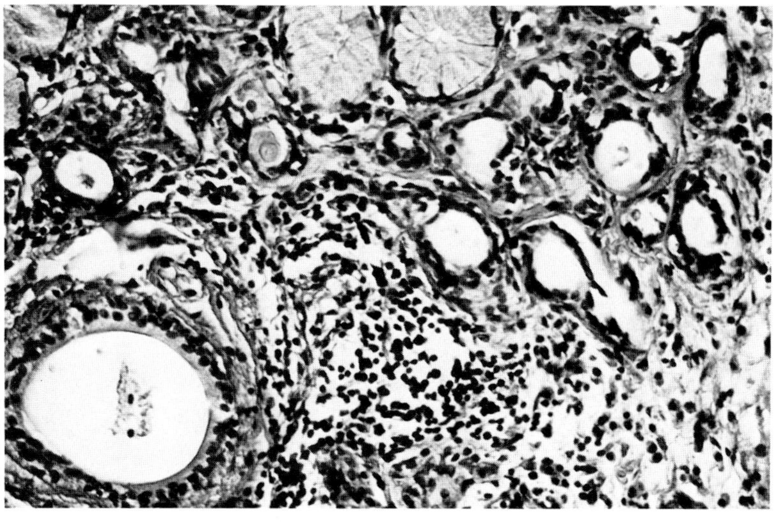

Figure 12.**69** Obstructive sialadenitis of a buccal gland in carcinoma: dilation of the duct, increased mucous congestion of the end pieces, extravasation of mucus, and interstitial inflammatory infiltrate. H & E, 160×.

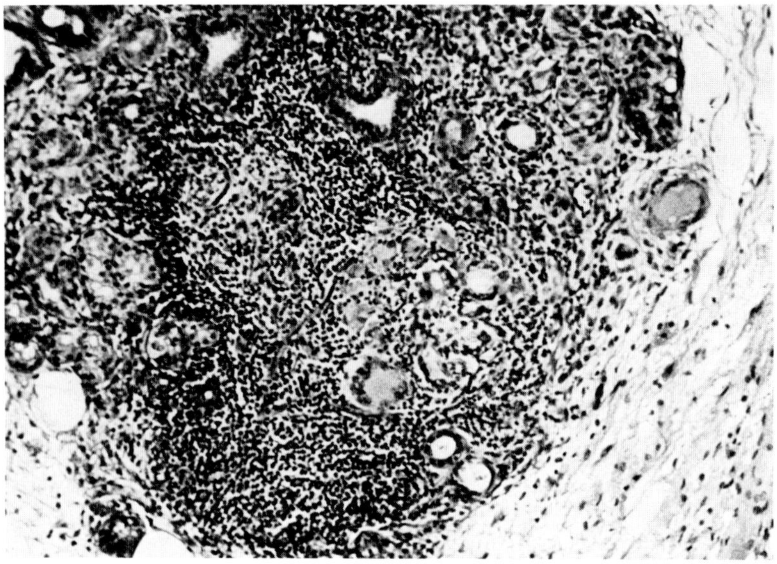

Figure 12.**70** Granulomatous cheilitis of the upper lip: tuberculoid granuloma with lymphocytes and multinuclear Langhans' giant cells. H & E, 160×.

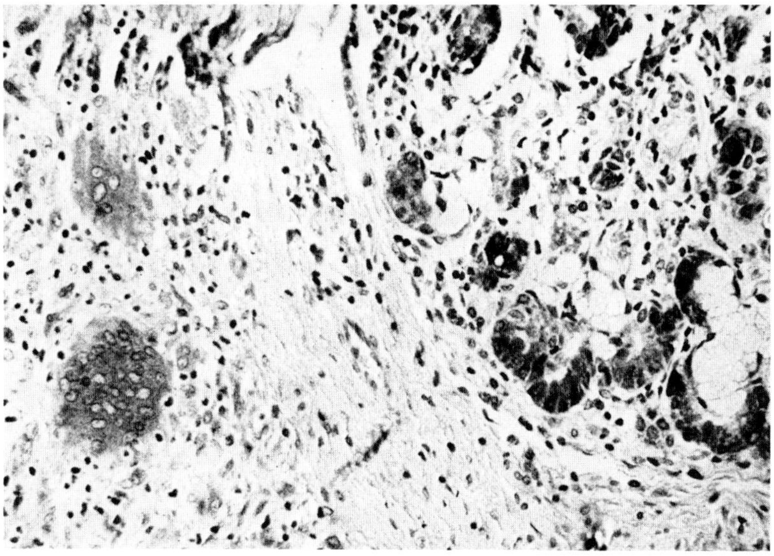

Figure 12.**71** Granulomatous cheilitis of the upper lip: granuloma with giant cells within the lobules of the gland. Lysozyme reaction, 250×.

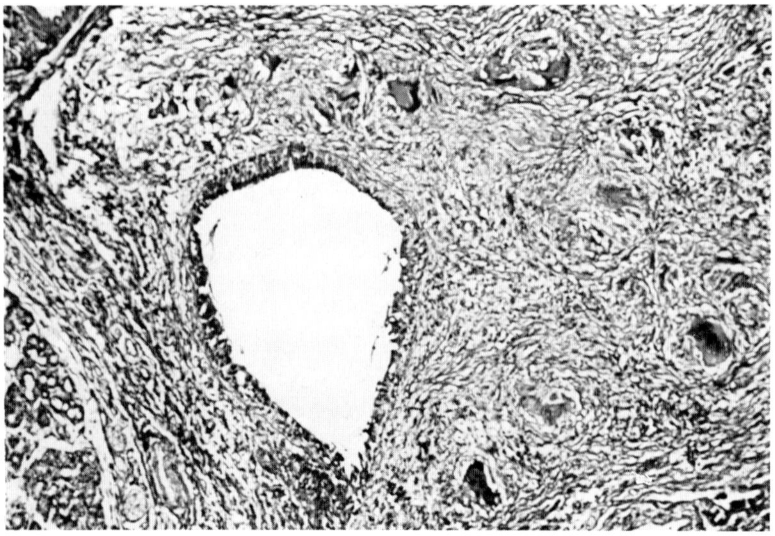

Figure 12.**72** Giant cell sialadenitis of the submandibular gland: periductal granuloma with multinuclear giant cells. H & E, 63×.

granuloma and an infiltrate of histiocytes, plasma cells, and lymphocytes. The infiltrate invades the connective tissue, the musculature, and also the local minor salivary glands. Recently, an association between granulomatous cheilitis and Crohn's disease of the gastrointestinal tract has been demonstrated in which Crohn's disease can be asymptomatic (Brook et al 1983). *Glossodynia* (Haneke 1978) is defined as a burning of the tongue, dryness of the mouth, and atypical depression; it is a differential diagnosis of Sjögren's syndrome. The minor salivary glands of the lower lip relatively often demonstrate extensive inflammation, including diffuse lymphocytic infiltration, loss of gland acini. interstitial fibrosis, and ductular proliferations. A pure case of glossodynia is distinguished from Sjögren's syndrome by the lesser degree of sialadenitis. (Luhn et al 1981).

References

Brook, I. M., D. J. King, I. D. Miller: Chronic granulomatous cheilitis and its relationship to Crohn's disease. Oral Surg. 56 (1983) 405

Haneke, E.: Psychische Aspekte der Glossodynie. Dtsch. med. Wschr. 103 (1978) 1302

Hornstein, O. P., E. Haneke: Granulomatöse Reaktionen der Haut. Verh. Dtsch. Ges. Path. 64 (1980) 180

Hornstein, O. P., H. Schuermann: Das sog. Melkersson-Rosenthal-Syndrom (einschl. Cheilitis granulomatosa Miescher). Ergebn. Inn. Med. Kinderheilk. 17 (1962) 190

Luhn, J.-P., K. Donath, E. Haneke: Veränderungen der Lippenspeicheldrüsen bei Glossodynie. Pathohistologische und morphometrische Analyse. HNO (Berl.) 29 (1981) 10

Miescher, G.: Über essentielle granulomatöse Makrocheilie (Cheilitis granulomatosa). Dermatologica (Basel) 91 (1945) 57

Seifert, G.: Mundhöhle, Mundspeicheldrüsen, Tonsillen und Rachen. In Doerr, W., E. Uehlinger: Spezielle pathologische Anatomie, Bd. 1. Springer, Berlin 1966 (S. 1)

Other Rare Forms of Inflammation

Granulomatous giant cell sialadenitis of the sublingual or submandibular glands (Seifert et al 1980) is an unusual form of sialadenitis caused by salivary calculi, tumors, or other diseases (Figs. 12.**72**,, 12.**73a, b**). Periductal granulomas with multinuclear foreign-body giant cells arise from dissolution of mucous acini or extravasation of

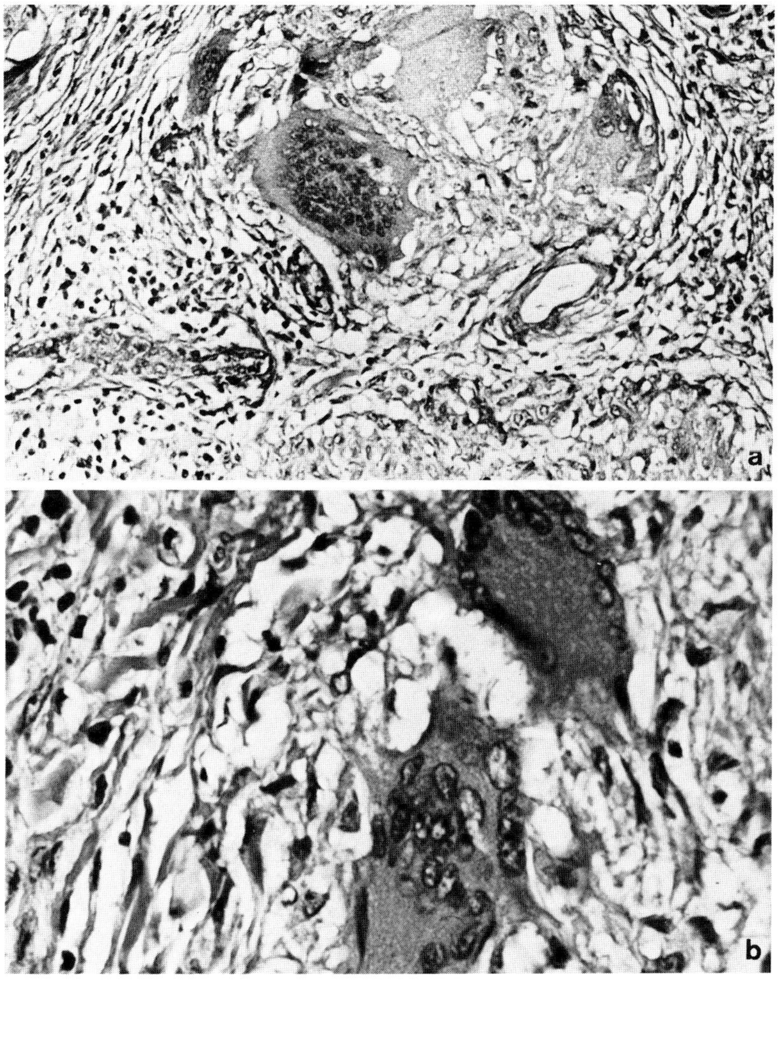

Figure 12.**73** Giant cell sialadenitis of the submandibular gland: granuloma formation with multinucleated foreign-body giant cells. H & E. **a** 160×, **b** 400×.

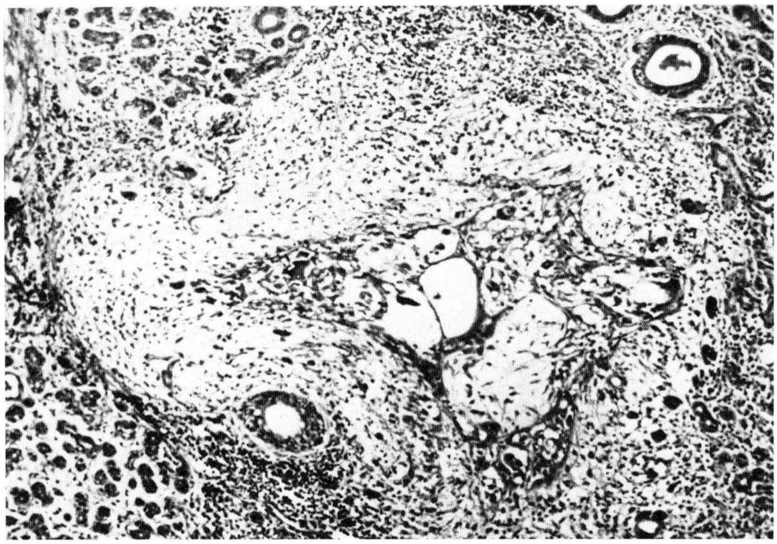

Figure 12.**74** Granulomatous infiltration of the parotid gland after sialography: periductal extrusion of mucus with development of inflammatory granulation tissue. H & E, 63×.

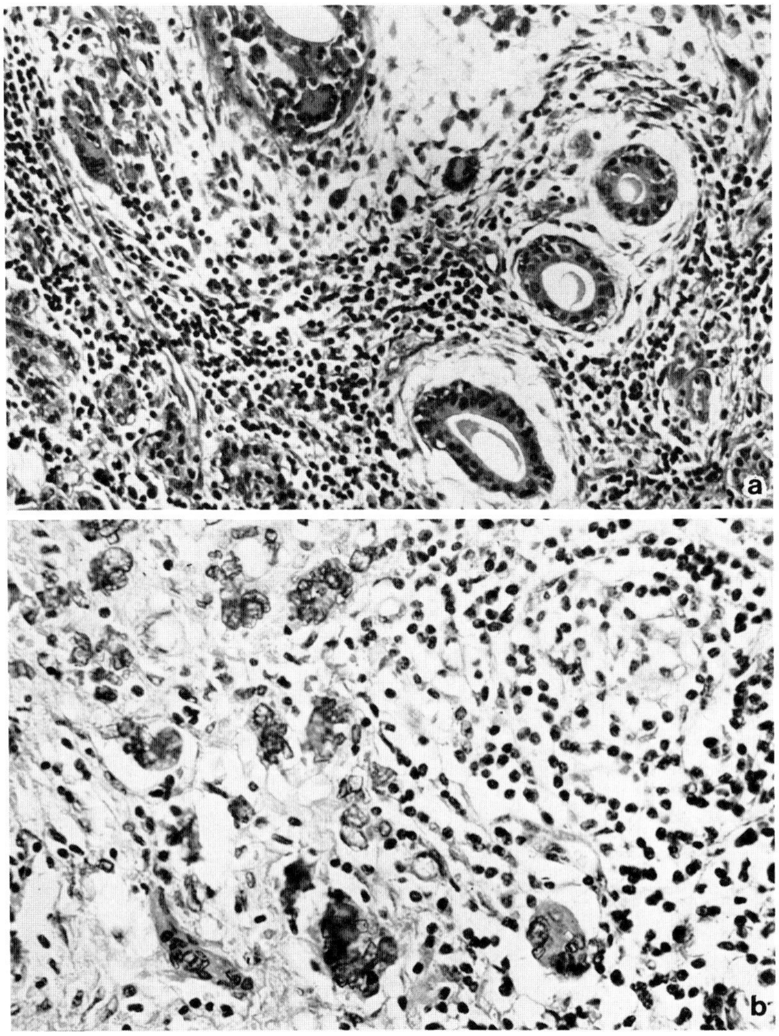

Figure 12.**75** Granulomatous parotitis after sialography:
a Periductal granuloma with giant cells. **b** Giant cell formation with inclusion of contrast medium.
H & E. **a** 160×, **b** 400×.

mucus from the duct system. The giant cells contain mucous vacuoles. The pathogenesis of these changes is similar to that of extravasation.

Contrast medium and mucus can be extravasated into the interstitium during *sialography:* a periductal foreign body granuloma develops as a result (Figs. 12.**74**, 12.**75a, b**). It contains remnants of contrast medium in the form of fine granular particles stained light brown in addition to masses of mucus. Scar tissue transformation of these granulomas and focal gland sclerosis occur later in this disease (Patey & Thackray 1970, Thackray & Lucas 1974). Similar granulomas are repeatedly observed in the stroma of tumors, especially cystadenolymphomas (Seifert et al 1980). These granulomas must be distinguished from tuberculous granulomas. The restitution of the glandular tissue after sialography with water- or lipid-soluble contrast media is being studied under experimental conditions (Qwarnstrom & Hand 1983, Qwarnstrom et al 1983).

References

Patey, D. H., A. C. Thackray: Infected adenolymphoma: A new parotid syndrome. Brit. J. Surg. 57 (1970) 569

Qwarnstrom, E. E., A. R. Hand: A morphologic study of the recovery of the rat submandibular gland after retrograde infusion. II. Lipid-soluble radiographic contrast medium. J. oral Path. 12 (1983) 430

Qwarnstrom, E. E., K.-A. Omnell, A. R. Hand: A morphologic study of the recovery of the rat submandibular gland after retrograde infusion. I. Water-soluble radiographic contrast medium. J. oral Path. 12 (1983) 417

Seifert, G., K. Donath, Chr. v. Gumberz: Granulomatöse Reaktionen der Speicheldrüsen. Klassifikation und Pathogenese. Verh. Dtsch. Ges. Path. 64 (1980) 250

Thackray, A. C., R. B. Lucas: Tumors of the Major Salivary Glands. Atlas of Tumor Pathology, 2. series, fascicle 10, Armed Forces Institute of Pathology, Washington 1974

13. Salivary and Branchial Cleft Fistulas

Salivary Gland Fistulas

Parotid fistulas arising from the parenchyma must be distinguished from those arising from the duct system. However, in both cases large or small ducts are damaged, allowing saliva to drain from sites other than the parotid papilla (Chilla 1981). Parotid fistulas may be due to serious ascending inflammation of the salivary gland parenchyma, to operations on the parotid gland, or to deep wounds of the lateral part of the face penetrating the parenchyma of the parotid gland. The latter are often accompanied by lesions of the peripheral branches of the facial nerve. Parenchymatous fistulas in which the larger ducts are not damaged usually close spontaneously, but spontaneous healing of an injury of one of the larger ducts is not to be expected.

The **treatment** of a parenchymatous fistula must be conservative to allow spontaneous healing. The healing period may be shortened by outlining the duct with methylene blue, excising the fistula,

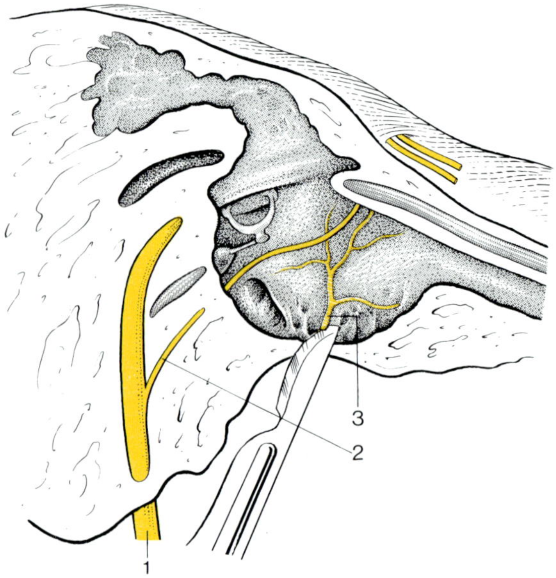

Figure 13.**1** Intratympanic division of the tympanic plexus. 1 = facial nerve, 2 = chorda tympani, 3 = tympanic plexus.

and closing the soft tissues over it in several layers.

The following method of treatment is advised for persistent salivary fistulas (Chilla 1981).

1. Supression of function of the parenchyma by:
   a) Drugs, for example parasympatholytic drugs until the fistula has healed
   b) Radiotherapy (Löhr & Vieten 1969, Pearson 1935, Reeves 1940)
   c) Denervation of the gland by:
   Division of the auriculotemporal nerve (Muler 1953, Leriche 1914)
   Tympanic neurectomy (Hashash et al 1978, Mandour et al 1976, Arulpragasam 1967)
   d) Ligature of the proximal end of the duct (Baron 1961, Morestin 1917).
2. Operations on the fistula:
   a) Excision and cover of the parotid capsule (Cook 1936)
   b) Reconstruction of the damaged parotid duct (Rehrmann 1958, Rehrmann & Reil 1974, de Vylder et al 1978, Glascock & Glascock 1937)
   c) Diversion of the fistula into the oral cavity (Fishler & Pogorel 1955)
3. Removal of the secreting parenchyma by partial or total parotidectomy (Redon 1955)

We have not had very convincing results from medical treatment with parasympatholytic drugs intended to suppress or reduce the parotid secretion.

We have also not used radiotherapy in doses of about 1500 rad (Löhr & Vieten 1969) for the treatment of parotid fistulas, because of the danger of a late radiation-induced carcinoma.

Parasympathetic denervation of the parotid gland by resection of the tympanic plexus (Fig. 13.**1**) reduces the secretory pressure in the duct system by reduction of the reflex salivary secretion. This may favor the healing of a fistula; the operation does not upset the patient and may be helpful. Mandour et al (1976) reported that they were able to control 20 parotid fistulas with this minor procedure.

We have no experience of division of the auriculotemporal nerve to denervate the gland.

If the parotid duct is divided completely, an attempt should obviously be made to reunite the ends using the operating microscope. The introduction of a fine plastic tube is recommended to maintain the patency of the duct temporarily during the healing phase. The results are dubious, because obliteration can occur easily after removal of the tube.

A further proposal is surgical conversion of the external duct fistula into an internal fistula. Mobilization and suture of the mobilized stump of the duct into the buccal mucosa may be successful for a defect in the buccal segment of the parotid duct. For fistulas in the masseteric part of the duct, reconstruction of the duct is the most reliable procedure (Rehrmann & Kiel 1974). Rehrmann (1958) constructed a duct from a free split-skin graft. A split flap from the buccal mucosa reflected around the edge of the masseter and sutured to the mobilized central stump of the duct is also recommended. It is of historic interest that Perthes (1917) created a new parotid duct by wrapping a split-skin graft around a silk suture and sewing this in place.

All these procedures are burdensome for the patient and their results uncertain. Retrograde bacterial infection, due to the shortness of the new duct, and the absent valvular mechanism lead to chronic recurrent parotitis.

The method proposed by Redon (1955) of removal of the fistula by superficial or total parotidectomy, with preservation of the facial nerve, is more certain.

Parenchymatous fistulas after superficial parotidectomy are occasionally incorrectly diagnosed as a seroma. The correct diagnosis may be established by aspirating fluid from the fluctuant area before a fistula has formed and measuring the amylase concentration of the fluid: 1000–6000 units/ml of amylase indicate that a salivary fistula will form, whereas a lower amylase content of 100–200 U/ml indicates the presence of a serum with slight admixture of saliva.

Branchial Cleft Fistula

Altmann (1951, 1965), Rankow (1968), Ungerecht (1962), König (1957), and Franz (1959) have emphasized that a congenital cervical fistula due to an anomaly of arrest of the first two branchial arches may open distally near the angle of the jaw at the level of the hyoid bone or may end blindly. Superiorly, there lies either a blind ending at the junction of the cartilaginous and bony parts of the external auditory meatus, or an open connection with the same structure. A rare variant has its cranial opening in the hypotympanum. These branchial cleft fistulas are lined by squamous epithelium. Clinically, they may present as a duplicate external meatus or as an accessory structure (Deneke 1959, Minnigerode & Haubrich 1965, Beck 1970, Stennert & Arold 1973), and finally they may also present as a combination of the two: the duplicate meatus irritates the surrounding tissue in such a way that a fistula forms, extending into the second branchial arch. An accessory anomaly is thus combined with an anomaly of arrested development. (Franz 1959). The term "duplicate meatus" is not clearly defined, and it cannot be distinguished from a congenital branchial cleft fistula either macroscopically or histologically (Franz 1959).

The duct of the fistula may contain hair, dysontogenetic cartilage and bone, glandular elements, and debris. Abscesses in the parotid area often result, and a fistula may form as a result of rupture through the skin of the cheek.

The branchial cleft fistulas run anterolateral to the posterior belly of the digastric muscle and anterior to the external carotid artery through the parotid gland, or closely related to it. The relation of the fistula to the facial nerve varies (Altmann 1951, Ungerecht 1962). If the ectoderm of the first branchial arch persists near the surface, a fistula may remain whose duct runs lateral to the nerve (Fig. 13.**2**). However, if a part of the ectoderm persists in the depth of the first branchial arch, the resulting fistula runs medial to the trunk of the facial nerve and its branches (Fig. 13.**3**). The suggested explanation for the variable position of these fistulas compared with the course of the facial nerve (Work 1972, Work & Proctor 1963, Denecke 1980) is that the muscles of the face that arise from the second branchial arch cross the first branchial arch in the course of their development and drag the fibers of the facial nerve with them (Denecke 1980). In our experience and that of Denecke (1980), intermediate forms of both variants are possible (Fig. 13.**4**) in which the track of the fistula penetrates between the cervicofacial and the temporofacial branches of the facial nerve (Miehlke 1973, Stennert & Arold 1973). The facial nerve is thus in great danger during inexpert attempts to remove the fistula.

Branchial cleft fistulas may also occasionally be accompanied by a hypoplasia of the parotid gland of similar genesis. In such cases, a small dimple may be found anterior to the tragus. This parotid hypoplasia further endangers the facial nerve, since the main trunk of the nerve and its branches

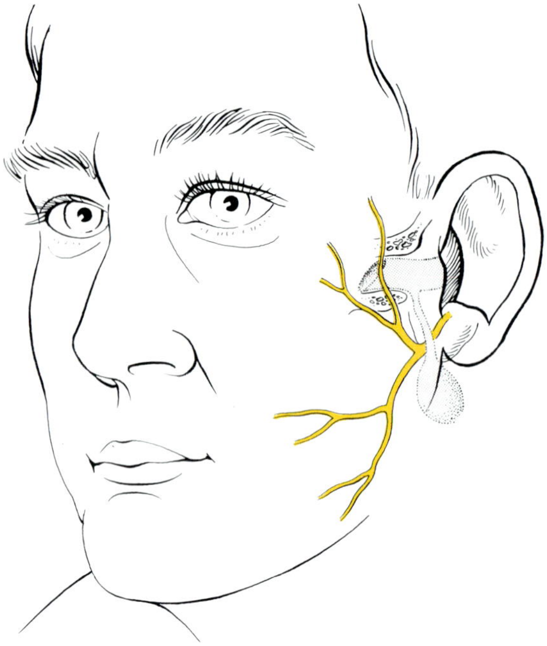

Figure 13.**2** Branchial cleft fistula running lateral to the trunk of the facial nerve. (Dokianakis.)

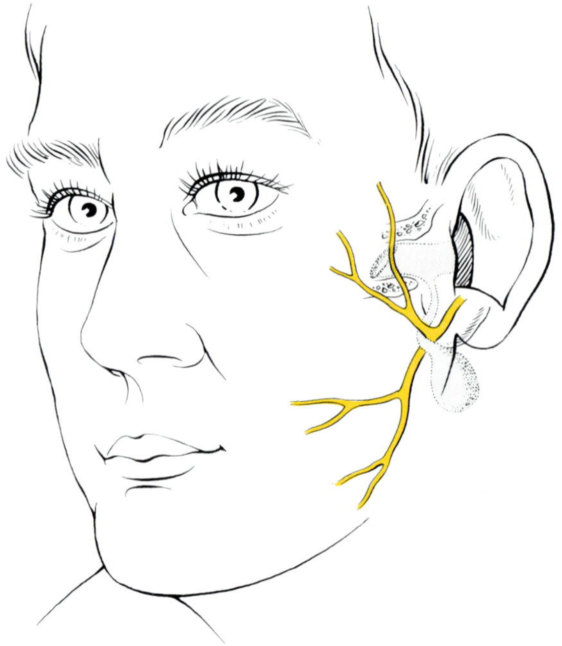

Figure 13.**4** Branchial cleft fistula running between the main branches of the facial nerve. (Dokianakis.)

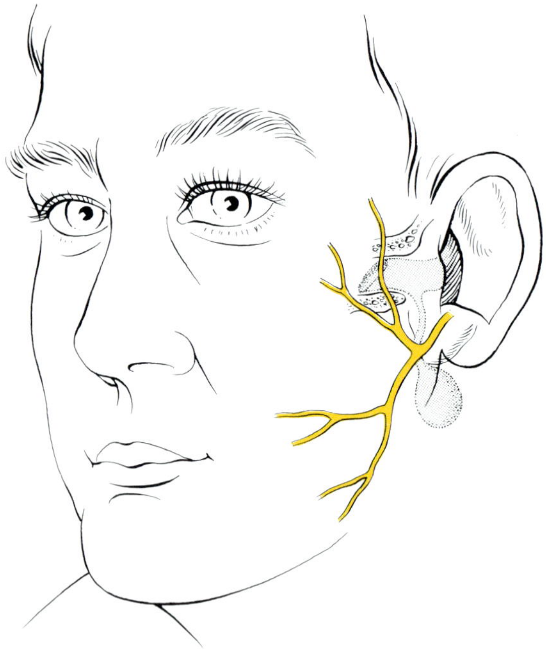

Figure 13.**3** Branchial cleft fistula running medial to the facial nerve trunk. (Dokianakis.)

lie immediately under the skin without any covering of parotid tissue, and the track of the fistula may cross over or under them.

Because of the double danger to which the facial nerve is exposed in the presence of such a fistula, we condemn the simple procedure of following the fistulous track with the hope of removing it. The first step must be exposure of the extratemporal course of the facial nerve, as in parotidectomy, that is, exposure of the facial nerve and its trunk and branches from the stylomastoid foramen, through the retromandibular fossa to its bifurcation and a little beyond (Chapter 22). The fistula can then be removed easily and safely from its origin in the external auditory meatus or the hypotympanum to its opening in the upper triangle of the neck, using an operating microscope with continuous control of the course of the facial nerve. The main branch is mobilized using the rubber band technique (see before). It must be emphasized again that any other type of procedure carries a great danger of damage to the facial nerve.

References

Altmann, F.: Malformations of the auricle and the external auditory meatus. A critical review. Arch. Otolaryng. 54 (1951) 115

Altmann, F.: Mißbildungen des Ohres. In Berendes, J., R. Link, F. Zöllner: HNO-Heilkunde, Bd. III/1. Thieme, Stuttgart 1965; 2. Aufl. 1979

Arulpragasam, A. C.: On the treatment of parotid fistula. J. Laryng. Otol. 81 (1967) 633

Baron, H. C.: Surgical correction of salivary fistula. Ann. Surg. 153 (1961) 545

Beck, Ch.: Zur Chirurgie der Gehörgangsdoppelung. HNO 18 (1970) 307

Chilla, R.: Chirurgie der Nerven im HNO-Bereich. Vegetative Hirnnervenstrukturen. Arch. Oto-Rhino-Laryng. 231 (1981) 353

Cook, J.: Treatment of parotid fistulas. Lancet 1936/I, 1239

Denecke, H. J.: Zur Chirurgie der Ohrmißbildungen unter Berücksichtigung des N. facialis. 43. Versammlung SW-deutscher HNO-Ärzte, Würzburg 1959
Denecke, H. J.: Die oto-rhino-laryngologischen Operationen im Mund- und Halsbereich. Springer, Berlin 1980
Fishler, H. W., B. S. Pogorel: Repair of parotid fistula. Arch. Otolaryng. 61 (1955) 331
Franz, H.: Über Gehörgangsduplikaturen. Z. Laryng. Rhinol 38 (1959) 16
Glascock, H., H. Glascock jun: Repair of traumatic fistulas of Stenon's duct. Surg. Gyn. Obstet. 65 (1937) 355
Hashash, M., F. State, H. J. Dessouky: Effects of tympanic neurectomy on experimentally induced parotid fistulae. J. Laryng. Otol. 92 (1978) 399
König, W.: Zur Kenntnis der (seltenen) congenitalen Ohr-Hals-Fisteln. HNO 6 (1957) 137
Leriche, R.: Behandlung der permanenten Parotisfisteln durch die Entnervung der Speicheldrüse. Zbl. Chir. 41 (1914) 754
Löhr, H., H. Vieten: Die Röntgentherapie der Speicheldrüsenerkrankungen. Fortschr. Kiefer- u. Gesichtschir. 6 (1969) 266
Mandour, M. A., M. M. El-Sheikh, F. El-Garem: Tympanic neurectomy for parotid fistula. Arch. Otolaryng 102 (1976) 327
Miehlke, A.: Surgery of the Facial Nerve. Urban & Schwarzenberg, München, und Saunders, Philadelphia 1973
Minnigerode, B., J. Haubrich: Angeborene echte Gehörgangsverdoppelung, eine seltene embryogenetische Überschußbildung. Z. Laryng. Rhinol. 44 (1965) 706
Morestin, H.: Contribution à l'étude du traitement des fistules salivaires consecutives aux blessures de guerre. Bull. Mem. Soc. Chir. (Paris) 43 (1917) 845
Muler, M.: Fistule parotidienne traitée par resection du nerf auriculo-temporal. Ann. Oto-laryng. (Paris) 70 (1953) 53
Pearson, R. S. B.: Recurrent swelling of parotid glands. Arch. Dis. Child 10 (1935) 363
Perthes, G.: Zur operativen Behandlung der Parotis-Fisteln nach Schußverletzungen. Zbl. Chir. 44 (1917) 13
Rankow, R. M.: Surgery of the Face, Mouth and Neck. Saunders, Philadelphia 1968
Redon, H.: Chirurgie des glandes salivaires. Masson, Paris 1955
Reeves, R. J.: Röntgentherapy of bilateral parotid fistula. Ann. J. Röntgen. 43 (1940) 425
Rehrmann, A.: Beseitigung einer Speichelfistel durch Neubildung des Ductus parotideus mit Spalthautlappen. Dtsch. Zahn- u. Kiefer-Heilkd. 28 (1958) 380
Rehrmann, A., B. Reil: Die Behandlung von Verletzungen des Ausführungsganges der Ohrspeicheldrüse. In Naumann, H. H., E. R. Kastenbauer: Plastisch-chirurgische Maßnahmen nach frischen Verletzungen. Thieme, Stuttgart 1974
Stennert, E., R. Arold: Der doppelte Gehörgang. HNO 21 (1973) 293
Ungerecht, K.: Die Gefährdung des N. facialis bei der operativen Behandlung der angeborenen Hals-Ohr-Fistel. HNO 10 (1962) 197
Vylder, de. J., J. Carlo, G. T. Stratigos: Early recognition and treatment of the traumatically transected parotid duct. J. oral Surg. 36 (1978) 43
Work, W. P.: Newer concepts of first branchial cleft defects. Laryngoscope 82 (1972) 1581
Work, W. P., C. A. Proctor: The otologist and first branchial cleft anomalies. Ann. Otol. (St. Louis) 72 (1963) 548

14. Interstitial Lesions and Tissue Infiltrates

Lipomatosis

Occasional fat cells may often be found within normal parotid tissue. The amount of fatty tissue increases in the older age groups, particularly in the parotid gland (Fig. 14.**1**), less often in the submandibular gland, and almost never in the sublingual gland. A pronounced interstitial lipomatosis of the parotid gland may be found in general adiposity, diabetes mellitus (Fig. 14.**2**), or hypertension. The growth of the fatty tissue may lead to a lipomatous pseudohypertrophy of the parotid gland. Unilateral focal fatty hyperplasia must be distinguished from intraglandular or subaponeurotic lipomas (page 307).

A compensatory growth of fatty tissue can occur in parenchymatous atrophy (see pages 109, 110).

Amyloidosis

Cords of homogeneous amyloid deposits may be found in the interstitium and the vessel walls in secondary amyloidosis (Fig. 14.**3a, b**). Secondary parenchymatous atrophy occurs in massive amyloid deposition.

Fibrosis and Sclerosis

Increase of the interstitial connective tissue is usually due to prior inflammation of the gland. This is especially true of the submandibular gland in chronic sclerosing sialadenitis. Slight hyperplasia of the connective tissue may be defined as fibrosis and more pronounced forms as sclerosis. The periductal connective tissue is especially affected. Periacinar fibrosis with resultant loss of the acini occurs if the process progresses within the lobules of the gland.

Cords of hyaline fiber swellings may be observed around the duct acini and vessels in the collagenoses, particularly lupus erythematosus (Seifert 1971).

Vascular Lesions

The vessels of the salivary glands may be involved in systemic disorders, such as arteriosclerosis, and arteritis. Secondary vascular lesions, such as sclerosis, occur in radiation sialadenitis and chronic sialadenitis of the submandibular gland especially.

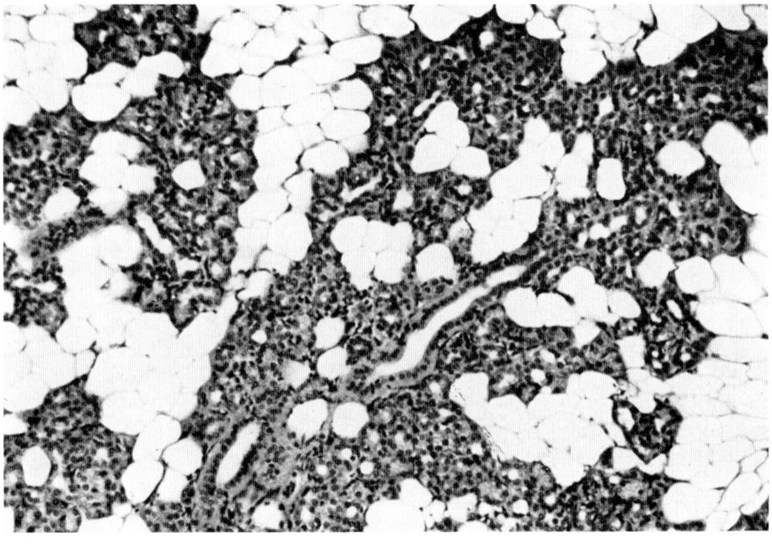

Figure 14.**1** Interstitial lipomatosis of the parotid gland: increased infiltration of the lobule by fat cells, and partial atrophy of the acini. H & E, 63×.

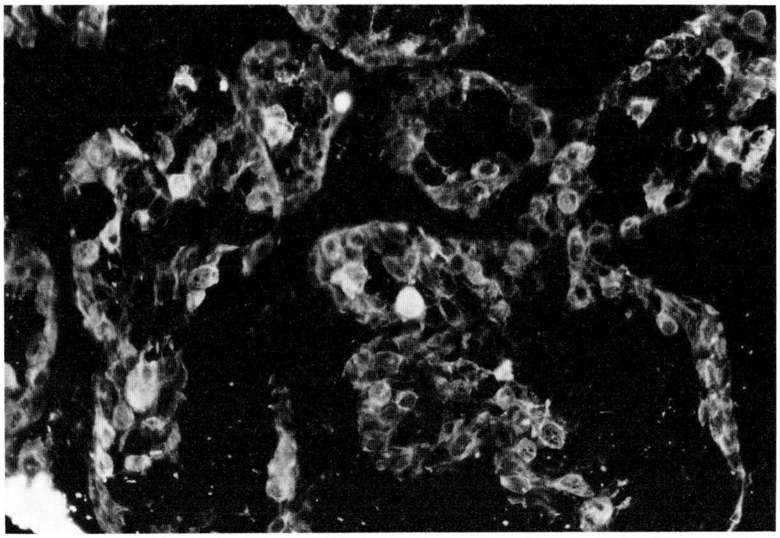

Figure 15.**1** Keratin in a mucoepidermoid tumor of the parotid gland. Immunofluorescence, 210×. (Caselitz et al 1982.)

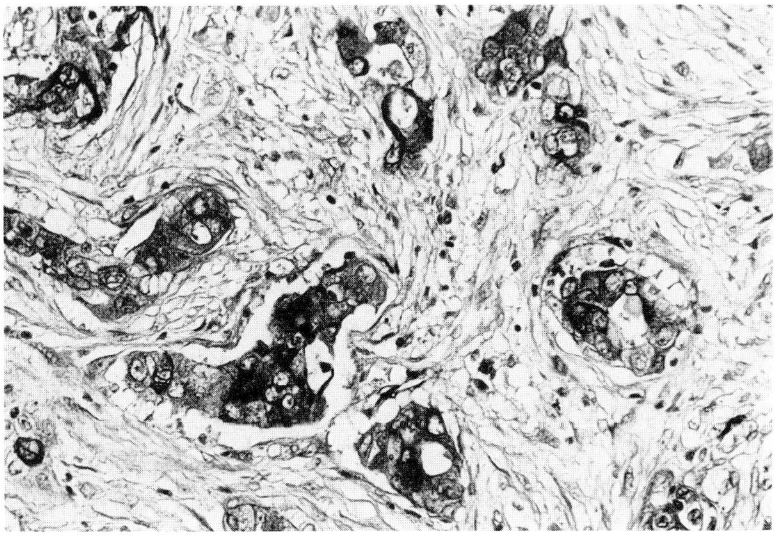

Figure 15.**2** Positive CEA in an adenocarcinoma of the parotid gland. Immunoperoxidase, 300×. (Caselitz et al 1981.)

Tumor Markers

Tumor markers have opened new horizons of tumor classification. Immunocytochemical methods (immunofluorescence and immunoperoxidase) demonstrate the components of the cytoskeleton, the membrane-bound antigens, and cytochemical cell products (Seifert 1982, Caselitz et al 1982a, 1982 b, Seifert & Caselitz 1985). The occurrence of these cell structures in normal salivary tissue has already been described (see page 21ff).

Components of the Cytoskeleton. Keratin may be demonstrated in numerous salivary tumors (cystadenolymphomas, pleomorphic adenomas, mucoepidermoid tumors, adenoid cystic carcinomas, adenocarcinomas, squamous cell carcinomas) as a marker of epithelial tumor cells (Fig. 15.**1**) (Caselitz et al 1981c, 1982a, 1982b, Becker et al 1983, Nathrath et al 1982). *Vimentin* marks the mesenchymal stromal cells, fibrocytes, endothelial cells, lymphocytes, Langerhans' cells, etc. The myoepithelial cells in pleomorphic adenomas and adenoid cystic carcinomas show a double marking with keratin and vimentin (Caselitz et al 1984b).

Cell Membrane Antigens. The *carcinoembryonic antigen* (CEA) is an oncofetal antigen that is important in the diagnosis of salivary gland tumors (Tables 15.**2**, 15.**3**). CEA may be demonstrated in glandular tumors, especially adenoid cystic carcinoma, adenocarcinoma, duct carcino-

Table 15.**2** Occurence of CEA and Lactoferrin in Parotid Tumors

Tumor Type	No.	CEA	Lactoferrin
Adenoid cystic carcinoma	4	3	2
Adenocarcinoma	13	10	8
Duct carcinoma	3	3	2
Mucoepidermoid tumor	2	2	2
Carcinoma ex pleomorphic adenoma	21	9	5
Squamous cell carcinoma	8	5	–
Anaplastic carcinoma	3	–	–
Total	54	32	19

ma, carcinoma ex pleomorphic adenoma, and furthermore in mucoepidermoid tumors, principally in mucus-forming areas of the tumor, and in well-differentiated squamous cell carcinomas, but not in anaplastic carcinomas (Caselitz et al 1981a, McDicken & Scott 1981). There is good correlation between the occurrence of CEA and lactoferrin in glandular tumors (Table 15.**2**). The tissue polypeptide antigen [TPA] can be demonstrated in glandular tumors, such as adenoid cystic carcinoma, adenocarcinoma and pleomorphic adenoma (Figs. 15.**4**, 15.**5**) and also in more solid epidermoid areas of mucoepidermoid tumors (Caselitz et al 1983a). The conclusion may thus be drawn that the solid epidermoid areas of mucoepidermoid tumors form the proliferative

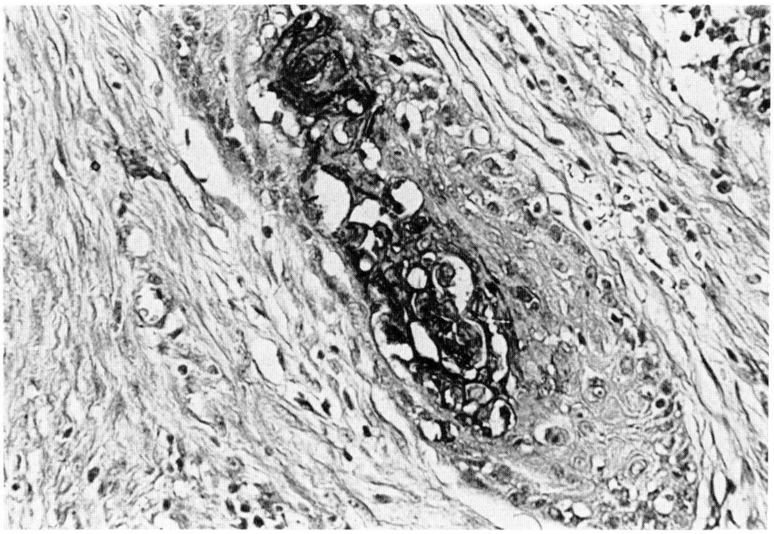

Figure 15.**3** CEA in a highly differentiated keratinizing squamous cell carcinoma of the parotid gland. Immunoperoxidase, 300×. (Caselitz et al 1981.)

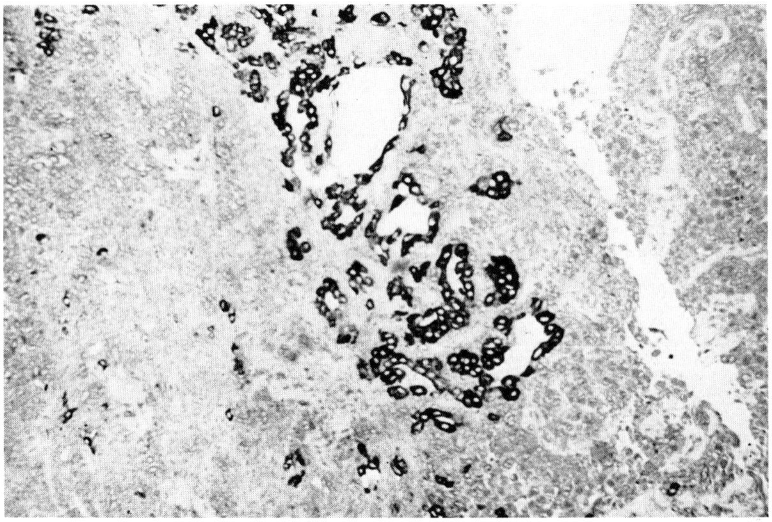

Figure 15.**4** TPA in a pleomorphic parotid adenoma. Special demonstration of tubular structures. Immunoperoxidase, 63×.

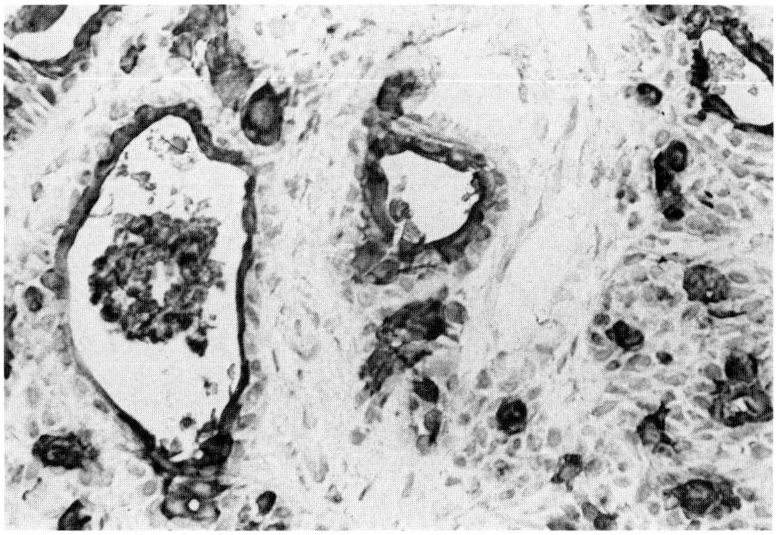

Figure 15.**5** TPA in an adenoid cystic carcinoma of the parotid gland: marking of cystic and cribriform structures. Immunoperoxidase, 160×.

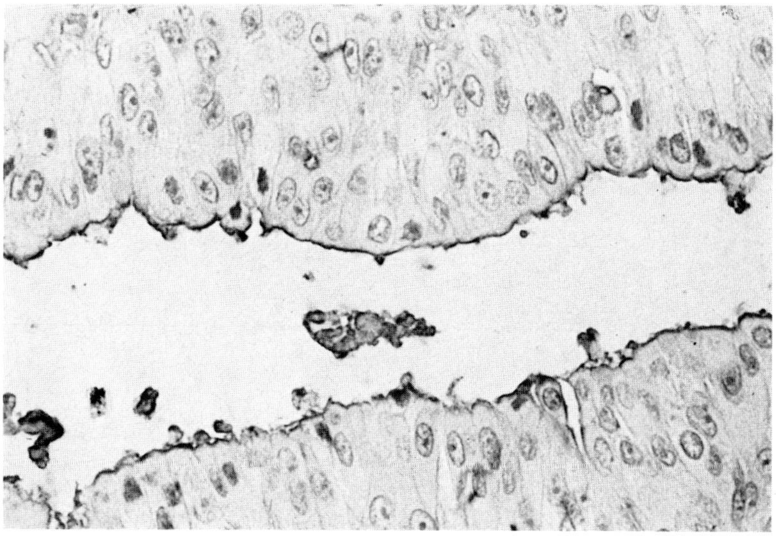

Figure 15.**6** Wheat germ agglutinin lectin on the apical cell membrane of a cystadenolymphoma of the parotid gland. Immunoperoxidase, 160×.

pool of the tumor. The *epithelial membrane antigen* (Gusterson et al 1982) marks the cell surface of ductal structures in pleomorphic adenomas, adenoid cystic carcinomas, adenocarcinomas, and mucoepidermoid tumors, but not the mesenchymal cells or acini. *S-100-protein* can be demonstrated in myoepithelial cells of pleomorphic adenomas especially (Hara et al 1983, Nakazato et al 1982). The *secretory component* can be demonstrated in the ductal structures of pleomorphic adenomas, but not in myoepithelial cells or acinar structures (Fantasia & Lally 1984, Korsrud & Brandtzaeg 1984). In 75% of pleomorphic adenomas, there exists a parallel positive expression of lactoferrin, with the secretory component as evidence of the histogenetic relationship of the tumor matrix to the terminal ducts (Korsrud & Brandtzaeg 1984a).

Lectin Receptors. Malignant cellular transformation is accompanied by changes of cell membrane structure (Fig. 15.**6**). These may be demonstrated by lectin receptors and by the expression of antigens and crypt antigens from the cell membrane (Caselitz & Seifert 1981). Peanut agglutinin (PNA) and helix pomatia agglutinin (HPA) have proved suitable as receptor substances for the classification of salivary tumors (Table 15.**3**). Glandular tumors, mucoepidermoid tumors, well-differentiated squamous cell carcinomas, and pleomorphic adenomas produce a positive lectin receptor reaction, whereas undifferentiated carcinomas do not.

Cell Products. These include *amylase* (Fig. 15.**7**) for the differentiation of acinic cell tumors (Caselitz et al 1983b) and *lactoferrin* (Figs. 15.**8a, b,** 15.**9a, b**), in glandular tumors (Caselitz et al

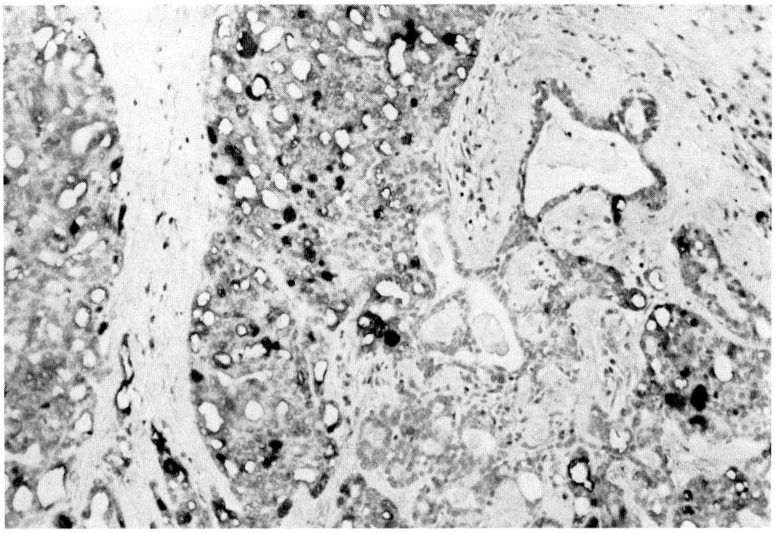

Figure 15.**7** Amylase in an acinic cell tumor of the parotid gland. Immunoperoxidase, 63×.

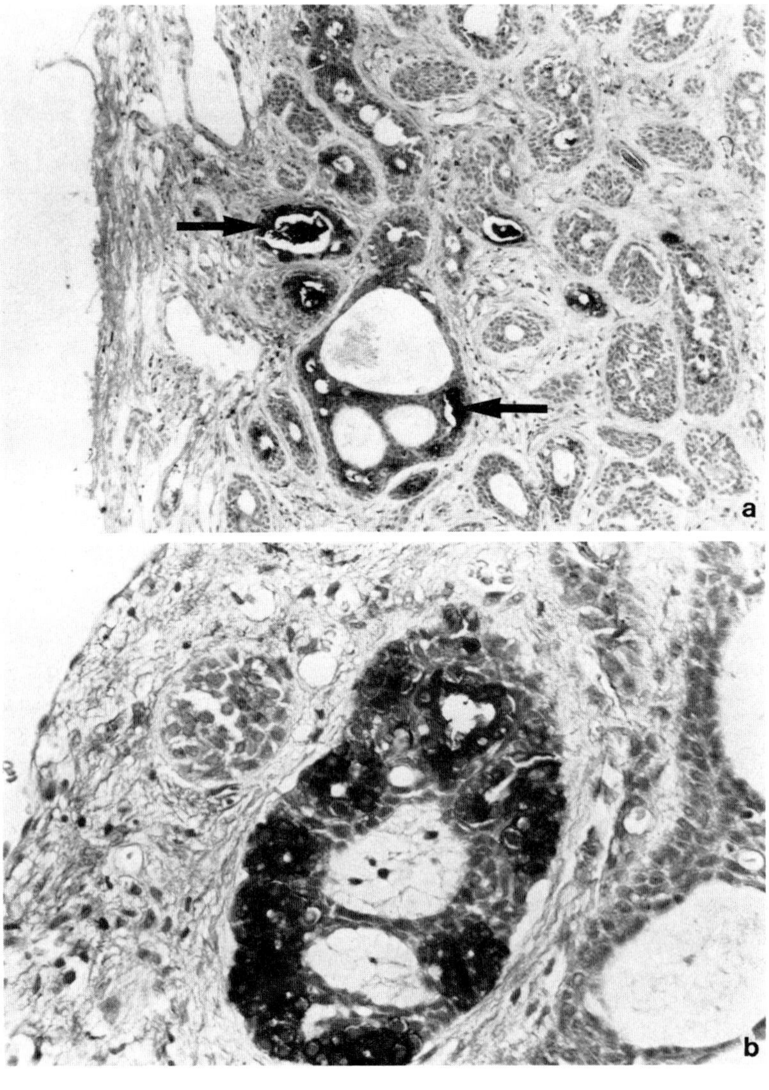

Figure 15.**8** Lactoferrin in an adenoid cystic carcinoma of the parotid gland: **a** Positive tumor cells in a cystic structure (arrows). **b** Clearly positive tumor cell nest in the center of the field. Immunoperoxidase.
a 120×, **b** 300×.
(Caselitz et al 1981.)

1981b). The epithelial cell elements of pleomorphic adenomas, but not the stromal cells, can be marked with antisera against human saliva, especially salivary proteins, (Vigliani & Stramignoni 1981).

Stromal Reaction. Salivary gland tumors show a variable stromal reaction (Fleischer et al 1980). Differentiation of plasma cells with respect to formation of immunoglobulins is possible using immunocytochemical techniques (Korsrud & Brandtzaeg 1984b), and it is also possible to characterize the lymphocyte population and the Langerhans' cells (page 23). The lymphoid stroma of the cystadenolymphoma may be subclassified using monoclonal antibodies (Fig. 15.**10a, b**) (Caselitz et al 1984a, see also page 201).

Table 15.**3** Occurence of PNA and HPA Lectins in Salivary Gland Carcinomas

Type of Carcinoma	No.	PNA*	HPA*
Adenocarcinoma	16	9	4
Adenoid cystic carcinoma	4	1	2
Duct carcinoma	2	2	1
Mucoepidermoid tumor	7	4	–
Squamous cell carcinoma	10	9	7
Carcinoma ex pleomorphic adenoma	21	16	10
Undifferentiated carcinoma	3	–	–
Total	63	41	24

* PNA = peanut agglutinin,
HPA = helix pomatia agglutinin

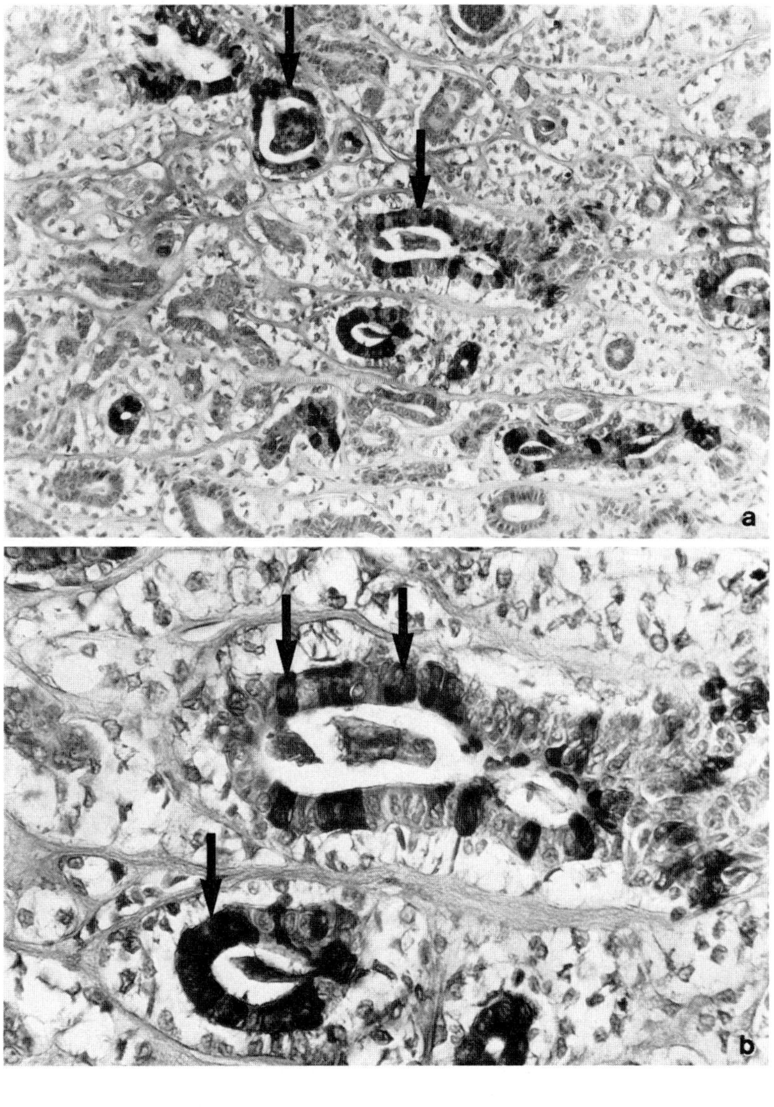

Figure 15.**9** Lactoferrin in a duct carcinoma of the parotid gland: tumor cells in the luminal part of the duct structures, with absence of staining of the clear cells on the outer surface of the ductular structures. Immunoperoxidase.
a 120×, **b** 300×.

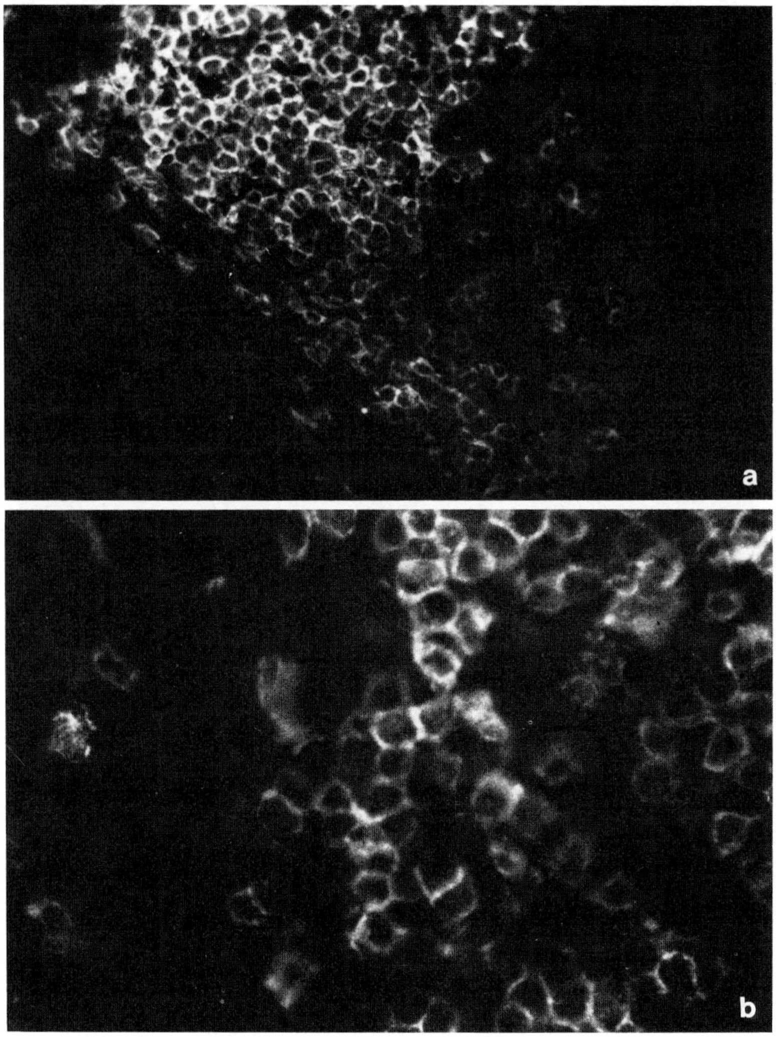

Figure 15.**10** Lymphocytes in the stroma of a cystadenolymphoma of the parotid gland: **a** T suppressor cells. Monoclonal antibodies (anti-leu 2a). **b** T lymphocytes. Monoclonal antibodies (anti-leu 1a) immunofluorescence. **a** 160×, **b** 400×.

Intercellular Components. Glycosaminoglycans may be demonstrated in the stroma of pleomorphic adenomas, as may be Factor VIII in the vessels, and laminin around the epithelial cell (Toida et al 1984). Adenoid cystic carcinomas have a marked laminin content, particularly on the inner surface of the pseudocysts and on the external surface of the trabecular cell bands.

Ultrastructure

Further criteria for the classification of tumors, particularly clear cell tumors (Seifert & Donath 1978), rest on the ultrastructural cellular differentiation of salivary tumors (Donath 1983). Particular cell types include undifferentiated duct cells, storage striated cells, epithelial cells, epidermoid cells, goblet cells, sebaceous cells, acinar cells, and disseminated endocrine cells. Clear cell salivary tumors must be differentiated from metastases, particularly of a renal carcinoma. Undifferentiated carcinomas must be distinguished from undifferentiated squamous carcinomas and primitive duct carcinomas (Donath et al 1982). Electron microscopy has led to the splitting off of several cell types of pleomorphic adenomas.

Other Methods of Classification

These include histochemistry (Quintarelli & Robinson 1967, Eversole 1972), DNA analysis by spectrophotometry (Eneroth & Zetterberg 1974), aspiration cytology (Droese et al 1977, Droese 1980), and immunocytochemical examination of the stromal reaction of salivary tumors (Fleischer et al 1980). In addition, the age grouping (for example, salivary gland tumors in childhood) and the question of bilateral or multiple tumors (see before) may also be included in the classification. The special differentiation of the mesenchymal stroma in individual tumors, particularly pleomorphic adenomas, will be considered later in greater detail.

References

Assor, D.: Bilateral carcinoma of the parotid, one cancer arising in a Warthin's tumor. Amer. J. clin. Path. 61 (1974) 270

Astacio, J. N.: Papillary cystadenoma lymphomatosum associated with pleomorphic adenoma of the parotid gland. Oral Surg. 38 (1974) 91

Bab, I. A., M. Ulmansky: Simultaneously occurring salivary gland tumors of different types. J. oral Surg. 37 (1979) 826

Becker, J., J. Caselitz, P. Reichert: Immunhistologische Untersuchung von adenoidzystischen Speicheldrüsenkarzinomen. Dtsch. Z. Mund-Kiefer-Gesichts-Chir. 8 (1984) 294

Becker, W., J. Haubrich, G. Seifert: Krankheiten der Kopfspeicheldrüsen. In Berendes, J., R. Link, F. Zöllner: Hals-Nasen-Ohren-Heilkunde in Praxis und Klinik, Bd. 3. Thieme, Stuttgart 1978

Behnke, E. E.: Unilateral multiple benign mixed tumours of the parotid gland. Laryngoscope 92 (1982) 1265

Carlsoo, B., T. Ekstrand: Unilateral multiple mixed tumours of the parotid gland. J. Laryng. 91 (1977) 629

Caselitz, J., G. Seifert: Immunhistologische Untersuchungen zum Verteilungsmuster von intrazytoplasmatischen Antigenen und Lektinrezeptoren bei Parotiskarzinomen. Verh. Dtsch. Ges. Path 65 (1981) 378

Caselitz, J., G. Seifert, T. Jaup: Tumor antigens in neoplasms of the human parotid gland. J. oral Path. 11 (1982a) 374

Caselitz, J., T. Jaup, G. Seifert: Immunohistochemical detection of carcinoembryonic antigen (CEA) in parotid gland carcinomas. Analysis of 52 cases. Virchows Arch. Path. Anat. 394 (1981a) 49

Caselitz, J., T. Jaup, G. Seifert: Lactoferrin and lysozyme in carcinomas of the parotid gland. A. comparative immunocytochemical study with the occurrence in normal and inflamed tissue. Virchows Arch. Path. Anat. 394 (1981b) 61

Caselitz, J., A. Salfelder, G. Seifert: Adenolymphoma: An immunohistochemical study with monoclonal antibodies against lymphocyte antigens. J. oral Pathol. 13 (1984a) 438

Caselitz, J., M. Osborn, G. Seifert, K. Weber: Intermediate-sized filament proteins (prekeratin, vimentin, desmin) in the normal parotid gland and parotid gland tumours. Immunofluorescence study. Virchows Arch. Path. Anat. 393 (1981c) 273

Caselitz, J., G. Seifert, B. Björklund, V. Björklund: Detection of tissue polypeptide antigen in salivary glands and salivary gland tumors. Appl. Pathol. 1 (1983a) 115

Caselitz, J., M. Osborn, J. Wustrow, G. Seifert, K. Weber: The expression of different intermediate-sized filaments in human salivary glands and their tumours. Path. Res. Pract. 175 (1982b) 266

Caselitz, J., G. Seifert, G. Grenner, R. Schmidtberger: Amylase as an additional marker of salivary gland neoplasms. An immunoperoxidase study. Path. Res. Pract. 176 (1983b) 276

Caselitz, J., J. Becker, G. Seifert, K. Weber, M. Osborn: Coexpression of keratin and vimentin filaments in adenoid cystic carcinomas of salivary glands. Virchows Arch. Path. Anat. 403 (1984b) 337

Donath, K.: Ultrastrukturelle Marker bei Speicheldrüsentumoren. Dtsch. Z. Mund-Kiefer-Gesichts-Chir. 7 (1983) 119

Donath, K., G. Seifert, E. Sunder-Plassmann: Ultrastrukturelle Subklassifikation undifferenzierter Parotiscarcinome. Analyse von 11 Fällen. J. Cancer Res. Clin. Oncol. 103 (1982) 75

Droese, M.: Punktionscytologie der Speicheldrüsenerkrankungen. Habil.-Schrift, Göttingen 1980

Droese, M., M. Tute, J. Haubrich: Punktionszytologie von Speicheldrüsentumoren. Z. Laryng. Rhinol. 56 (1977) 703

Eneroth, C. M., A. Zetterberg: Microspectrophotometric DNA analysis of malignant salivary gland tumours. Acta otolaryng. 77 (1974) 289

Evans, R. W., A. H. Cruickshank: Epithelial Tumours of the Salivary Glands. Saunders, Philadelphia 1970

Eversole, L. R.: Histogenic classification of salivary gland tumors. Arch. Path. (Chic.) 92 (1971) 434

Eversole, L. R.: The histochemistry of mucosubstances in human minor salivary glands. Arch. oral Biol. 17 (1972) 1225

Fantasia, J. E., E. T. Lally: Localization of free secretory component in pleomorphic adenomas of minor salivary gland origin. Cancer 53 (1984) 1786

Fleischer, I., J. Caselitz, Th. Löning, G. Seifert: Histological and immunocytochemical examinations of the stroma reaction in carcinomas of the parotid gland. Analysis of 52 cases. J. Cancer Res. Clin. Oncol. 96 (1980) 193

Ferlito, A.: Bilateral synchronous trabecular adenocarcinoma of the parotid gland. ORL (Basel) 40 (1978) 120

Gadient, St. E., B. Kalfayan: Mucoepidermoid carcinoma arising within a Warthin's tumor. Oral Surg. 40 (1975) 391

Gaillard, A., P. Nicouleau, D. Jacquemaire, N. Le Neel, L. Cousin: Cystadenolymphomes multiples des parotides et de la levre supérieure. Rev. Stomat. 82 (1981) 282

Gaynor, E. B., R. Hershberg: Unilateral multiple tumours of the parotid gland. J. Laryng. 90 (1976) 295

Gläser, A.: Geschwülste der Kopfspeicheldrüsen. In Gläser, A.: Klinische Pathologie der Geschwülste, Lieferung 3. Thieme, Leipzig 1979 (S. 85)

Gusterson, B., R. Lucas, M. Ormerod: Distribution of epithelial membrane antigen in benign and malignant lesions of the salivary glands. Virchows Arch. Path. Anat. 397 (1982) 227

Hales, B., J. E. Hansen: Bilateral simultaneous Warthin's tumor in a woman. Southern Med. J. 70 (1977) 257

Hara, K., M. Ito, J. Takeuchi, S. Iijima, T. Endo, H. Hidaka: Distribution of S-100b protein in normal salivary glands and salivary gland tumors. Virchows Arch. Path. Anat. 401 (1983) 237

Hughes, E. S.: Multiple parotid tumors. Brit. med. J. 1956/I, 332

Iannaccone, P.: Multiple primary tumors. Four distinct head and neck tumors. Arch. Pathol. 99 (1975) 270–272

Ibi, A., T. Yokobayashi, T. Kawasaki, T. Nakajima: Bilateral Warthin's tumor: Report of case and review of Japanese literature. J. oral Surg. 39 (1981) 362

Ibrahim, N. B. M., J. C. Briggs: Salivary gland pleomorphic adenoma and malignant lymphoma. Histopathology 7 (1983) 445

Isacsson, G., M. Shear: Intraoral salivary gland tumors: A retrospective study of 201 cases. J. oral Path. 12 (1983) 57

Jend-Rossmann, I.: Pathomorphologische Klassifikation von Tumoren der Submandibularis und Sublingualis. Analyse von 188 Fällen. Diss. Hamburg 1980

Jensen, P. St., E. Husted: Cystadenolymphoma (Warthin's tumor) of the parotid gland. Scand. J. plast. reconstr. Surg. 4 (1970) 114

Kavka, S. J.: Bilateral simultaneous Warthin's tumors. Arch. Otolaryng. 91 (1970) 302

Korsrud, F. R., P. Brandtzaeg: Immunofluorescence study of secretory epithelial markers in pleomorphic adenomas. Virchows Arch. Path. Anat. 403 (1984a) 291

Korsrud, F. R., P. Brandtzaeg: Immunohistochemical characterization of cellular immunoglobulins and epithelial marker antigens in Warthin's tumor. Human Pathol. 15 (1984b) 361

Kleinsasser, O.: Einteilung, Morphologie und Verhalten der epithelialen Speicheldrüsentumoren. HNO (Berl.) 17 (1969) 197

Levin, J. M., D. W. Robinson, F. Lin: Acinic cell carcinoma. Collective review, including bilateral cases. Arch. Surg. 110 (1975) 64

Lumerman, H., P. Freedman, P. Caracciolo, P. S. Remigio: Synchronous malignant mucoepidermoid tumor of the parotid gland and Warthin's tumor in adjacent lymph node. Oral Surg. 39 (1975) 953

Man, A., L. Zaidel: Monomorphic adenoma and adenolymphoma in the same parotid gland. Israel J. Med. Sci. 16 (1980) 136

McDicken, I. W., J. Scott: The presence and distribution of carcinoembryonic antigen in tumors of human minor salivary glands. J. oral Path. 10 (1981) 296

Nakazato, Y., J. Ishizeki, K. Takahashi, H. Yamaguchi, T. Kamei, T. Mori: Localization of S-100 protein and glial fibrillary acidic protein-related antigen in pleomorphic adenoma of the salivary glands. Lab. Invest. 46 (1982) 621

Nathrath, W. B. J., P. D. Wilson, L. K. Trejdosiewicz: Immunohistochemical localisation of keratin and luminal epithelial antigen in myoepithelial and luminal epithelial cells of human mammary and salivary gland tumours. Path. Res. Pract. 175 (1982) 279

Nelson, D. W., R. D. Nichols, G. Fine: Bilateral acinus cell tumors of the parotid gland. Laryngoscope 88 (1978) 1935

Pontilena, N., R. M. Rankow: Coexisting benign mixed tumor and mucoepidermoid carcinoma of the parotid gland. Ann. Otol. 88 (1979) 327

Quintarelli, G., L. Robinson: The glycosaminoglycans of salivary gland tumors. A histochemical characterization and a critical evaluation. Amer. J. Pathol. 51 (1967) 19

Scheffer, P., A. M. Roucayrol, M. C. Schnirer: Cystadenolymphomes parotidiens plurifocaux. Rev. Stomat. 82 (1981) 279
Schröder, M., M. Droese: Doppelseitiges tubuläres Speichelgangkarzinom der Glandula parotis. Z. Laryng. Rhinol. 56 (1977) 907
Seifert, G.: Klassifikation der epithelialen Speicheldrüsentumoren. Verh. Dtsch. Ges. Path. 62 (1978) 549
Seifert, G.: Der Einsatz von Tumormarkern bei der Diagnostik von Speicheldrüsentumoren. Wien. klin. Wschr. 94 (1982) 372
Seifert, G., J. Caselitz: Markers of oral and salivary gland tumors. Immunocytochemical investigations. Cancer Detect. Prevent. 8 (1985) in Druck
Seifert, G., K. Donath: Die Morphologie der Speicheldrüsenerkrankungen. Arch. Oto-Rhino-Laryng. 213 (1976a) 111
Seifert, G. K. Donath: Classification of the pathohistology of diseases of the salivary glands. Review about 2600 cases of the salivary gland register. Beitr. Pathol. 159 (1976b) 1
Seifert, G., K. Donath: Über das Vorkommen sog. heller Zellen in Speicheldrüsentumoren. Ultrastruktur und Differentialdiagnose. Z. Krebsforsch. 91 (1978) 165
Seifert, G., H. G. Bull, K. Donath: Histologic subclassification of the cystadenolymphoma of the parotid gland. Virchows Arch. Path. Anat. 388 (1980a) 13
Seifert, G., M. Heckmayr, K. Donath: Carcinome in papillären Cystadenolymphomen der Parotis. Definition und Differentialdiagnose. Z. Krebsforsch. 90 (1977) 25
Seifert, G. H. Rieb, K. Donath: Klassifikation der Tumoren der kleinen Speicheldrüsen. Pathohistologische Analyse von 160 Tumoren. Z. Laryng. Rhinol. 59 (1980b) 379
Smith, J. F., F. M. Fesmire: The benign papillary cystadenoma lymphomatosum. Oral Surg. 27 (1969) 95
Tanaka, N., W. C. Chen: A case of bilateral papillary cystadenoma lymphomatosum (Warthin's tumor) of the parotid complicated with a mucoepidermoid tumor. Gann 44 (1953) 229
Thackray, A. C., R. B. Lucas: Tumors of the major salivary glands. Atlas of Tumor Pathology, 2. ser. fasc. 10. Armed Forces Institute of Pathology, Washington 1974
Thackray, A. C., L. H. Sobin: Histological typing of salivary gland tumours. World Health Organization, Geneva 1972
Thompson, A. S., H. C. Bryant jr.: Histogenesis of papillary cystadenoma lymphomatosum (Warthin's tumor) of the parotid gland. Amer. J. pathol. 26 (1950) 807
Toida, M., J. Takeuchi, K. Hara, M. Sobue, K. Tsukidate, K. Goto, N. Nakashima: Histochemical studies of intercellular components of salivary gland tumors with special reference to glycosaminoglycan, laminin and vascular elements. Virchows Arch. Path. Anat. 403 (1984) 15
Trejo, I. H., T. R. Harwood, J. C. Goldstein, G. W. Summers: Oxyphil adenoma four years after a benign mixed tumor. Arch. Otolaryng. 96 (1972) 570
Turnbull, A. D., E. L. Frazell: Multiple tumors of the parotid glands. Amer. J. Surg. 118 (1969) 787
Vigliani, R., A. Stramignoni: Cytologic localization of antigens from human saliva in pleomorphic adenomas of salivary glands. Cancer (Philad.) 48 (1981) 293
Volmer, J.: Multiple unilaterale Tumoren der Glandula parotis. Zbl. allg. Path. path. Anat. 126 (1982) 327
Weimert, T. A., W. P. Work: Bilateral asynchronous mixed tumors of the parotid gland. Arch. Otolaryng. 102 (1976) 702
Williams, C.: Bilateral parotid neoplasms. Plast. Reconstr. Surg. 66 (1980) 448

Clinical Findings

Epithelial tumors are the most common neoplasms of the major and minor glands. There are numerous forms of tumor that previously were very difficult to classify histologically. This difficulty has now been largely resolved by numerous investigations. Increased knowledge of these tumors has had enormous influence on the correct treatment (Miehlke 1973, Naumann 1974, Conley 1975).

About 80% of epithelial tumors affect the parotid gland, 5–10%, the submandibular gland, and 5–6%, the palatal glands. Most of these tumors are benign. In most large series (Eneroth 1971), benign tumors are four times more common than malignant. The incidence of salivary gland tumors is 40 per million per year (Eneroth 1976).

The age and sex distribution of salivary gland tumors varies so much that firm conclusions cannot be drawn, although the following guidelines may be stated.

- The nonepithelial tumors, such as hemangioma and lymphangioma, occur mainly in children; 95% of parotid tumors in childhood are hemangiomas (Seifert 1965).
- In adults the great majority of tumors (95%) are epithelial in origin.
- Epithelial tumors are encountered at all ages, but are rare in patients less than the age of 20 years.

Malignant tumors are exceedingly rare in the adolescent, much the most common being the mucoepidermoid tumor (Kauffman & Stout 1963).

- Malignant tumors have a peak age incidence between 40 and 60 years.
- Pleomorphic adenomas mainly present between the ages: 40 and 50 years.
- Adenoid cystic carcinomas occur mainly between 50 and 60 years.
- Of cystadenolymphomas, 90% arise in men, but there is no clear sex difference for pleomorphic adenomas. Well-differentiated mucoepidermoid tumors, adenoid cystic carcinomas, and acinic cell tumors are more common in women.

A salivary gland tumor may be localized or diffuse, mobile or fixed, painless or painful, may affect only a specific part of the gland, or may affect the entire body of the gland. The function of the facial nerve may be affected by the tumor, because of the close anatomic relationships between the gland and the nerve. A partial or complete paralysis of the facial nerve provides important information about the nature of the tumor. Facial paralysis is almost exclusively observed in malignant tumors. A sialogram may show a displacement of the duct system. These tumors may be cold or hot on scanning, the cystadenolymphoma being the typical example of a tumor with high uptake of isotope.

All the methods of investigation just described take second place to histologic diagnosis, the only certain foundation for correct treatment. Two possibilities are available: aspiration cytology or intraoperative frozen section. If there is the slightest doubt about the results of the frozen section, the operation must be abandoned to avoid an unnecessarily mutilating procedure based on a false diagnosis.

References

Conley, J.: Salivary Glands and the Facial Nerve. Thieme, Stuttgart 1975

Eneroth, C. M.: Salivary gland tumors in the parotid gland, submandibular gland and the palate region. Cancer (Philad.) 27 (1971) 1415

Eneroth, C. M.: Die Klinik der Kopfspeicheldrüsentumoren. Arch. Oto-Rhino-Laryng. 213 (1976) 61

Kauffman, S. L., A. P. Stout: Tumors of the main salivary glands in children. Cancer 16 (1963) 1317

Miehlke, A.: Surgery of the Facial Nerve. Urban & Schwarzenberg, München; Saunders, Philadelphia 1973

Naumann, H. H.: Kopf- und Halschirurgie, Bd. 2, Gesicht und Gesichtsschädel. Thieme, Stuttgart 1974

Seifert, G.: Die Speicheldrüsengeschwülste im Kindesalter. Z. Kinderchir. 2 (1965) 285

TNM System

The TNM classification of salivary tumors follows the basic principles for other tumors. The T category ranges from T_1 to T_4 with increasing size of the tumor. The N category relates to the regional lymph node metastases: N_0 = no nodes, N_1 = homolateral nodes, N_2 = mobile contra- or bilateral nodes, N_3 = fixed lymph node metastases. The M category relates to distant metastases: M_0 = no metastases, M_1 = metastases present, the lung being the site most commonly affected by malignant salivary tumors.

So far, there are no generally recognized rules for defining the extent of the primary tumor (T stage). The working group on clinical oncology of the German Ear, Nose and Throat Society has suggested the following classification based solely on the extent of the tumor:

T_1 = a tumor of 2 cm or less in its greatest extent
T_2 = a tumor more than 2 cm but not more than 4 cm in its greatest extent
T_3 = tumor measuring more than 4 cm in its greatest extent or extending beyond the organ.

The prognostic value of this T classification has so far not been investigated.

Spiro et al drew up a classification in 1975 for malignant salivary gland tumors, which also has three T categories, but which takes into account the mobility of the tumor, ulceration of the skin, and the function of the facial nerve (Fig. 15.**11**). They were able to prove the prognostic value of this classification based on a series of 288 patients treated for malignant salivary gland tumors between 1939 and 1968. Levitt et al (1981) carried out a retrospective multicenter study of the fac-

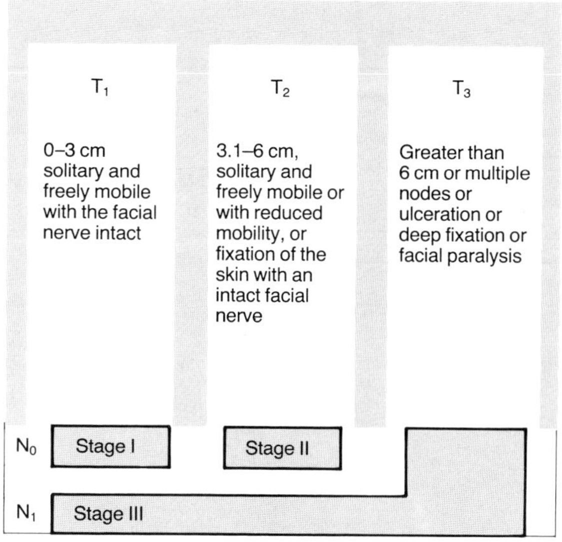

Figure 15.**11** T categories and staging of malignant salivary tumors. (Spiro et al.)

Table 15.**4** TNM Categories and Stage Classification for Malignant Salivary Tumors (Levitt et al). Local Extension Indicates Extension of the Tumor to Surrounding Structures, such as Bone, Skin and Other Soft Tissues, and also Invasion of the Intraglandular Segment of the Facial Nerve

T_1	Tumor with a diameter of 0.1–2 cm, no local extension
T_2	Tumor with a diameter of 2.1–4 cm, no local extension
T_3	Tumor with a diameter of 4.1–6 cm, no local extension
T_{4a}	Tumor diameter greater than 6 cm, no local extension
T_{4b}	Tumor of any diameter with local extension
N_0	No evidence of regional lymph node metastases (patient with palpable but nonsuspect regional lymph nodes are included)
N_1	Evidence of regional lymph node metastasis (included are palpable and suspect regional lymph nodes)
M_0	No distant metastis
M_1	Distant metastasis present

Stage I	$T_1N_0M_0$
	$T_2N_0M_0$
Stage II	$T_3N_0M_0$
Stage III	$T_1N_1M_0$
	$T_2N_1M_0$
	$T_{4a}N_0M_0$
	$T_{4b}N_0M_0$
Stage IV	
	$T_3N_1M_0$
	$T_{4a}N_1M_0$
	$T_{4b}N_1M_0$
	all M_1

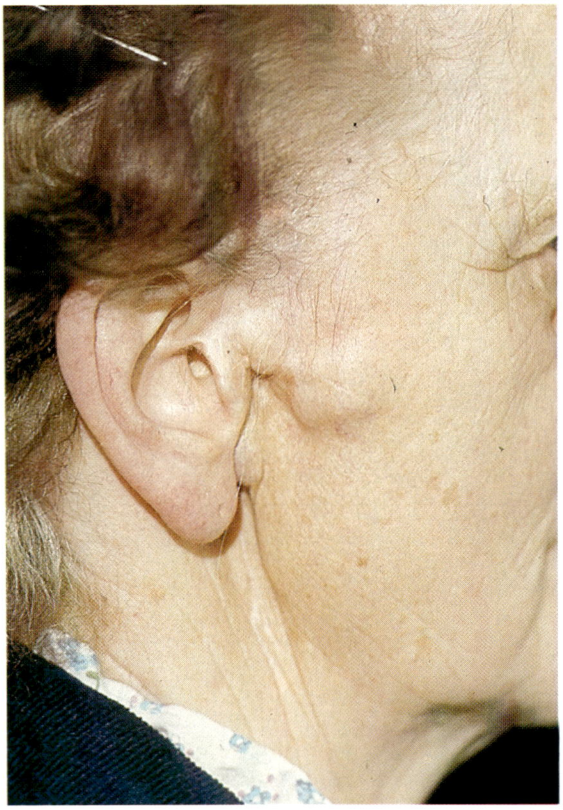

Figure 15.**12** Recurrent pleomorphic adenoma of the parotid gland in a 69-year-old woman who had undergone several operations.

tors influencing the prognosis of 861 patients with malignant salivary gland tumors. Invasion of the tumor into surrounding structures, such as the facial nerve, the skin, bones, and soft tissue, including the retromandibular fossa and the sternocleidomastoid muscle, were particularly significant. Local extent of tumor has a decisive influence on the prognosis and is therefore included in the four T categories (Table 15.**4**). Except for invasion of the intraglandular segment of the facial nerve, the presence of a local extension indicates extension of the tumor beyond the boundaries of the organ, which is classified as T_4. The classifications suggested by Spiro et al (1975) and by Levitt et al (1981) for the TNM classification of malignant tumors correlate well with the prognosis. It would be welcome if one of these two schemes achieved general acceptance.

References

Levitt, S. H., R. B. McHugh, O. Gómez-Marin, V. J. Hyames, E. H. Soule, E. W. Strong, A. H. Sellers, J. E. Woods, O. M. Guillamondegui: Clinical staging system for cancer of the salivary gland: A retrospective study. Cancer 47 (1981) 2712

Spiro, R. H., A. G. Huvos, E. W. Strong: Cancer of the parotid gland. A clinicopathologic study of 288 primary cases. Amer. J. Surg. 130 (1975) 452

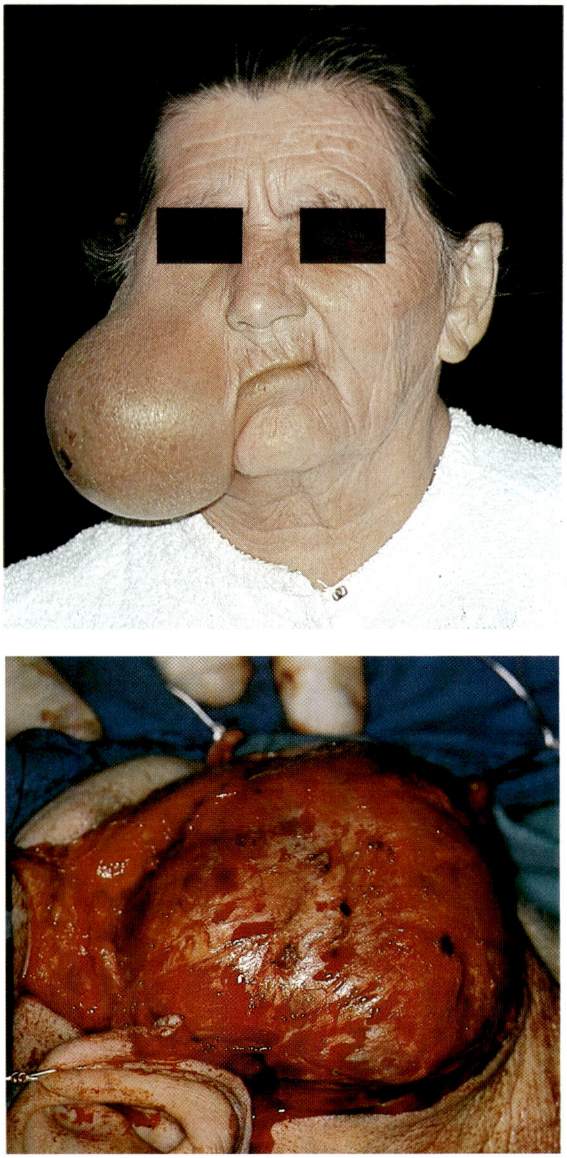

a

b

Figure 15.**13** **a** Pleomorphic adenoma of the right parotid gland present for 20 years. **b** View of the operative field.

Pleomorphic Adenoma

Clinical Data

The term "pleomorphic adenoma" indicates the histologic diversity of the tumor, at the same time indicating its epithelial origin. For many decades, the biologic behavior of pleomorphic adenoma was the subject of controversy. We now know from large series (Eneroth 1964, 1965, 1976) that none of the criteria of malignancy or semimalignancy is satisfied by pleomorphic adenoma. Neither the varying cell content nor the cylindromatous tissue structures of the tumor support the argument of possible malignancy, as clinical observations clearly show.

Even less does the multifocal nature of the tumor indicate malignancy. A true multifocal tumor is very rare (Eneroth 1964, 1965). In most cases the tumor consists of lobules joined by fine connections not visible to the naked eye. The multifocal nature of a recurrent pleomorphic adenoma is well known (Fig. 15.**12**). In many cases, this is due to spillage of tumor tissue. However, every surgeon knows that the capsule may be torn, allowing spillage of tumor, even with the most delicate operative technique. Our careful observations have shown that recurrence of tumor is very rare in these cases, if the operative field is subjected to thorough toilet by aspiration.

Paralysis of the facial nerve by pleomorphic adenoma is very rare. The facial nerve appears to be extremely resistant to pressure or traction from even the largest tumor (Fig. 15.**13a, b**).

Histologic Subclassification

Despite its diverse nature, pleomorphic adenoma (Figs. 15.**14**–15.**16**) shows certain patterns characterized by two criteria: Differentiation of the epithelial cells, and the amount and properties of the stroma. Pleomorphic adenomas may be subdivided into four types with respect to these two architectural patterns (Seifert et al 1976: Table 15.**5**):

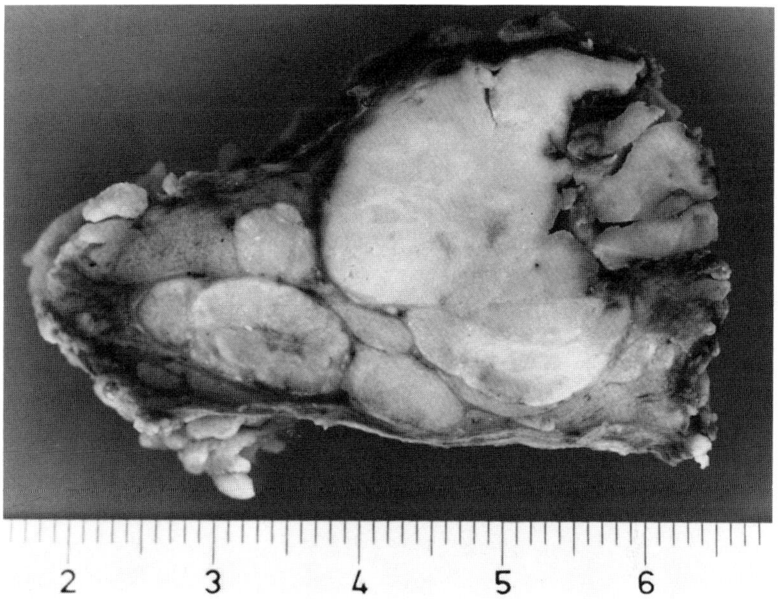

Figure 15.**14** Pleomorphic adenoma of the parotid gland showing a relatively compact tumor nodule clearly demarcated from the remaining glandular tissue.

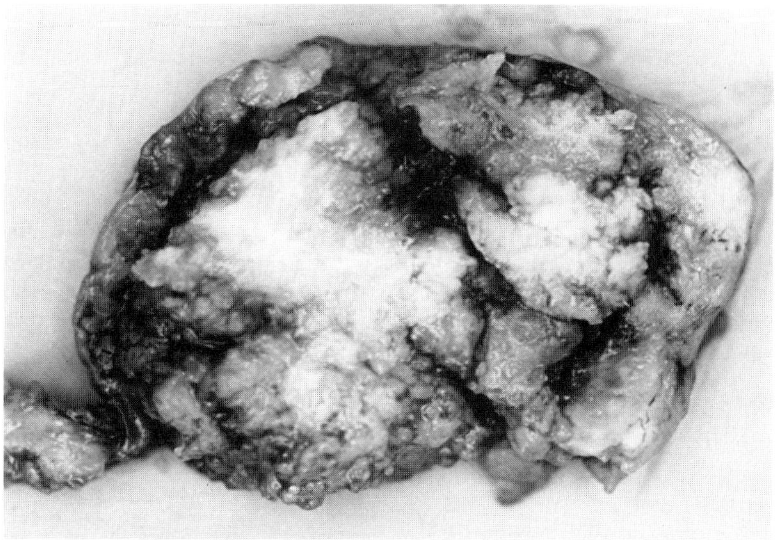

Figure 15.**15** Pleomorphic adenoma of the parotid gland: tumor nodules with inclusion of cystic areas and a margin of parotid tissue.

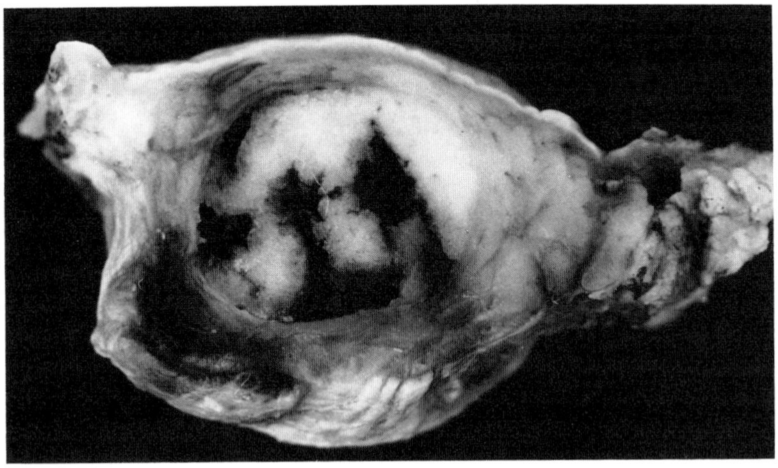

Figure 15.**16** Pleomorphic adenoma of the palatal glands presenting as a mucosal swelling: cystic areas within the tumor.

Table 15.**5** Subclassification of Pleomorphic Parotid Adenoma (Seifert et al)

Subtype	Frequency (%)	Proportion of Stroma (%)	Stromal Differentiation	Epithelial Differentiation
1	30.5	30–50	Mucoid	Duct and myoepithelial cells Epidermoid cells Solid and tubular cystic cells
2a	37.5	80	Mucoid	As subtype 1
2b	2.5	80	Chondroid	As subtype 1
2c	5.0	80	Mucoid-chondroid	As subtype 1
2d	0.5	80	Fascicular	As subtype 1
2e	8.5	80	Hyalin-fibrous	As subtype 1
3	9.0	20–30	Subtype 2	As subtype 1
4	6.5	20–30	Subtype 2	As subtype 1 but with some monomorphic differentiation

Type 1 is the classic tumor type in which the stroma constitutes 30–50% of the tumor mass (Fig. 15.**17a, b**). The epithelium forms solid trabecular, tubular, or cystic structures consisting of epithelial cells of varying differentiation. These include duct epithelium, myoepithelial cells, epidermoid cells, and other cell forms. The epithelium and stroma are not sharply demarcated from each other. The peripheral epithelial bands merge into the stroma like a swarm of bees. The stroma shows mainly a mucoid differentiation and contains much acid mucopolysaccharide. The tumor is usually limited by connective tissue structures of salivary tissue without the formation of a continuous capsule. There is very little cellular stromal reaction. About 30% of all pleomorphic adenomas show a type I pattern.

Type 2 may be defined as a pleomorphic adenoma rich in stroma (Figs. 15.**18**–15.**20**). This type includes 55% of all pleomorphic adenomas. The stroma is mucoid in structure and constitutes 80% of the tumor. Chondroid or mixed mucoid-chondroid stromal areas are rarer (Fig. 15.**21a, b**). A fascicular arrangement of the stroma is extremely rare; it is constructed of spindle-shaped cell bands and must be differentiated from neural tumors (Fig. 15.**22a, b**). An osseous pattern may also occur on occasions. The stroma may show degenerative changes with hyalin-fibrous architecture in longstanding tumors or after radiotherapy (Fig. 15.**23**). The epithelial differentiation is varied as in type I.

Type 3 is a pleomorphic adenoma rich in cells but poor in stroma; the latter only makes up 20% of

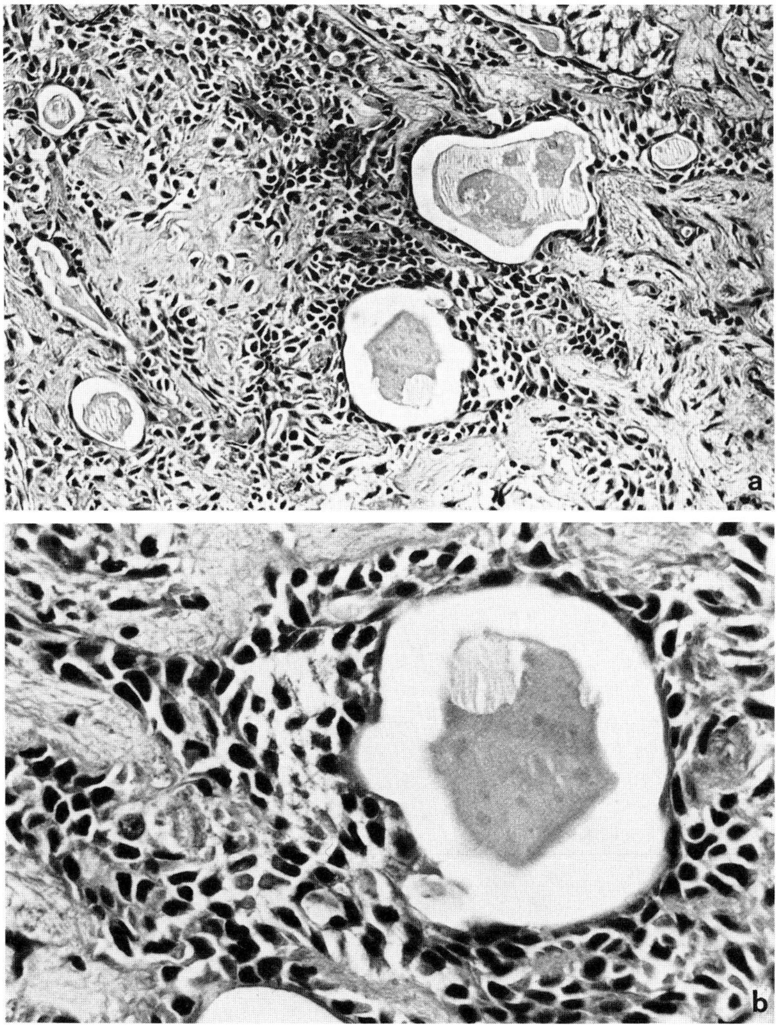

Figure 15.**17** Pleomorphic adenoma (type 1) showing epithelial components with a poorly demarcated microcystic and trabecular structures, and spongy expansion of the epithelium (**b**). Astra blue. **a** 160×, **b** 400×.

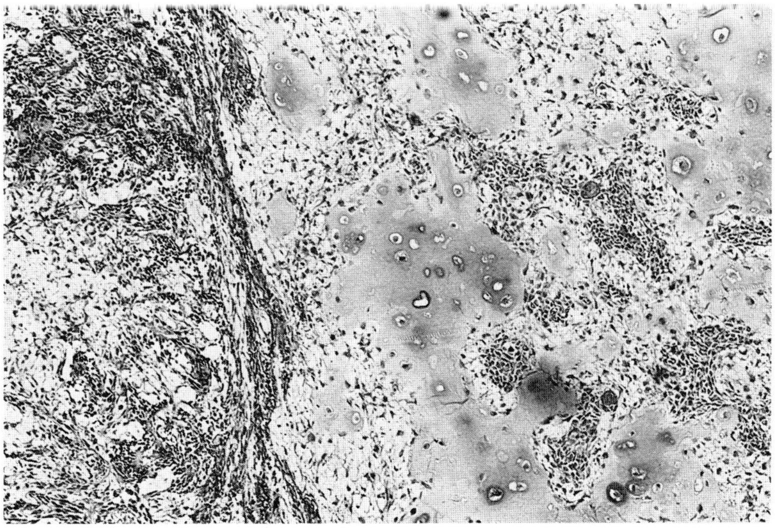

Figure 15.**18** Pleomorphic adenoma (type 2): a richly developed mucoid and chondromatous stroma. Astra blue, 63×.

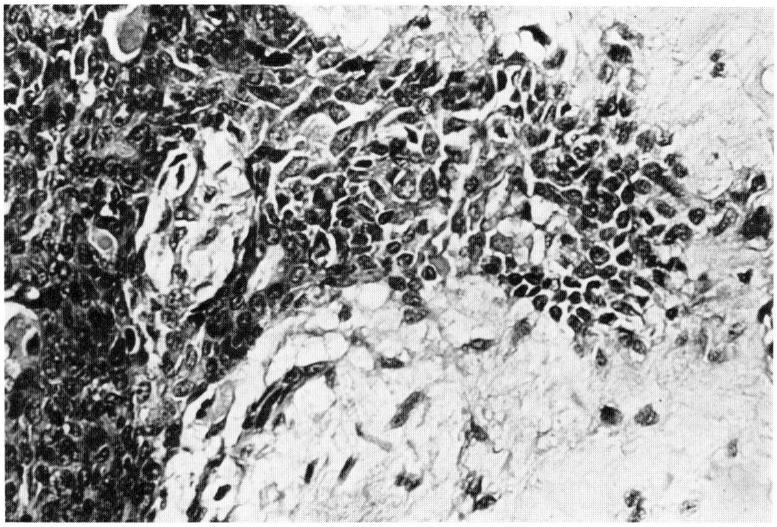

Figure 15.**19** Pleomorphic adenoma (type 2): extension of the partially spindle-shaped epithelial cells into the mucoid stroma. H & E, 250×.

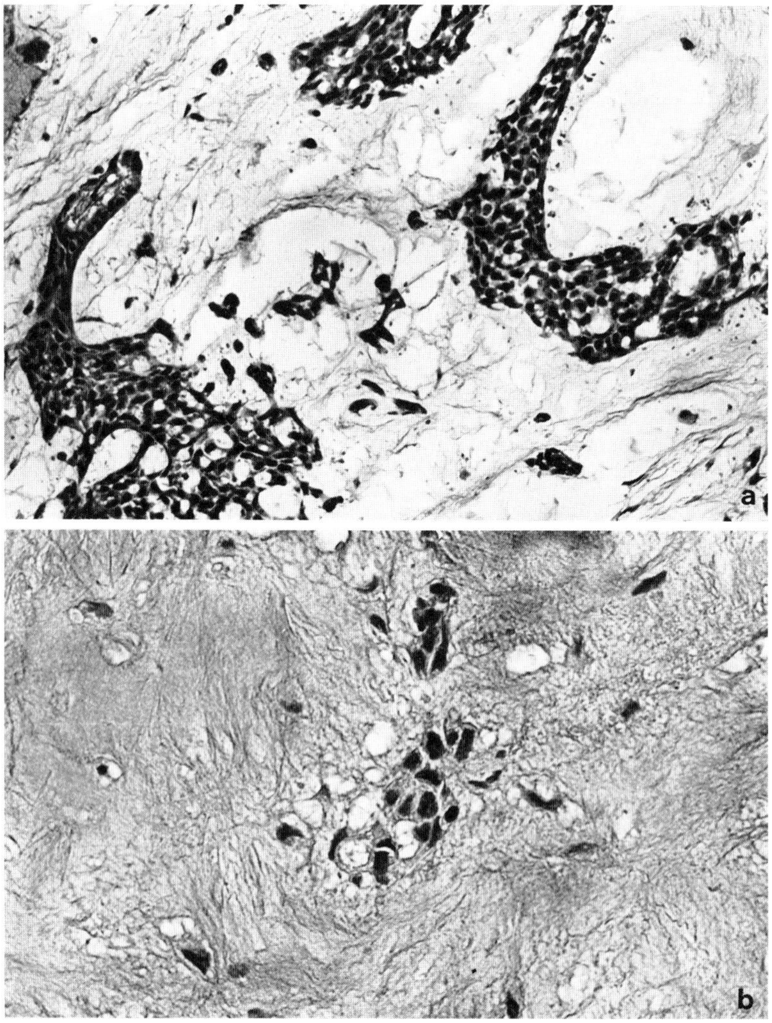

Figure 15.**20** Pleomorphic adenoma (type 2): **a** Epithelial complex not clearly demarcated from the mucoid stroma. H & E, 160×. **b** Mucoid stroma with infiltration by spindle-shaped myoepithelial cells. Astra blue, 400×.

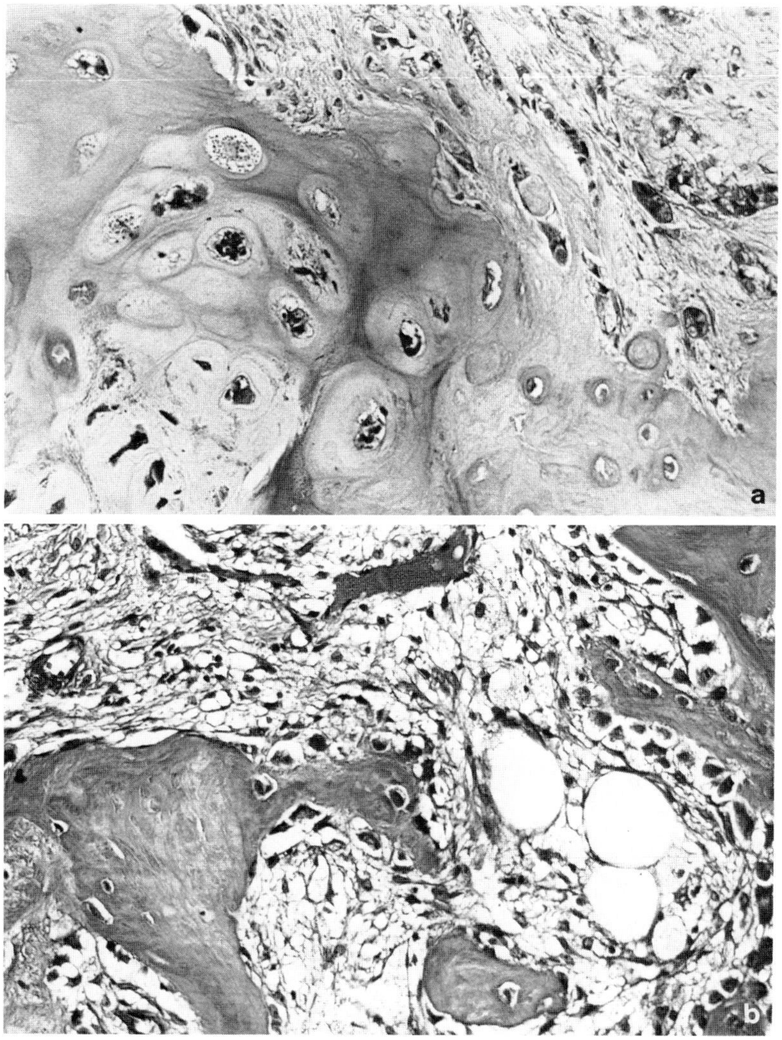

Figure 15.**21** Pleomorphic adenoma (type 2): **a** Chondroid stroma. PAS, 160×. **b** Osseous stroma. H & E, 160×.

the tumor (Figs. 15.**24**, 15.**25a, b**). The diverse differentiation of the epithelium and the stroma resembles that of type 2. About 9% of all tumors fall into type 3.

Type 4 is also an adenoma rich in cells but poor in stroma, as in type 3, but with the difference that the epithelial component at some points is uniformly differentiated, resembling a monomorphic adenoma (Figs. 15.**26a, b**,, 15.**27**). An important characteristic in differential diagnosis is the mucoid stromal component, which is absent in monomorphic adenomas. Of all pleomorphic adenomas, 6.5% fall in type 4. The peak age incidence of type 4 lies in the seventh decade, a decade higher than that for types 1–3.

Subtypes 3 and 4 may be summarized as pleomorphic adenomas poor in stroma, which constitute about 15.5% of all pleomorphic adenomas of the major glands. In contrast, 35% of pleomorphic adenomas of the minor glands fall into subtypes 3 and 4 (Seifert et al 1980). Almost 50% of carcinomas ex pleomorphic adenomas arise from subtypes 3 and 4. This finding justifies the recommendation that all pleomorphic adenomas poor in stroma, particularly in patients in the older age groups, should be followed carefully for the possible development of a carcinoma (Seifert et al 1977). Recurrences of pleomorphic adenomas, on the other hand, are more common in subtype 2, which is rich in stroma.

Duct epithelium and myoepithelial cells occur in more than 75% of cases with *cellular differentiation* of the epithelial tumor component. The duct cells form primitive ducts buds, narrow duct bands, or epithelial complexes resembling inter-

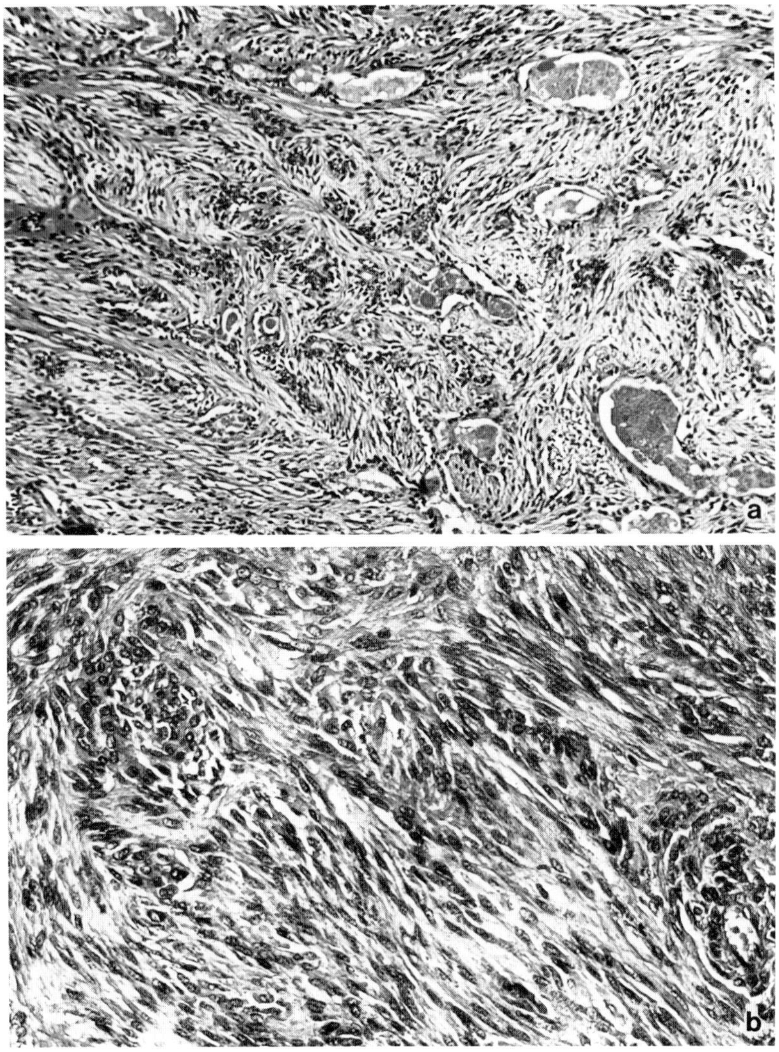

Figure 15.**22** Pleomorphic adenoma (type 2): fascicular stroma. H & E. **a** 160×, **b** 400×.

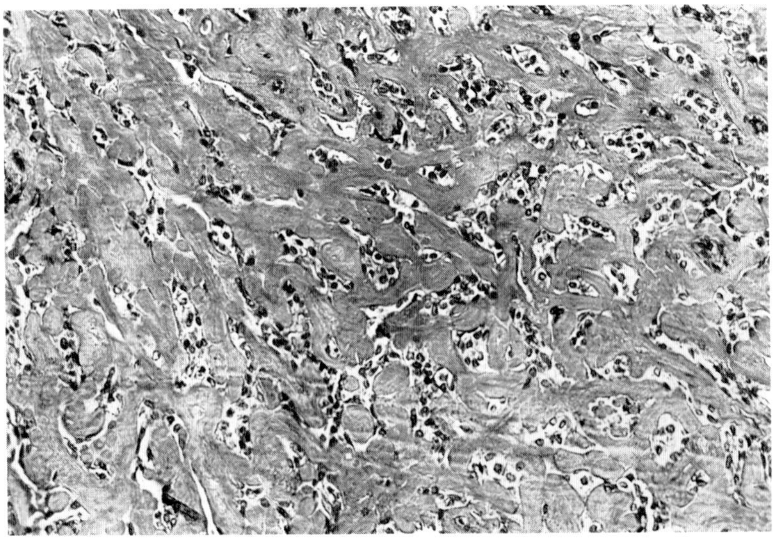

Figure 15.**23** Pleomorphic adenoma (type 2): hyaline stroma. H & E, 160×.

Figure 15.**24** Pleomorphic adenoma (type 3): cell-rich epithelial area with scanty stromal component. H & E, 63×.

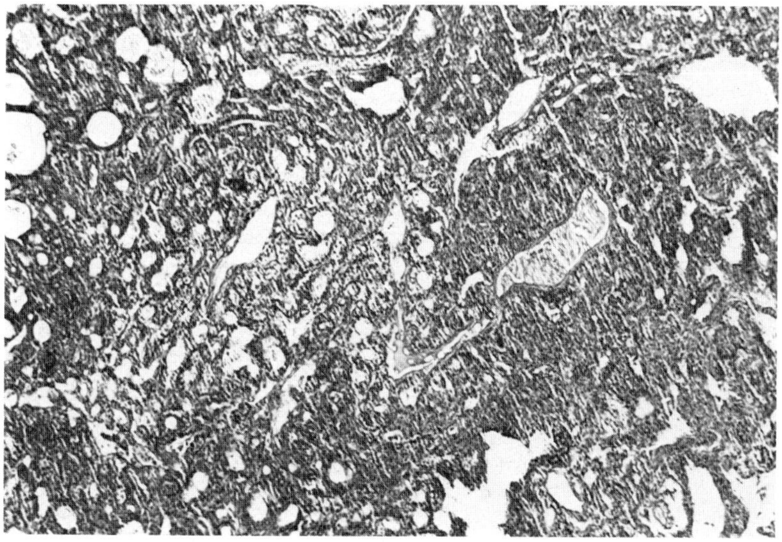

Figure 15.**25** Pleomorphic adenoma (type 3): **a** Microcystic structures. H & E, 160×. **b** Solid and trabecular structures. Astra blue, 160×.

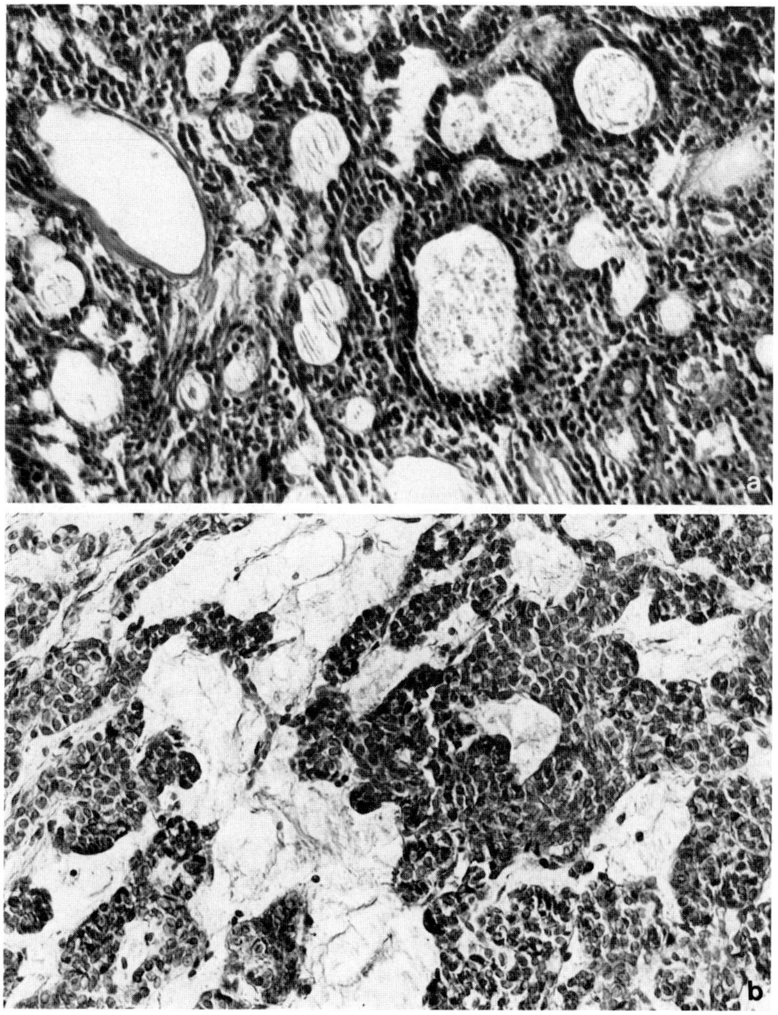

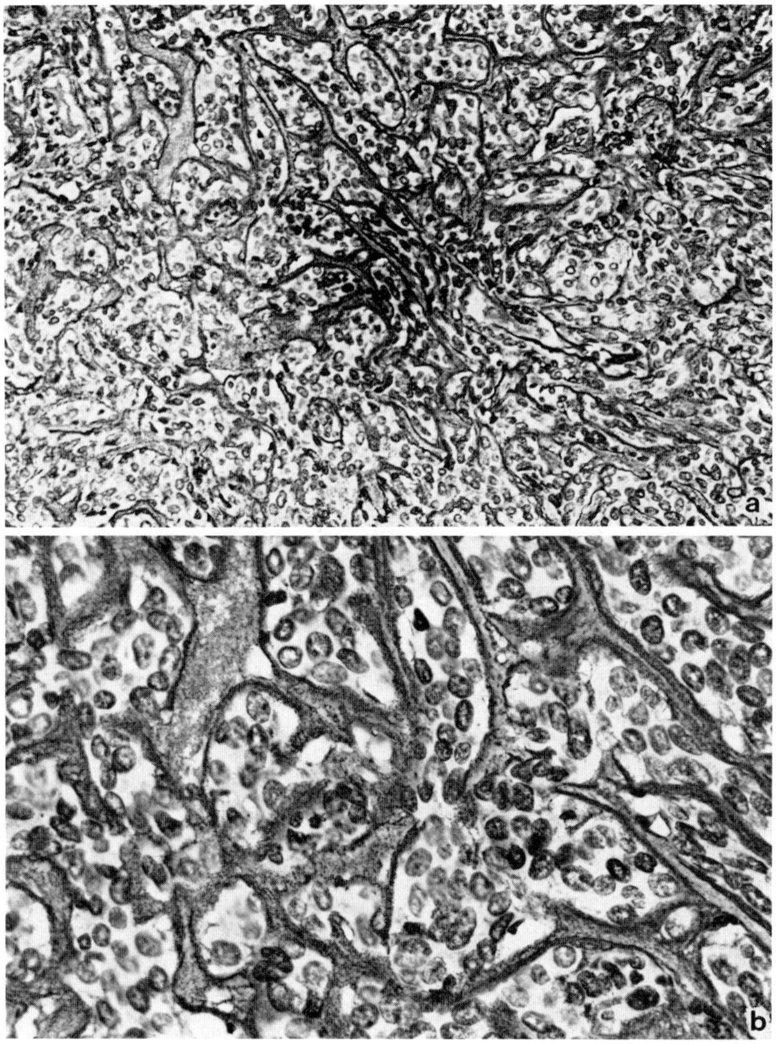

Figure 15.**26** Pleomorphic adenoma (type 4): trabecular clear cell structures separated by a hyaline stroma. Gomori. **a** 160×, **b** 400×.

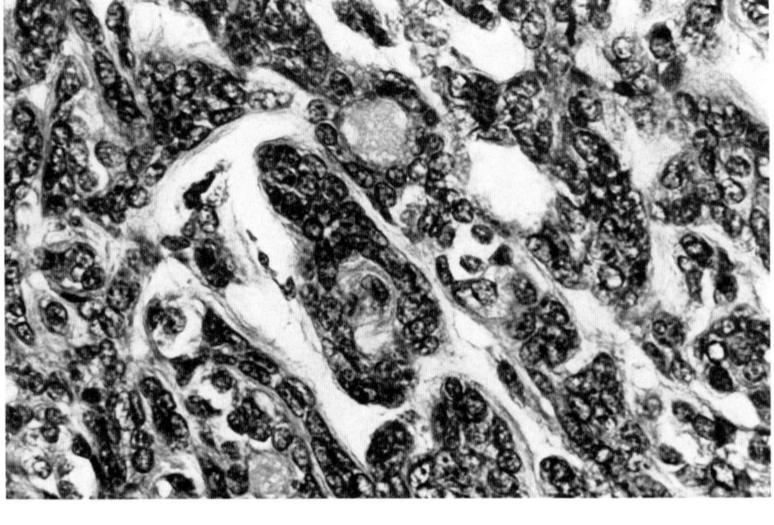

Figure 15.**27** Pleomorphic adenoma (type 4): relatively monotonous trabecular and tubular formations. H & E, 400×.

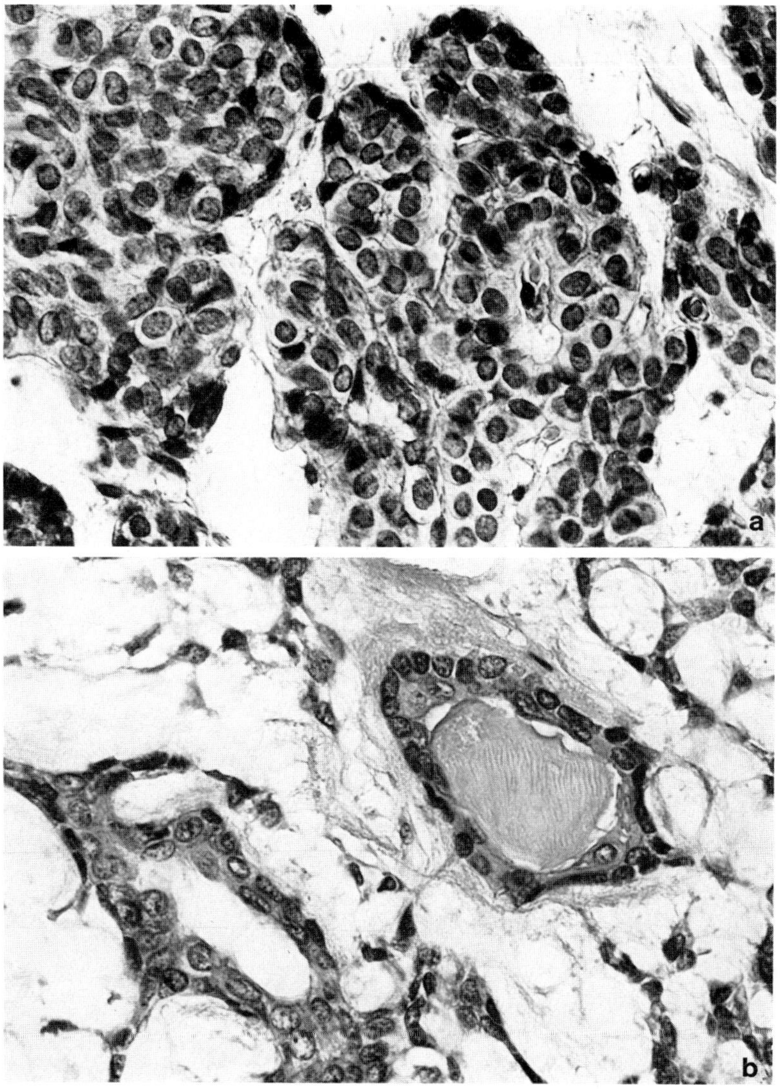

Figure 15.**28** Cellular differentiation in a pleomorphic adenoma: **a** Primitive duct buds. **b** Duct units with transition to spindle-shaped structures. H & E. **a**, **b** 400×.

calated ducts (Fig. 15.**28a, b**). The myoepithelial cells usually possess a clear cytoplasm and a more spindle cell-like structure. Epidermoid cell units develop relatively more often in 70% of cases (Fig. 15.**29**), but keratinization is much less common, being found in only 2.5% of cases. Striated duct epithelium (Figs. 15.**30a, b**, 15.**31**), oncocytes, basal cells, or sebaceous epithelium are rare forms of differentiation. Plasmacytoid cells (Fig. 15.**32**) or hyaline cells are particular forms of differentiation of modified myoepithelial cells (Buchner et al 1981) and can lead to confusion with plasmacytomas or other tumors. Tyrosine crystals are also occasionally described in pleomorphic adenomas (Thomas & Hutt 1983).

Electron microscopy has provided further conclusions about the cellular differentiation and stromal properties of the pleomorphic adenoma (Seifert & Donath 1976, Bienengräber 1983). Duct cells and epithelial cells constitute the main mass of tumor cells. Myoepithelial cells contain myofilaments, epidermoid cells contain desmosomes, and duct cells contain granules or other cell organelles. Less characteristic epithelial cells are classified as indifferent or transitional cells.

On the whole, duct cells of the intercalated duct type and myoepithelial cells form the actual tumor matrix (Shirasuno et al 1980). A particular proliferative activity, the ability to undergo epidermoid differentiation and the induction action to mucoid stromal transformation, are ascribed to the myoepithelial cells especially (Dardick et al 1982, 1983). The duct cells of pleomorphic adenoma also show ultrastructural findings similar to the intercalated duct epithelium, such as a positive phosphatase reaction and secretory

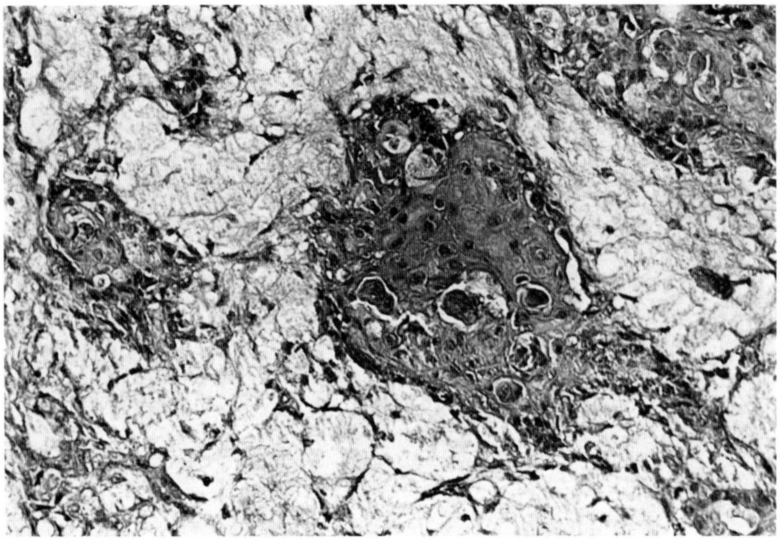

Figure 15.**29** Epidermoid differentiation in a pleomorphic adenoma. Astra blue, 400×.

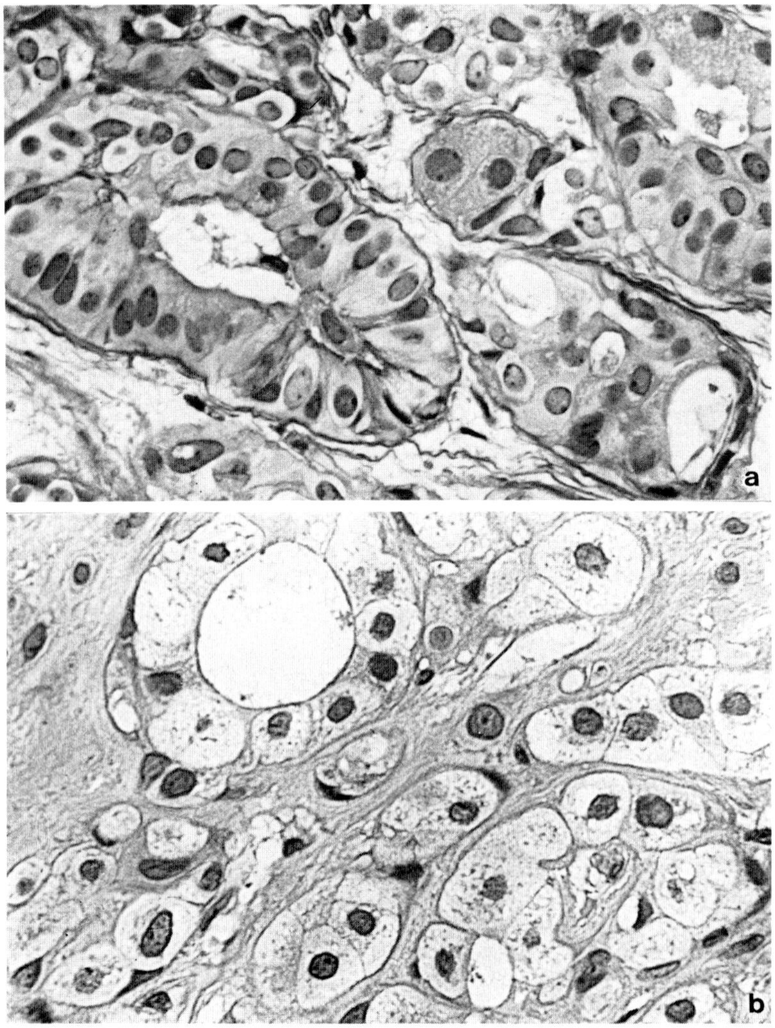

Figure 15.**30** Ductular structures in a pleomorphic adenoma:
a Structures resembling striated ducts. **b** Clear cell ductular structures. Semithin sections. Astra blue, **a**, **b** 400×.

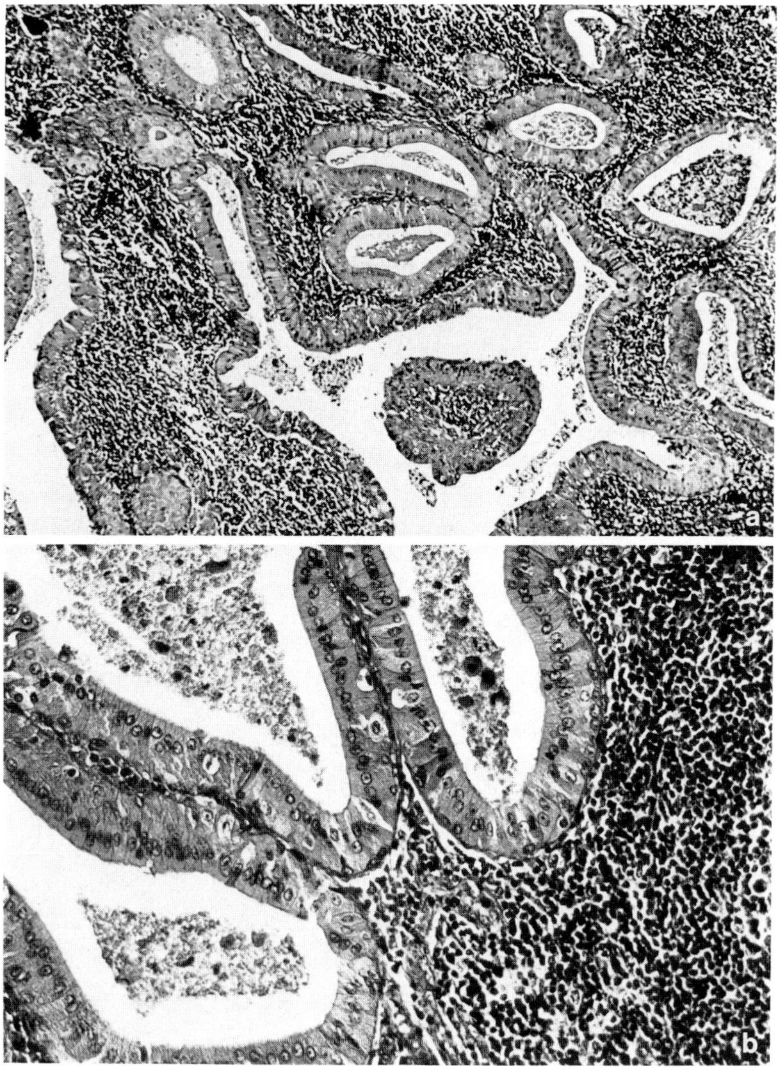

Figure 15.**37** Subtype 1 of cystadenolymphoma: cyst limited by double layer of oncocytes with a typical lymphoid stroma. H & E. **a** 63×, **b** 160×.

consist partly of friable, grayish yellow masses and partly of thin fluid mucous secretion. Because of its macroscopic appearance and its site in the upper part of the neck, the tumor is occasionally confused with a branchial cyst or a liquifying tuberculous lymphadenopathy. Small tumors in the early phases of development may masquerade as regional lymph nodes. This type of microcystadenolymphoma is indeed often of found coincidentally during histologic examination of a parotid removed surgically.

Histopathology. The tumor consists of an epithelial, monomorphic, mostly oncocytic component and a lymphoid stroma with follicles of the type seen in a lymph node (Fig. 15.**36a, b**). Four different *subtypes* of cystadenolymphoma may be distinguished, depending on the ratio of the two tissue components and on the epithelial differentiation (Seifert et al 1980).

Subtype I is the classic type of cystadenolymphoma (Fig. 15.**37a, b**), with a ratio of epithelium to stroma of 1 : 1; 77% of all cystadenolymphomas are in subtype 1. The monomorphic tumor cells are arranged in a double row and possess an acidophilic fine granular cytoplasm (Fig. 15.**38a, b**). The epithelium forms papillary structures in the lumen of micro- or macrocysts. The luminal epithelium demonstrates an apocrine secretion. The lumen of the cysts contains an acidophil secretion, with occasional desquamated epithelium, lymphocytes and macrophages, or crystalline deposits (David & Buchner 1978). The epithelial cords are separated from the lymphoid stroma by a basement membrane. Occasional mucus-forming goblet cells (Fig. 15.**39a, b**) with concentration of secretion in the cytoplasm, circumscribed areas of squamous metaplasia (Fig. 15.**40**), or a combination of both types of epithelial metaplasia may be demonstrated within the

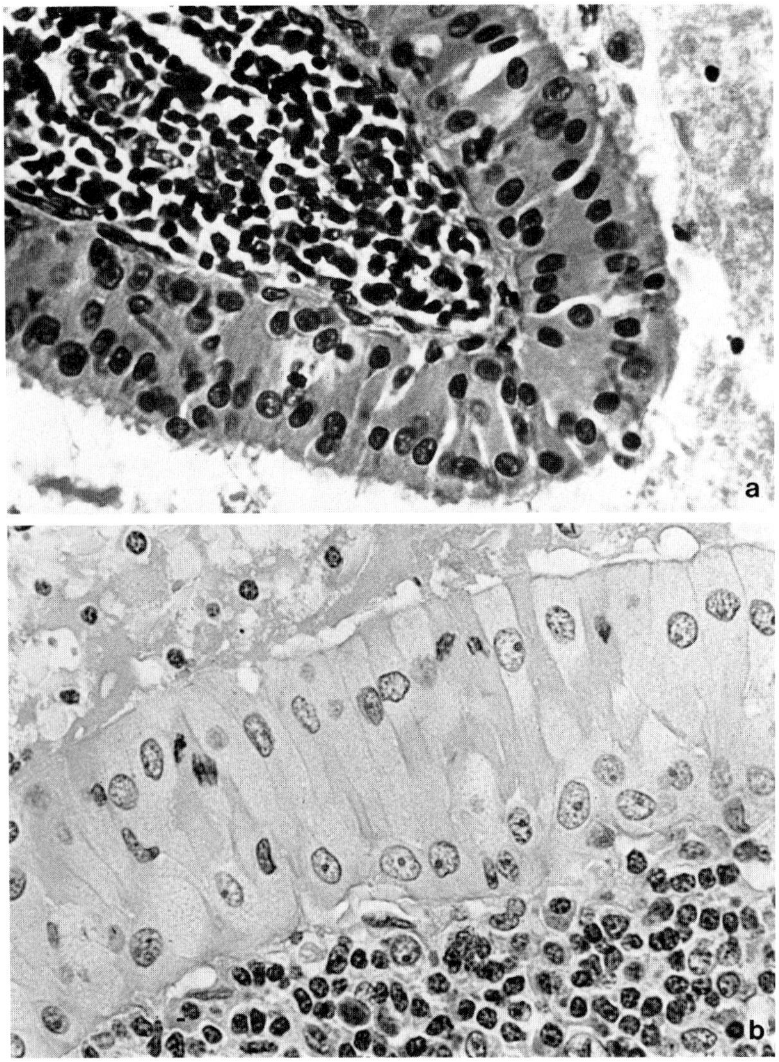

Figure 15.**38** Cystadenolymphoma subtype 1: **a** Double layers of oncocytes with fine granular cytoplasm surrounded by a lymphoid stroma. **b** Semithin section, basal and luminal arrangement of cell nuclei. H & E. **a**, **b** 400×.

oncocytic differentiated epithelium. Foci of marked oncocytic epithelial proliferation may even develop into microadenomas. The lymphoid stroma (see later) resembles the structure of a regional lymph node (Fig. 15.**41**) with a cellular composition of lymphocytes, plasma cells, mast cells, and macrophages. Secondary follicles with follicular center are formed.

Subtype 2 is lacking in stroma (Fig. 15.**42a, b**). Epithelial tumor components make up 70–80% of the tumor mass, and 13.5% of cases fall into subtype 2. At some points, the structure of the tumor resembles an oncocytoma, but differs in that a focal lymphoid stromal component is always developed. The other structural characteristics of subtype 2, such as oncocytic cell forms, focal metaplasia of squamous epithelium, or goblet cells, resemble subtype 1.

In *subtype 3*, the lymphoid stroma makes up 70–80% of the tumor mass (Fig. 15.**43a, b**). Only 2% of all cystadenolymphomas show this pattern. Subtype 3 occurs exclusively in men with a slightly lower average age than that of subtypes 1 and 2. The richly developed lymphoid stroma contains numerous active lymph follicles with large follicular centers. The remaining structures resemble subtype 1.

Subtype 4. This metaplastic subtype comprises 7.5% of all cystadenolymphomas. The characteristics are widespread replacement of the oncocytic differentiation by squamous cell metaplasia and degenerative changes, such as necrosis, pseudocysts, hyaline areas, and focal reduction of the lymphoid stroma (Figs. 15.**44a, b**, 15.**45a, b**). In 20–50% of patients, there is history of irradiation to the parotid area. Women are more commonly represented in subtype 4 than in cystadenolymphomas as a whole.

Composition of the Lymphoid Stroma. Morphometry (Nikai & Schröder 1984) shows that

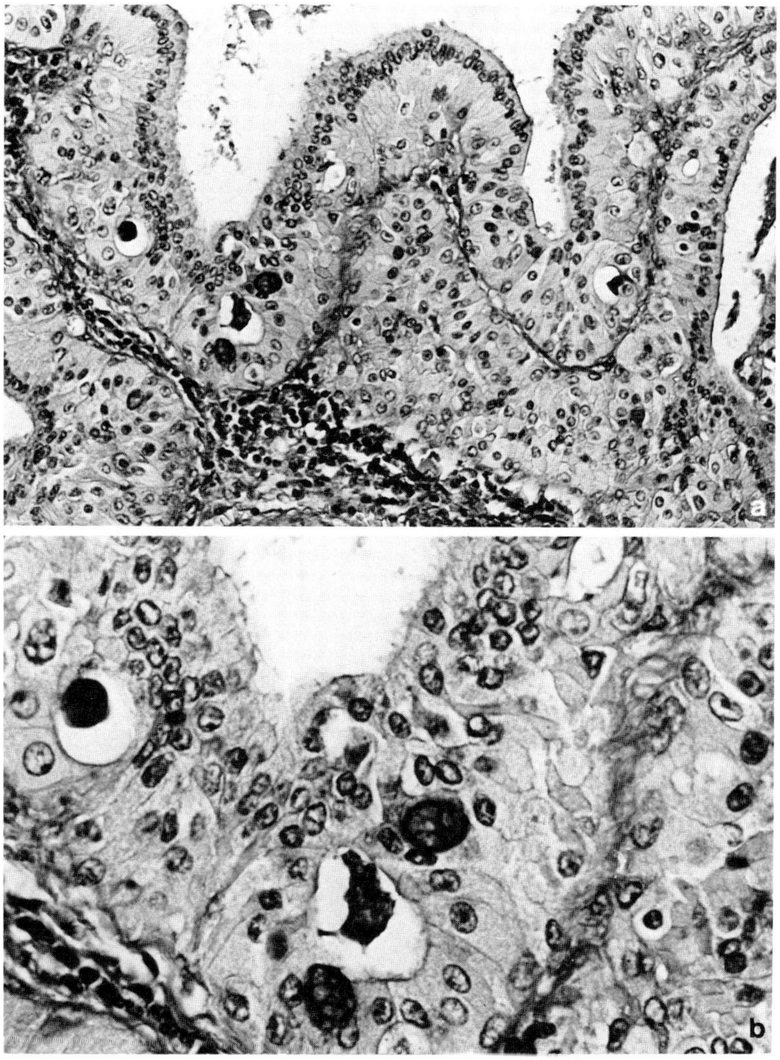

Figure 15.**39** Cystadenolymphoma subtype 1: goblet cell metaplasia with formation of mucus between the oncocytic cell masses. PAS. **a** 160×, **b** 400×. (Seifert et al 1980.)

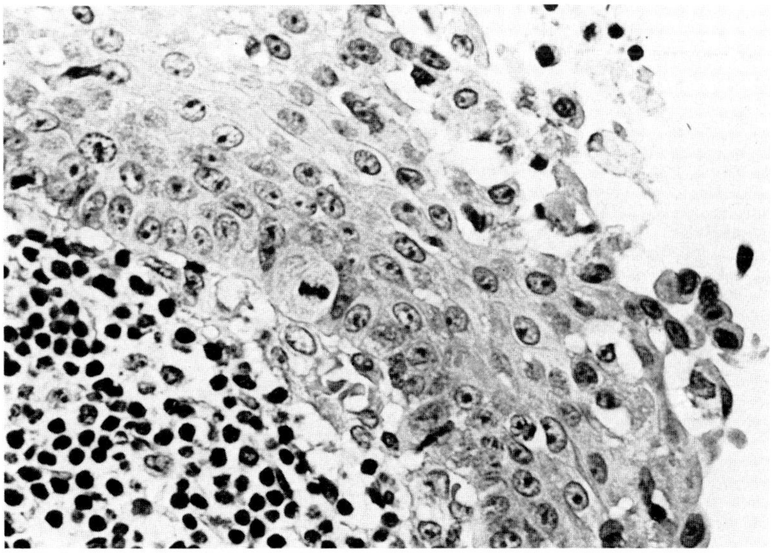

Figure 15.**40** Cystadenolymphoma subtype 1 showing focal squamous metaplasia. H & E, 400×.

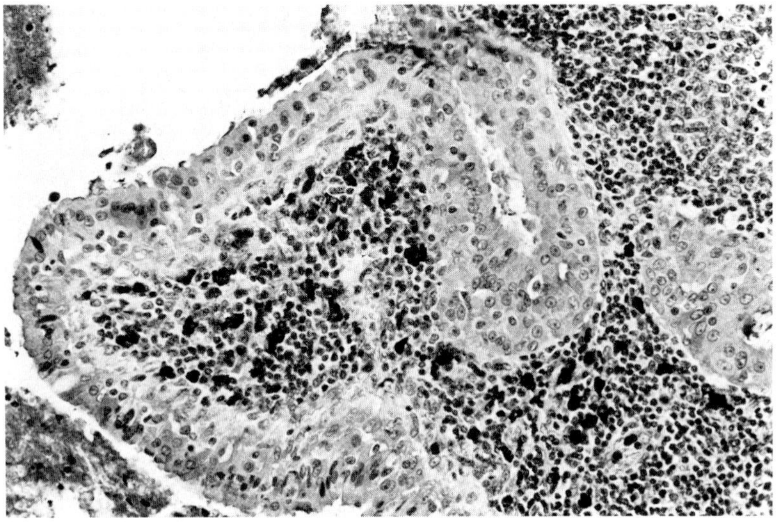

Figure 15.**41** Cystadenolymphoma subtype 1 showing a collection of IgA-containing plasma cells in a lymphoid stroma close to an oncocytic epithelium. Immunoperoxidase, 160×.

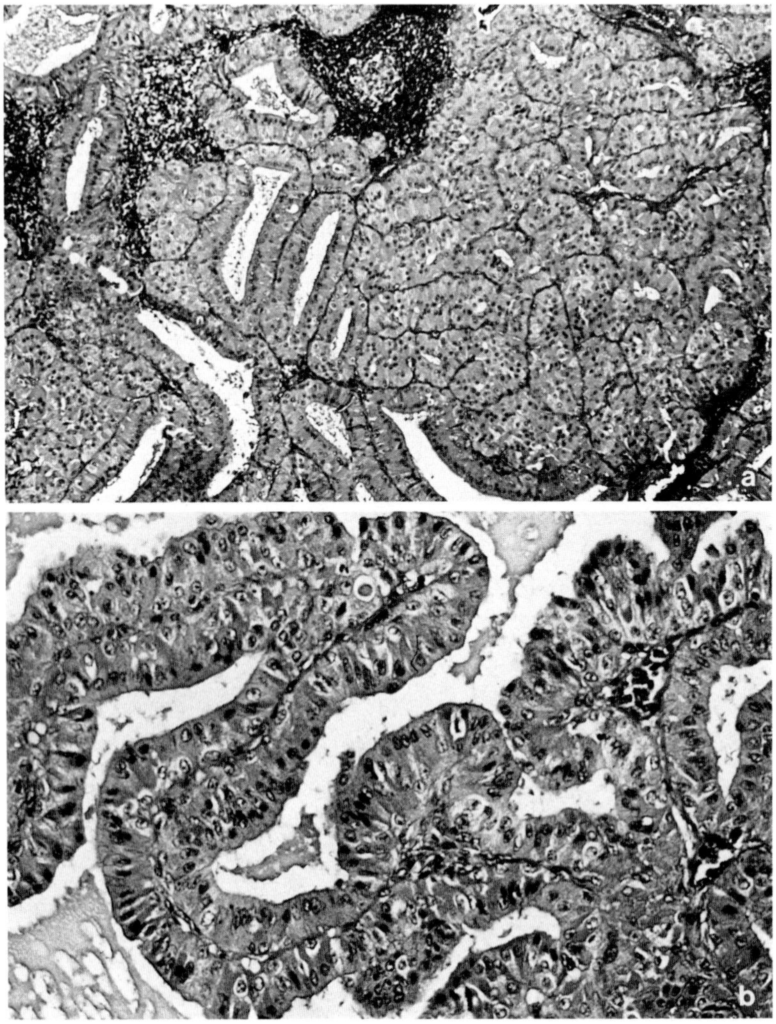

Figure 15.**42** Cystadenolymphoma subtype 2 consisting mainly of oncocytic cell cords and a scarce lymphoid stroma. H & E. **a** 63×, **b** 160×. (Seifert et al 1980.)

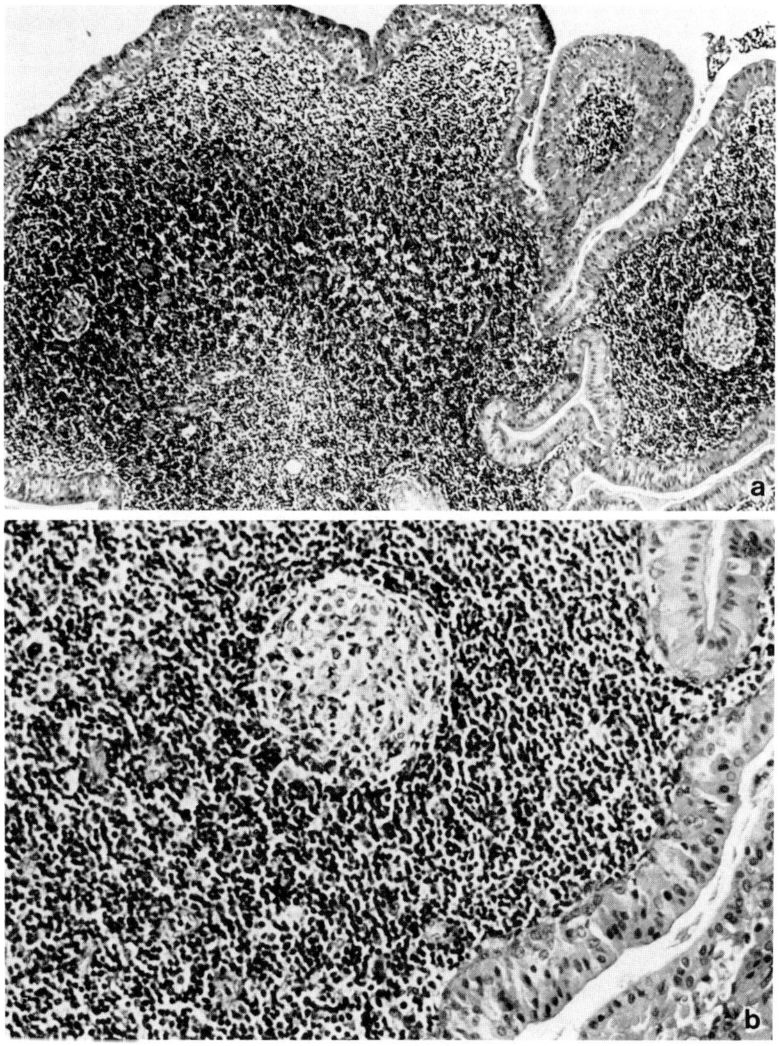

Figure 15.**43** Subtype 3 of cystadenolymphoma consisting mainly of lymphoid stroma with lymphoid follicles. H & E. **a** 63×, **b** 160×. (Seifert et al 1980.)

the main components of the lymphoid stroma include small (69%) and medium-to-large lymphocytes (19%). Further components in decreasing order of frequency include fibroblasts (5%), macrophages (3%), plasma cells (2%), blast-forming B lymphocytes (2.5%), and T lymphocytes (0.5%). Of the B lymphocytes, 48.5% contain IgG, 38% IgA, 9% IgM, 3.5% IgD, and 0.5% IgE (Korsrud & Brandtzaeg 1984). A polyclonal distribution pattern of light chains is present. Mast cells contain IgE (Caselitz et al 1984a).
A further subclassification of the lymphoid stroma may be achieved by monoclonal antibodies (Caselitz et al 1984b). B lymphocytes are mainly localized in the lymphoid follicles and between the oncocytic tumor cells. T helper cells are three times more common than T suppressor cells in the T lymphocytes, but T killer cells or Langerhans' cells are uncommon. The distribution pattern of lymphocytes resembles that of a lymph node and supports the hypothesis that cystadenolymphomas arise by inclusion of salivary parenchyma within a lymph node. The marker pattern of the epithelial tumor components, such as demonstration of IgA, secretory components, lactoferrin, CEA etc. resembles that of a striated duct (Korsrud & Brandtzaeg 1984; see also page 183).

Changes of the Lymphoid Stroma. The lymphoid stroma reacts like a regional lymph node because of its architecture. This includes the formation of a granuloma consisting of foreign body giant cells, macrophages, foam cells, histiocytes, and cholesterol or mucus particles (Fig. 15.**46a, b**). The cellular composition of this granuloma indicates that the mucous granuloma resembles the extravasation mucocele or the resorptive granuloma after previous surgery or radiation. The pigment deposits in the macrophages are mainly lysosomal breakdown products of mitochondria of the oncocytic cells (Buchner & David 1977). The granuloma may be confused with true tuber-

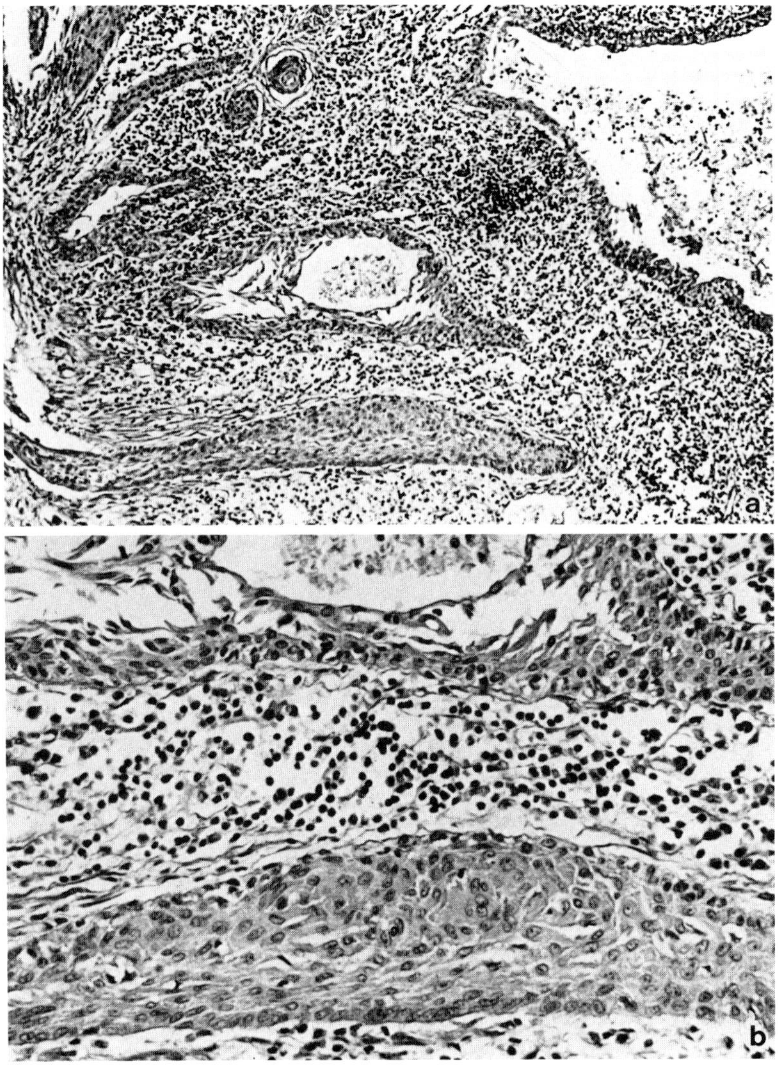

Figure 15.**44** Cystadenolymphoma subtype 4 showing squamous cell metaplasia of the oncocytic epithelium. H & E. **a** 63×, **b** 160×. (Seifert et al 1980.)

culosis because of its tuberculoid pattern. Involvement of the lymphoid stroma by productive-exsudative miliary tuberculosis is possible (Fig. 15.**47a, b**), but is very rare (Bucciarelli 1969). Tumor metastases (Fig. 15.**48a, b**) or malignant lymphomas may occasionally be observed in the lymphoid stroma. These neoplastic lesions must be distinguished from second tumors in the tissue surrounding a cystadenolymphoma.

Electron Microscopy. The apical oncocytic cells show similar structural characteristics to the neoplastic oncocytes in other oncocytic tumors. These include permeation of the cytoplasm with mitochondria, which are characterized by long, densely layered cristae mitochondriales, giant mitochondria, and mitochondrial enzymes and lysosomes (Tandler 1966, Kim et al 1973, Brocheriou et al 1981). The basal, more pyramid-shaped cells occasionally contain crystalloids (Tandler & Shipkey 1964).

Malignant Transformation *(see pages 172 and 269)*. The development of secondary carcinoma in preexisting benign cystadenolymphoma is very rare (Seifert et al 1977, Fleischer et al 1980). The histologic types include adenocarcinoma (Nakashima et al 1983, Moosavi et al 1980), squamous carcinoma (Baker et al 1980, Damjanov et al 1983), or undifferentiated carcinoma. Some of these tumors may be radiation induced.

Concomitant Tumors (*see page 172*). Of cystadenolymphomas 7.5% are bilateral and 4% are multifocal. There is also a striking coincidence with other tumors, including pleomorphic adenomas (Astacio 1974), mucoepidermoid tumors (Gadient & Kalfayan 1975, Lumerman et al 1975), carcinoma (Assor 1974, Volmer 1982), or malignant lymphoma (Miller et al 1982). In our material, 3% of all cystadenolymphomas were associated with other tumors, including parotid carcinoma, basal cell carcinoma, malignant lym-

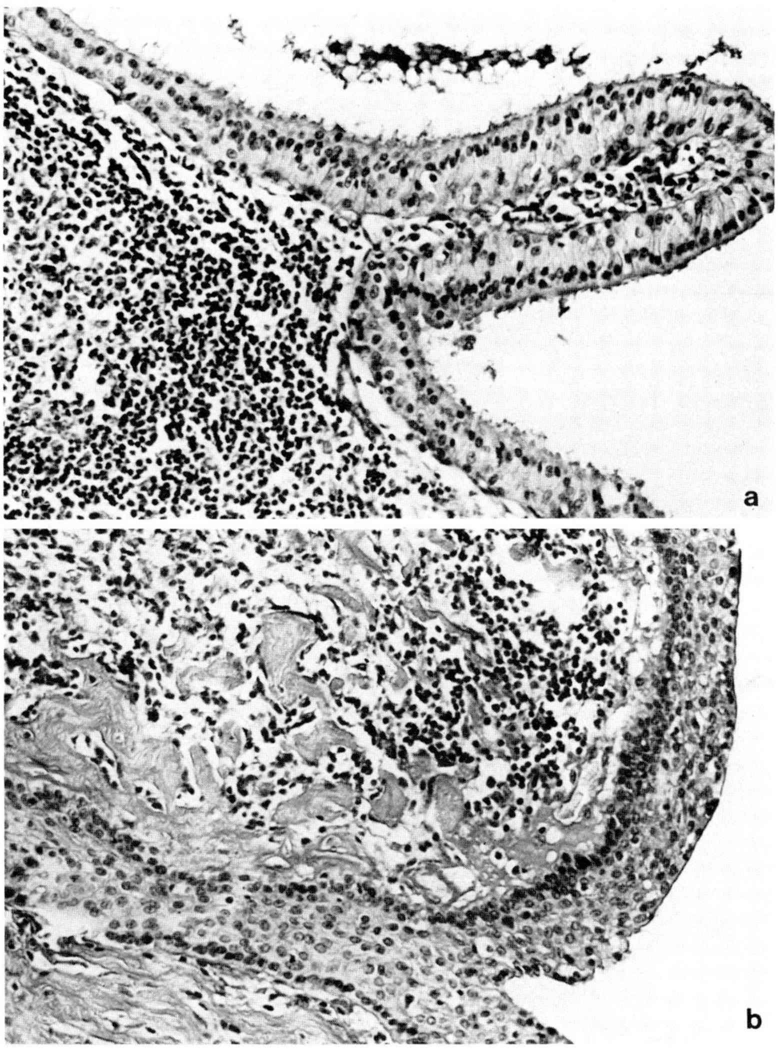

Figure 15.**45** Cystadenolymphoma subtype 4. **a** Rests of oncocytic epithelium. **b** Squamous metaplasia and hyaline stromal transformation. PAS. **a**, **b** 160×. (Seifert et al 1980.)

phoma, and carcinoma of the head and neck, including the larynx. In our experience, previous irradiation may be an etiologic factor.

Differential Diagnosis. Subtype 1 presents no difficulties in differential diagnosis. Subtype 2, which is poor in stroma, may be distinguished from an oncocytoma or an oncocytic cystic duct adenoma by the demonstration of the lymphoid stromal component of the cystadenolymphoma. The metaplastic subtype 4 must be distinguished from sebaceous adenoma (see later), from mucoepidermoid tumor, from squamous cell carcinoma, and from necrotizing sialometaplasia (Gnepp 1981). These may be confused, especially on aspiration cytology (Lindberg & Ackermann 1976, Zajicek et al 1976, Droese 1978). Nonneoplastic lesions that also must be distinguished include duct and lymphoepithelial cysts (pages 95 and 98) and chronic myoepithelial sialadenitis in Sjögren's syndrome (page 148ff) (Seifert et al 1980).

Pathogenesis. Numerous arguments support the view that cystadenolymphomas arise from parenchymatous inclusions in intra- or periglandular lymph nodes (Pape 1963, Kleinsasser et al 1966). Parenchymatous inclusions in the parotid lymph nodes are a common finding (see Chapters 2 and 3); the duct component persists longer and demonstrates oncocytic metaplasia with increasing age. The tumor usually lies in the lower pole of the parotid or in the neighboring lymph nodes, so that there is usually a tissue connection between the marginal gland tissue, the lymph nodes, and the cystadenolymphoma, which can be demonstrated by histologic examination. The bilateral occurrence (see also page 172) and the reaction pattern of the lymphoid stroma that resembles that of a lymph node also support this hypothesis.

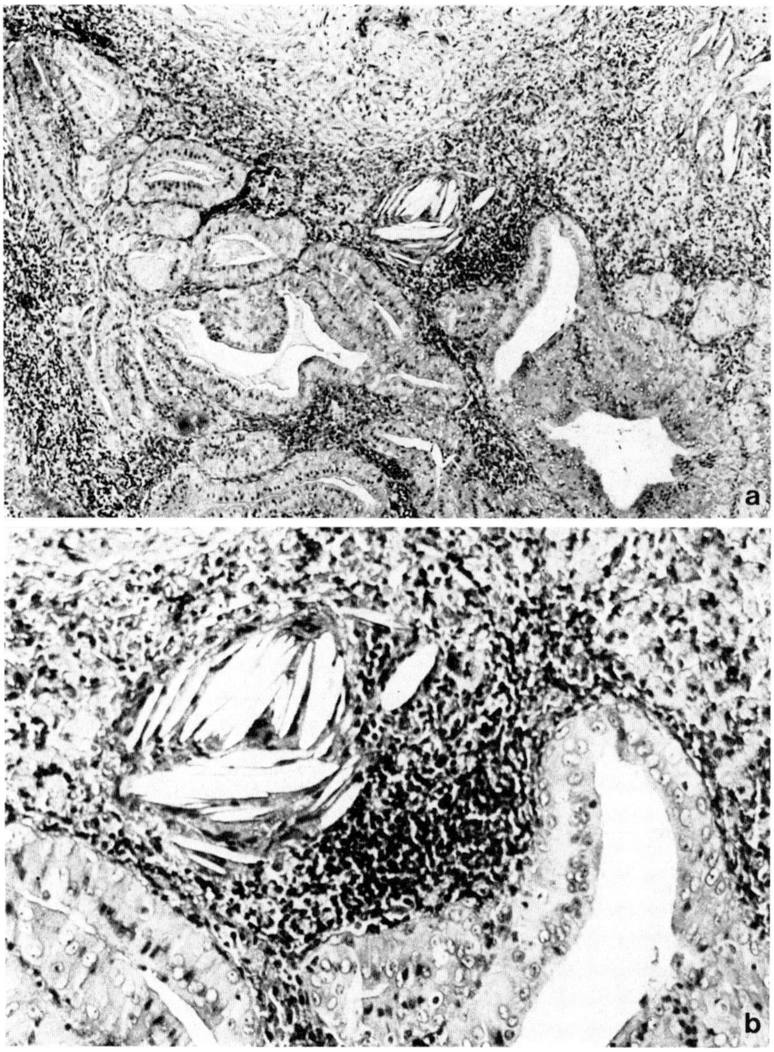

Figure 15.**46** Cystadenolymphoma showing giant cell granuloma with cholesterol crystals close to an oncocytic cell nest. H & E. **a** 160×, **b** 400× (Seifert et al 1980.)

The lymphoid stroma is dominated by the B lymphocyte (Cossman et al 1977, Hsu et al 1981, Howard et al 1982, Caselitz et al 1984b). Subtype 3, which is rich in stroma, possibly represents an early stage that may develop by epithelial proliferation of subtype 1 or 2. The frequent finding of mast cells in the epithelial-rich areas of the cystadenolymphoma is probably a feature of the proliferative activity of the tumor epithelium, since mast cells possess a mitogenic effect (Caselitz et al 1984a). The rare occurrence of cystadenolymphomas in the submandibular gland (Kurreja & Jain 1971, Glaeser 1979), the tonsil (Fahmy 1973), or the lower lip (Veronesi & Corbetta 1960) may be explained by the fact that the lymphoid tissue in these regions lies in close contact with the overlying epithelium. The neoplastic potential of the oncocytic proliferation may also be demonstrated by the presence of CEA in the proliferation foci (Korsrud & Brandtzaeg 1979). The oncocytic cells show a positive keratin reaction, whereas the stromal cells show a positive vimentin reaction (Caselitz et al 1982). The hypothesis (Allegra 1971) that cystadenolymphoma represents an immune disease of delayed cellular type, similar to Hashimoto's lymphocytic thyroiditis, and that the lymphoid stromal cells represent an immunologic reaction to the oncocytic cell proliferation is not supported by the evidence available to date.

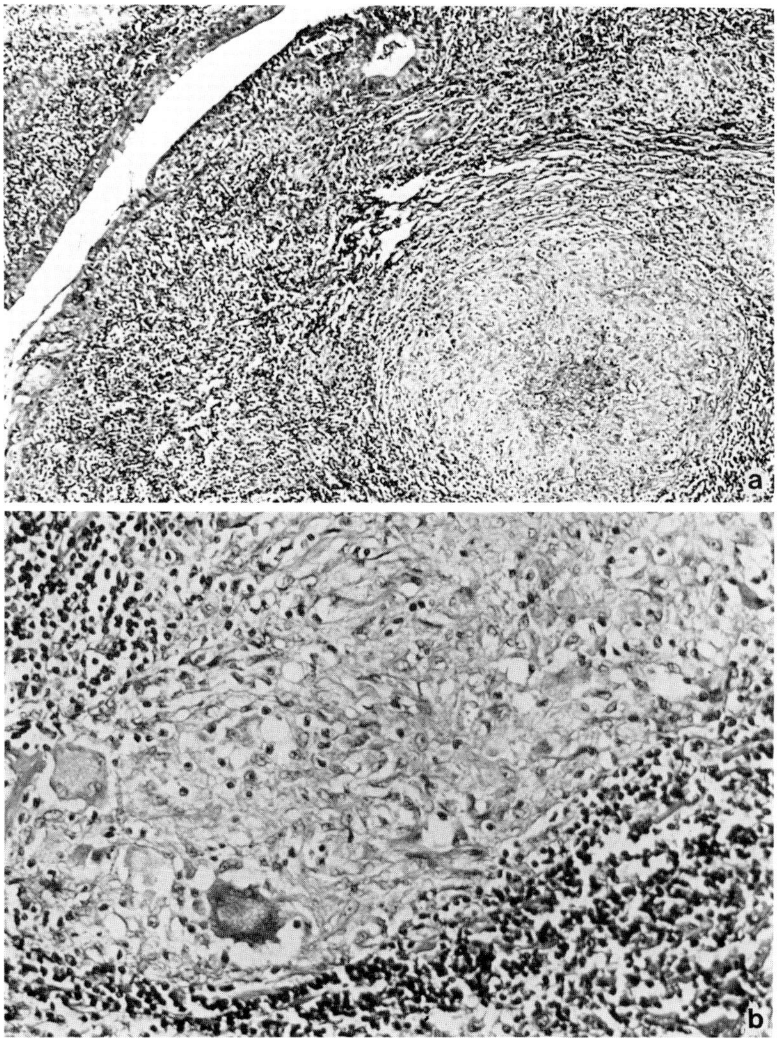

Figure 15.**47** Cystadenolymphoma showing a tuberculous granuloma in the lymphoid stroma with Langhans' giant cells and epithelioid cells. H & E. **a** 63×, **b** 160×.

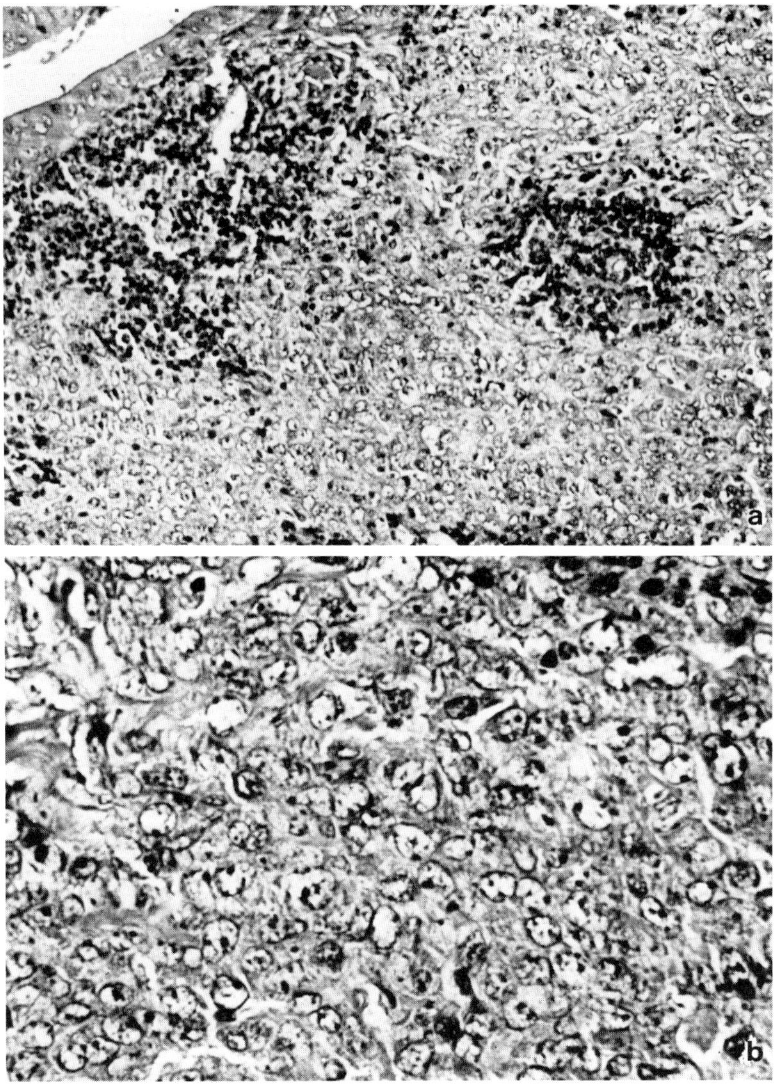

Figure 15.**48** Cystadenolymphoma showing a metastasis of an undifferentiated carcinoma in the lymphoid stroma. H & E. **a** 160×, **b** 400×.

Duct Adenoma

Duct adenomas are the most frequent monomorphic adenomas after the cystadenolymphomas, constituting almost 20% of all monomorphic adenomas (Table 15.**6**). If basal cell adenomas are included, this figure increase to 25%.

Site. More than 70% of duct adenomas arise in the parotid gland, the remainder in the minor glands (Levine et al 1981), in particular those of the upper lip (Seifert & Schultz 1979). Rarer sites are the buccal mucosa and palate. A few cases have been reported in the lower lip, the floor of the mouth (Seifert et al 1980, Mintz et al 1982), and the submandibular gland (Mintz et al 1982).

Table 15.**6** Classification of Monomorphic Salivary Adenomas in the Salivary Gland Register (1965–1982) in 549 Patients

Type of Tumor	No.	%
Cystadenolymphoma	400	72.5
Duct adenoma	106	19.0
Basal cell adenoma	24	4.5
Oncocytoma	10	2.0
Sebaceous adenoma	3	0.5
Other adenomas	6	1.5
Total	549	100.0

Macroscopic Appearances. This tumor is on average 1–1.5 cm in size and is separated from the gland parenchyma by a fibrous capsule (Fig. 15.**49**). The peak·age incidence is in the seventh decade, and 65% of these tumors occur in women.

Histopathology. Three forms of duct adenoma may be distinguished, depending on the predominant architecture (Seifert & Schultz 1979, Crumpler et al 1976, Nelson & Jacoway 1973, Mintz et al 1982).

The *trabecular duct adenoma* consists of cords of three or four layers (Fig. 15.**50a, b**). Basal cells lie on the external surface in a polar orientation and are clearly demarcated from the surrounding stroma by a basal membrane. Less differentiated intermediate duct epithelium lies within the cell cord and it may be termed "transformation cells." A sparse stroma is developed between the epithelial cords, but it does not have a mucoid component as it does in pleomorphic adenoma.

The *tubular duct adenoma* imitates the pattern of salivary ducts and has a duct lumen (Fig. 15.**51a, b**). The luminal cell layer consists of narrow, darkly stained duct epithelium whose architecture

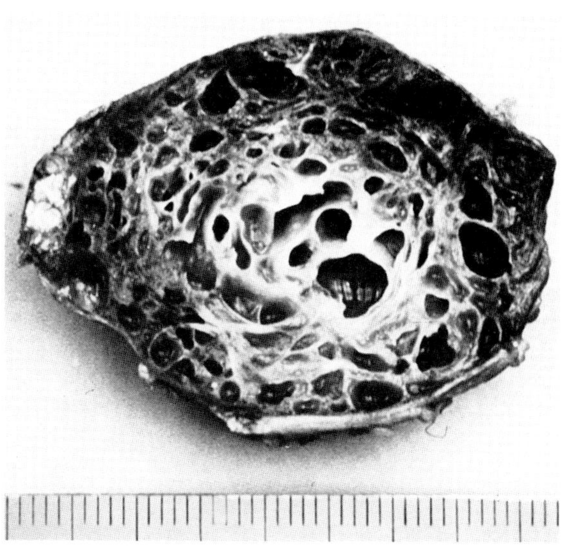

Figure 15.**49** Cystic duct adenoma of the parotid gland showing multiple cysts on the cut surface.

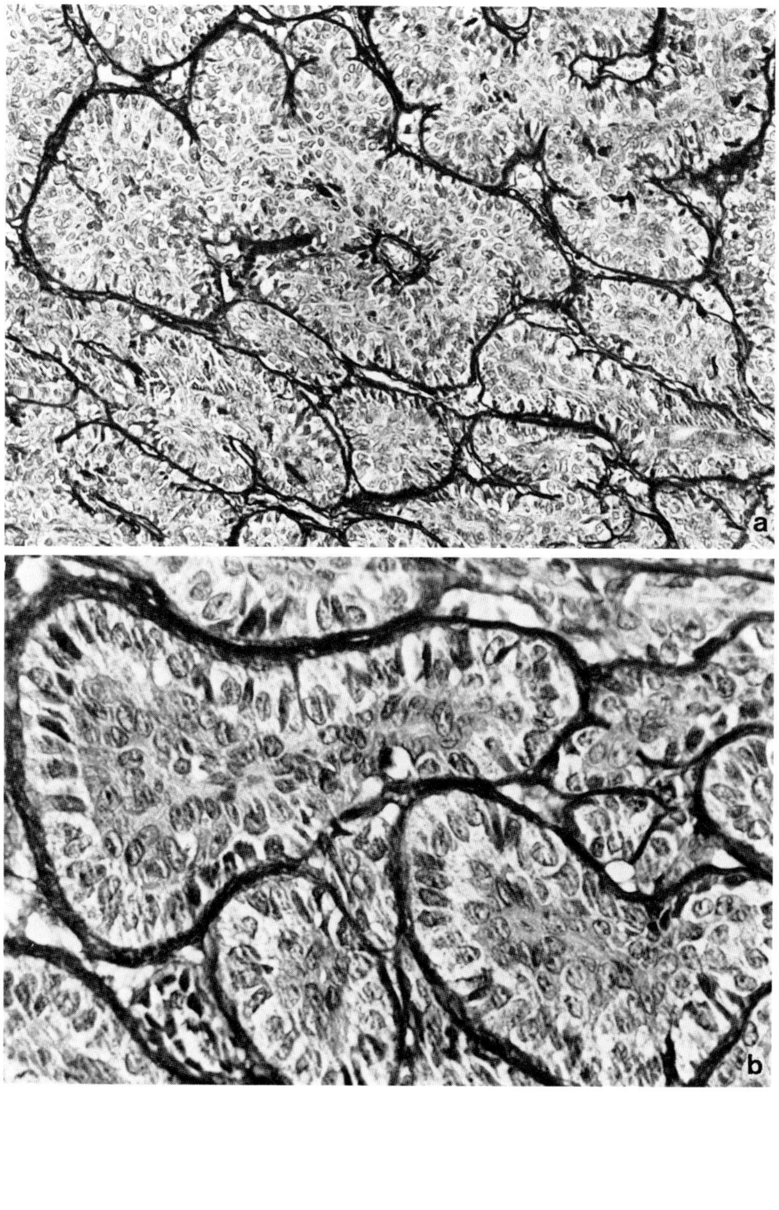

Figure 15.**50** Trabecular type of duct adenoma: **a** PAS-positive material on the external surface of the duct epithelial units. **b** Structure of the trabeculae consisting of polar-arranged basal cells and intermediate duct cells on the inside. PAS. **a** 160×, **b** 400×. (Seifert et al 1979.)

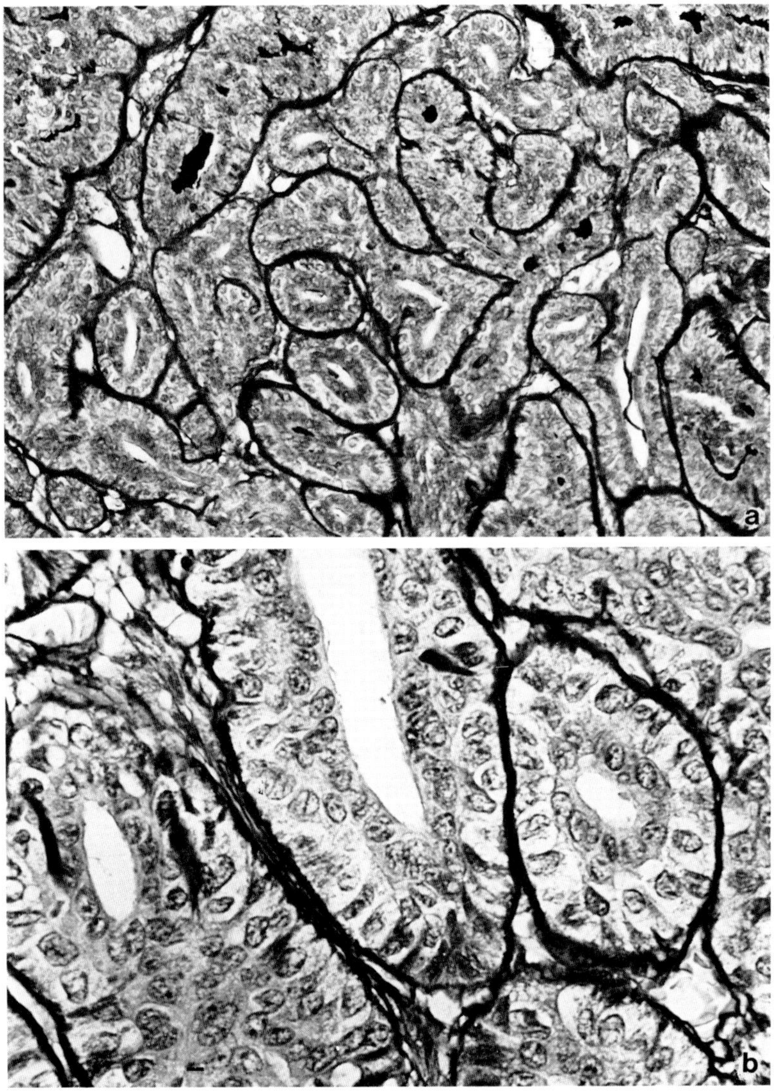

Figure 15.**51** Tubular type of duct adenoma: duct lumen bounded by dark epithelial cells, an external layer of basal reserve cells, and clear cytoplasm. PAS. **a** 160×, **b** 400×. (Seifert et al 1979.)

is similar to that of the intercalated duct epithelium. On the outer surface lie cells with a broader cytoplasm that is modestly transluscent. PAS-positive secretion is found in the duct lumen. The ductlike epithelial structures are limited externally by a basal membrane. The stroma is sparsely developed and demonstrated occasional hyaline transformation.

The *cystic duct adenoma* may be solitary or multiple (Fig. 15.**52a, b**). PAS-positive secretion is found in the cyst lumen, which may sometimes contain crystalline secretory particles in the form of spheroliths or microliths. In degenerative tumors, the cysts also contain desquamated epithelium, blood, or resorptive cell collections with inclusion of foam cells and macrophages. The epithelium of the cyst wall is arranged in two or more layers consisting of the same cell types as the trabecular and duct adenomas. Occasionally, oncocytic differentiation may be found similar to the architecture of the intercalated duct. Fingerlike or papilliferous protrusions of papillary structures into the cyst lumen may be found at some points. The connective tissue stroma between the epithelial structures occasionally shows degenerative changes with focal collections of lymphocytes.

The *cell types* of duct adenoma imitate various cell forms of the duct system, including oncocytic cell forms (Fig. 15.**53**) similar to the striated ducts, small dark cells, similar to the intercalated ducts, and basal reserve cells bounded externally by a PAS-positive basal membrane. The transformation cells especially in the trabecular formations resemble cell forms that occur in the embryonal development of the salivary ducts (see Chapter 3).

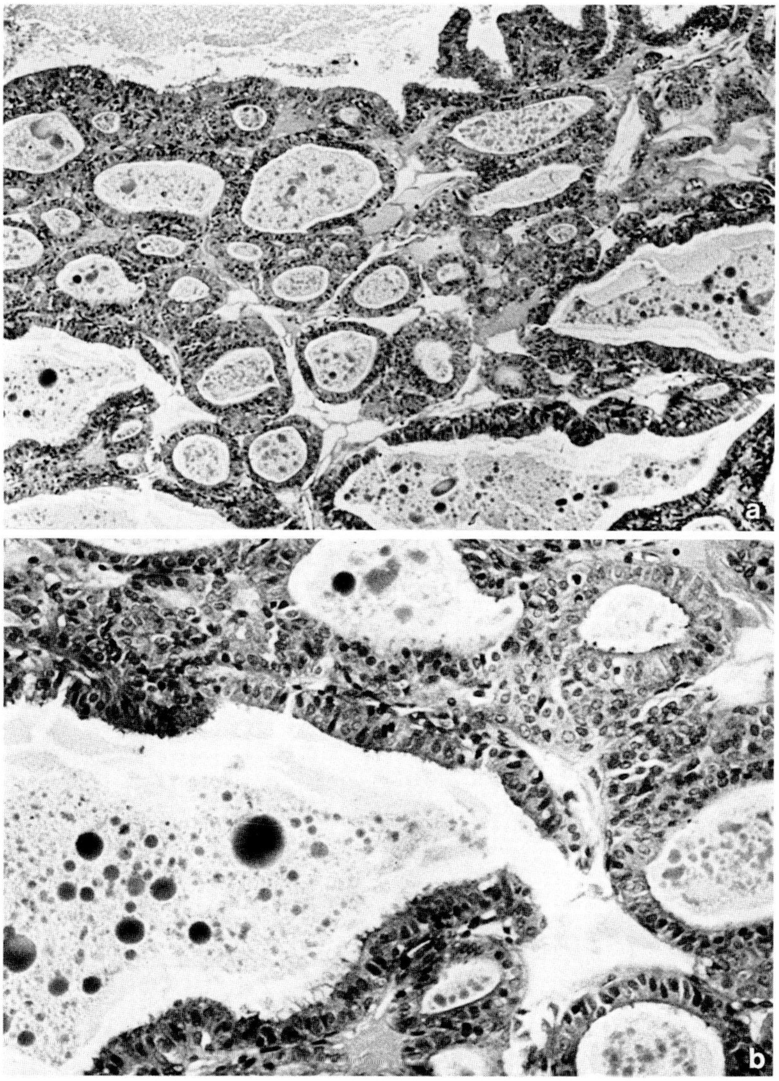

Figure 15.**52** Cystic type of duct adenoma: cysts bounded by multilayered ductal epithelium with secretory particles in the lumen. Giemsa. **a** 63×, **b** 160×.

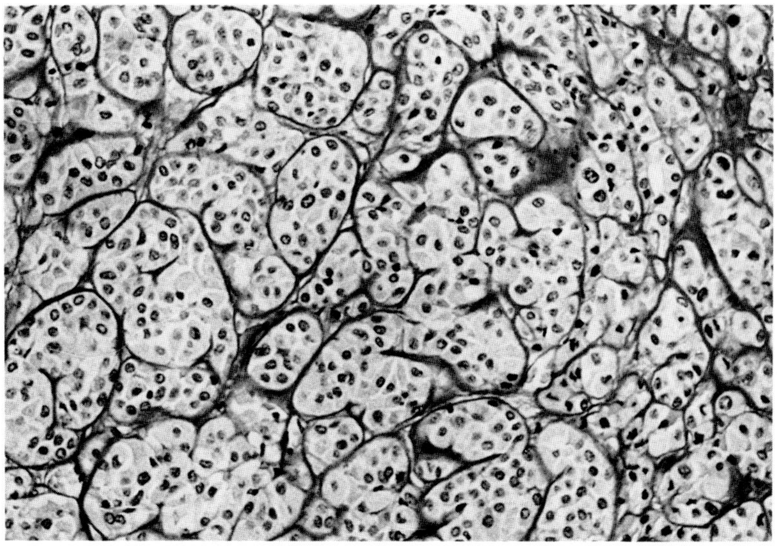

Figure 15.**53** Duct adenoma showing trabecular cell cords of oncocytic cells. PAS, 160×.

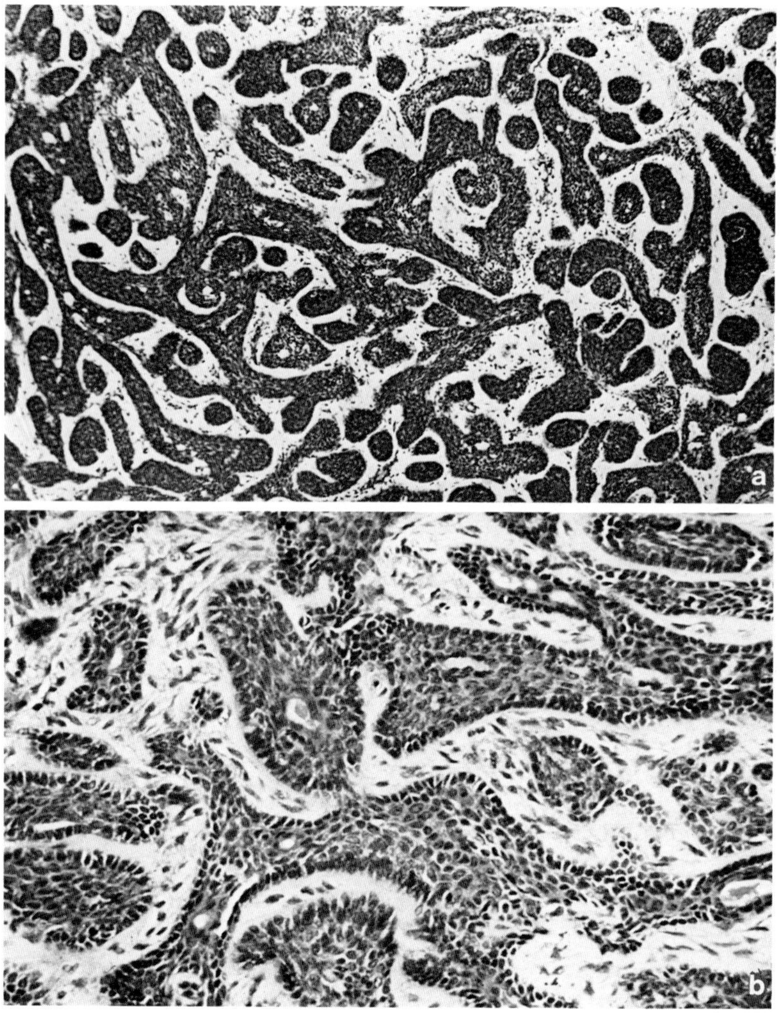

Figure 15.**54** Basal cell adenoma of the parotid gland: **a** Solid and trabecular cell cords. **b** Clear demarcation from the connective tissue. H & E. **a** 63×, **b** 130×.

The cytologic pattern of duct adenoma does not include squamous metaplasia or mucus-forming goblet cells.

Pathogenesis. The different architecture of the individual segments of the duct system, that is, intercalated and striated ducts and intra- and interlobular ducts, are reproduced in duct adenomas, as in the embryonal development of the duct system. Trabecular duct formations resemble the stage of development reached in the 12th embryonal week, whereas tubular structures with a lumen correspond to a later period of development. The ductal epithelium may differentiate into trabecular, tubular, and cystic structures. These include basal reserve cells, intermediate or transformation cells, intercalated and striated duct epithelium, primitive duct epithelium, and clear cell forms (Seifert & Donath 1978, see Chapter 2). The differences of differentiation between the parotid gland and the minor glands result from the different structure of the ducts in the individual glands. Trabecular, tubular, or cystic epithelial units can occur within the same tumor. If basal cells predominate, the tumor is termed a "basal cell adenoma," but in our opinion this is a particular form of duct adenoma that will be discussed separately because of its relative frequency.

Differential Diagnosis. In differential diagnosis, it is particularly important to distinguish *pleomorphic adenomas with scanty stroma (type 4).* Pleomorphic adenomas with scanty stroma are always characterized by areas that possess a mucoid or hyalin stroma with an ill-defined boundary to the epithelial tumor component. In addition, the stroma of pleomorphic adenomas contains a spindle-shaped cell type that is absent from the stroma of monomorphic adenomas. The practical importance of distinguishing these tumors is that the pleomorphic adenoma, especially subtype 4, has a greater tendency to recur and to undergo malignant transformation, a prop-

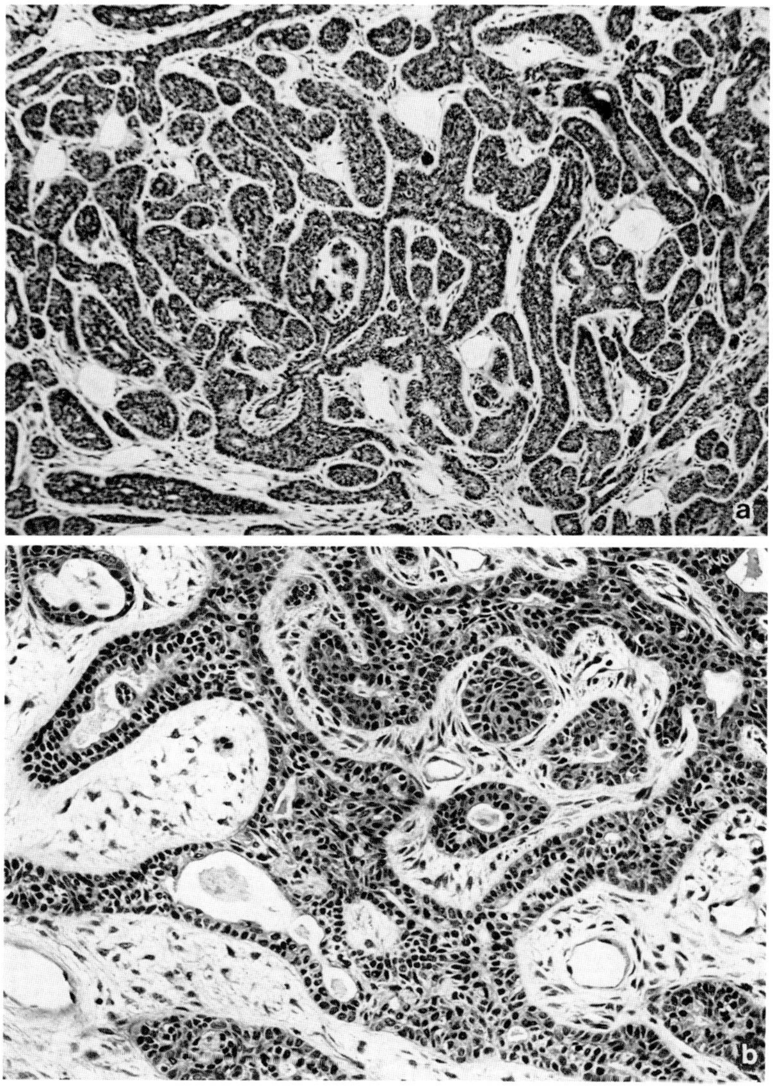

Figure 15.**55** Basal cell adenoma of the parotid gland. **a** Basal cell cords clearly defined from the stroma with no mucoid stromal transformation as in pleomorphic adenoma. **b** Local formation of narrow duct lumen. H & E. **a** 63×, **b** 160×.

erty that has so far not been claimed for monomorphic adenoma. *Cystadenomas* (Harrison 1974), which affect the minor salivary glands particularly, should be included with the cystic duct adenomas, since they demonstrate no difference in prognosis or treatment. Duct tumors with predominant *papillary differentiation* may also be termed *sialadenoma papilliferum* (Abrams & Finck 1969, Freedman & Lumerman 1978, Drummond et al 1978, Nasu et al 1981, Shirasuna et al 1984), *intraductal papilloma* (Abbey 1975), or *inverted ductal papilloma* (White et al 1982). These are all variations of differentiation of the duct system. The differential diagnosis of other monomorphic adenomas will be discussed later.

Basal Cell Adenoma

Of basal cell adenomas, 70% arise in the parotid gland (Kleinsasser & Klein 1967, Strauss et al 1981). Minor salivary gland tumors mainly affect the upper lip (Fantasia & Neville 1980). The peak age incidence lies in the seventh decade.

Histopathology. The tumors are formed of uniformly differentiated basal cells forming solid trabecular structures (Fig. 15.**54a, b**) and occasional tubular (Figure 15.**55a, b**) or cystic structures. About 60% of all basal cell adenomas demonstrate solid trabecular structures and more than 30%, tubular formations (Nagao et al 1982). On the other hand, papillary epithelial structures are rare. The following characteristics are typical (Fig. 15.**56a, b**): clear separation of the tumor cells from the stroma by a PAS-positive basal membrane, a pallisade polar arrangement of the

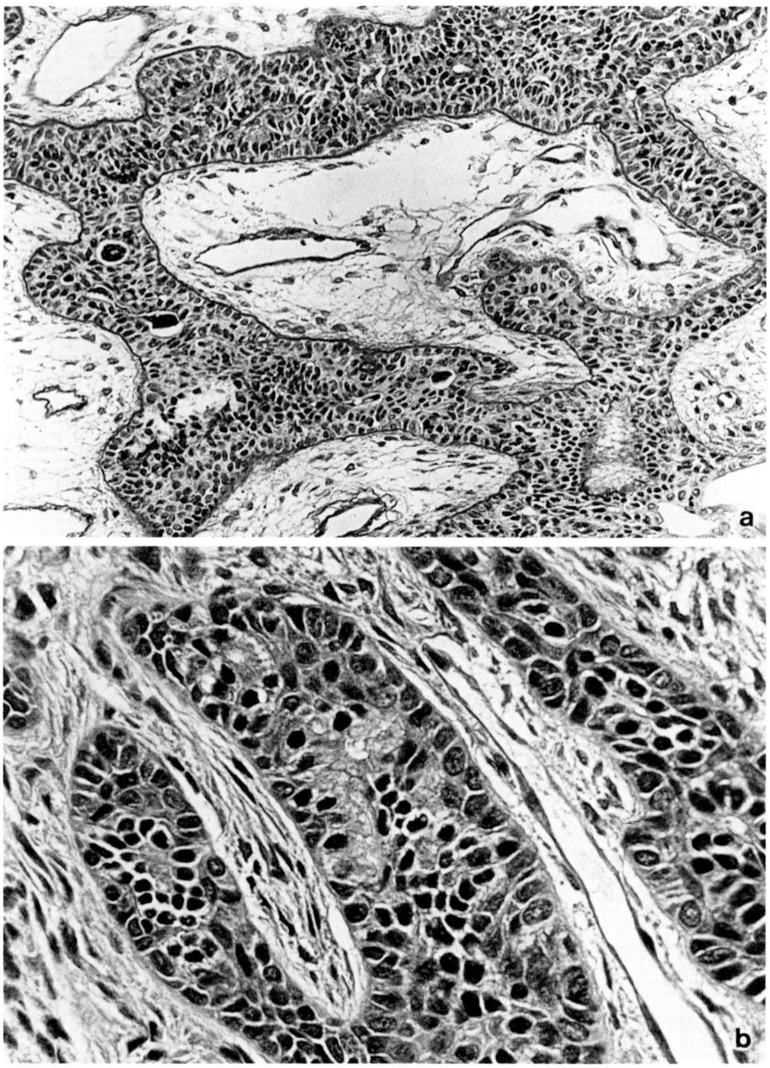

Figure 15.**56** Basal cell adenoma of the parotid gland. **a** Individual duct lumen with PAS-positive secretion. PAS, 160×. **b** Polar arrangements of basal cells on the external surface with a network arrangement of internal cells. H & E, 400×.

peripheral cell layer, and anchoring to the basement membrane by desmosomes (Hübner et al 1971). Mucous stromal transformation is absent. The stroma may be highly vascularized (Bernacki et al 1974) and occasionally contain rich elastic fibers (Nagao et al 1982).

Electron Microscopy. A multilayered basal membrane envelops the basal cells. Desmosomes and cytoplasmic interdigitations are developed between the cells. Glandlike lumens with microvilli are developed at some points. Other cells resemble the architecture of intermediate prickle cells that contain tonofilaments in the cytoplasm (Nagao et al 1982). More highly differentiated epithelium, secretory granules, and microfilaments have been described also (Jao et al 1976). Opinions differ about the presence or absence of myoepithelial cells (Nagao et al 1982, Hübner et al 1971).

Pathogenesis. The cell forms of the basal cell adenoma also occur in the duct adenoma. The terms previously used for basal cell adenoma, such as "trabecular adenoma," "canalicular adenoma," "basiloma," and "tubular-solid adenoma," testify to its similarity to duct adenoma. Kleinsasser (1969) points out that one stage of the embryonic development of the parotid gland is repeated in the basal cell adenoma. Segmental differentiation similar to that of a basal cell adenoma is found in numerous duct adenomas (Chaudhry et al 1983). It is therefore reasonable to regard basal cell adenoma as being merely a variant of a duct adenoma. Only those tumors showing the basal cell characteristics throughout the tumor should be classified as basal cell adenomas, whereas tumors of partial basal cell type should be classified as duct adenomas (Seifert & Schultz 1979). If the hyaline basal membrane is pronounced, comparisons may also be drawn with the tumors of skin appendages (Headington et al 1977, Batsakis & Brannon 1981, Reingold et al 1977). Multifocal basal cell adenomas of the dermal type are occasionally accompanied by dermal cylindromas and indicate a possible predisposition (Herbst & Hutz 1984).

Oncocytoma

Oncocytoma is a typical but very rare salivary tumor, forming only 2% of monomorphic adenomas (Table 15.**6**). Fewer than 0.5% of epithelial salivary tumors are oncocytomas. Numerous reports have appeared since the original description by Hamperl (1931) (Askew et al 1971, Balogh & Roth 1965, Blanck et al 1970, Carlsöö et al 1979, Gray et al 1976, Gruenfeld & Jorstad 1976, Hamperl 1937 & 1962, Hastrup et al 1982, Hübner et al 1967, Meza-Chávez 1949, Tandler et al 1970). Characteristically, the oncocytoma occurs in women in the seventh to eighth decades, almost always arises in the parotid gland, is usually benign, and grows slowly.

Macroscopic Appearances. The oncocytoma has an average size of 3–4 cm, is clearly encapsulated, and has a brownish, lobular, cut surface (Fig. 15.**57**). Oncocytomas are almost always solitary, although focal oncocytic hyperplasia may be observed outside the tumor capsule.

Histology. The oncocytes form solid and trabecular structures and, more rarely, microcysts (Fig. 15.**58**). The ductlike structures contain PAS-positive secretion. The individual oncocytes possess a swollen granular acidophillic cytoplasm with dis-

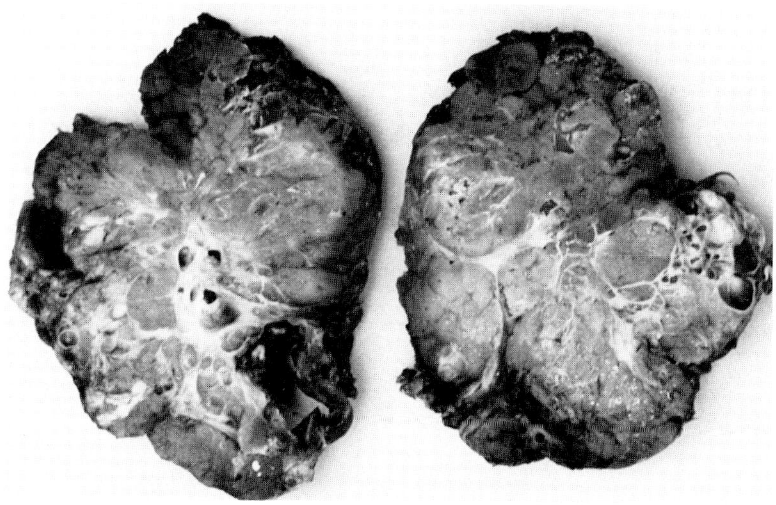

Figure 15.**57** Oncocytoma of the parotid gland with a lobular cut surface with a few septa.

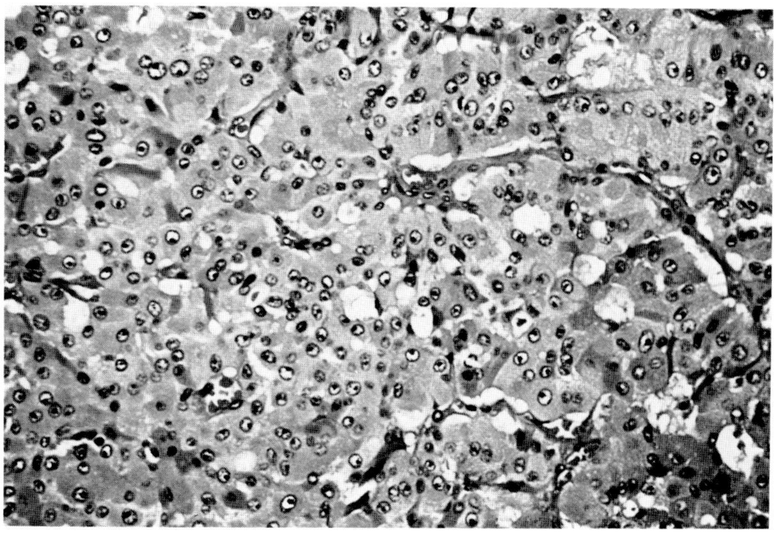

Figure 15.**58** Oncocytoma of the parotid gland with solid and trabecular cell cords with granular cytoplasm. H & E, 250×.

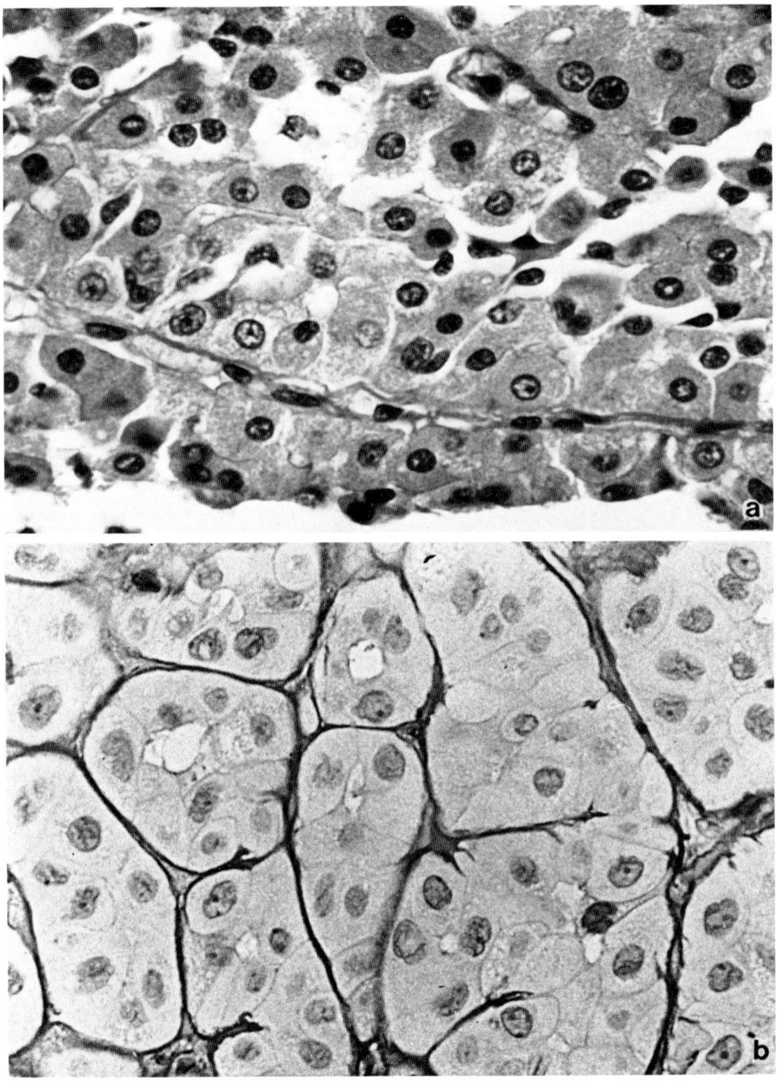

Figure 15.**59** Oncocytoma of the parotid gland. **a** Typical oncocytic cell masses with granular cytoplasm. H & E, 400×. **b** Semithin sections: swollen cytoplasm with clear cell boundaries. An external PAS-positive basement membrane. PAS, 400×.

tinct cell boundaries (Fig. 15.**59a, b**). The nuclei are small and somewhat pyknotic. Clear cell oncocytes are also found occasionally (Becker et al 1982). Degenerative changes with hyaline transformation and occasional lymphocytic infiltration are sometimes found in the stroma, but a well-developed lymphoid stromal component, as is typical of a cystadenolymphoma, is absent. Septa are present within the walls of large oncocytomas. The surrounding gland tissue shows a focal obstructive sialadenitis with duct dilation, retention of secretion, and periductal lymphocytic infiltration, and occasionally also focal adenomatous oncocytic hyperplasia (see also page 109).

Electron Microscopy. The tumor cells contain numerous mitochondria with prolonged cristae mitochondriales and a partially lamellar internal structure (Fig. 15.**60a, b**). The mitochondria show marked variation in size, including giant mitochondria, and also a form with a discuslike structure or fusion of mitochondria (Tandler et al 1970, Seifert & Donath 1976). Glycogen deposits are also found occasionally. Enzyme histochemistry shows that the tumor cells contain oxidative and hydrolytic mitochondrial enzymes, in particular phosphatases and esterases.

Pathogenesis. The oncocytoma derives from the duct system, particularly the striated duct. The relationship between oncocytomas, cystadenomas, and duct adenomas finds expression in the fact that an oncocytic cell differentiation dominates in oncocytomas and cystadenolymphomas, but is also present focally in duct adenomas. All oncocytic types of salivary tumors are more common in the older age groups. The common origin from the duct system expresses

Figure 15.**60** Oncocytoma of the parotid gland. **a** Electron microscopic section of a tumor cell with numerous mitochondria (M). K = cell nucleus. **b** Giant mitochondria with lamellar internal structure. **a** 7200×, **b** 19 800× (Seifert & Donath 1976.)

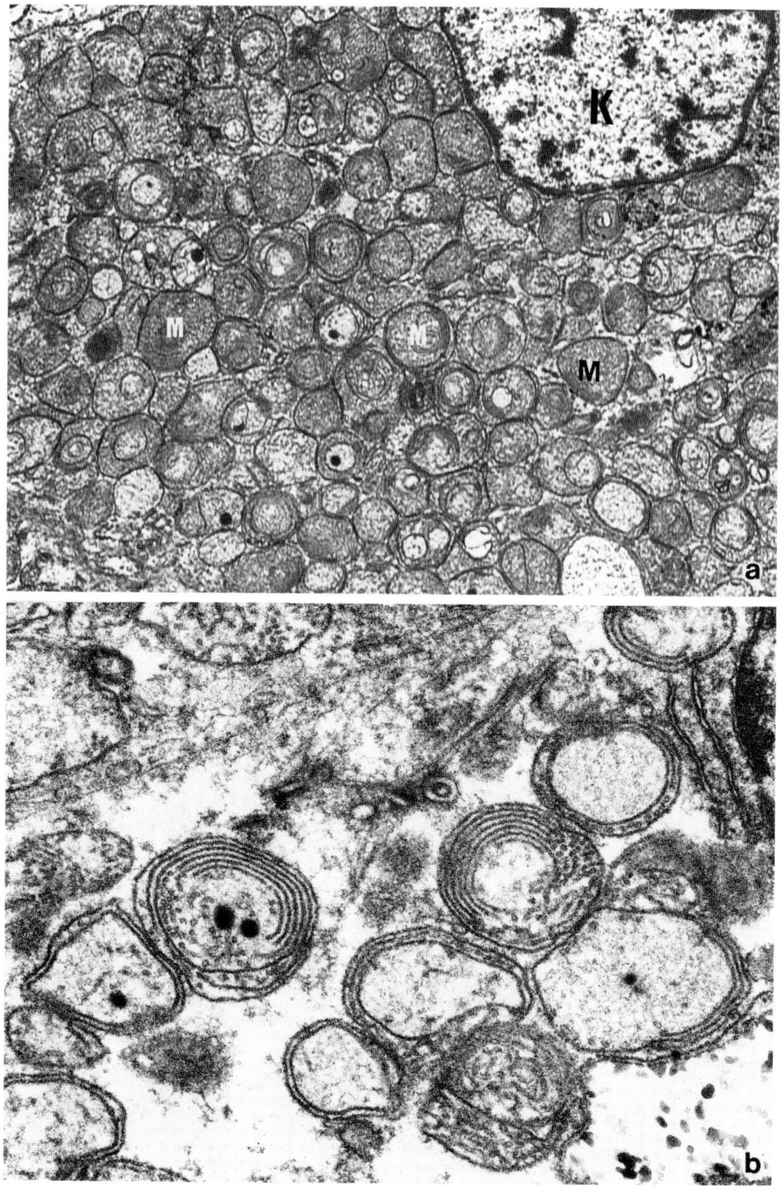

itself in the ultrastructural and enzyme histochemical characteristics of the tumor cells.

Oncocytic differentiation can also occur in other salivary tumors, such as pleomorphic adenoma and adenocarcinoma (Seifert et al 1980, Seifert & Schultz 1979). A few cases of malignant metastasizing oncocytoma have been described (Mair & Johannessen 1972, Seifert & Donath 1976).

Sebaceous Adenoma

Sebaceous adenomas are rare, constituting 0.5% of all monomorphic adenomas. Like the cystadenolymphoma, they lie almost exclusively in the parotid gland (Schmid & Albrich 1973, Baratz et al 1976, Kleinsasser 1964, Wuketich & Kittinger 1966, Assor 1970, Wasan 1971, Fleming & Morrice 1973, Kunze 1979, Cameron & Stenram 1979, Gnepp & Sporck 1980), but they may occur very rarely in the submandibular or minor salivary glands (Gnepp & Brannon 1984).

Histology. The architecture of the sebaceous adenoma resembles that of a cystadenolymphoma. The sebaceous cells form solid acinar and ductlike structures surrounded by a lymphoid stroma (Figs. 15.**61**–15.**63**). The tumor cells can be distinguished from oncocytes by a Sudan-positive fat deposit in the cytoplasm, almost complete absence of mitochondria, and a content of lipid drops and desmosomes demonstrated by electron

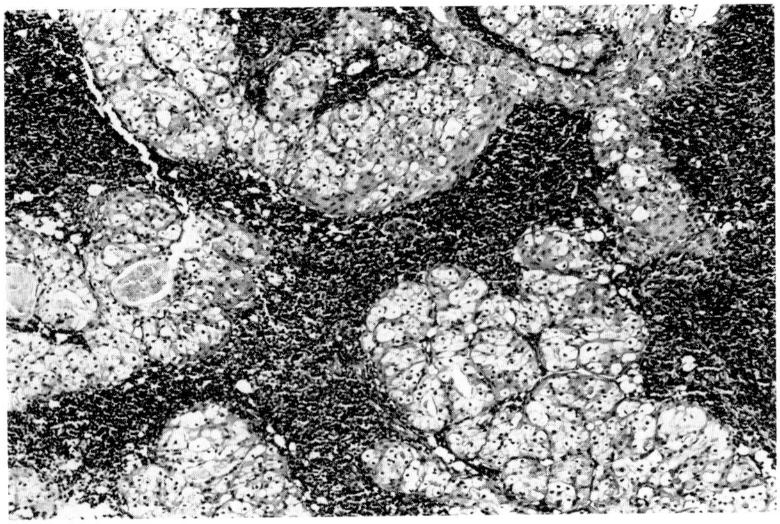

Figure 15.**61** Sebaceous adenoma of the parotid gland showing acinar clear cell nests in a lymphoid stroma. H & E, 63×.

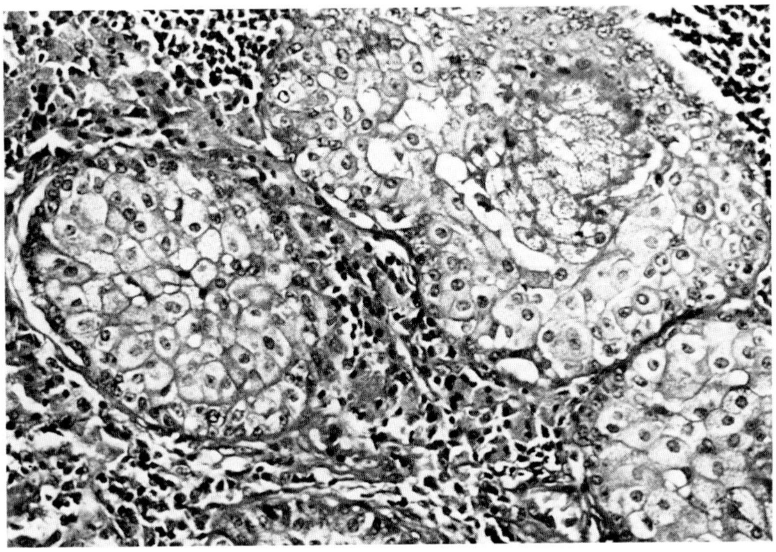

Figure 15.**62** Sebaceous cell adenoma of the parotid gland: clumps of cells with honeycombed cytoplasm. H & E, 160×.

microscopy (Tschen & McGavran 1979). Occasional squamous metaplasia can cause confusion with metaplastic cystadenolymphoma.

Pathogenesis. Like the cystadenolymphoma, the sebaceous adenoma may derive from parenchymatous inclusions in the parotid lymph nodes. The presence of sebaceous metaplasia has already been mentioned (page 106). Sebaceous foci can also occur in other tumors, such as pleomorphic adenoma and mucoepidermoid tumor. Sebaceous carcinomas are very rare (Seifert & Donath 1976, Silver & Goldstein 1966, Kleinsasser et al 1970, Zechner & Albegger 1973, Shulman et al 1973, Akhtar et al 1973). Lipid droplets in the cytoplasm, desmosomes, and microvilli are characteristics of this tumor, but tonofilaments are absent (page 270).

Clear Cell Adenoma

Numerous terms have been used to describe the rare clear cell adenoma, including hypernephroid adenoma, parathyroid-like adenoma, glycogen-rich adenoma, and myoepithelial adenoma. This multiplicity of terms demonstrates that the cytologic classification of this tumor is controversial (Seifert & Donath 1978, Batsakis 1980b). The tumor mainly arises in the parotid gland (Papache et al 1982), but also from the minor glands, particularly those of the palate (Goldman & Klein 1972, Saksela et al 1972, Kahn & Schoub 1973, Luna et al 1973, Stromeyer et al 1975, Sciubba & Goldstein 1976, Seifert & Schulz 1979, Chaudhry et al 1982, 1983a).

Histology. The architecture resembles that of trabecular duct adenoma. The tumor cells form

Bucciarelli, E.: Adenolinfoma e tuberculosi cliciamente primitiva della parotide. Lav. Anat. Patol. Perugia 29 (1969) 139
Buchner, A., R. David: Pigmented cells in adenolymphoma (Warthin's tumor). J. oral Pathol. 6 (1977) 106
Cameron, W. R., U. Stenram: Adenoma of parotid gland with sebaceous and oncocytic features. Cancer (Philad.) 43 (1979) 1429
Carlsöö, B., S. Domeij, H. F. Helander: A quantitative ultrastructural study of a parotid oncocytoma. Arch. Path. Lab. Med. 103 (1979) 471
Caselitz, J., M. Osborn, J. Wustrow, G. Seifert, K. Weber: The expression of different intermediate-sized filaments in human salivary glands and their tumours. Path. Res. Pract. 175 (1982) 266
Caselitz, J., A. Salfelder, G. Seifert: Adenolymphoma: An immunohistochemical study with monoclonal antibodies against lymphocyte antigens. J. oral Pathol. 13 (1984b) 438
Caselitz, J., A. Salfelder, G. Seifert: Mast cells in cystadenolymphomas, Klin. Wschr. 62 (1984a) 284
Chaudhry, A. P., S. Satchidanand, R. Peer, L. S. Cutler: Myoepithelial cell adenoma of the parotid gland. Cancer (Philad.) 49 (1982) 288
Chaudhry, A. P., L. S. Cutler, S. Satchidanand, G. Labay, M. Sunder Raj, Ch.-Ch. Lin: Glycogen-rich tumor of the oral minor salivary glands. A histochemical and ultrastructural study. Cancer (Philad.) 52 (1983a) 105
Chaudhry, A. P., L. S. Cutler, S. Satchidanand, G. Labay, M. Sunder Raj, Ch.-Ch. Lin: Monomorphic adenomas of the parotid glands. Their ultrastructure and histogenesis. Cancer (Philad.) 52 (1983b) 112
Cossman, J., M. J. Deegan, J. G. Batsakis: Warthin's tumor. B-lymphocytes within the lymphoid infiltrate. Arch. Path. Lab. Med. 101 (1977) 354
Crumpler, C., J. C. Scharfenberg, R. J. Reed: Monomorphic adenomas of salivary glands. Trabecular-tubular, canalicular, and basaloid variants. Cancer (Philad.) 38 (1976) 193
Daley, T. D., D. G. Gardner, M. S. Smout: Canalicular adenoma: not a basal cell adenoma. Oral Surg. 57 (1984) 181
Damjanov, I., E. M. Sneff, A. N. Delerme: Squamous cell carcinoma arising in Warthin's tumor of the parotid gland. A light, electron microscopic, and immunohistochemical study. Oral Surg. 55 (1983) 286
David, R., A. Buchner: Corpora amylacea in adenolymphoma (Warthin's tumor). Amer. J. clin. Pathol. 69 (1978) 173
Donath, K., H. Dietrich, G. Seifert: Entwicklung und ultrastrukturelle Cytodifferenzierung der Parotis des Menschen. Virchows Arch. Path. Anat. 378 (1978) 297
Droese, M.: Zytologische Diagnose und Differentialdiagnose des Adenolymphoms. Verh. Dtsch. Ges. Path. 62 (1978) 327
Drummond, J. F., J. S. Giansanti, W. R. Sabes, C. R. Smith: Sialadenoma papilliferum of the oral cavity. Oral Surg. 45 (1978) 72
Eneroth, C.-M.: Die Klinik der Kopfspeicheldrüsentumoren. Arch. Oto-Rhino-Laryng. 213 (1976) 61
Eversole, L. R.: Histogenic classification of salivary tumors. Arch. Pathol. 92 (1971) 433
Fahmy, S.: Adenolymphoma of the tonsillar fossa. J. Laryngol. 87 (1973) 675
Fantasia, J. E., A. S. Miller: Papillary cystadenoma lymphomatosum arising in minor salivary glands. Oral Surg. 52 (1981) 411
Fantasia, J. E., B. W. Neville: Basal cell adenomas of the minor salivary glands. A clinicopathologic study of seventeen new cases and a review of the literature. Oral Surg. 50 (1980) 433
Fleischer, I., J. Caselitz, Th. Löning, G. Seifert: Histological and immunocytochemical examinations of the stromal reaction in carcinomas of the parotid gland. Analysis of 52 cases. Cancer Res. Clin. Oncol. 96 (1980) 193
Fleming, K. A., I. Morrice: Sebaceous lymphadenoma of the parotid gland: A report of a case. J. Path. 110 (1973) 259
Freedman, P. D., H. Lumerman: Sialadenoma papilliferum. Oral Surg. 45 (1978) 88
Gadient, St. E., B. Kalfayan: Mucoepidermoid carcinoma arising within a Warthin's tumor. Oral Surg. 40 (1975) 391
Gardner, D. G., T. D. Daley: The use of the terms monomorphic adenoma, and canalicular adenoma as applied to salivary gland tumors. Oral Surg. 56 (1983) 608
Gläser, A.: Geschwülste der Kopfspeicheldrüsen. In Gläser, A.: Klinische Pathologie der Geschwülste, Lieferung 3. Thieme, Leipzig 1979 (S. 85)
Gnepp, D. R., R. Brannon: Sebaceous neoplasms of salivary gland origin. Report of 21 cases. Cancer (Philad.) 53 (1984) 2155
Gnepp, D. R.: Warthin's tumor exhibiting sebaceous differentiation and necrotizing sialometaplasia. Virchows Arch. Path. Anat. 319 (1981) 267
Gnepp, D. R., T. Sporck: Benign lymphoepithelial parotid cyst with sebaceous differentiation. Cystic sebaceous lymphadenoma. Amer. J. clin. Pathol. 74 (1980) 683
Goldman, R. L., H. Z. Klein: Glycogen-rich adenoma of the parotid gland. An uncommon benign clear-cell tumor resembling certain clear-cell carcinoma of salivary origin. Cancer (Philad.) 30 (1972) 749
Gray, S. R., J. I. Cornog, I. S. Leo: Oncocytic neoplasms of the salivary glands. A report of fifteen cases including two malignant oncocytomas. Cancer (Philad.) 38 (1976) 1306
Greer, R. O.: Inverted oral papilloma. Oral Surg. 36 (1973) 400
Gruenfeld, G. E., L. H. Jorstad: Adenoma of the parotid gland: Oncocyte tumor. Amer. J. Cancer 26 (1936) 571
Hamperl, H.: Onkocyten und Geschwülste der Speicheldrüsen. Virchows Arch. Path. Anat. 282 (1931) 724
Hamperl, H.: Über das Vorkommen von Onkocyten in verschiedenen Organen und ihren Geschwülsten. Virchows Arch. Path. Anat. 298 (1937) 327
Hamperl, H.: Das Onkocytom der Speicheldrüsen. Z. Krebsforsch. 64 (1962) 427
Harrison, J. D.: Cystic adenoma of a minor salivary gland: a histochemical study. J. Path. 114 (1974) 29
Hastrup, N., P. Bretlau, A. Krogdahl, M. Melchiors: Oncocytomas of the salivary glands. J. Laryng. Otol. 96 (1982) 1027
Headington, J. T., J. G. Batsakis, T. F. Beals, T. E. Campbell, J. L. Simmons, W. D. Stone: Membranous basal cell adenomas of parotid gland, dermal cylindromas, and trichoepitheliomas: Comparative histochemistry and ultrastructure. Cancer (Philad.) 39 (1977) 2460
Herbst, E. W., W. Utz: Multifocal dermal-type basal cell adenomas of parotid glands with co-existing dermal cylindromas. Virchows Arch. Path. Anat. 403 (1984) 95
Howard, D. R., C. Bagley, J. G. Batsakis: Warthin's tumor: A functional immunologic study of the lymphoid cell component. Amer. J. Otolaryng. 371 (1982) 15
Hsu, S.-M., P.-L. Hsu, R. N. Nayak: Warthin's tumor: An immunohistochemical study of its lymphoid stroma. Human Pathol. 12 (1981) 251
Hübner, G., O. Kleinsasser, H. J. Klein: Zur Feinstruktur der Basalzelladenome der Speicheldrüsen. Ein Beitrag zur Zelldifferenzierung in Speicheldrüsengeschwülsten. Virchows Arch. Path. Anat. 353 (1971) 333
Hübner, G., F. Paulussen, O. Kleinsasser: Zur Feinstruktur und Genese d. Onkocyten. Virchows Arch. Path. Anat. 343 (1967) 34
Jao, W., P. C. Keh, M. A. Swerdlow: Ultrastructure of the basal cell adenoma of the parotid gland. Cancer (Philad.) 37 (1976) 1322
Johnston, C. A., C. Toker: Syringomatous tumors of minor salivary gland origin. Human Pathol. 13 (1982) 182
Kahn, L. B., L. Schoub: Myoepithelioma of the palate. Histochemical and ultrastructural observations. Arch. Path. (Chic.) 95 (1973) 209
Kim, S. K., L. Weatherbee, C. E. Nasjleti: Lysosomes in the epithelial component of Warthin's tumor. Arch. Path. (Chic.) 95 (1973) 56
Kleinsasser, O.: Über das Sebaceolymphom der Parotis. Mschr. Ohrenheilk. 98 (1964) 318
Kleinsasser, O.: Einteilung, Morphologie und Verhalten der epithelialen Speicheldrüsentumoren. HNO (Berl.) 17 (1969) 197
Kleinsasser, O., H. J. Klein: Basalzelladenome der Speicheldrüsen. Arch. klin. exp. Ohr.-, Nas.- u. Kehlk.-Heilk. 189 (1967) 302
Kleinsasser, O., G. Hübner, H. J. Klein: Talgzellcarcinom der Parotis. Arch. klin. exp. Ohr.-, Nas.- u. Kehlk.-Heilk. 197 (1970) 59
Kleinsasser, O., H. J. Klein, E. Steinbach, G. Hübner: Onkozytäre adenomartige Hyperplasien, Adenolymphome und Onkozytome der Speicheldrüsen. Arch. klin. exp. Ohr-, Nas.- u. Kehlk.-Heilk. 186 (1966) 317
Korsrud, F. R., P. Brandtzaeg: Immunohistochemical characterization of cellular immunoglobulins and epithelial marker antigens in Warthin's tumor. Human Pathol. 15 (1984) 361
Korsrud, F. R., P. Brandtzaeg: Immunohistochemical studies on the epithelial and lymphoid components of Warthin's tumor. Acta otolaryngol., Suppl. 360 (1979) 221
Kunze, P.: Talgdrüsenlymphadenom der Glandula parotis. Zbl. allg. Path. u. path. Anat. 123 (1979) 210
Kurreja, H. K., H. K. Jain: Adenolymphoma of submandibular salivary gland. J. Laryngol. 85 (1971) 1201

Levine, J., D. J. Krutchkoff, E. Eisenberg: Monomorphic adenoma of minor salivary glands: Reappraisal and report of nine new cases. J. oral Surg. 39 (1981) 101
Lindberg, L. G., M. Ackerman: Aspiration cytology of salivary gland tumors: Diagnostic experience from six years of routine laboratory work. Laryngoscope 86 (1976) 584
Lumerman, H., P. Freedman, P. Caracciolo, P. S. Remigio: Synchronous malignant mucoepidermoid tumor of the parotid gland and Warthin's tumor in adjacent lymph node. Oral Surg. 39 (1975) 953
Luna, M. A., B. Mackay, J. Gamez-Araujo: Myoepithelioma of the palate. Report of a case with histochemical and electron microscopic observations. Cancer (Philad.) 32 (1973) 1429
Mair, I. W. S., Th. A. Johannessen: Benign and malignant oncocytoma of the parotid gland. Laryngoscope 82 (1972) 638
Meza-Chávez, L.: Oxyphilic granular cell adenomas of the parotid gland (oncocytoma). Report of five cases and study of oxyphilic granular cells (oncocytes) in normal parotid gland. Amer. J. Pathol. 25 (1949) 523
Miller, R., E. T. Yanagihara, A. A. Dubrow, R. J. Lukes: Malignant lymphoma in a Warthin's tumor. Report of a case. Cancer (Philad.) 50 (1982) 2948
Mintz, G. A., A. M. Abrams, R. J. Melrose: Monomorphic adenomas of the major and minor salivary glands. Report of twenty-one case and review of the literature. Oral Surg. 53 (1982) 375
Moosavi, H., Ch. K. Ryan, St. Schwartz, J. A. Donnelly: Malignant adenolymphoma. Human Pathol. 11 (1980) 80
Nagao, K., O. Matsuzaki, H. Saiga, I. Sugano, H. Shigematsu, T. Kaneko, T. Katoh, T. Kitamura: Histopathologic studies of basal cell adenoma of the parotid gland. Cancer (Philad.) 50 (1982) 736
Nakashima, N., K. Goto, J. Takeuchi: Malignant papillary cystadenoma lymphomatosum. Light and electron microscopic study. Virchows Arch. Path. Anat. 399 (1983) 207
Nasu, M., M. Takagi, G. Ishikawa: Sialadenoma papilliferum. Report of case. J. oral Surg. 39 (1981) 367
Nelson, J. F., J. R. Jacoway: Monomorphic adenoma (canalicular type). Report of 29 cases. Cancer (Philad.) 31 (1973) 1511
Nesland, J. M., J. Olafsson, M. Sobrinho-Simoes: Plasmacytoid myoepithelioma of the palate. A case report with ultrastructural findings and review of the literature. J. oral Pathol. 10 (1981) 14
Nikai, H., H. E. Schroeder: Stereologic analysis of the lymphoid stroma in parotid adenolymphoma. J. oral Pathol. 13 (1984) 295
Papache, R. M., B. Bodelet, J. C. Guedenet: Adenome a cellules claires de la parotide. Considérations anatomo-cliniques à propos d'un cas. J. Franc. Otorhinolaryng. 31 (1982) 191
Pape, H.-D.: Das papilläre Zystadenolymphom. Ein Bericht über 20 Fälle. Stoma (Heidelberg) 15 (1963) 189
Reingold, I. M., L. E. Keasbey, J. H. Graham: Multicentric dermal-type cylindroma of the parotid glands in a patient with florid turban tumor. Cancer (Philad.) 40 (1977) 1702
Saksela, E., J. Tarkkanen, J. Wartiovaara: Parotid clear-cell adenoma of possible myoepithelial origin. Cancer (Philad.) 30 (1972) 742
Schmid, K. O., W. Albrich: Die Bedeutung der Talgzellen und Talgdrüsen für Parotisgeschwülste. Virchows Arch. Path. Anat. 359 (1973) 239
Sciubba, J. J., R. B. Brannon: Myoepithelioma of salivary glands: Report of 23 cases. Cancer (Philad.) 49 (1982) 562
Sciubba, J. J., B. H. Goldstein: Myoepithelioma. Review of the literature and report of a case with ultrastructural confirmation. Oral Surg. 42 (1976) 328
Seifert, G.: Mundhöhle, Mundspeicheldrüsen, Tonsillen und Rachen. In Doerr, W., E. Uehlinger: Spezielle pathologische Anatomie, Bd. 1. Springer, Berlin 1966 (S. 1)
Seifert, G., K. Donath: Die Morphologie der Speicheldrüsenerkrankungen. Arch. Oto-Rhino-Laryng. 213 (1976) 111
Seifert, G., K. Donath: Über das Vorkommen sog. Heller Zellen in Speicheldrüsentumoren. Z. Krebsforsch. 91 (1978) 165
Seifert, G., C.-P. Schulz: Das monomorphe Speichelgangadenom. Klassifikation und Analyse von 79 Fällen. Virchows Arch. Path. Anat. 383 (1979) 77
Seifert, G., H. G. Bull, K. Donath: Histologic subclassification of the cystadenolymphoma of the parotid gland. Analysis of 275 cases. Virchows Arch. Path. Anat. 388 (1980a) 13
Seifert, G., M. Heckmayr, K. Donath: Carcinome in papillären Cystadenolymphomen der Parotis. Definition und Differentialdiagnose. Z. Krebsforsch. 90 (1977) 25
Seifert, G., H. Rieb, K. Donath: Klassifikation der Tumoren der kleinen Speicheldrüsen. Pathohistologische Analyse von 160 Tumoren. Z. Laryng. Rhinol. 59 (1980b) 379
Shirasuna K., K. Watatani, T. Miyazaki: Ultrastructure of a sialadenoma papilliferum. Cancer 53 (1984) 468
Shulman, J., J. Waisman, D. Morledge: Sebaceous cell carcinoma of the parotid gland. Arch. otolaryngol. 98 (1973) 417
Silver, H., M. A. Goldstein: Sebaceous cell carcinoma of the parotid region. A review of the literature and a case report. Cancer (Philad.) 19 (1966) 1773
Strauss, M., A. Abt, P. Mahataphongse, G. H. Conner: Basal cell adenoma of the major salivary glands. Arch. Otolaryngol. 107 (1981) 120
Stromeyer, F. W., R. C. Haggitt, J. F. Nelson, J. M. Hardmann: Myoepithelioma of the minor salivary gland origin. Light and electron microscopical study. Arch. Path. 99 (1975) 242
Tandler, B.: Warthin's tumor: electron microscopic studies. Arch. otolaryng. (Chic.) 84 (1966) 68
Tandler, B., F. H. Shipkey: Ultrastructure of Warthin's tumor. II. Crystalloids. J. Ultrastruct. Res. 11 (1964) 306
Tandler, B., R. V. Hutter, R. A. Erlandson: Ultrastructure of oncocytoma of the parotid gland. Lab. Invest. 23 (1970) 567
Tschen, J. A., M. H. McGavran: Sebaceous lymphadenoma. Ultrastructural observations and lipid analysis. Cancer (Philad.) 44 (1979) 1388
Veronesi, U., L. Corbetta: Adenolymphoma of the lower lip. Acta oto-laryng. 52 (1960) 1
Volmer, J.: Multiple unilaterale Tumoren der Glandula parotis. Zbl. allg. Pathol. u. path. Anat. 126 (1982) 327
Wasan, S. M.: Sebaceous lymphadenoma of the parotid gland. Cancer (Philad.) 28 (1971) 1019
White, D. K., A. S. Miller, R. K. McDaniel, B. N. Rothman: Inverted ductal papilloma: A distinctive lesion of minor salivary gland. Cancer (Philad.) 49 (1982) 519
Wilson, D. F., B. W. Robinson: Oral inverted ductal papilloma. Oral Surg. 57 (1984) 520
Wuketich, St., G. Kittinger: Lymphadenoma sebaceum der Parotis. Arch. klin. exp. Ohr-, Nas.- u. Kehlk.-Heilk. 187 (1966) 836
Zajicek, J., C.-M. Eneroth, P. Jakobsson: Aspiration biopsy of salivary gland tumors. VI. Morphologic studies on smears and histologic sections from mucoepidermoid carcinoma. Acta Cytol. 20 (1976) 35
Zechner, G., K. W. Albegger: Talgdrüsencarcinom der Parotis. Arch. klin. exp. Ohr.-, Nas.- u. Kehlk.-Heilk. 205 (1973) 119

Clinical Aspects of Malignant Salivary Gland Tumors

Malignant tumors of the major and minor salivary glands are uncommon. In Sweden, they are estimated to form 0.3% of all malignant tumors (Eneroth 1976). More than 80% of these malignant tumors arise in the parotid gland, 10% in the submandibular gland, and another 10% in the minor glands (Chilla et al 1983, Eneroth 1976, Thompson 1982). The ratio of malignant to benign tumors is 1 : 4, but varies from gland to gland. In Eneroth's series (1971), only 13% of all parotid tumors were malignant. This proportion increased to 32% for submandibular tumors and to 56% for tumors of the palate.

Whereas the clinical aspects of the less malignant salivary tumors, such as the highly differentiated acinic cell and mucoepidermoid tumors, resemble those of benign tumors, such as pleomorphic adenoma and cystadenolymphoma (Fig. 15.**68**), the symptoms and signs of the more aggressive variants almost always indicate their malignant nature. Rapid growth and pain should lead to a

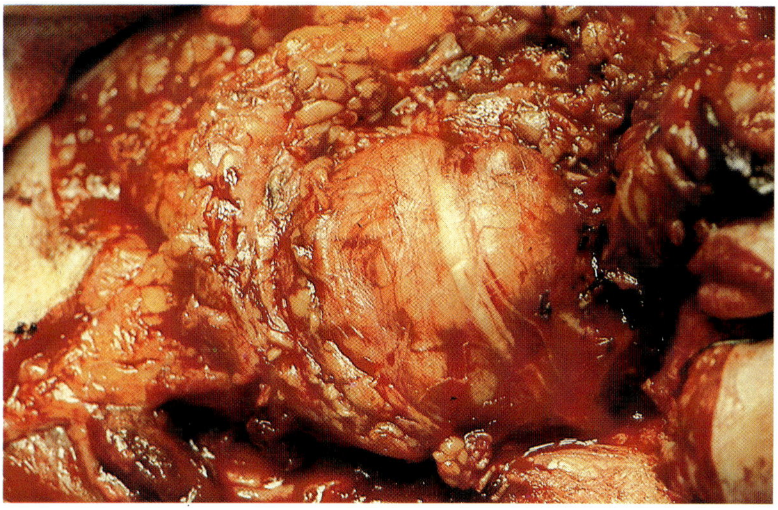

Figure 15.**68** Duct carcinoma of the parotid gland: a well-encapsulated and mobile tumor of the deep lobe without a facial paralysis.

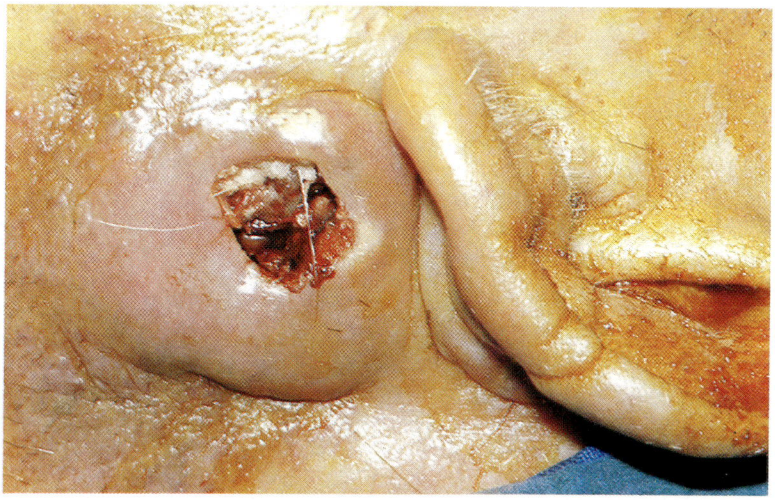

Figure 15.**69** Ulcerating squamous cell carcinoma of the parotid gland.

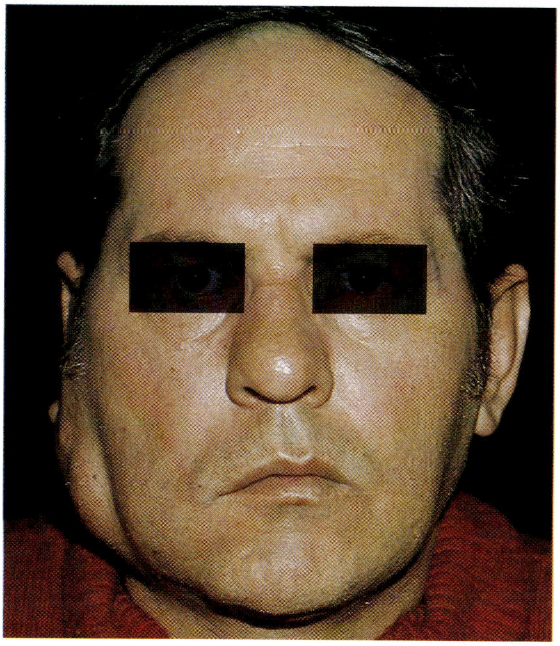

Figure 15.**70** Carcinoma in a longstanding pleomorphic adenoma with paralysis of the right facial nerve.

suspicion of malignancy, although these symptoms are not specific of malignancy (Chilla 1983). Reduced mobility or fixation and extension of the tumor beyond the boundaries of the salivary gland support this suspicion, which becomes a certainty in the presence of ulceration (Fig. 15.**69**) or facial nerve paralysis in the case of a parotid tumor (Fig. 15.**70**). Spontaneous facial paralysis in a parotid tumor inevitably indicates malignancy. In our series, facial paralysis did not occur in patients with well-differentiated acinic cell and mucoepidermoid tumors, whereas the proportion of paralysis in undifferentiated carcinomas and solid adenoid cystic carcinomas was 60 and 68%, respectively (Table 15.**7**). A preoperative facial paralysis is a very unfavorable prognostic sign (see pages 282, 283).

Table 15.**7** Frequency of Preoperative Facial Paralysis in Malignant Parotid Tumors (Göttingen Series, 1965–1975)

	%
Well differentiated acinic cell tumors	0
Well differentiated mucoepidermoid tumors	0
Duct carcinoma	0
Poorly differentiated acinic cell tumor	17
Cribriform adenoid cystic carcinoma	20
Poorly differentiated mucoepidermoid tumors	33
Carcinoma ex pleomorphic adenoma	36
Adenocarcinoma	40
Tubular adenoid cystic carcinoma	40
Squamous cell carcinoma	58
Undifferentiated carcinoma	60
Solid adenoid cystic carcinoma	67

We have found aspiration cytology (see page 56), supplemented by a frozen section examination during the operation, to be the most certain method of confirming the diagnosis and planning treatment. Biopsy (page 59) is now only used in doubtful cases, if a strong suspicion of malignancy is not confirmed by cytology.

Sialographic criteria of malignancy, such as flow of the contrast medium into the lymphatic pathways of the parotid gland (Som & Shugar 1981), isotope scanning (McGuirt & McCabe 1977), and computed tomography (Bryan et al 1982) are of secondary diagnostic significance. Computed tomography may be especially useful in the assessment of the deep extension of salivary tumors, particularly that of a parotid tumor into the infratemporal fossa (Golding 1982).

References

Bryan, R. N., P. H. Miller, R. I. Ferreyro, R. B. Sessions: Computed tomography of the major salivary glands. Amer. J. Roentgenol. 139 (1982) 547

Chilla, R.: Kavernöses Hämangiom im M. masseter. Ein Beitrag zur Differentialdiagnose des schmerzhaften Parotistumors. HNO 31 (1983) 88

Chilla, R., R. Casjens, U. Eysholdt, M. Droese: Maligne Speicheldrüsentumoren. Der Einfluß von Histologie und Lokalisation auf die Prognose. HNO 31 (1983) 286

Eneroth, C.-M.: Salivary gland tumors in the parotid gland, submandibular gland, and the palate region. Cancer 27 (1971) 1415

Eneroth, C.-M.: Die Klinik der Kopfspeicheldrüsentumoren. Arch. Oto-Rhino-Laryng. 213 (1976) 61

Golding, S.: Computed tomography in the diagnosis of parotid gland tumours. Brit. J. Radiol. 55 (1982) 182

McGuirt, W. F., B. F. McCabe: Limitations of parotid scans. Ann. Otol. 86 (1977) 247

Som, P. M., J. M. A. Shugar: Parotolymphatic backflow: a new sign of malignancy. Ann. Otol. 90 (1981) 64

Thompson, St. H.: Malignant salivary gland tumours. J. Dent. Ass. South Africa 37 (1982) 561

Acinic Cell Tumors

Acinic cell tumors form 2% of the material of the Salivary Gland Register (see Table 15.**1**); 90% of the tumors lie in the parotid gland, and they are much less common in the submandibular gland (Gläser 1979) or the minor glands (Chen et al 1978, Abrams & Melrose 1978, Ferlito 1980, Murphy & Corio 1981, Fermont 1979, Perzin & LiVolsi 1979, Gardner et al 1980, Keane et al 1982, Inoue et al 1984). This tumor is more common in women, with a peak age incidence in the fifth to sixth decades. The term "acinic cell tumor" in the WHO classification expresses the fact that it is difficult to assess the degree of malignancy by histologic criteria alone. The term "acinic cell tumor" therefore is to be preferred to others, such as carcinoma or adenoma.

Clinical Appearances. The tumor usually presents as a round, well-encapsulated swelling. In the early stages it cannot be distinguished from benign tumors, so that previously it was thought that it remained benign in its entire clinical course. However, it is now known that this is not true, because the acinic cell tumor infiltrates locally and tends to recur (Fig. 15.**71**). Preoperative fa-

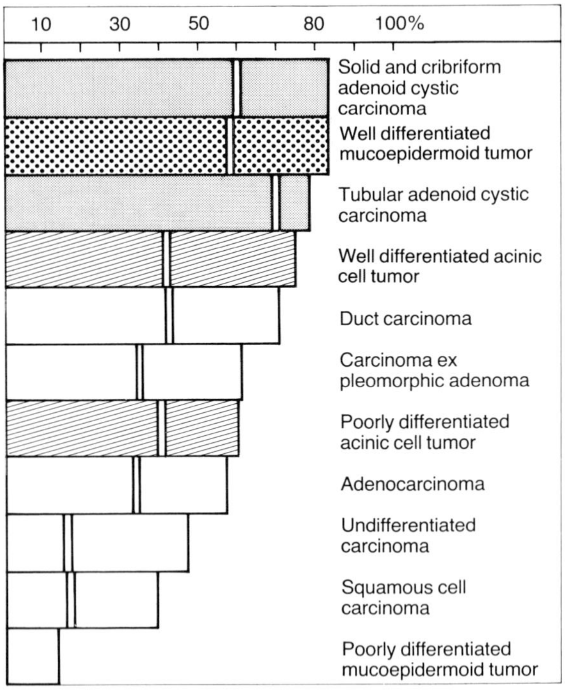

Figure 15.**71** Local recurrences of malignant salivary tumors in the authors' series (1965 – 1975). The full length of each bar represents the overall recurrence rate, and the left-hand segment, the number of multiple recurrences.

cial paralysis is occasionally observed in poorly differentiated tumors (Table 15.**7**). In our experience, both poorly and well-differentiated acinic cell tumors may occasionally metastasize to lymph nodes and by the bloodstream (Fig. 15.**72a, b**).

Histology. The tumor is characterized by an acinic epithelial complex whose cytoplasm demonstrates a fine granular or honeycomb appearance (Fig. 15.**73**). Secretory granules of varying amounts may be demonstrated in the cytoplasm by the PAS reaction (Fig. 15.**74a, b**). Immunocytochemistry shows that the tumor cells contain amylase (Caselitz et al 1983), but amylase granules are not present in all tumor cells and the distribution varies within the cell groups (Fig. 15.**7**). Ductular and microcystic structures containing secretion (Figs. 15.**75a, b,** 15.**76**) occur in addition to the acinic cell complexes. The clear cell variant is a particular form of the acinic cell tumor (Fig. 15.**77a, b**).

The clear cell structures may be interpreted as intracellular secretory disorders similar to the sialadenoses (Seifert & Donath 1978). Ellis and Corio (1983) distinguished four histologic types: solid acinar, microcystic, papillary cystic, and follicular, the dominant being the microcystic type.

They also differentiated five different cell types: acinic cells, intercalated duct cells, vacuolized cells, clear cells, and nonspecific gland cells, but emphasize that several different types of differentiation may be found in the same tumor. Ductular differentiation with intercalated duct cells predominate in acinic cell tumors that metastasize (Fig. 15.**78**).

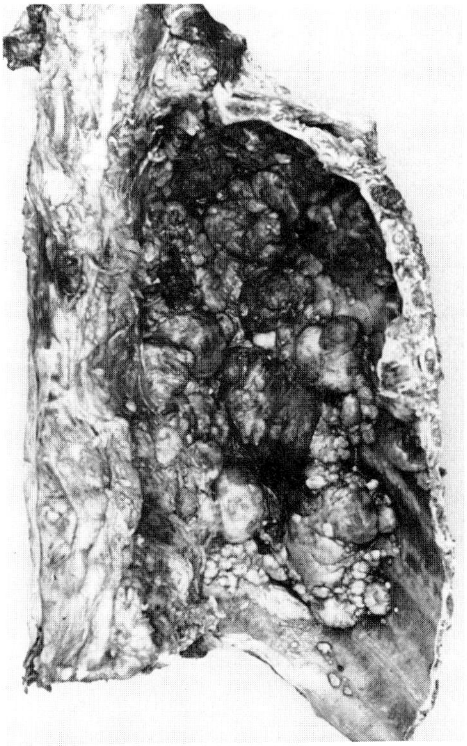

Figure 15.**72** Metastasizing acinic cell tumor (primary operation on the left parotid in 1966, recurrence and death in 1973). **a** Extensive pleural deposits on the left side.

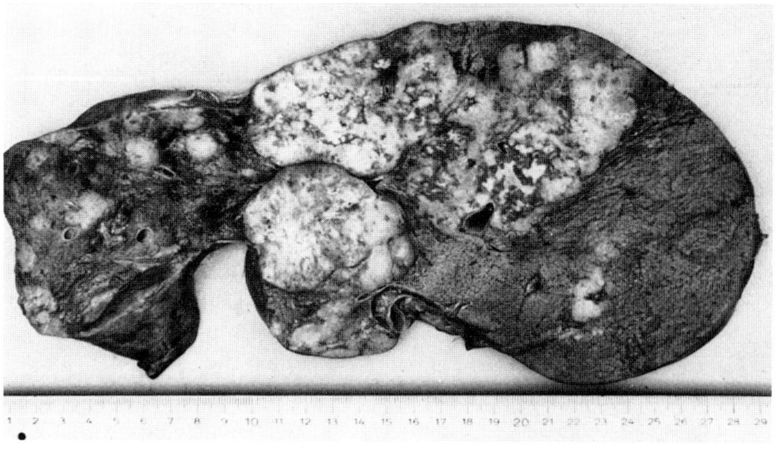

Figure 15.**72b** Multiple liver metastases.

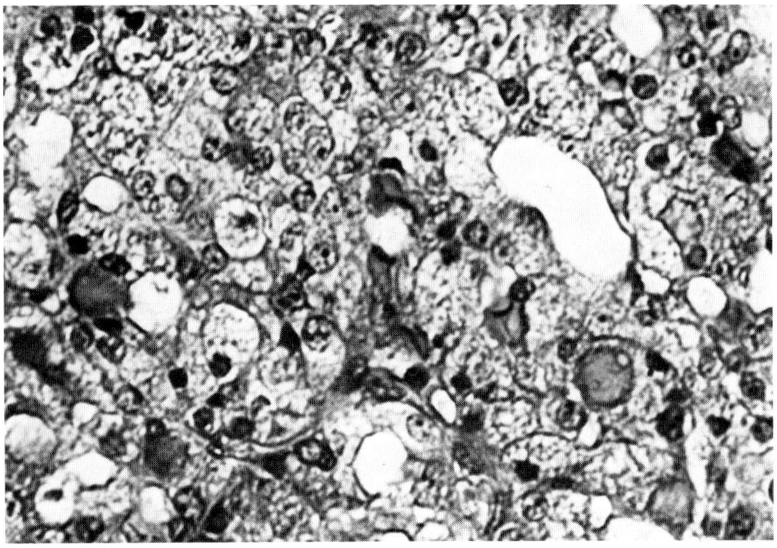

Figure 15.**73** Acinic cell tumor of the parotid gland showing acinic cell complexes with deposits of secretion. H & E, 400×.

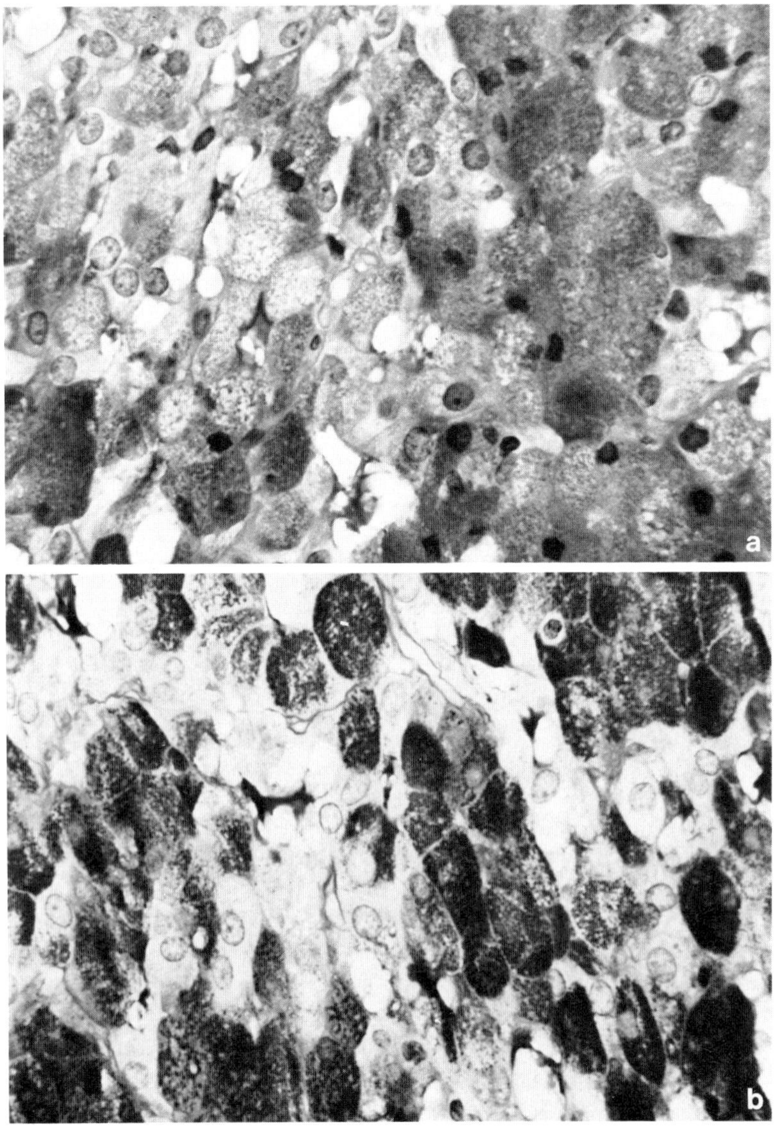

Figure 15.**74** Acinic cell tumor of the parotid gland. **a** Fine granular nature of the cytoplasm. H & E. **b** PAS-positive secretory granules in the cytoplasm. PAS. **a**, **b** 400×.

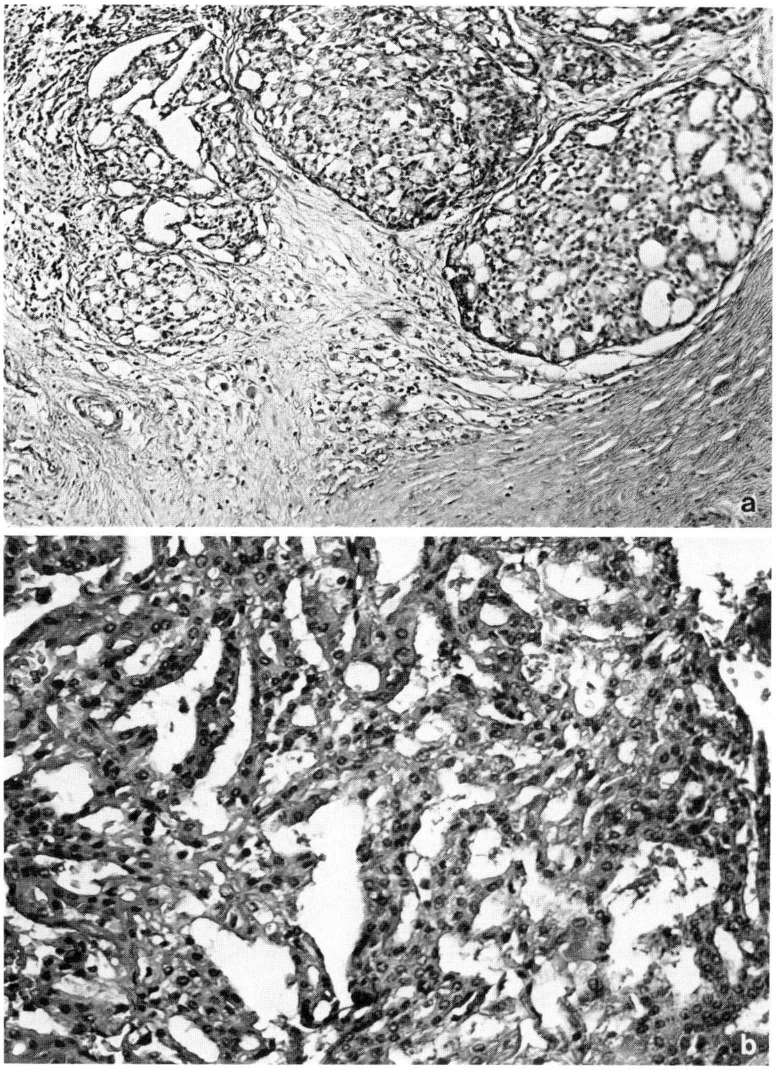

Figure 15.**75** Acinic cell tumor of the parotid gland showing neighboring acinic and ductular structures. H & E. **a** 63×, **b** 160×.

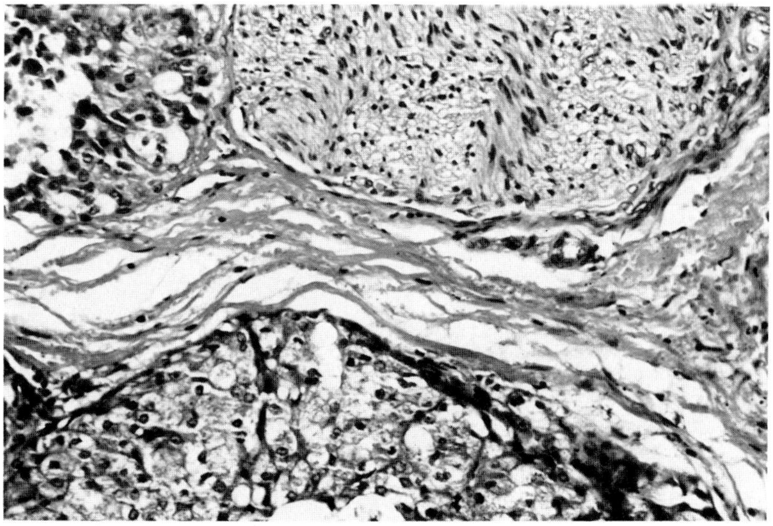

Figure 15.**76** Acinic cell tumor of the parotid gland showing perineural infiltration. H & E, 160×.

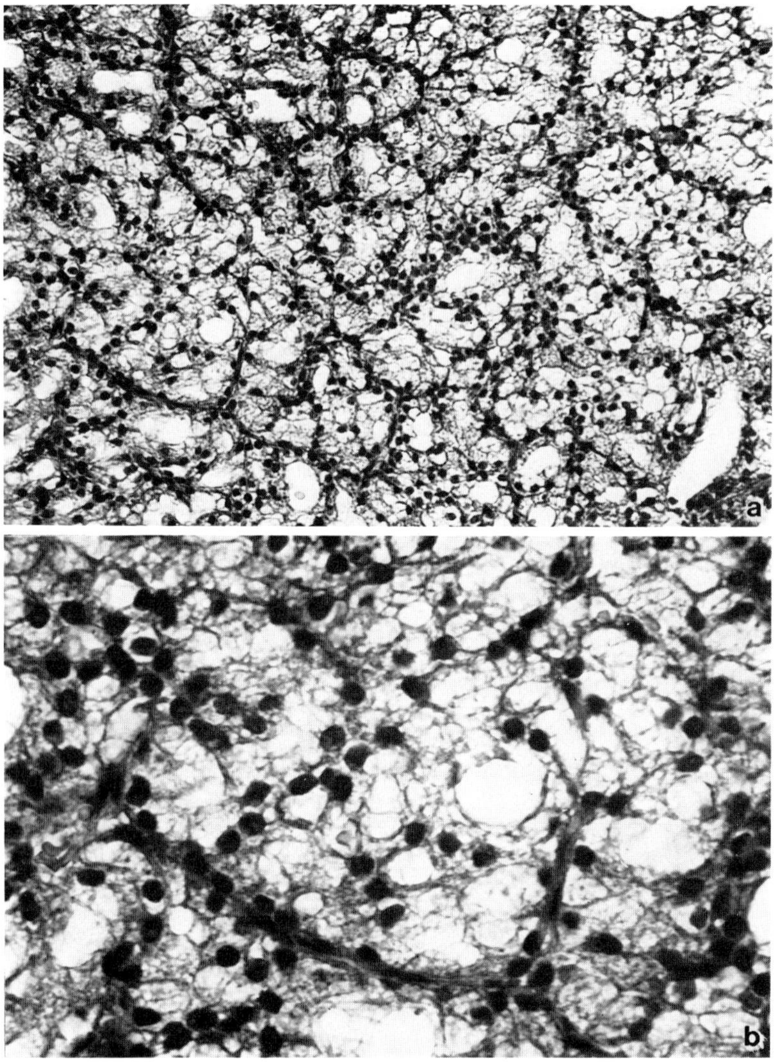

Figure 15.**77** Acinic cell tumor of the parotid gland showing a clear cell variant. H & E. **a** 160×, **b** 400×.

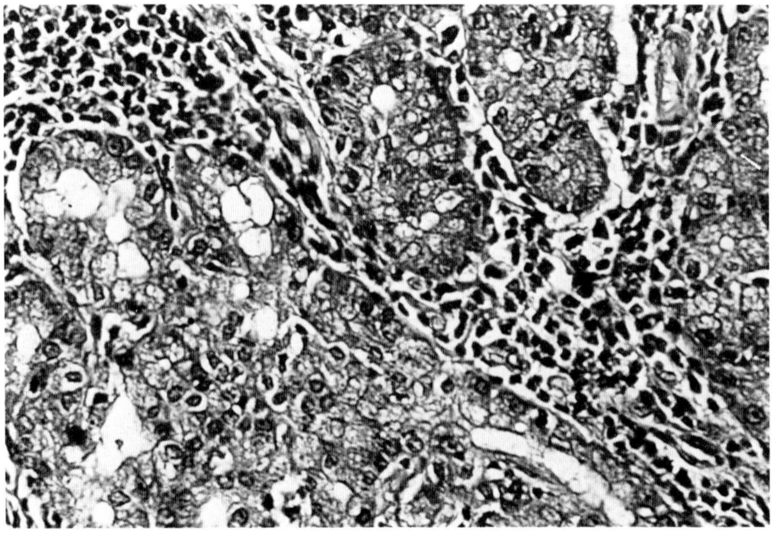

Figure 15.**78** Lymph node metastases of an acinic cell tumor of the parotid gland consisting mainly of ductular structures. H & E, 160×.

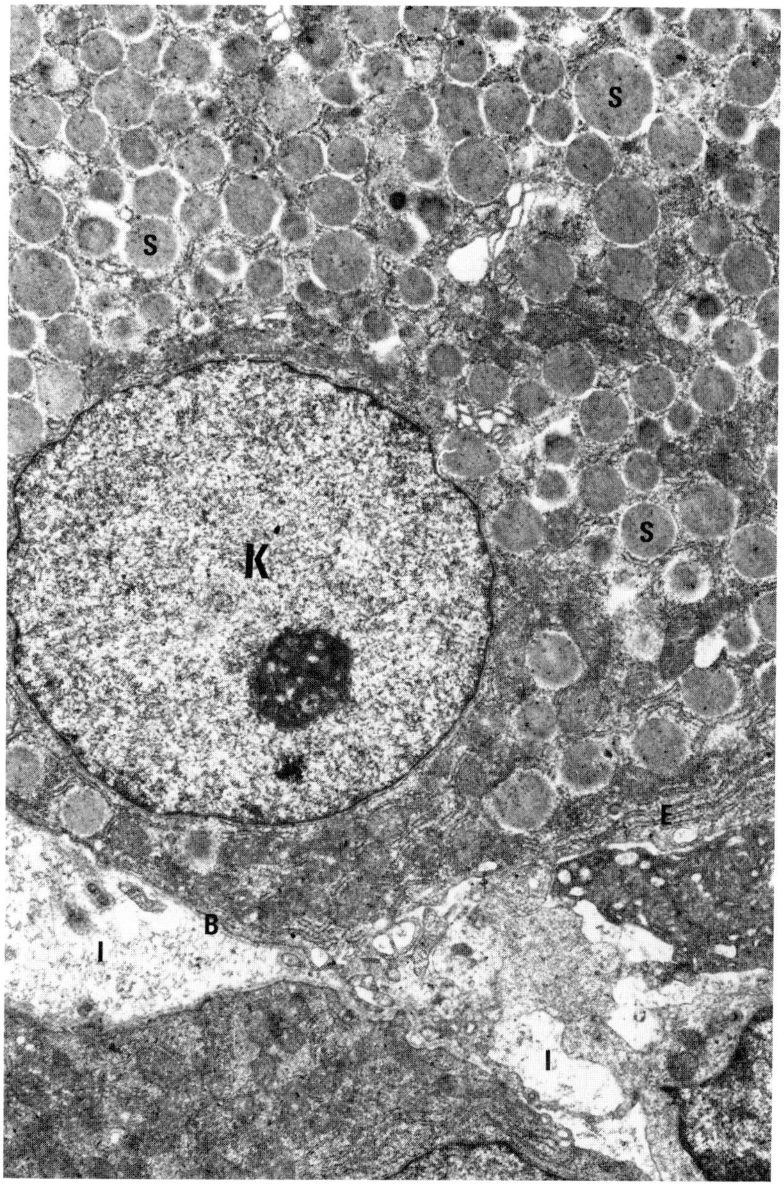

Figure 15.**79** Electron microscopic section of an acinic cell tumor of the parotid gland showing acinic differentiated tumor cells with secretory granules. S = secretory granule, E = endoplasmic reticulum, K = cell nucleus, B = basal cell bounding membrane, I = interstitium. 8500×. (Seifert & Donath 1976.)

Electron Microscopy. The acinic cell units resemble the structure of the acinic cells of the gland parenchyma (Fig. 15.**79**). The characteristics include formation of an endoplasmic reticulum, the development of Golgi apparatus, and the inclusion of secretory granules of varying size and optical density (Echevarria 1967, Hübner et al 1968, Hirtzler et al 1969, Bloom & Henriksson 1977, Erlandson & Tandler 1972, Kay & Schatzki 1972, Micheau & Lacour 1971, Seifert & Donath 1978). The ultrastructural characteristics, particularly of the clear cell variant, include an intracellular abnormality of protein synthesis manifested by marked modification of the secretory granules and the formation of granular vesicles. Ductular differentiation, but usually no myoepithelial cells, are found in acinic cell tumors.

Pathogenesis. The acinic cell tumor develops from the boundary zone between the intercalated duct system and the acini. This region of the gland possesses a well-developed regenerative capacity that is mainly expressed in the acinic cell tumor by acinar differentiation, but also by the development of primitive terminal ductal structures.

Prognosis. It is difficult to forecast the behavior of an individual case, since local infiltration and metastases can occur, even if the tumor does not show pronounced cellular atypia (Perzin & LiVolsi 1979). The presence or absence of a tumor capsule is also not a certain criterion. Local recurrences are recorded in 20% of cases, regional lymph node metastases in 10%, and death due to distant metastases in about 6% (Spiro et al 1978, Jack 1981, Ellis & Corio 1982). The histologic classification into a *well-differentiated form* with low-grade malignancy and into a *poorly differentiated form* with high-grade malignancy (Batsakis et al 1979, Evans & Cruikshank 1970, Ungerecht 1975) correlates well with the prognosis (see page 281ff). The prognosis is worse for poorly differentiated tumors. Well-differentiated tumors are more common than poorly differentiated tumors. The latter formed 35% of our series. A further parameter is the extent of the tumor at the time of the operation, particularly if the tumor also demonstrates a high degree of mitotic activity (Perzin & LiVolsi 1979).

The tumor may be bilateral (Levin et al 1975, see also page 172). Ectopic ACTH production by metastases in lung and liver is also recorded rarely (Lilian et al 1970).

Differential Diagnosis. The acinic cell tumor must be distinguished from adenocarcinoma and clear cell tumors (Seifert & Donath 1978). Without exact knowledge of the source of the tissue, it may be difficult to distinguish between an acinic cell tumor with lymphoid stromal components and a lymph node metastases of an acinic cell tumor. The cytologic diagnosis of an acinic cell tumor generally presents no difficulty.

Confusion with cystadenolymphoma is possible if the aspirate is rich in lymphocytes and partially oncocytic differentiated cells, in addition to acinar cells (Lindenberg & Akerman 1976, Droese 1980). The acinar adenolymphoma described by Geiler (1957) obviously represented a lymph node metastasis from an acinic cell tumor and not a special form of an adenolymphoma. The tumor cells in this case formed typical acinar and clear cell structures surrounded by a lymphoid stroma.

Surgical Treatment. The surgical treatment of acinic cell tumors depends on their degree of histologic differentiation. For well-differentiated tumors, treatment schedule I (page 278ff) should be followed, that is, superficial or total parotidectomy with preservation of the facial nerve or partial resection with reconstruction of the nerve, depending on the site of the tumor (Conley's "big-little" operation). We do not use postoperative radiation therapy.

Total parotidectomy, if necessary with resection and reconstruction of the facial nerve (group 2 of the therapy schedule), followed by radiotherapy is recommended for poorly differentiated tumors.

References

Abrams, A. M., R. J. Melrose: Acinic cell tumors of minor salivary gland origin. Oral Surg. 46 (1978) 220

Batsakis, J. G., E. K. Chinn, T. A. Weimert, W. P. Work, C. J. Krause: Acinic cell carcinoma: a clinicopathologic study of thirty-five cases. J. Laryng. 93 (1979) 325

Bloom, G. D., R. Henriksson: Some ultrastructural features of acinic cell carcinoma. J. Laryng. 91 (1977) 947

Caselitz, J., G. Seifert, G. Grenner, R. Schmidtberger: Amylase as an additional marker of salivary gland neoplasms. An immunoperoxidase study. Path. Res. Pract. 176 (1983) 276

Chen, S.-Y., R. B. Brannon, A. S. Miller, D. K. Withe, S. P. Hooker: Acinic cell adenocarcinoma of minor salivary glands. Cancer (Philad.) 42 (1978) 678

Droese, M.: Punktionscytologie der Speicheldrüsenerkrankungen. Habil.-Schrift, Göttingen 1980

Echevarria, R. E.: Ultrastructure of the acinic cell carcinoma and clear cell carcinoma of the parotid gland. Cancer (Philad.) 20 (1967) 563

Ellis, G. L., R. L. Corio: Acinic cell adenocarcinoma. A clinicopathologic analysis of 294 cases. Cancer (Philad.) 52 (1983) 542

Erlandson, R. A., B. Tandler: Ultrastructure of acinic cell carcinoma of the parotid gland. Arch. Path. 93 (1972) 130

Evans, R. W., A. H. Cruickshank: Epithelial Tumours of the Salivary Glands. Saunders, Philadelphia 1970

Ferlito, A.: Acinic cell carcinoma of minor salivary glands. Histopathology 4 (1980) 331

Fermont, D. C.: Acinic cell carcinoma of intraoral minor salivary gland origin. J. Laryng. 93 (1979) 423

Gardner, D. G., M. E. A. Bell, R. K. Wesley, G. P. Wysocki: Acinic cell tumors of minor salivary glands. Oral Surg. 50 (1980) 545

Geiler, G.: Zur Pathogenese der Adenolymphome. Virchows Arch. Path. Anat. 330 (1957) 172

Gläser, A.: Geschwülste der Kopfspeicheldrüsen. In Gläser, A.: Klinische Pathologie der Geschwülste, Lieferung 3. Thieme, Leipzig 1979 (S. 85)

Hirtzler, R., B. Oberman, M. Kulis, N. Ljubesic: Acinuszelladenocarcinome der Speicheldrüsen: Bericht über 4 Fälle mit elektronenmikroskopischer Bearbeitung von 2 Geschwülsten. Arch. klin. exp. Ohr.-, Nas.- u. Kehlk.-Heilk. 195 (1969) 68

Hübner, G., H. J. Klein, O. Kleinsasser: Zur Feinstruktur und Genese der Azinuszelltumoren der Glandula Parotis. Virchows Arch. Path. Anat. 345 (1968) 1

Inoue, T., M. Shimono, T. Yamamura, I. Saito, O. Watanabe, H. Kawahara: Acinic cell carcinoma arising in the glossopalatine glands: A report of two cases with electron microscopic observations. Oral Surg. 57 (1984) 398

Jack, G. A.: Irradiation of metastatic acinic cell carcinoma of the parotid gland. Cancer (Philad.) 48 (1981) 1557

Kay, S., P. F. Schatzki: Ultrastructure of acinic cell carcinoma of the parotid salivary gland. Cancer (Philad.) 29 (1972) 235

Keane, W. M., J. C. Denneny, J. P. Atkins, F. McBrearty: Acinic cell carcinoma of the oral cavity. Otolaryngol. Head Neck Surg. 90 (1982) 696

Levin, J. M., D. W. Robinson, F. Lin: Acinic cell carcinoma. Collective review, including bilateral cases. Arch. Surg. 110 (1975) 64

Lilian, M., R. D. Gourley, A. E. Kitabchi: Acinic cell adenocarcinoma of the parotid gland with ectopic production of adrenocorticotropic hormone. Amer. J. Med. 49 (1970) 529

Lindenberg, L. G., M. Akerman: Aspiration cytology of salivary gland tumors: diagnostic experience from six years of routine laboratory work. Laryngoscope 86 (1976) 584

Micheau, Ch., J. Lacour: Epithelioma acineux de la parotide. Ann. Anat. Path. 16 (1971) 173

Murphy, J. B., K. L. Corio: Acinic cell adenocarcinoma of the buccal mucosa: Report of case. J. oral Surg. 39 (1981) 357

Perzin, K. H., V. A. LiVolsi: Acinic cell carcinomas arising in salivary glands. A clinicopathologic study. Cancer. (Philad.) 44 (1979) 1434

Seifert, G., K. Donath: Über das Vorkommen sog. heller Zellen in Speicheldrüsentumoren. Ultrastruktur und Differentialdiagnose. Z. Krebsforsch. 91 (1978) 165

Spiro, R. H., A. G. Huvos, E. W. Strong: Acinic cell carcinoma of salivary origin. A clinicopathologic study of 67 cases. Cancer (Philad.) 41 (1978) 924

Ungerecht, K.: Diagnostik und Therapie der Parotiserkrankungen. Münch. med. Wschr. 116 (1975) 439

Mucoepidermoid Tumors

Mucoepidermoid tumors form 5% of all salivary tumors (Table 15.**1**), two thirds affecting the parotid gland and the remaining third, the minor glands (Jakobsson et al 1968, Micheau et al 1972, Bhashar & Bernier 1962, Brocheriou & Seghir 1974, Healey et al 1970, Eneroth 1976, Lentrodt & Hafke 1974, Spiro et al 1978, Smitheringale et al 1981, Sciubba et al 1980). Mucoepidermoid tumors arise two to three times more often from the minor glands than from the major glands, in all reported series and in our material (Seifert et al 1980). About 2% of all mucoepidermoid tumors arise within the facial skeleton, more often in the mandible than in the maxilla (Gingell et al 1984). These central mucoepidermoid tumors might originate from pluripotent odontogenic epithelium. One mucoepidermoid tumor arising in parotid lymph nodes has been recorded (Schulze & Kleinsasser 1978).

Mucoepidermoid tumors form 10.5% of minor gland tumors and are thus the third most common type, being exceeded by pleomorphic adenomas (45%) and adenoid cystic carcinomas (22%). The favorite site is the palate (40–50%) and the floor of the mouth (20%), but the tumor may also occur in the tongue and cheek (Chomette et al 1982). The peak age incidence is in the fifth decade, with a slight preponderance for women.

Clinical Aspects. A mucoepidermoid tumor of low-grade malignancy presents as a circumscribed nodule. It grows slowly and does not cause pain. Facial paralysis did not occur in any of the cases reported by Foote and Frazell (1953). We too

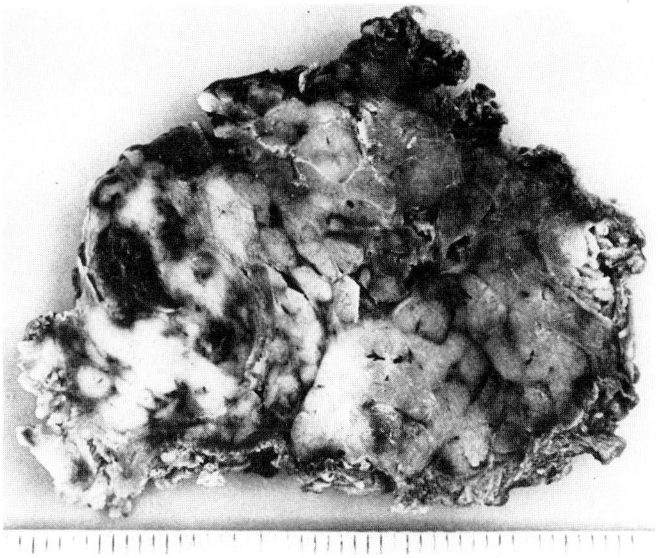

Figure 15.**80** Mucoepidermoid tumor of the parotid gland showing solid, rather speckled tumor nodules.

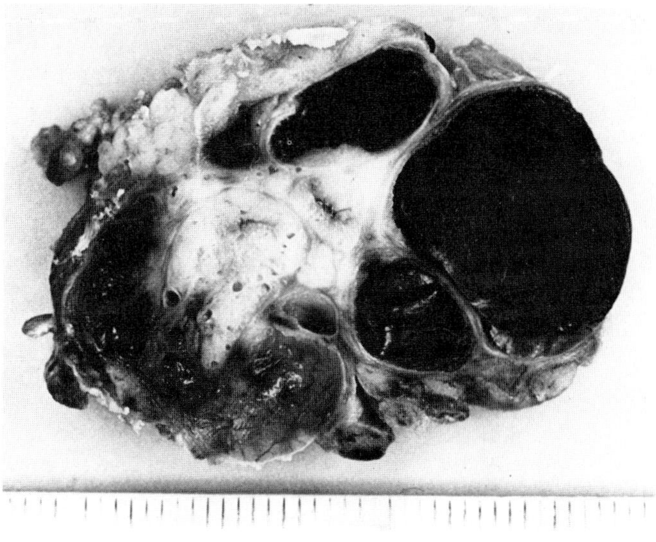

Figure 15.**81** Cystic mucoepidermoid tumor of the parotid gland.

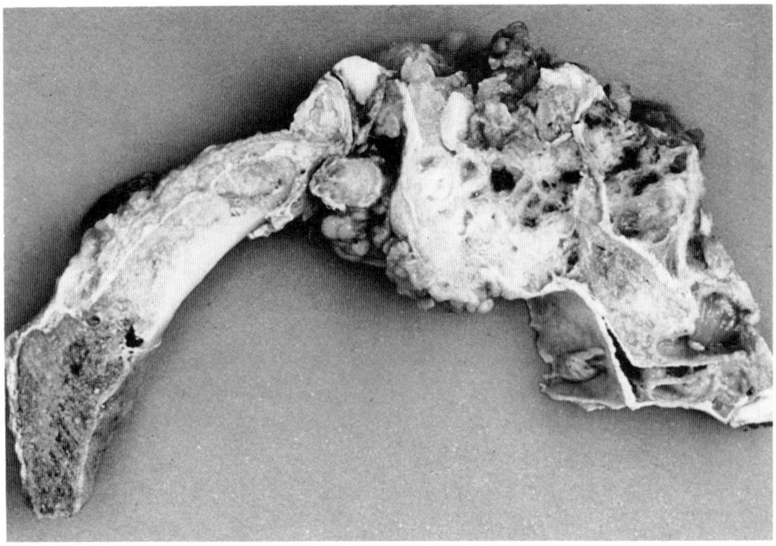

Figure 15.**82** Infiltration of the mandible by a mucoepidermoid tumor of the parotid gland.

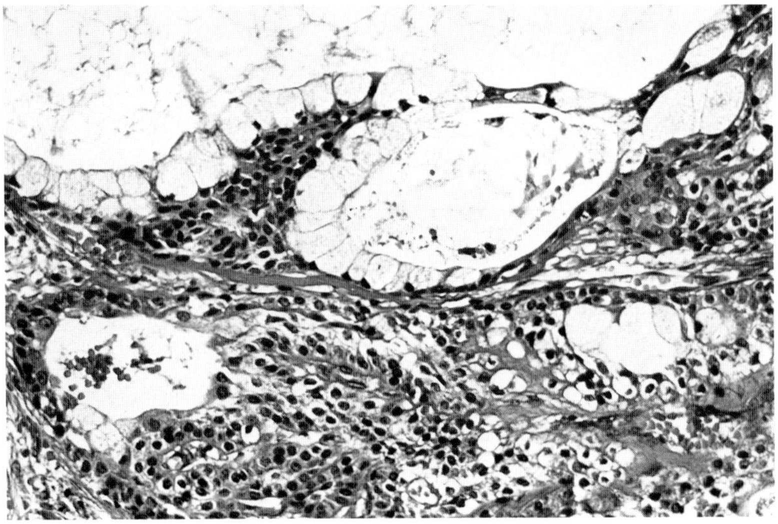

Figure 15.**83** Mucoepidermoid tumor of the parotid gland showing epidermoid cell complexes and mucus-filled cysts with goblet cells. H & E, 160×.

have only seen facial paralysis in high-grade tumors (Table 15.**7**). This tumor often causes pain. Its limits are usually ill defined and the tumor is of reduced mobility. Neither lymph node or blood-borne metastases are observed in well-differentiated mucoepidermoid tumors, whereas lymph node metastases predominate in poorly differentiated tumors. These metastases were accompanied by local recurrence in more than half of our patients.

Macroscopic Appearances. Mucoepidermoid tumors demonstrate irregular boundaries, and have an average size of 3–5 cm (Figs. 15.**80**–15.**82**). The surface is partly solid and partly replaced by large cysts that contain a mucous secretion and also blood. The well-differentiated types may resemble cystic duct adenoma or a mucous cyst.

Histology. The architecture is divided into two cell types: a solid cell group consisting of prickle cells and mucus-forming goblet cells (Figs. 15.**83**–15.**85**). Typical intercellular bridges are developed between the prickle cells. Some of the mucus-forming cells are distributed diffusely and some are arranged in groups between the epidermoid cell cords. Acid and neutral mucopolysaccharides can be demonstrated in the cytoplasm. Larger mucus-filled cysts are predominantly limited by mucus-forming cells. Histochemistry shows the mucus to be heterogenous (Eversole

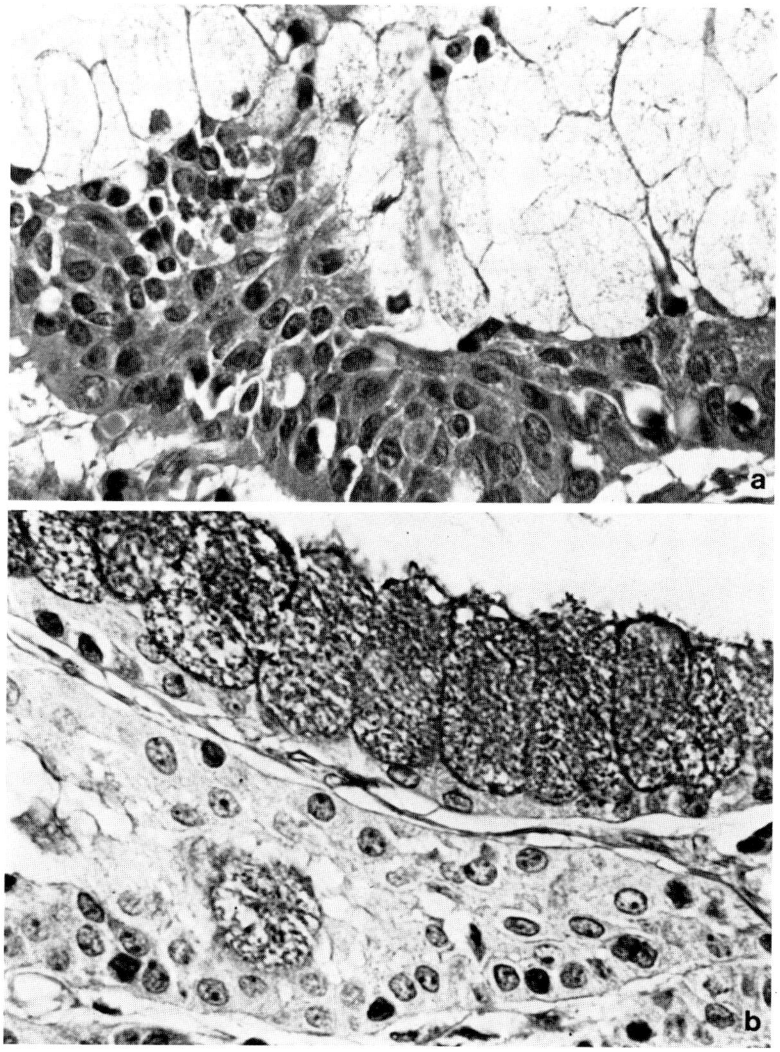

Figure 15.**84** Mucoepidermoid tumor (same case as 15.**83**): juxtaposition of epidermoid cells and mucus-forming goblet cells. **a** H & E, **b** PAS. **a**, **b** 400×.

1972). Similar criteria for differentiation are provided by an aspiration biopsy (Zajicek et al 1976).

The clear cell variant of mucoepidermoid tumor is an unusual type of differentiation (Fig. 15.**86a, b**).

Electron Microscopy. Three cell types may be distinguished (Chen 1979): typical epidermoid prickle cells with tonofilaments and desmosomes, mucus-forming cells with mucous vacuoles, and intermediate poorly differentiated cells with glycogen granules in the cytoplasm. Small hollow spaces are bounded by microvilli and contain secretory particles (Hübner & Kleinsasser 1970, Sugar & Toth 1967, Seifert & Donath 1978, Nicolatou et al 1979, Chomette et al 1982). Other features include clear cell structures with glycogen granules and oncocytic areas (Sidhu & Waldo 1975) rich in mitochondria. Poorly differentiated tumor cells are rich in ribosomes and demonstrate an increased activity of alkaline phosphatase and ATPase (Chomette et al 1982).

Pathogenesis. Mucoepidermoid tumors arise from the duct system, particularly the central segment. Goblet cell metaplasia may be demonstrated in this region even in tumor-free salivary glands (see page 108).

Prognosis. Several *subclassifications* have been put forward for the assessment of prognosis (Eneroth 1976). Mucoepidermoid tumors demonstrating typical epidermoid structures, a richness of mucus-forming areas with macro- and microcysts (Fig. 15.**87a, b**) are assigned to the well-differentiated (low-grade) category. The mucus-forming part constitutes more than 50% of the tumor mass. The high-grade or poorly differentiated tumors consist mainly of epidermoid cell units and sparsely distributed mucus-forming

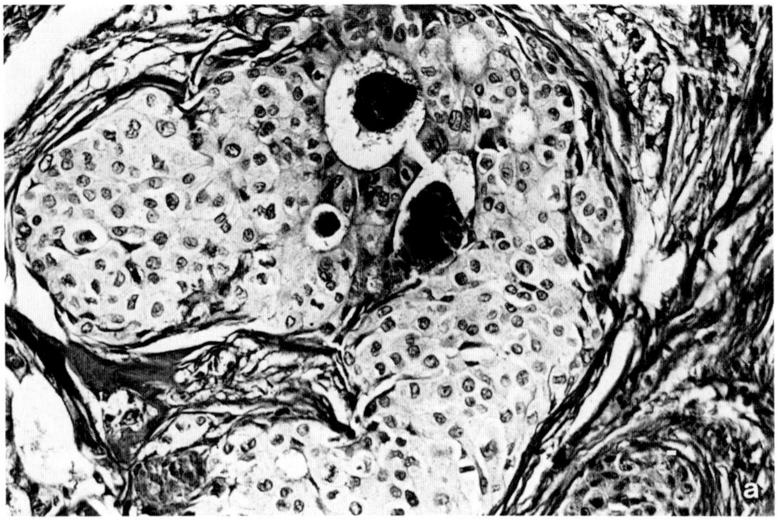

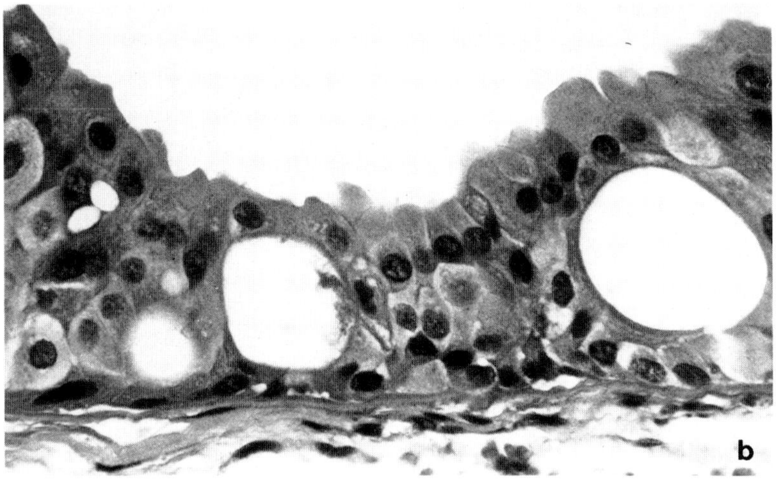

Figure 15.**85** Mucoepidermoid tumor of the parotid gland: **a** Solid epidermoid cell complex with inclusion of mucus-filled microcysts. PAS, 160×. **b** Detail of a section with small mucous cysts between epidermoid cells. H & E, 400×.

cells, constituting at most 10% of the tumor (Figs. 15.**88a, b,** 15.**89a, b**). Tumors demonstrating microcysts and mucus-forming cells that constitute more than 10% of the tumor mass may be classified as intermediate (Haenisch 1979). In our own material, 65% were low-grade tumors and about 17.5% each fell in the intermediate and high-grade categories (Seifert et al 1980). The well-differentiated tumors, including the clear cell and oncocytic variants, have a high 5-year survival of more than 95%, whereas the poorly differentiated tumors have a survival of only 25% (Chomette et al 1982). Poorly differentiated mucoepidermoid tumors that also demonstrate an intense invasive propensity have a particularly poor prognosis (Accetta et al 1984). Despite the high degree of differentiation, 10–40% recur (Eversole 1970, Melrose et al 1973). Metastases contain predominantly epidermoid cell clumps (Saksela et al 1971) (Fig. 15.**90**). Immunocytochemistry (Fig. 15.**5**) confirms that the epidermoid tumor component contains the proliferation antigen TPA localized in the cell membrane and the endoplasmic reticulum; the mucus-forming areas contain tumor-associated CEA (Seifert 1982). From this, it can be concluded that the epidermoid cells form the active proliferative pool in mucoepidermoid tumors.

In our experience, the *prognosis* of mucoepidermoid tumors depends even more on the histologic differentiation than it does for the acinic cell tumor. Whereas the highly differentiated (low-grade) mucoepidermoid tumors should be classified in the group of malignant tumors with a favorable prognosis (group I, page 281ff), the poorly differentiated mucoepidermoid tumors (high-grade type) belong in the unfavorable group III with a 5 year survival of only 40% (Fig. 15.**135**).

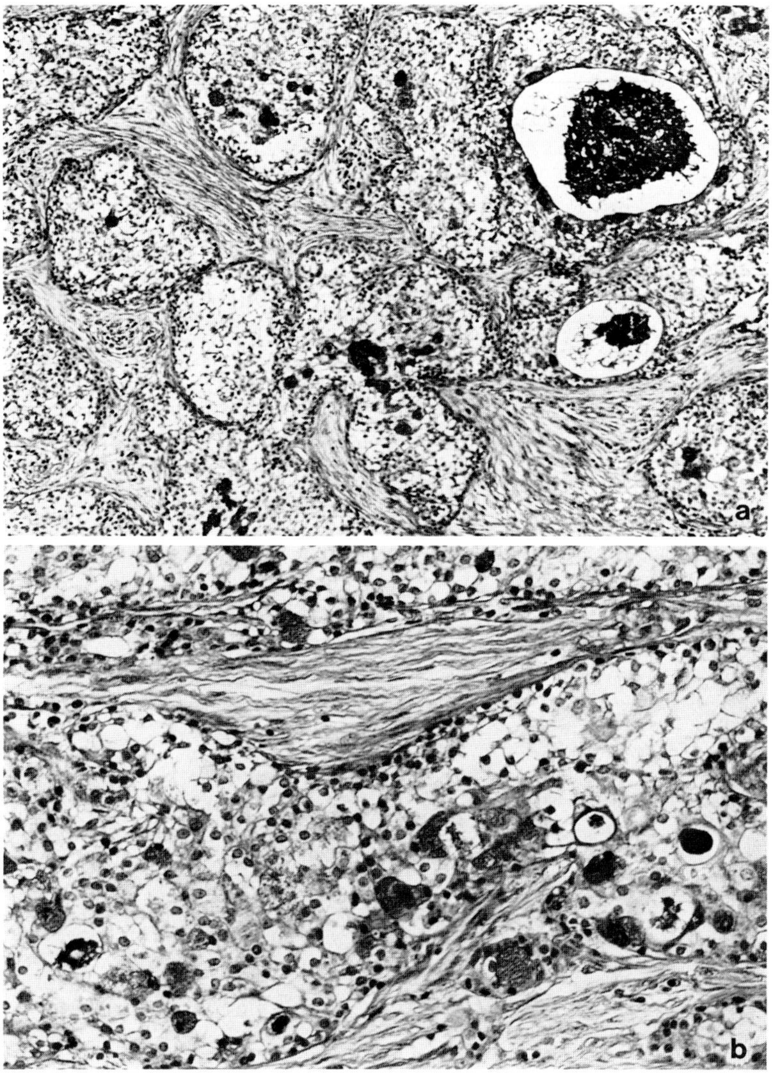

Figure 15.**86** Clear cell variant of a mucoepidermoid tumor of the parotid gland. Mucous cysts and goblet cells between epidermoid clear cell nests. PAS. **a** 63×, **b** 160×.

Differential Diagnosis. Mucoepidermoid tumors must be distinguished from sebaceous tumors, squamous cell carcinoma, and clear cell tumors. The cytology of mucoepidermoid tumors may be confused with that of metaplastic cystadenolymphoma and necrotizing sialometaplasia (page 104ff).

Surgical Treatment. The treatment of a mucoepidermoid tumor is determined by its extent (TNM stage) and by its degree of differentiation. These correlate with each other. Depending on their site, low-grade mucoepidermoid tumors are treated by superficial or total parotidectomy; the facial nerve is preserved or partially resected and reconstructed (group 2 of the treatment schedule in Table 15.11). Total resection of the facial nerve is almost never required for this tumor. However, the surgeon must take care not to carry out an inadequate operation, particularly for a high-grade tumor. Inadequate procedures, such as enucleation of the tumor, considerably worsen the prognosis.

We regard postoperative radiation therapy as unnecessary for low-grade tumors, particularly because mucoepidermoid tumors are, at best, poorly radiosensitive (Jacobsson & Eneroth 1970, Stewart et al 1945).

Surgery for high-grade (poorly differentiated) mucoepidermoid tumors must be radical (groups 2 and 3 of the treatment schedule, Table 15.**11**). This requires a total parotidectomy with partial or complete sacrifice of the facial nerve (group 3 of the treatment schedule), combined with a neck dissection for lymph node metastases. Reconstruction of the facial nerve is indicated if frozen section shows that the margins are clear of tumor. We regard postoperative radiotherapy as being essential for high-grade tumors.

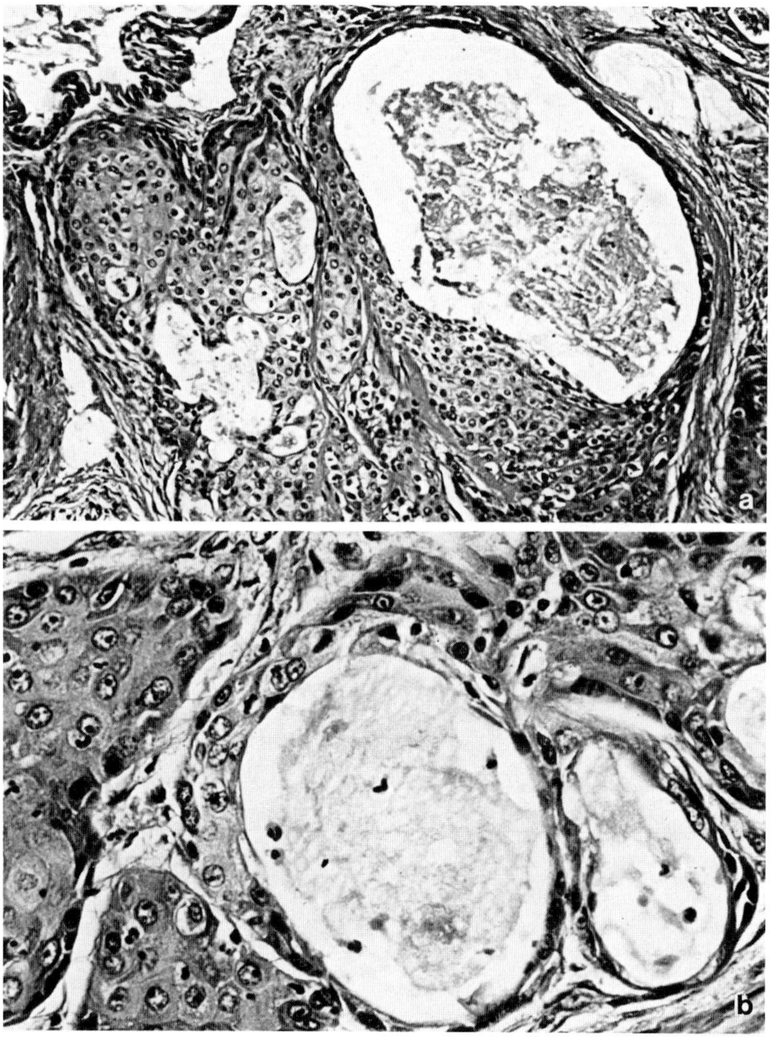

Figure 15.**87** Well-differentiated mucoepidermoid tumor: cysts filled with mucus lying between the epithelial masses. H & E. **a** 160×, **b** 400×.

References

Accetta, P. A., G. F. Gray, R. M. Hunter, L. Rosenfeld: Mucoepidermoid carcinoma of salivary glands. Arch. Path. Lab. Med. 108 (1984) 321

Bhashar, S. N., J. L. Bernier: Mucoepidermoid tumors of major and minor salivary gland. Clinical features, histology, variation, natural history and results of treatment for 144 cases. Cancer (Philad.) 15 (1962) 801

Brocheriou, Cl., M. Seghir: Les tumeurs mucoepidermoides des glandes salivaires. A propos de 30 observations. Rev. Stomat. (Paris) 75 (1974) 1039

Chen, S. Y.: Ultrastructure of mucoepidermoid carcinoma in minor salivary glands. Oral Surg. 47 (1979) 247

Chomette, G., M. Auriol, Y. Tereau, J. M. Vaillant: Les tumeurs mucoepidermoides des glandes salivaires accessoires. Dénombrement. Etude clinico-pathologique, histoenzymologique et ultrastructurale. Ann. Pathol. (1082) 29

Eneroth, C.-M.: Die Klinik der Kopfspeicheldrüsentumoren. Arch. Oto-Rhino-Laryng. 213 (1976) 61

Foote, F. W., E. L. Frazell: Tumours of the major salivary glands. Cancer (Philad.) 6 (1953) 1065

Eversole, L. R.: Mucoepidermoid carcinoma: Review of 815 reported cases. J. Oral Surg. 28 (1970) 490

Eversole, L. R.: Glycoprotein heterogeneity in mucoepidermoid carcinoma. A histochemical evaluation. Arch. Otolaryngol. 96 (1972) 426

Gingell, J. C., T. Beckerman, B. A. Levy, L. A. Snider: Central mucoepidermoid carcinoma. Review of the literature and report of a case associated with an apical periodontal cyst. Oral Surg. 57 (1984) 436

Haenisch, H.: Pathohistologische Subklassifikation der Mukoepidermoidtumoren. Analyse von 61 Fällen. Diss. Hamburg 1979

Healey, E. W., K. H. Perzin, L. Smith: Mucoepidermoid carcinoma of salivary gland origin. Classification, clinical-pathologic correlation, and results of treatment. Cancer (Philad.) 26 (1970) 368

Hübner, G., O. Kleinsasser: Zur Feinstruktur und Genese des Mukoepidermoidtumors der Speicheldrüsen. Virchows Arch. Path. Anat. 349 (1970) 281

Jakobsson, P. A., C.-M. Eneroth: Variations in radiosensitivity of various types of malignant salivary gland tumors. Acta otolaryng., Suppl. 263 (1970) 186

Jakobsson, P. A., C. Blanck, C.-M. Eneroth: Mucoepidermoid carcinoma of the parotid gland. Cancer (Philad.) 22 (1968) 111

Lentrodt, J., G. Hafke: Beitrag zur Klinik und insbesondere zur Dignität der Mukoepidermoidtumoren der Speicheldrüsen. Dtsch. zahnärztl. Z. 29 (1974) 615

Melrose, R. J., A. M. Abrams, F. V. Howell: Mucoepidermoid tumors of the intraoral minor salivary gland: A clinicopathologic study of 54 cases. J. Oral Pathol. 2 (1973) 314

Micheau, C., J. Lacour, J. Genin, J. Bucere: Tumeurs mucoepidermoides de la parotide et de la cavité buccale. Ann. Anat. Path. 17 (1972) 59

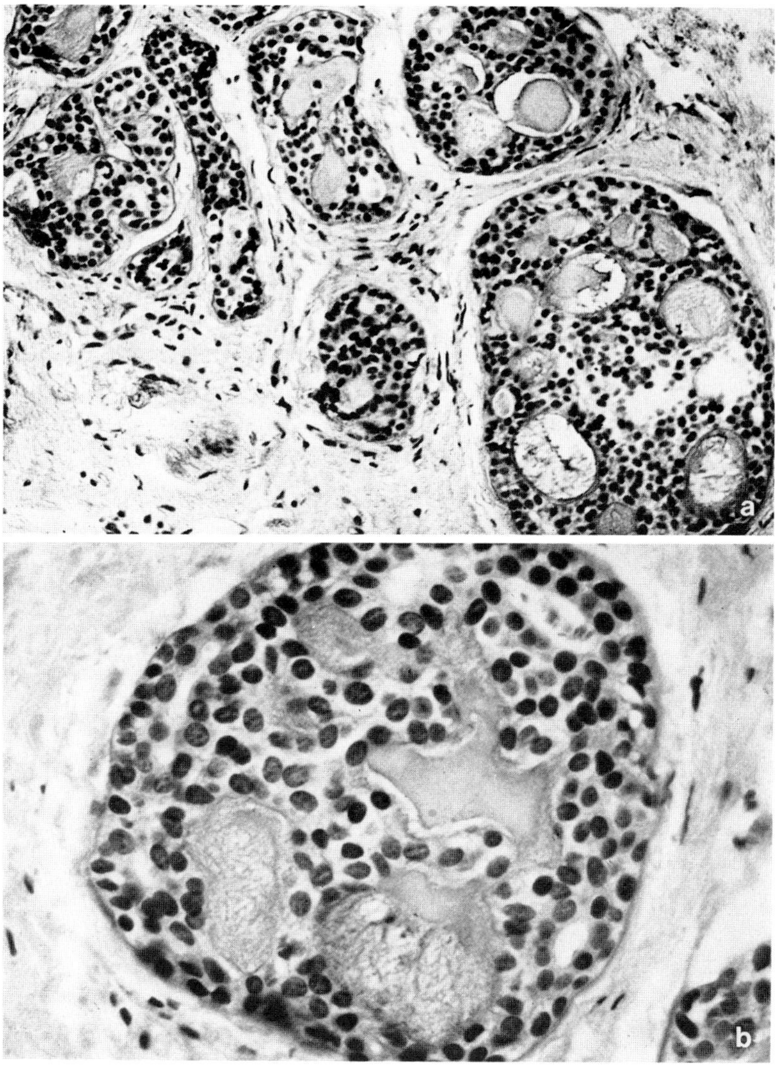

Figure 15.**98** Adenoid cystic carcinoma of the palate: granular-cribriform cell nests. Astra blue. **a** 160×, **b** 400×. (Seifert et al 1980.)

tubules is bounded by multilayered cuboidal cells (Fig. 15.**101**). Circumscribed cribriform areas are also seen occasionally. About 20–30% of adenoid cystic carcinomas show a tubular architecture.

The *solid or basaloid type* (Fig. 15.**102a, b**) is constructed of solid narrow cubical cells that often possess small foci of necrosis in the center of the cell masses. The small basophil epithelial cells are characterized by chromatin-dense cell nuclei that demonstrate numerous mitoses. Cribriform areas with sievelike spaces containing mucoid material are scattered sparsely between the solid islands of cell nests. The solid basaloid architecture comprises 20% of all cases.

There is a positive correlation between the *histologic architecture and the clinical prognosis* (Chilla et al 1980, Chomette et al 1982, Gamel & Font 1982). The tubular type possesses the best prognosis for recurrence or metastases (only 14% after 5 years), the cribriform type, a modest prognosis (36% after 5 years), and the solid basaloid type with necrotic inclusions has the worst prognosis, with 70% of recurrences or metastases after 5 years. The 8-year survival in the tubular type is 100%, in the cribriform type, 67%, and in the solid basaloid type, only 32%. The tubular differentiated adenoid cystic carcinoma of the minor glands has the best prognosis both for survival and recurrence.

Cytology. The characteristics of aspiration cytology are the presence of the epithelial cell cords and spherical secretory particles (Eneroth & Zajieck 1969, Droese 1980, Plakfer & Nosher 1983). The tumor cells have a diploid or tetraploid DNA content (Kino et al 1973).

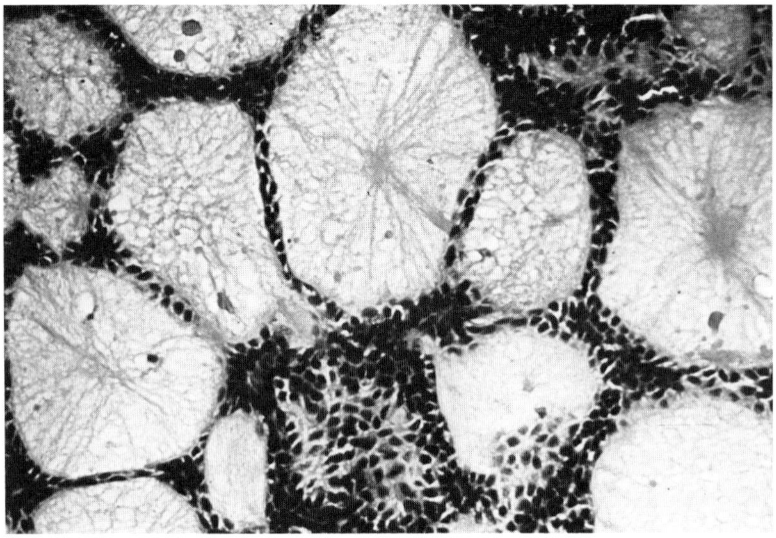

Figure 15.**99** Type 1 adenoid cystic carcinoma. Stellate arrangement of mucoid material in the glandular structures. H & E, 400×.

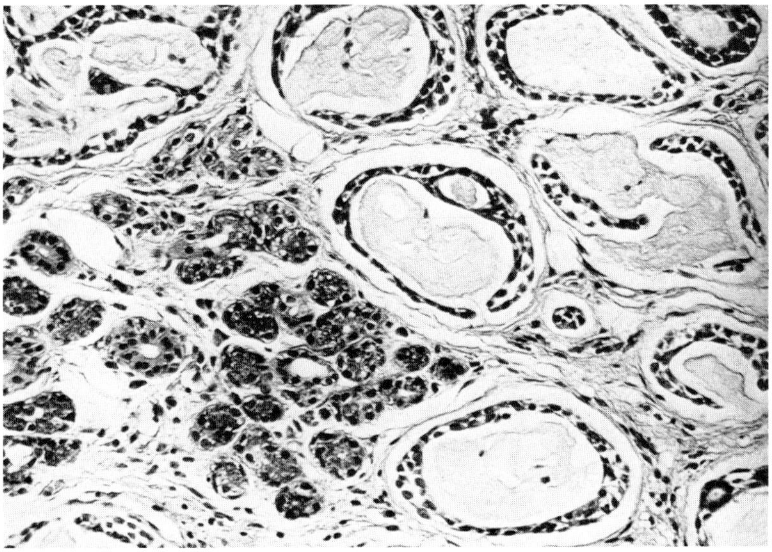

Figure 15.**100** Adenoid cystic carcinoma of the parotid gland, cribriform type: extension within the gland. H & E, 160×.

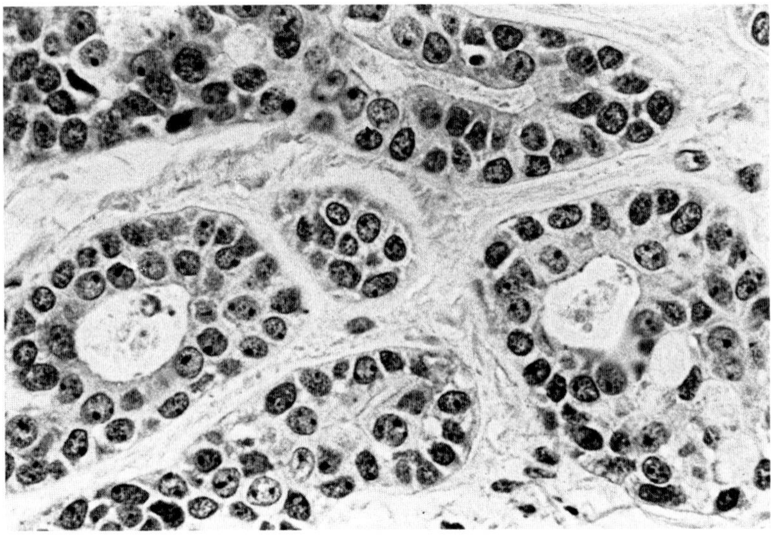

Figure 15.**101** Tubular type of adenoid cystic carcinoma showing limitation of tubules demarcated by multilayered cubical cells. Semithin section. Masson-Goldner, 400×.

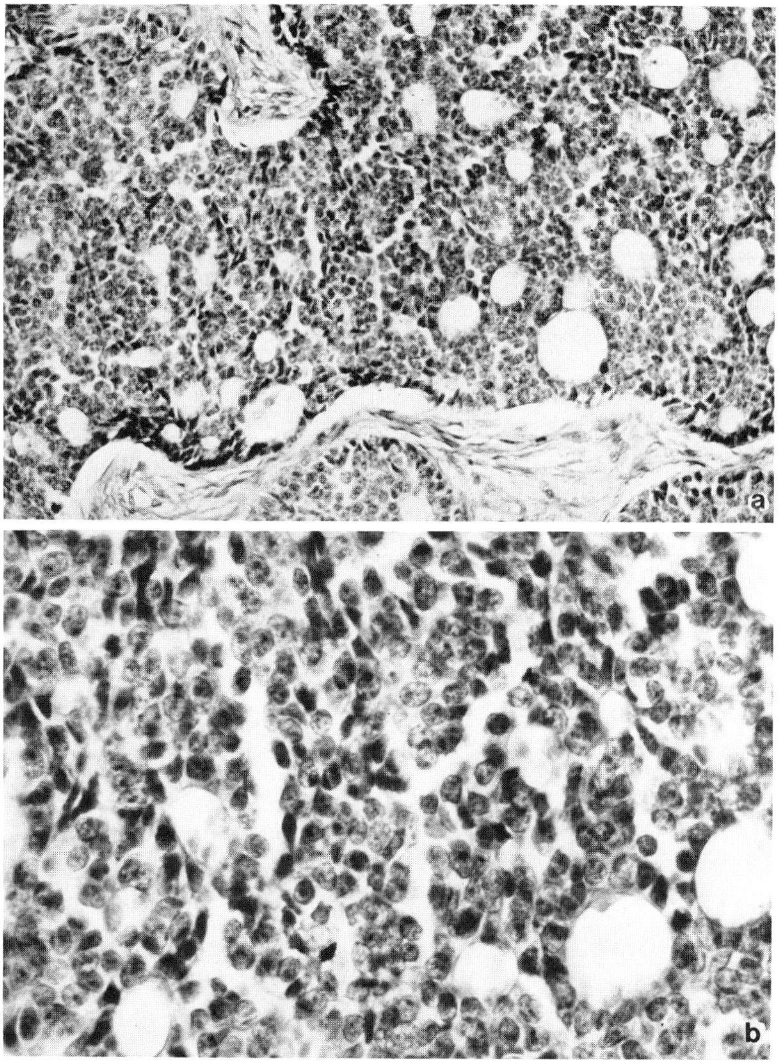

Figure 15.**102** Basaloid type of adenoid cystic carcinoma consisting mainly of solid cell nests with inclusion of occasional cribriform areas. PAS. **a** 160×, **b** 400×. (Seifert et al 1980.)

Electron Microscopy. There are two predominant cell types. The first is a poorly differentiated small ductal epithelium, containing numerous ribosomes and few other cell organelles (Hübner et al 1969, Tandler 1971, Chisholm et al 1975, Murao 1980, Chomette et al 1982, Bienengräber 1981, Lawrence & Mazur 1982). The second is the myoepithelial cell with myofilaments in the cytoplasm. Epidermoid cells are also occasionally seen. The hollow spaces demonstrated by light microscopy are shown to be pseudocysts containing basal membrane substances, mucopolysaccharide particles, and fibrillar substances with inclusions of collagen fiber elements. A true narrow lumen is also developed, bounded by epithelial cells with microvilli and containing epithelial secretory material. All epithelial cell types possess oxidative enzymes. A clear enzyme activity for acid phosphatase, alkaline phosphatase, and leucine aminopeptidase is present at the edge of the pseudocysts. The occurrence of tyrosine-rich crystalloids in an adenoid cystic carcinoma of the palatal glands has been described as a rarity (Gould et al 1983).

Pathogenesis. Adenoid cystic carcinoma arises from the terminal duct system. Cytochemistry demonstrates both keratin and vimentin in the tumor cells (Caselitz et al 1984). There are similarities of cellular architecture between adenoid cystic carcinoma and duct carcinoma (Daley & Dardick 1983). Apparently, the tumor structure represents an intermediate embryonic stage of development of the salivary duct (Chomette et al 1982).

Prognosis. Numerous factors are important, including the site (minor gland tumors have a better prognosis), the histologic type (see before), the size of the primary tumor, and the presence of metastases. Of cases arising in the parotid gland,

10% demonstrate lymph node metastases, compared with 34% of submandibular tumors (Bosch et al 1980, Chilla et al 1981). Blood-borne metastases have a predilection for the lung and liver (Haguenauer et al 1972, Bundi 1974).

Treatment. Although we have managed a relatively large number of patients, we find it very difficult to define the appropriate treatment for an adenoid cystic carcinoma (Chilla et al 1980, 1981). It is possible that surgery or radiotherapy do not influence the patient's ultimate fate, although the outcome depends to some extent on the histologic type (solid, cribriform, or tubular).

The first operation should be as extensive as possible, with a wide margin of healthy tissue, at least to postpone the ultimate outcome. On the other hand, because of the ultimate futility of all treatment, there is an ethical duty to make the remaining life span of the patient as tolerable as possible. The operation should be so designed that severe disfigurement is avoided and that the function of the facial skeleton and the masticatory apparatus are preserved as much as possible. The justification for reconstruction needs careful consideration for each patient.

We have compared our material with that of Blanck et al (1967) with respect to radicality of the procedure. Blanck et al (1967) reported 35 patients from the years 1921–1958, of whom only three treated by a total parotidectomy. In 31 patients, only a local excision was carried out. Of our 20 patients with adenoid cystic carcinoma of the parotid gland, only seven were submitted to a primary total parotidectomy and the others, to a secondary total parotidectomy. However, our determinate survival rate after 5 and 12 years of 76% and 33% compares remarkably well with that of Blanck et al (1967) of 73% and 39%. A primary radical procedure also had almost no effect on the determinate survival rate in our patients. It should be added that the patients referred to us usually have an advanced tumor.

The comparison described here of the Göttingen series with that of Blanck et al (1967) addresses the problem directly. Obviously, the influence of treatment, whether it be a local excision or whether it be extremely radical with a wide margin, is very little. Also, a full tumor dose of radiation therapy postoperatively has not achieved any improvement in survival in our series, rather the reverse (Chilla et al 1981). Blanck et al (1967) claimed a small nonsignificant increase in survival of those patients who underwent postoperative irradiation. In the light of this fact, it must be asked whether the therapeutic goal can best be achieved by long-established procedures, such as radiation and surgery, by extending the radicality of the procedure, or whether the procedure should be less radical, that is, less mutilating, without sacrifice of the facial nerve. We have already emphasized (Chilla et al 1981) that this is a question that is difficult to answer given the rarity of the tumor, the various preconditions, and the protracted course of the disease. The decision must therefore be taken after assessing each individual patient. We have thus developed the following therapeutic concepts:

1. If a patient presents with a small adenoid cystic carcinoma up to 2.5 cm in size, it is to be hoped that the disease can be controlled or at least the patient's fate may be delayed for many years by an extremely comprehensive radical operation. The appropriate surgical strategy is a total parotidectomy with sacrifice of the facial nerve. The surrounding structures (mandible, skin, the mastoid process, the external auditory meatus, the muscles, etc.) must be resected with a wide margin of healthy tissue. We then decide in the individual case whether reconstruction of the facial nerve is justifiable, taking into account the patient's age and social circumstances. Further reconstructive procedures using distant skin flaps (deltopectoral or musculocutaneous flaps) may be undertaken.
2. Extensive surgery is not applicable to those patients whose adenoid cystic carcinomas have already become widely extensive and in whom it is difficult to be certain that a radical excision with a healthy margin can be achieved.
3. Extensive surgery is also not applicable for all recurrences of adenoid cystic carcinoma.

We limit ourselves to a simple excision of the tumor for patients in categories 2 and 3, that is, a total parotidectomy with sacrifice of the facial nerve without reconstruction of the nerve, since this would provide a pathway for spread of the expected recurrence after a purely local circumscribed procedure.

Naturally, the question remains whether the supraradical surgical concept described for the first category could not be restricted to a less mutilating procedure, particularly for an adenoid cystic carcinoma demonstrating a predominantly tubular histologic pattern, which has a clinically less malignant course. This question must be asked repeatedly, because patients with adenoid cystic carcinoma are often still young or at most middle aged and are faced with a long and difficult course.

In our view, it is therefore justifiable in young or middle-aged patients with a small adenoid cystic carcinoma of the tubular type arising from the superficial lobe of the parotid gland to carry out a less extensive operation than outlined in category 1, after careful consideration of all the findings. The concept is thus as follows: a total parotidectomy with sacrifice of individual peripheral branches of the facial nerve, if they lie close to the tumor, with preservation of the trunk of the facial nerve and the unendangered portion of the facial nerve fibers. The fibers that are sacrificed are not reconstructed.

The reader will doubtless sense that we are on very uncertain ground. The surgeon is advised to have close contact with the histopathologist. In the individual case, an attempt should always be made to reach a decision, taking into account the histologic variant (solid, cribriform, or tubular), since these variations have a considerable effect on the prognosis. It requires great experience to reach the correct decision and to adhere to it.

Postoperative high voltage radiotherapy is much discussed. The radiosensitivity of adenoid cystic carcinoma requires further clarification. It is often assumed that adenoid cystic carcinomas are not radiocurable and are thus not radionsensitive (Berdal et al 1970, Conley & Dingman 1974, Eneroth 1977, Grahne et al 1977, Leafstedt et al 1971, Mora et al 1961, Scherer et al 1972). We have been unable to confirm the prolongation of survival in our own patients (Chilla et al 1980, 1981).

The place of polychemotherapy for adenoid cystic carcinoma has not yet been clarified. Occasional reports of regression of the tumor or its metastases after polychemotherapy using 5-fluorouracil, doxorubicin, or mitomycin C require further investigation (Budd & Groppe 1982).

References

Adkins, K. F., T. J. Daley: Elastic tissues in adenoid cystic carcinomas. Oral Surg. 38 (1974) 562

Belson, T. P., R. J. Toohill, S. L. Chobanian, R. H. Lehmann, J. W. Grossman, T. C. Malin: Adenoid cystic carcinoma of the submaxillary gland. Laryngoscope 92 (1982) 497

Berdal, P., D. de Besche, E. Mylius: Cylindroma of salivary glands. Acta Otolaryng. 263 (1970) 170

Bienengräber, V.: Ultrastruktur des adenoid-zystischen Karzinoms als ein Malignitätsmerkmal. Arch. Geschwulstforsch. 51 (1981) 262

Billroth, T.: Beobachtungen über Geschwülste der Speicheldrüsen. Virchows Arch. Path. Anat. 17 (1859) 357

Blanck, C., C.-M. Eneroth, F. Jacobsson, P. Å. Jacobsson: Adenoid cystic carcinoma of the parotid gland. Acta Radiol. 6 (1967) 177

Bosch, A., J. H. Brandenburg, K. W. Gilchrist: Lymph node metastases in adenoid cystic carcinoma of the submaxillary gland. Cancer (Philad.) 45 (1980) 2872

Budd, G. Th., C. W. Groppe: Adenoid cystic carcinoma of the salivary gland. Sustained complete response to chemotherapy. Cancer (Philad.) 51 (1983) 589

Bundi, R. S.: A cribriform cylindroma with metastases. Brit. J. Radiol. 47 (1974) 506

Caselitz, J., J. Becker, G. Seifert, K. Weber, M. Osborn: Coexpression of keratin and vimentin filaments in adenoid cystic carcinomas of salivary glands. Virchows Arch. Path. Anat. 403 (1984) 337

Chilla, R., R. Schrot, U. Eysholdt, M. Droese: Adenoid cystic carcinoma of the head and neck. Controllable and uncontrollable factors in treatment and prognosis. ORL 42 (1980) 346

Chilla, R., R. Schrot, U. Eysholdt, M. Droese: Über die therapeutische Beeinflußbarkeit adenoid-zystischer Karzinome im Parotisbereich. HNO (Berl.) 29 (1981) 118

Chisholm, D. M., J. P. Waterhouse, E. Kraucunas, J. J. Sciubba: A qualitative and quantitative electronmicroscopic study of the structure of the adenoid cystic carcinoma of human minor salivary glands. J. Oral path. 4 (1975) 103

Chomette, G., M. Auriol, P. Tranbaloc, J. M. Vaillant: Adenoid cystic carcinoma of minor salivary glands. Analysis of 86 cases. Clinico-pathological, histoenzymological and ultrastructural studies. Virchows Arch. Path. Anat. 395 (1982) 289

Conley, J., R. L. Dingman: Adenoid cystic carcinoma in the head and neck (cylindroma). Arch. Otolaryng. 100 (1974) 81

Daley, T. D., I. Dardick: An unusual parotid tumor with histogenetic implications for salivary gland neoplasms. Oral Surg. 55 (1983) 374

Droese, M.: Punktionscytologie der Speicheldrüsenerkrankungen. Habil.-Schrift, Göttingen 1980

Eby, L. S., D. S. Johnson, H. W. Baker: Adenoid cystic carcinoma of the head and neck. Cancer (Philad.) 29 (1972) 1160

Eneroth, C.-M.: Die Klinik der Kopfspeicheldrüsentumoren. Arch. Oto-Rhino-Laryng. 213 (1976) 61

Eneroth, C.-M.: Frequenz, Prognose und Behandlung der Speicheldrüsentumoren. HNO-Praxis 2 (1977) 159

Eneroth, C.-M., J. Zajicek: Aspiration biopsy of salivary gland tumors. IV. Morphologic studies on smears and histologic sections from 45 cases of adenoid cystic carcinoma. Acta cytol. (Baltimore) 13 (1969) 59

Eneroth, C.-M., L. Hjertman, G. Moberger, J. Wersall: Ultrastructural characteristics of adenoid cystic carcinoma of salivary glands. Arch. klin. exp. Ohr.-, Nas.- u. Kehlk.-Heilk. 192 (1968) 358

Evans, R. W., A. H. Cruickshank: Epithelial Tumours of the Salivary Glands, Saunders. Philadelphia 1970

Facchetti, F., A. Buffoli, L. Olivetti, E. Viva: Il carcinoma adenoide cistico delle ghiandiole salivari minori. Importanza prognostica di alcuni fattori istopatologici. Pathologica 75 (1983) 725

Gamel, J. W., R. L. Font: Adenoid cystic carcinoma of the lacrimal gland. The clinical significance of a basaloid histologic pattern. Human Pathol. 13 (1982) 219

Gould, A. R., L. V. van Arsdall, S. J. Hinkle, W. R. Harris: Tyrosine-rich crystalloids in adenoid cystic carcinoma: histochemical and ultrastructural observations. J. oral Path. 12 (1983) 478

Grahne, B., C. Laurén, L. Holsti: Carcinoma adenoides cysticum im Kopf- und Halsbereich. HNO-Praxis 2 (1977) 181

Haguenauer, G., J. Kermarec, J. Batime, R. Souquet, J. Pernod: Les metastases pulmonaires des cylindromes des glandes salivaires. A propos de trois observations. Poumon coeur 28 (1972) 389

Hübner, G., O. Kleinsasser, H. J. Klein: Zur Feinstruktur und Genese der Cylindrome der Speicheldrüsen. Weitere Untersuchungen zur Rolle myoepithelial differenzierter Zellen in Speicheldrüsengeschwülsten. Virchows Arch. Path. Anat. 347 (1969) 296

Kino, I., R. M. Richart, R. Lattes: Nuclear DNA in salivary gland tumors. II. Adenoid cystic carcinoma. Arch. Path. (Chic.) 95 (1973) 325

Lawrence, J. B., M. T. Mazur: Adenoid cystic carcinoma: A comparative pathologic study of tumors in salivary gland, breast, lung, and cervix. Human Pathol. 13 (1982) 916

Leafstedt, S. W., J. F. Gaeta, K. Sako, F. C. Marchetta, D. P. Shedd: Adenoid cystic carcinoma of major and minor salivary glands. Amer. J. Surg. 122 (1971) 756

Marsh, W. L., M. Sh. Allen: Adenoid cystic carcinoma. Biologic behavior in 38 patients. Cancer (Philad.) 43 (1979) 1463

Mora, J. J., S. M. Becker, L. W. Brady, V. B. Rambo: Adenoid cystic carcinoma – a clinicopathological study. Cancer 14 (1961) 1235

Murao, T.: Ultrastructure of adenoid cystic carcinoma arising in the salivary gland of a child. Acta Pathol. Jpn. 30 (1980) 631
Nochomovitz, L. E., L. B. Kahn: Adenoid cystic carcinoma of the salivary gland and its histologic variants. A clinicopathologic study of 30 cases. Oral Surg. 44 (1977) 394
Perzin, K. H., P. Gullane, A. C. Clairmont: Adenoid cystic carcinoma arising in salivary glands. A correlation of histologic features and clinical course. Cancer (Philad.) 42 (1978) 265
Plakfer, J., J. L. Nosher: Fine needle aspiration of liver with metastatic adenoid cystic carcinoma. Acta cytol. (Baltimore) 27 (1983) 323
Scherer, E., G. Lehmann, M. John: Beitrag zur Strahlentherapie der Zylindrome im Kopf- und Halsbereich. Strahlentherapie 143 (1972) 361
Seaver, P. R., P. G. Kuehn: Adenoid cystic carcinoma of the salivary glands. A study on ninety-three cases. Amer. J. Surg. 137 (1979) 449
Seifert, G., H. Rieb, K. Donath: Klassifikation der Tumoren der kleinen Speicheldrüsen. Pathohistologische Analyse von 160 Tumoren. Z. Laryng. Rhinol. 59 (1980) 379
Spiro, R. H., A. G. Huvos, E. W. Strong: Adenoid cystic carcinoma of salivary origin. A clinicopathologic study of 242 cases. Amer. J. Surg. 128 (1974) 512
Tandler, B.: Ultrastructure of adenoid cystic carcinomas of salivary gland origin. Lab. Invest. 24 (1971) 504

Adenocarcinoma

Of all carcinomas in the Salivary Tumor Register, 14% were adenocarcinomas (Table 15.**8**). The peak age incidence is in the seventh decade. More than 50% arise in the parotid gland (Fig. 15.**103**), about 10% in the submandibular or sublingual glands, and about 20% in the minor salivary glands (Seifert et al 1980, Crocker et al 1970, Brocheriou et al 1975, Stene & Koppang 1978, Spiro et al 1982). In the minor salivary glands, the palate is the predominant site, followed by the buccal mucosa, the tongue, and the floor of the mouth (David & Buchner 1978, Russell & Nelson 1978, Allen et al 1974. In our series, 65% occurred in women.

Clinical Aspects. Adenocarcinomas resemble other high-grade malignant carcinomas in producing restricted or absent mobility, pain, and invasion of nerves (page 281ff). A preoperative facial paralysis occurred in 40% of our patients. Lymph node metastases are the preferred route of spread for adenocarcinomas (Fig. 15.**104**). In our series, 60% ultimately metastasized to lymph nodes, whereas 30% produced blood-borne metastases, exclusively to the lung.

Histology. Adenocarcinomas form a heterogeneous group with varying degrees of differentiation (Stene & Koppang 1980, Gläser 1979, Blanck 1974, Evans & Cruikshank 1970, Spiro et al 1982). Based on our study of 59 adenocarcinomas (Schulz 1984), three subtypes may be distinguished, depending on the predominant histologic picture: solid, tubular, and papillary adenocarcinoma. The *solid subtype*, which comprises only 5% of these tumors, is marked by moderately differentiated glandular structures with inclusion of occasional trabecular and tubular structures. Mucus formation does not occur. Fifty percent of these patients have lymph node metastases. The *tubular subtype* comprises 50% of all adenocarcinomas (Figs. 15.**105**–15.**108**). The tubular structures resemble primitive ductal structures and may be dilated to form microcysts containing mucous secretion. Lymph node metastases arise in 20% of these patients. Cytochemical reactions are useful in distinguishing metastases from thyroid carcinoma, which they can resemble. The thyroglobulin reaction of this tumor is negative. A *papillary subtype* is found in 30% of cases (Figs. 15.**109,** 15.**110**). The papillary structures are often

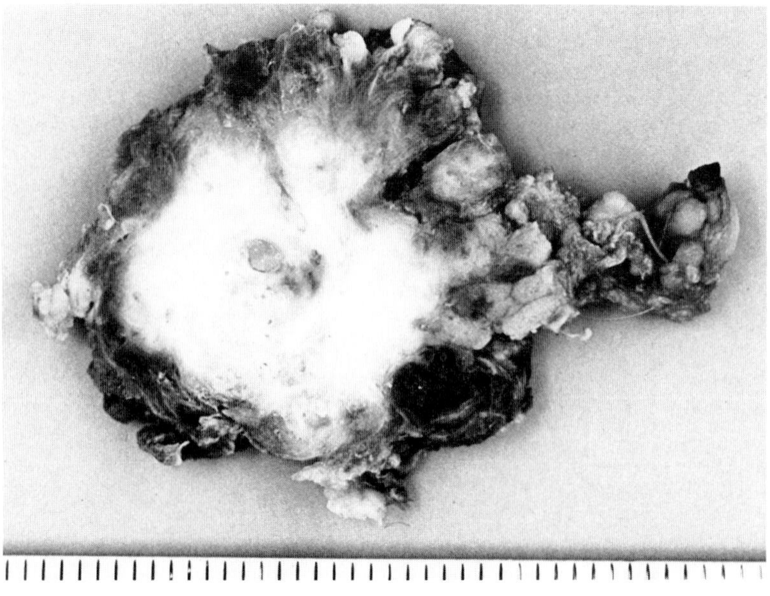

Figure 15.**103** Adenocarcinoma of the parotid gland with extensive destruction of the gland structure.

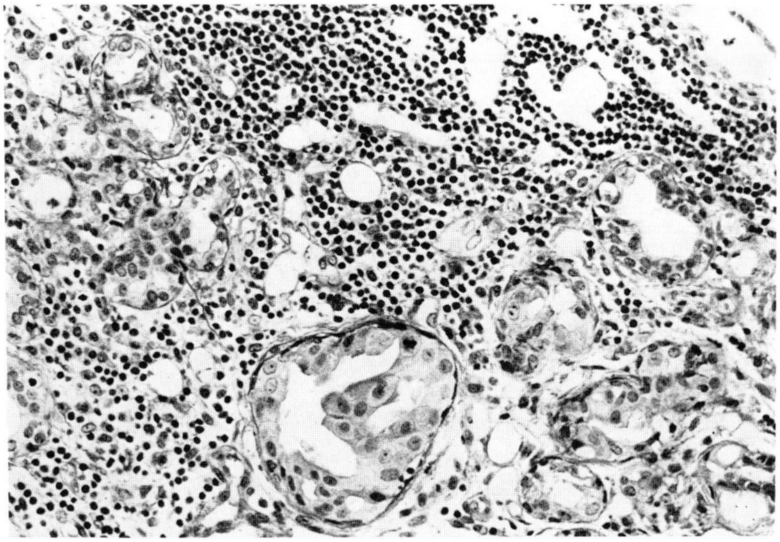

Figure 15.**104** Lymph node metastasis of an adenocarcinoma of the parotid gland. H & E, 160×.

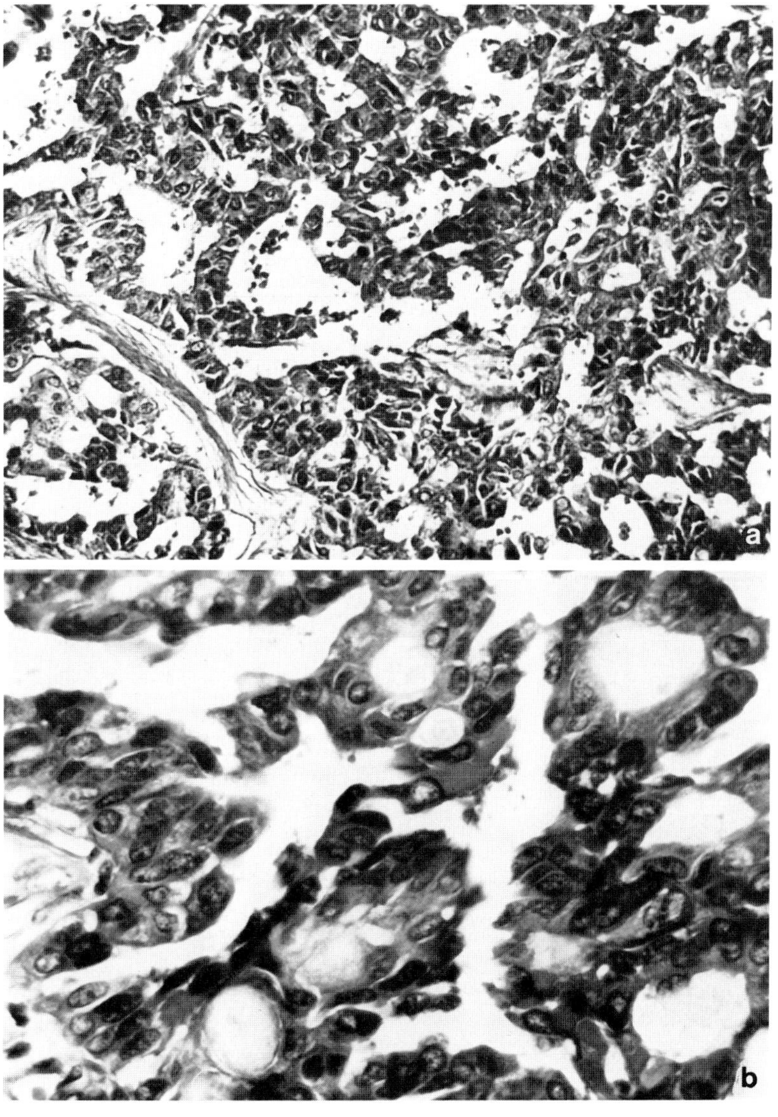

Figure 15.**105** Tubular adenocarcinoma of the parotid gland. H & E. **a** 160×, **b** 400×.

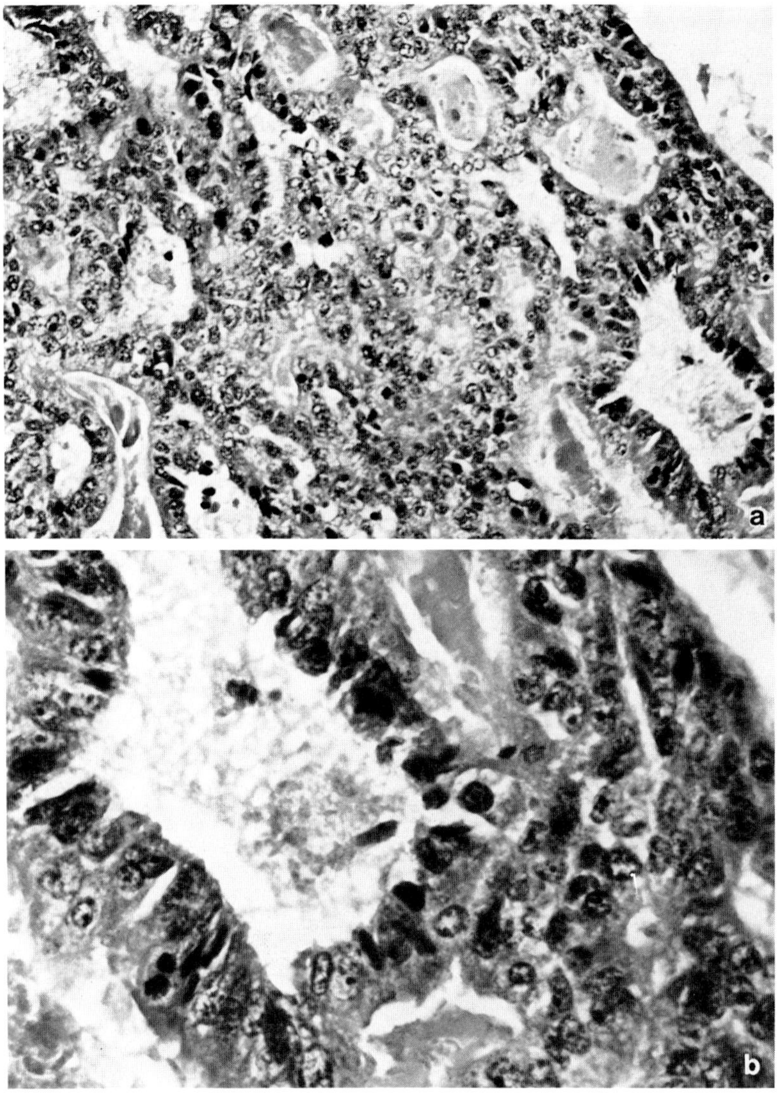

Figure 15.**106** Tubular adenocarcinoma of the apical lingual gland: primitive gland structure with inclusion of microcysts. H & E. **a** 160×, **b** 400×. (Seifert et al 1980.)

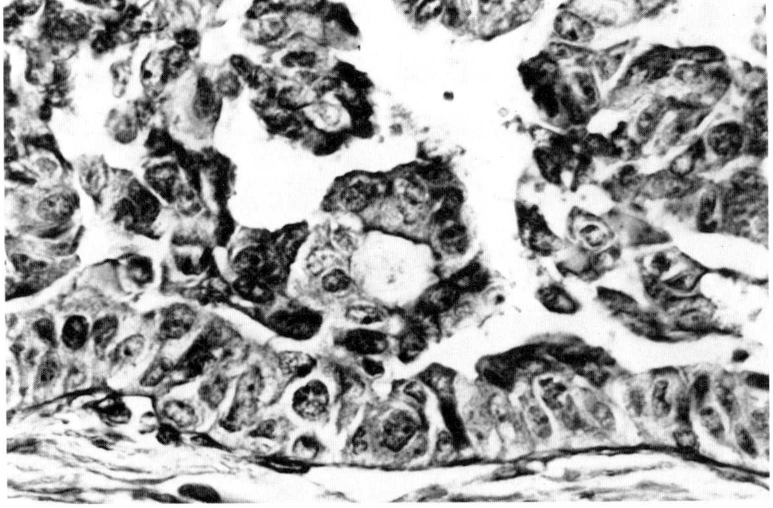

Figure 15.**107** Tubular adenocarcinoma of the parotid gland: irregular arrangement of glandular epithelium with formation of primitive duct structures. PAS, 400×.

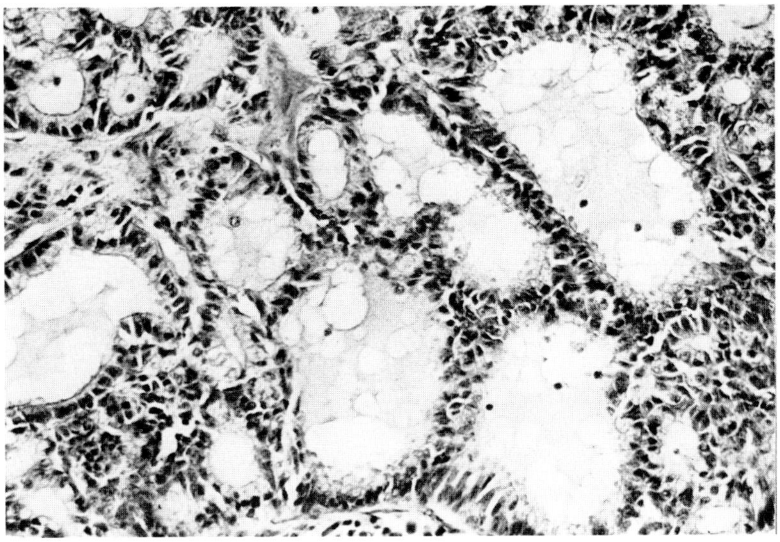

Figure 15.**108** Microcystic relatively well-differentiated adenocarcinoma of the submandibular gland. H & E, 160×.

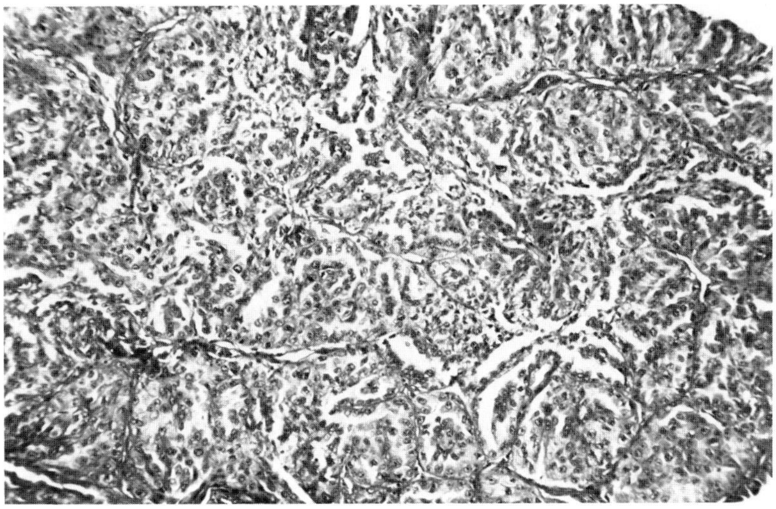

Figure 15.**109** Papillary adenocarcinoma of the parotid gland. H & E, 63×.

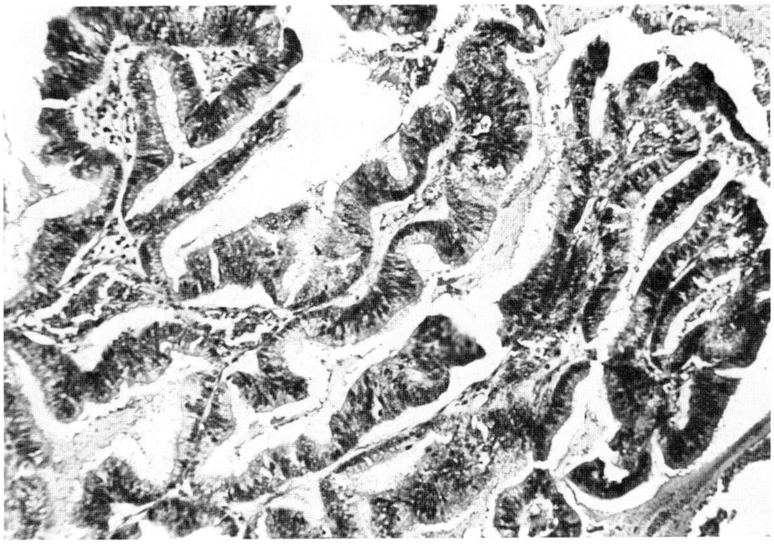

Figure 15.**110** Papillary adenocarcinoma of the parotid gland: formation of papillary structures by multilayered tumor epithelium. H & E, 160×.

accompanied by cysts and formation of mucus. In contrast to the other two subtypes, a papillary adenocarcinoma is more common (45%) outside the parotid gland, particularly in the minor glands. Lymph node metastases occur in 30% of patients. The thyroglobulin reaction to distinguish the tumor from metastases of a papillary thyroid carcinoma was always negative. Formation of acid mucopolysaccharides in the lumen of adenocarcinoma is an important criterion for distinguishing it from other tumors, for example, metastases of thyroid carcinoma (Fisher & Hellström 1962). The cytologic pattern shows a wide spectrum reflecting the varying degrees of differentiation of the duct system. Small undifferentiated polygonal tumor cells and highly differentiated cylindrical cells with some oncocytic differentiation are found. The tumors demonstrate an infiltrative growth pattern, (Blanck et al 1971) often with a marginal cellular stromal reaction. Evans and Batsakis (1984) described an unusual entity of a polymorphic adenocarcinoma of the minor salivary glands with varying degree of differentiation (solid, tubular, papillary, cribriform, and fascicular) and cellular polymorphism (clear cell, oncocytic, or mucinous), but without nuclear atypia or increased frequency of mitoses. The degenerative changes, such as calcification, necrosis, and hyalinization resemble those of an adenocarcinoma of low-grade malignancy. Tumor markers are described on page 173ff. David and Kim (1982) described the electron microscopic features of beta fibrillary bodies (amyloid) in low-grade carcinomas. Dahm and Minderjahn (1983) described the unusual finding of a pseudosarcomatous stromal differentiation. The lobular carcinoma is described on page 274 (Freedman & Lumerman 1983).

Prognosis. Prognosis depends on the size of the tumor and its site. Adenocarcinomas of the minor salivary glands carry a better prognosis with respect to life and frequency of metastases (Stene & Koppang 1980, Spiro et al 1973). A classification of the grade of adenocarcinoma has been suggested (Spiro et al 1982, Blanck 1974), but we were unable to confirm any influence of the differentiation on prognosis in our own series. The patients with adenocarcinoma were all classified in group III (see page 282) with a 5-year survival of about 40%. The adenocarcinomas thus belong to the same prognostic group as poorly differentiated mucoepidermoid tumors and squamous cell carcinomas.

Differential Diagnosis. The typical adenocarcinoma must be distinguished from adenoid cystic carcinoma, from well-differentiated mucoepidermoid tumors, from duct carcinomas, and also from tumor metastases of an nonoral primary carcinoma.

Treatment. Adenocarcinoma is treated by total parotidectomy. In many cases this must be extended to a radical parotidectomy, that is, with the resection of the facial nerve (see page 278). We have used postoperative radiation therapy for all our patients despite the relatively low radiosensitivity of this tumor.

References

Allen, M. S., G. S. Fitz-Hugh, W. L. Marsh: Low-grade papillary adenocarcinoma of the palate. Cancer (Philad.) 33 (1974) 153

Batsakis, J. G., G. R. Pinkston, M. A. Luba, R. M. Byers, J. J. Sciubba, G. W. Tillery: Adenocarcinomas of the oral cavity: a clinicopathologic study of terminal duct carcinomas. J. Laryng. Otol. 97 (1983) 825

Blanck, C.: Carcinoma of the parotid gland. Morphology and long term prognosis. Acta Universitatis Uppsaliensis, Uppsala 1974

Blanck, C., C.-M. Eneroth, P. A. Jakobsson: Mucus-producing adenopapillary (non-epidermoid) carcinoma of the parotid gland. Cancer (Philad.) 28 (1971) 676

Brocheriou, C., P. Laudenbach, A. Bakir, M. Seghir: Les tumeurs des glandes salivaires accessoires. Etude de 116 cas. Arch. Anat. Path. 23 (1975) 117

Crocker, D. J., C. J. Cavalaris, R. Finch: Intraoral minor salivary gland tumours. Report of thirty-eight cases. Oral Surg. 29 (1970) 60

Dahm, H. H., A. Minderjahn: Zur pseudosarkomatösen Differenzierung von Adenokarzinomen der Glandula parotis. Dtsch. Z. Mund-Kiefer-Gesichts-Chir. 7 (1983) 275

David, R., A. Buchner: Amyloid stroma in a tubular carcinoma of palatal salivary gland. A histochemical and ultrastructural study. Cancer (Philad.) 41 (1978) 1836

David, R., K. M. Kim: Beta-fibrillary bodies in low-grade adenocarcinoma of parotid gland. A histochemical and ultrastructural study. Human Pathol. 13 (1982) 1028

Evans, H. L., J. G. Batsakis: Polymorphous low-grade adenocarcinoma of minor salivary glands. A study of 14 cases of a distinctive neoplasm. Cancer (Philad.) 53 (1983) 935

Evans, R. W., A. H. Cruickshank: Epithelial Tumours of the Salivary Glands. Saunders, Philadelphia 1970

Freedman, P. D., H. Lumerman: Lobular carcinoma of intraoral minor salivary gland origin. Report of twelve cases. Oral Surg. 56 (1983) 157

Fisher, E. R., H. R. Hellström: Differential diagnosis of papillary carcinomas of thyroid and salivary gland origin. Amer. J. clin. Path. 37 (1962) 633

Gläser, A.: Geschwülste der Kopfspeicheldrüsen. In Gläser, A.: Klinische Pathologie der Geschwülste, Lieferung 3. Thieme, Leipzig 1979 (S. 85)

Mills, S. E., Th. A. Garland, M. S. Allen jr.: Low-grade papillary adenocarcinoma of palatal salivary gland origin. Amer. J. Surg. Pathol. 8 (1984) 367

Russel, E. A., J. F. Nelson: Adenocarcinoma of the palate. Diagnosis and management. Oral Surg. 45 (1978) 528

Schulz, J. P.: Pathomorphologische Klassifikation der Adenokarzinome der Speicheldrüsen. Analyse von 59 Fällen. Diss. Hamburg 1984

Seifert, G.: Mundhöhle, Mundspeicheldrüsen, Tonsillen und Rachen. In Doerr, W., E. Uehlinger: Spezielle pathologische Anatomie, Bd. 1. Springer, Berlin 1966 (S. 1)

Seifert, G., H. Rieb, K. Donath: Klassifikation der Tumoren der kleinen Speicheldrüsen. Pathohistologische Analyse von 160 Tumoren. Z. Laryng. Rhinol. 59 (1980) 379

Spiro, R. H., A. G. Huvos, E. W. Strong: Adenocarcinoma of salivary origin. Clinicopathologic study of 204 patients. Amer. J. Surg. 144 (1982) 423

Spiro, R. H., L. G. Koss, S. I. Hadju, W. W. Strong: Tumors of minor salivary gland origin. A clinicopathological study of 492 cases. Cancer (Philad.) 31 (1973) 117

Stene, T., St. Koppang: Intraoral adenocarcinomas. J. oral Path. 10 (1981) 216

Squamous Cell Carcinoma

Squamous cell carcinoma can invade the salivary glands either from the skin of from the mucosa (Chapter 18), it can metastasize to the salivary glands (Chapter 17), or it may arise primarily in the gland itself. In all large series, primary squamous cell carcinomas comprise about 10% of all salivary malignancies (Table 15.**8**). Elderly men, with a peak age incidence in the eighth decade, are principally affected. A preoperative facial paralysis occurs in 58% of patients (Table 15.**7**), and this proportion is only exceeded by that in undifferentiated and solid adenoid cystic carcinomas.

The tumor is generally hard, partially or completely fixed, poorly demarcated, and metastasizes early to the cervical lymph nodes. Squamous carcinoma thus lies at the opposite end of the spectrum from adenoid cystic carcinoma, which metastasizes later and then usually by the bloodstream (Figure 15.**111**).

Histology. The tumor architecture largely resembles that of squamous cell carcinoma of other sites (Batsakis et al 1976). The spectrum ranges from highly keratinized, well-differentiated squamous cell carcinomas to moderately or poorly differentiated carcinomas without keratinization (Fig. 15.**112**). The tumor grows rapidly, infiltrates the gland parenchyma, invades the surrounding soft tissues and metastasizes early to lymph nodes.

About 40% of patients have regional lymph node metastases (Gläser 1979). Blood-borne metastases are less common. The recurrence rate is more than 50%, and the 5-year survival is 20–30%.

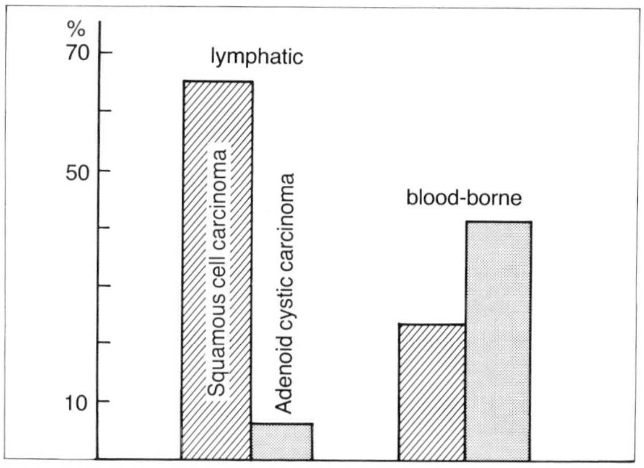

Figure 15.**111** Frequency of lymphatic and blood-borne metastases in squamous cell carcinoma and adenoid cystic carcinoma. The proportions are based on the patients seen in the Göttingen Clinic between 1965 and 1975.

Pathogenesis. The tumor takes origin from the larger ducts, which often demonstrate squamous metaplasia (page 107). The high glycosaminoglycan content of the squamous carcinoma (Takeuchi et al 1981) is also evidence of origin from the duct system. In tissue culture, the tumor cells demonstrate good differentiation with tonofilaments, desmosomes, and synthesis of large amounts of glycosaminoglycans. The glycosamine content is higher than in other salivary gland tumors, such as pleomorphic adenoma and adenoid cystic carcinoma.

Differential Diagnosis. Squamous cell carcinoma must be differentiated from poorly differentiated mucoepidermoid tumors, carcinoma ex pleomor-

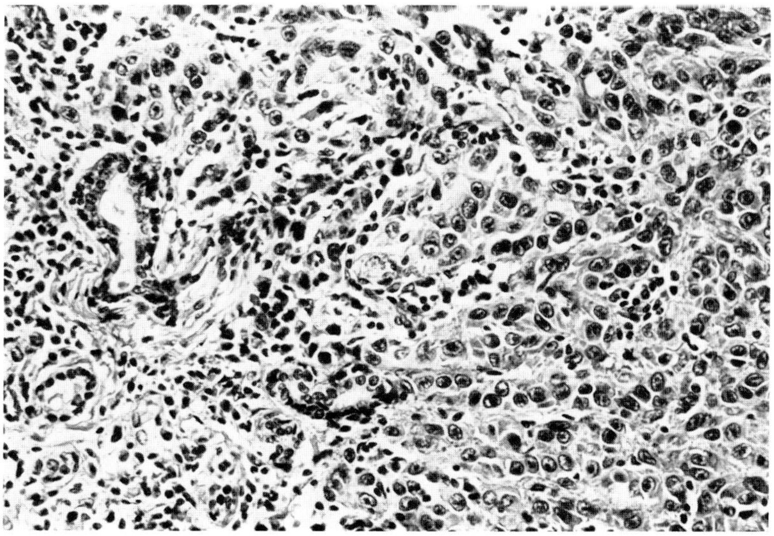

Figure 15.**112** Undifferentiated nonkeratinizing squamous cell carcinoma of the parotid gland: destruction of the glandular tissue. H & E, 160×.

phic adenoma, and from metastases of other primary extraglandular squamous cell carcinomas. The squamous cell carcinoma belongs to group III with respect to prognosis, that is, with a 5-year survival of 40% (page 282). It is thus in the group of tumors with the second worst prognosis.

Treatment. Treatment consists usually of radical parotidectomy, combined, if necessary, with radical neck dissection. The surgeon may elect to preserve the facial nerve or at least some of its branches depending on the site of the tumor and the age of the patient. Since the patients are often old and in poor general condition, the extent of the procedure must be compromised more often than for other salivary malignancies. This applies also to the various techniques for reconstruction of the facial nerve which we have now abandoned in favour of other cosmetic and functional procedures such as tarsorrhaphy and masseteric graft which achieves the required result more quickly. All squamous cell carcinomas should be submitted to postoperative radiation therapy.

References

Batsakis, J. G., K. D. Macclatchea, M. Johns, J. Regazi: Primary squamous cell carcinoma of the parotid gland. Arch. Otolaryng. 102 (1076) 355

Gläser, A.: Geschwülste der Kopfspeicheldrüsen. In Gläser, A.: Klinische Pathologie der Geschwülste, Lieferung 3. Thieme, Leipzig 1979 (S. 85)

Takeuchi, J., M. Sobue, E. Sato, M. Yoshida, N. Uchibori, K. Miura: A high level of glycosaminoglycan-synthesis of squamous cell carcinoma of the parotid gland. Cancer (Philad.) 47 (1981) 2030

Carcinoma ex Pleomorphic Adenoma

Definition. The definition proposed by WHO of “carcinoma in a pleomorphic adenoma” (Thackray & Sobin 1972) expresses more clearly than the old term “malignant transformation of a mixed tumor” the fact that a carcinoma is present in addition to the pleomorphic adenoma and that the carcinoma has developed within a preexisting adenoma. A carcinoma in a pleomorphic adenoma thus embraces the situation, in which a second tumor with all the criteria of malignancy develops in a pleomorphic adenoma that is usually longstanding. The criteria of malignancy include the cytologic and histologic characteristics of anaplasia, abnormal mitoses, infiltration, a progressive course, and metastases (Kleinsasser & Klein 1968, Moberger & Eneroth 1968, Eneroth et al 1968, Koblin & Blessing 1972, Eneroth & Zetterberg 1974, Micheau et al 1973, Heckmayr & Seifert 1977, Grymer et al 1982).

Clinical Aspects. The typical history is of sudden growth of a pleomorphic adenoma or of a recurrent tumor. The tumor is often very large when treatment is initiated and demonstrates reduced mobility. The development of facial paralysis, not due to a previous operation, is a warning signal. This sign was present in 36% of our patients before operation and had often led the patient to his doctor. Also, 50% of our patients developed lymph node metastases (Table 15.**9**) closely associated with local recurrence of tumor (Fig. 15.**70**), and 20% had in addition blood-borne metastases to the lungs. Carcinoma ex pleomorphic adenoma belongs with undifferentiated carcinoma in group IV (page 282), with a 5-year survival rate of about 25%.

Carcinoma ex pleomorphic adenoma constitutes 3–4% of salivary tumors in all large series (Eneroth et al 1968, Seifert & Donath 1976). In our series of patients operated on for a pleomorphic adenoma, 5.5% had a carcinoma ex pleomorphic adenoma, compared with 3% in Eneroth's series (1965). This difference may be due to the fact that a quarter of our patients are referred for a recurrent tumor. The peak age incidence lies in the seventh to eighth decades, that is, one to two decades older than for benign pleomorphic adenoma (Seifert et al 1977). The tumor affects men and women equally.

Table 15.**9** Lymph Node and Distant Metastases of Malignant Salivary Tumors (Göttingen Series 1965–1975). The percentage Figures Relate to the Entire Course of the Disease of All Patients in Each Tumor Group

Tumor Type	Lymph Node Metastases	Distant Metastases
Acinic cell tumor		
Well differentiated	36	0
Poorly differentiated	50	27
Adenocarcinoma	62	29
Adenoid cystic carcinoma		
Tubular	0	36
Cribriform	4	58
Solid	33	67
Mucoepidermoid tumor		
Well differentiated	0	0
Poorly differentiated	50	25
Carcinoma ex pleomorphic adenoma	57	22
Squamous cell carcinoma	65	23
Duct carcinoma	43	14
Undifferentiated carcinoma	64	21

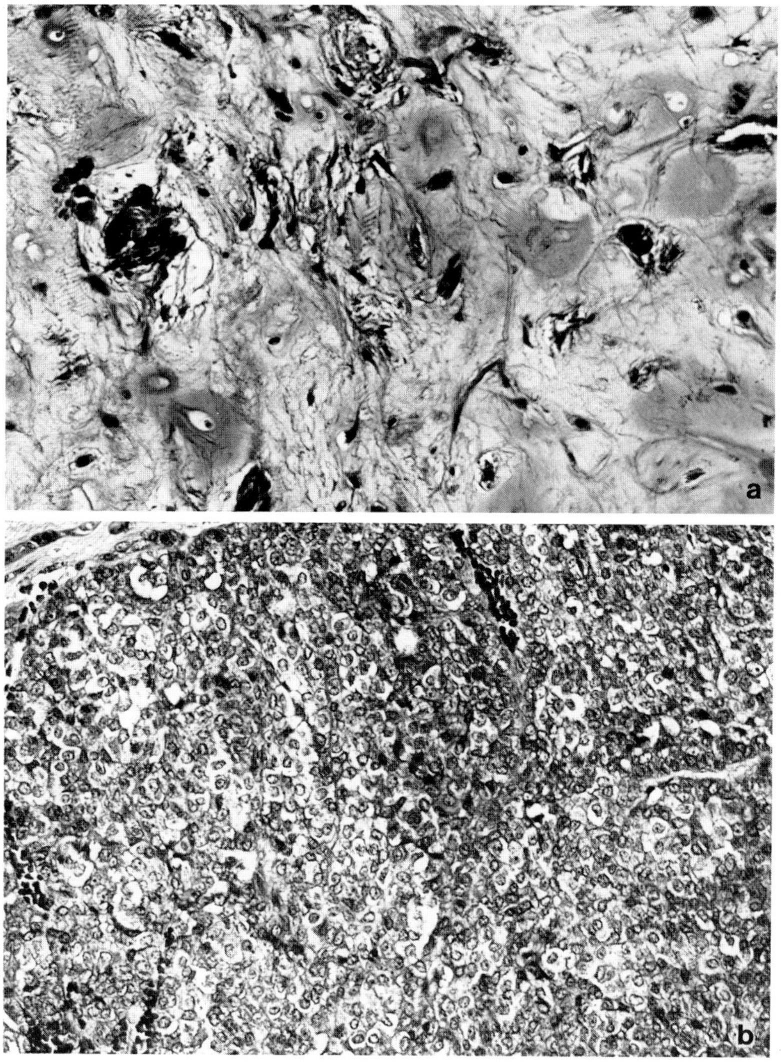

Figure 15.**113** Undifferentiated solid carcinoma in a pleomorphic adenoma of the palate: **a** Remnants of pleomorphic adenoma. **b** Solid carcinoma. H & E. **a, b** 160×.

Eighty percent of these tumors lie in the parotid gland, 10% in the submandibular gland, and 10% in the minor glands, particularly the palatal glands.

Histopathology. Several different types of carcinoma may be distinguished in carcinoma ex pleomorphic adenoma (Seifert et al 1977, Nagao et al 1981, Kleinsasser & Klein 1968, Spiro et al 1977, Saksela et al 1970, LiVolsi & Perzin 1977). All forms of epithelial tumors are observed with the exception of acinic cell tumors. The most frequent are undifferentiated carcinomas, forming more than 30% (Figs. 15.**113**–15.**115**), and adenocarcinoma, forming more than 25% (Figs. 15.**116a, b,** 15.**117a, b**).

Mucoepidermoid tumors (Fig. 15.**118a, b**), adenoid cystic carcinomas (Figs. 15.**119a, b** 15.**120a, b**) and squamous cell carcinoma (Fig. 15.**121a, b**) form 10% each (Seifert et al 1977). If one compares the frequency of specific forms of carcinoma arising in a pleomorphic adenoma with the frequency of carcinoma in the salivary glands without a preexisting pleomorphic adenoma, it appears that mucoepidermoid carcinoma and adenoid cystic carcinoma are less common than in the entire collection of salivary carcinomas, whereas adenocarcinoma and undifferentiated carcinomas are more common. Adenocarcinomas and undifferentiated carcinomas carry a worse prognosis with respect to frequency of recurrence and metastases (Figs. 15.**122,** 15.**123a, b**) and tumor progression. Occasionally, different patterns may be seen within the same tumor, for example, adenocarcinoma with mucoepidermoid tumor, or squamous cell carcinoma and adenocarcinoma (Fig. 15.**124a, b**). Carcinosarcoma is rarer.

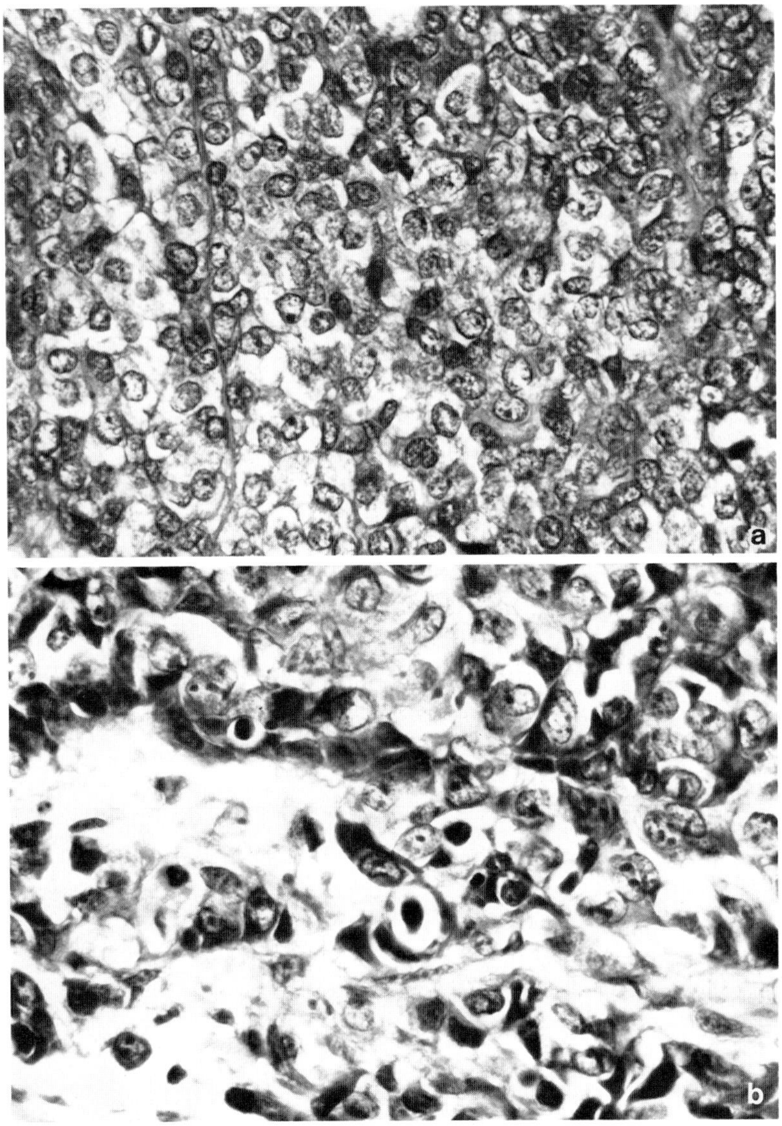

Figure 15.**114** Undifferentiated solid carcinoma in a pleomorphic adenoma: **a** A section from 15.**113**. **b** Undifferentiated carcinoma in a pleomorphic adenoma. H & E. **a**, **b** 400×.

Electron Microscopy. The epithelial structures, such as undifferentiated duct epithelium, immature myoepithelial cells, and epidermoid cells, resemble those of pleomorphic adenoma (Nagao 1981). A further peculiarity is characteristic of the *stromal component* of the preexisting pleomorphic adenoma. In pleomorphic adenomas without secondary carcinoma, the subtype poor in stroma forms 15% (page 184), but in the carcinoma group, almost 50%. From this, it follows that pleomorphic adenomas poor in stroma should be followed up carefully, for the possible development of a secondary carcinoma.

The *frequency of malignancy* shows a correlation between the length of history of the pleomorphic adenoma and the development of a carcinoma (Eneroth 1976). The risk of developing malignancy is only about 1.6% up to 5 years, but increases to 9.6% after more than 15 years.

In 87% of our patients, the carcinoma only developed after one or more recurrences of a benign pleomorphic adenoma. The average latent interval was 16 years. Only 13% arose in patients who had not previously been operated on for a pleomorphic adenoma, and the average life span of the tumor was 7 years.

As a pleomorphic adenoma ages, the number of *tetraploid cells* increases (Eneroth & Zetterberg 1974). Investigations of the malignant transformation of cells in pleomorphic adenoma by DNA flow cytophotometry produce similar results (Thorud et al 1981). The analysis was carried out on fine needle aspirates. This finding is evidence that a new cell population can develop in a pre-

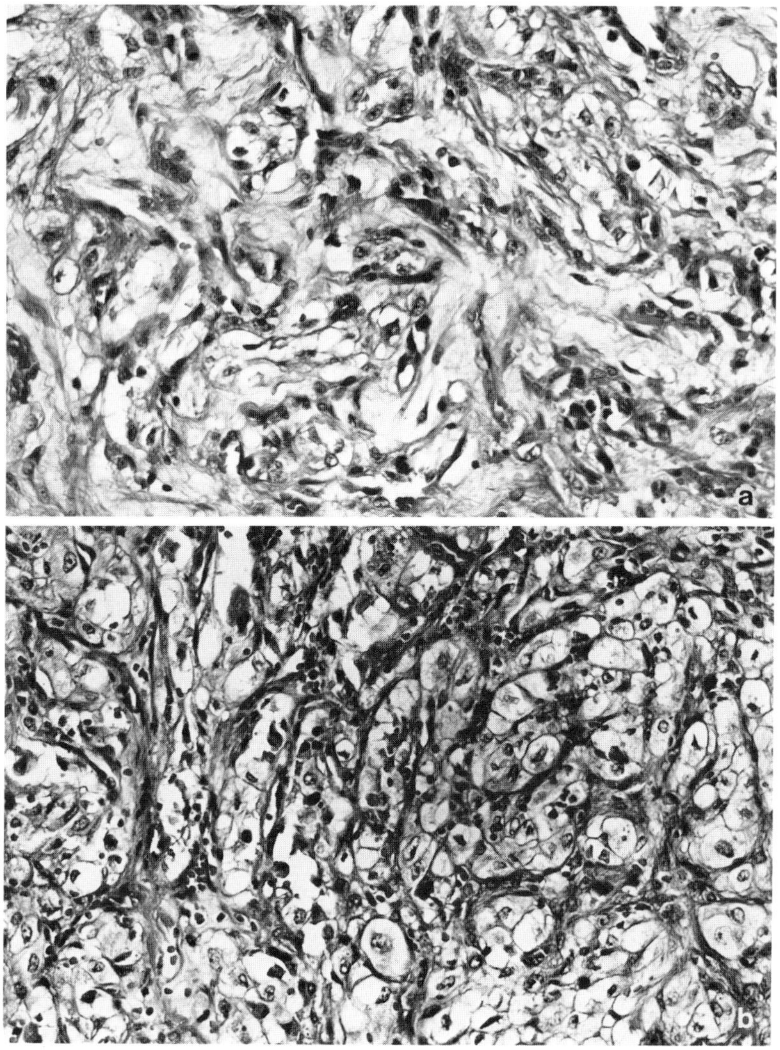

Figure 15.**115** Undifferentiated clear cell carcinoma in a pleomorphic adenoma in the parotid gland: **a** Remnants of the pleomorphic adenoma. **b** Clear cell carcinoma. H & E. **a**, **b** 160×.

existing pleomorphic adenoma with increasing age, which finally can lead to the development of a secondary carcinoma in a pleomorphic adenoma. The size of the tumor also plays a role: if the diameter of the tumor exceeds 5 cm, the chance of developing a carcinoma increases sharply (Nagao et al 1981). Carcinomas are also said to arise more frequently in deep lobe tumors (Spiro et al 1977).

The term *carcinoma in situ* in pleomorphic adenoma requires specific interpretation (LiVolsi & Perzin 1977). This term indicates that tumor areas in a pleomorphic adenoma are characterized by pronounced cellular atypia and proliferative activity with increased mitoses, but the tumor has not transgressed the boundaries of a preexisting pleomorphic adenoma and therefore does not demonstrate infiltration of the surrounding tissue. This indicates that this type of focal and circumscribed neoplastic proliferation may be removed completely by surgery. Since neither lymph node nor blood-borne metastases are present at this stage, removal achieves the same favorable prognosis achieved by early treatment of other forms of carcinoma in situ. Extended radical surgery with radical neck dissection is not indicated for this type of tumor.

Treatment. Depending on the site of the tumor, treatment of a carcinoma in a pleomorphic adenoma consists of radical parotidectomy, if necessary combined with neck dissection, or extended surgery, including removal of the ascending ramus of the mandible and of the mastoid process with postoperative radiation therapy. Reconstruction of the facial nerve is seldom indicated because of the poor prognosis of this tumor. Reconstructive procedures for cosmetic and functional rehabilitation present a compromise that rapidly renders the results of facial nerve paralysis tolerable for the patient.

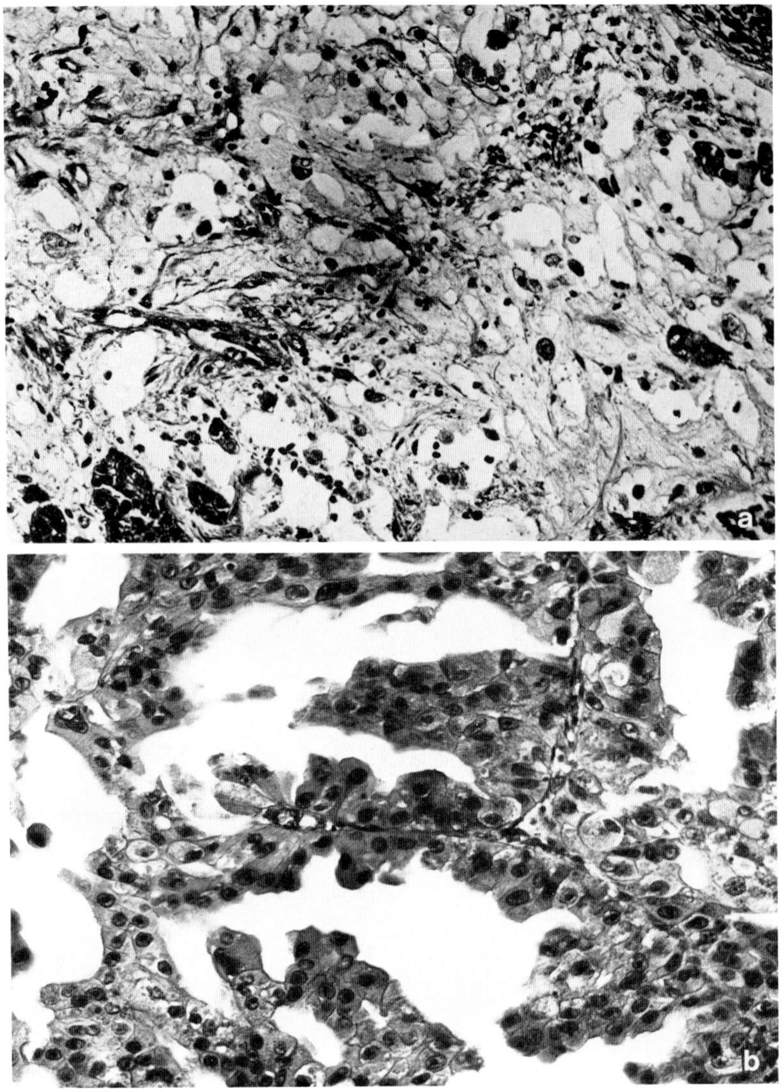

Figure 15.**116** Moderately differentiated partially papillary adenocarcinoma in a pleomorphic adenoma of the parotid: **a** Remnants of the pleomorphic adenoma. **b** Microcystic tumor structures. H & E. **a**, **b** 160×.

References

Eneroth, C.-M.: Mixed tumors of major salivary glands. Prognostic role of capsular structure. Ann. Otol. 74 (1965) 944

Eneroth, C.-M.: Die Klinik der Kopfspeicheldrüsentumoren. Arch. Oto-Rhino-Laryng. 213 (1976) 61

Eneroth, C.-M., C. Blanck, P. Ä. Jakobsson: Carcinoma in pleomorphic adenoma of the parotid gland. Acta oto-laryng. 66 (1968) 477

Eneroth, C.-M., A. Zetterberg: Microspectrophotometric DNA analysis of malignant salivary gland tumours. Acta oto-laryng. 77 (1974) 289

Grymer, L. F., K. Joergensen, C. Lund: Carcinoma in a calcified pleomorphic adenoma of the submandibular gland. J. Laryng. 96 (1982) 373

Heckmayr, M., G. Seifert: Metastasen bei pleomorphen Speicheldrüsenadenomen. Z. Laryng. Rhinol. 56 (1977) 19

Kleinsasser, O., H. J. Klein: Sekundäre Carcinome in primär gutartigen Mischtumoren der Speicheldrüsen. Arch. klin. exp. Ohr.-, Nas.- u. Kehlk.-Heilk. 190 (1968) 272

Koblin, I., M. H. Blessing: Die malignen Mischtumoren der großen und kleinen Speicheldrüsen. Dtsch. Z. Zahn-, Mund- u. Kieferheilk. 58 (1972) 225

LiVolsi, V. A., K. H. Perzin: Malignant mixed tumors arising in salivary glands. I. Carcinomas arising in benign mixed tumors: A clinicopathologic study. Cancer (Philad.) 39 (1977) 2209

Micheau, C., J. Lacour, R. Gerard-Marchant: Association tumeur mixte-epithelioma de la parotide. A propos de 23 cas. Arch. Anat. Path. 21 (1973) 251

Moberger, J. G., C.-M. Eneroth: Malignant mixed tumors of the major salivary glands. Special reference to the histological structure in metastases. Cancer (Philad.) 21 (1968) 1198

Nagao, K., O. Matsuzaki, H. Saiga, I. Sugano, H. Shigematsu, T. Kaneko, T. Katoh, T. Kitamura: Histopathologic studies on carcinoma in pleomorphic adenoma of the parotid gland. Cancer (Philad.) 48 (1981) 113

Saksela, E., J. Tarkkanen, A. Kohonen: The malignancy of mixed tumors of the parotid gland. A clinicopathological analysis of 70 cases. Acta oto-laryng. 70 (1970) 62

Seifert, G., K. Donath: Die Morphologie der Speicheldrüsenerkrankungen. Arch. Oto-Rhino-Laryng. 213 (1976) 111

Seifert, G., J. Schulz, K. Donath: Pathomorphologische Subklassifikation der Carcinome in pleomorphen Speicheldrüsenadenomen. Analyse von 38 Fällen. HNO (Berl.) 25 (1977) 337

Spiro, R. H., A. G. Huvos, E. W. Strong: Malignant mixed tumor of salivary origin. A clinicopathologic study of 146 cases. Cancer (Philad.) 39 (1977) 388

Thackray, A. C., L. H. Sobin: Histological Typing of Salivary Gland Tumours. World Health Organization. Geneva 1972

Thorud, E., E. A. Rolstad, F. Lexow: Malignancy in pleomorphic adenomas of the parotid gland. DNA flow cytometric analysis of the fine needle aspiration biopsies. Acta path. microbiol. immunol. scand. Sect A. Suppl. 274 (1981) 458

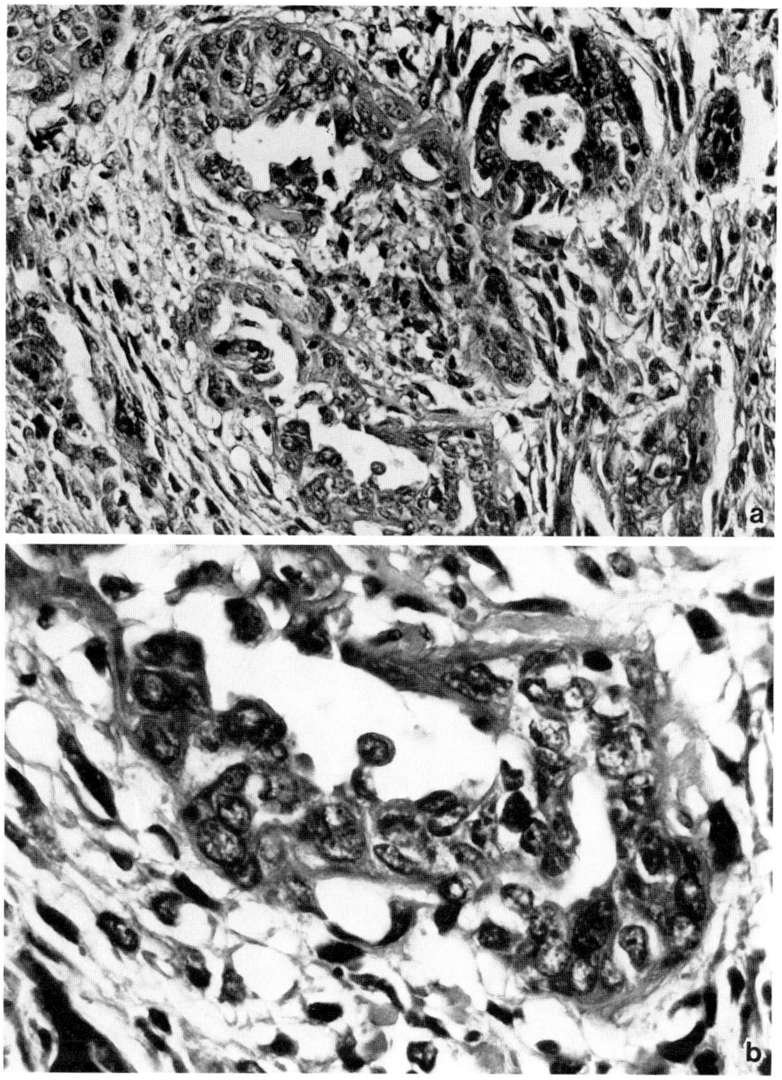

Figure 15.**117** Undifferentiated carcinoma in a pleomorphic adenoma of the parotid gland. H & E. **a** 160×, **b** 400×.

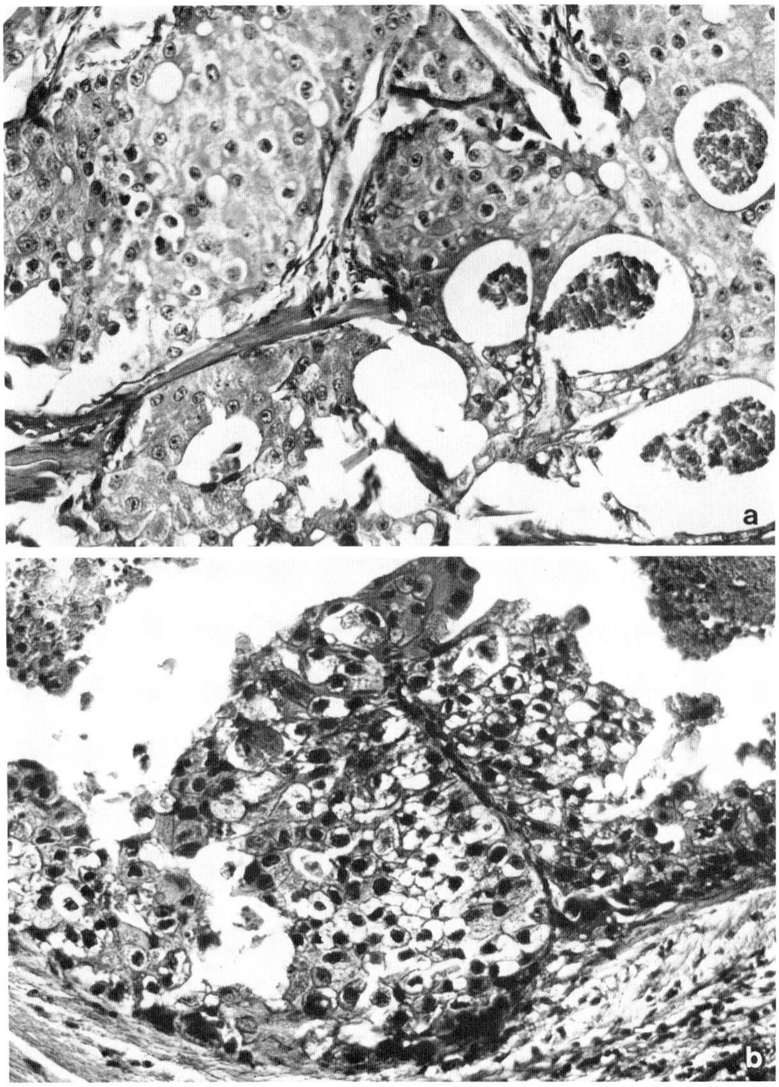

Figure 15.**118** Moderately differentiated mucoepidermoid tumor in a pleomorphic parotid adenoma: **a** Epidermoid masses with inclusions of microcysts. **b** Epidermoid partially clear cell nests with inclusion of mucus-forming cells. H & E. **a**, **b** 160×.

Figure 15.**119** Basaloid adenoid cystic carcinoma in a pleomorphic parotid adenoma: **a** Remnants of the pleomorphic adenoma. **b** Invasive basaloid cell nests with perineural spread. H & E. **a**, **b** 160×.

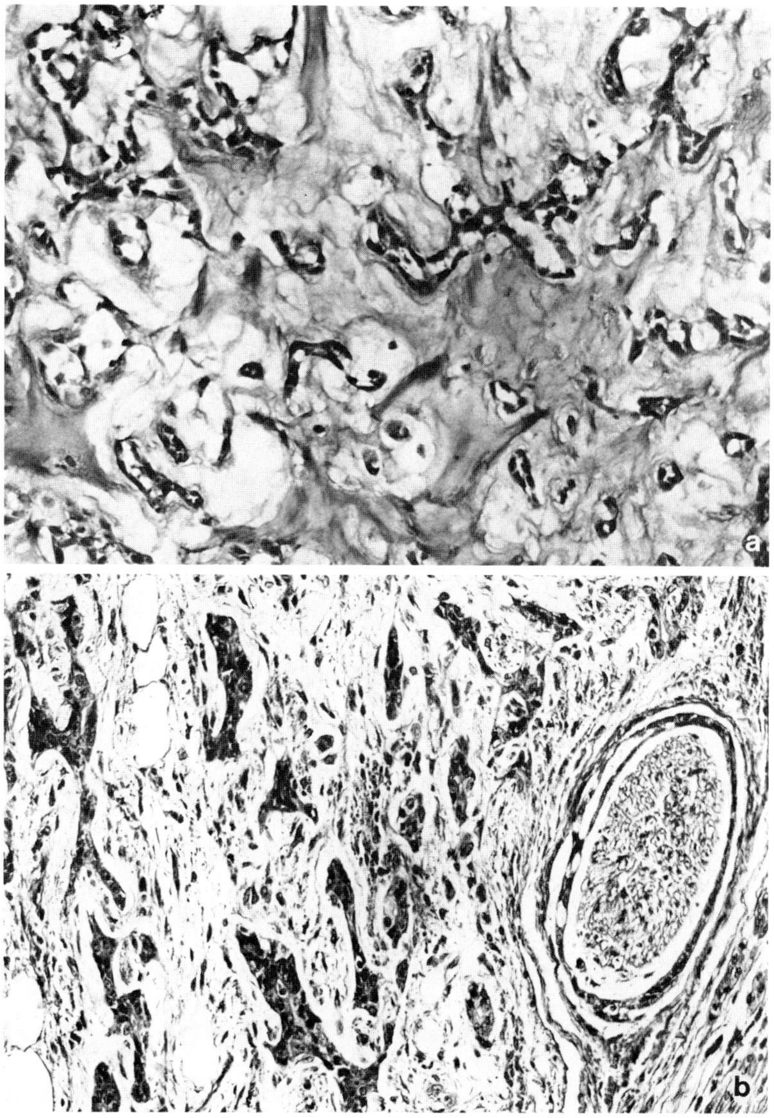

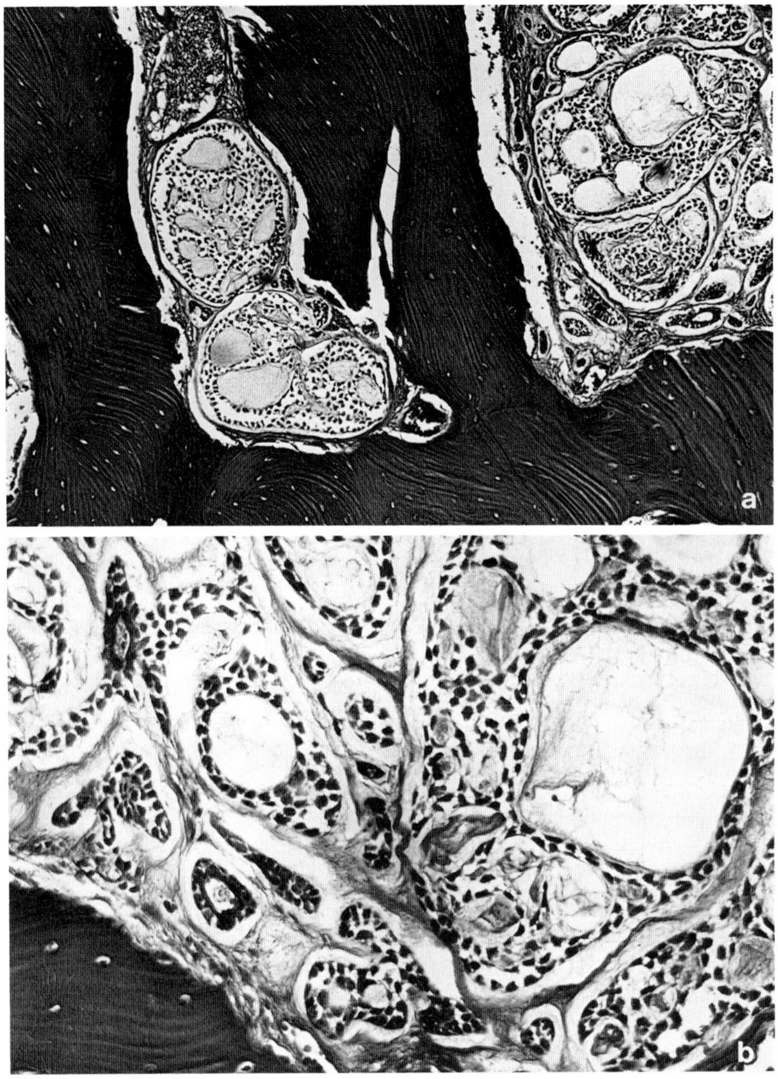

Figure 15.**120** Cribriform adenoid cystic carcinoma in a pleomorphic adenoma of the palate: extension in the osseous canals of the maxilla. H & E. **a** 63×, **b** 160×.

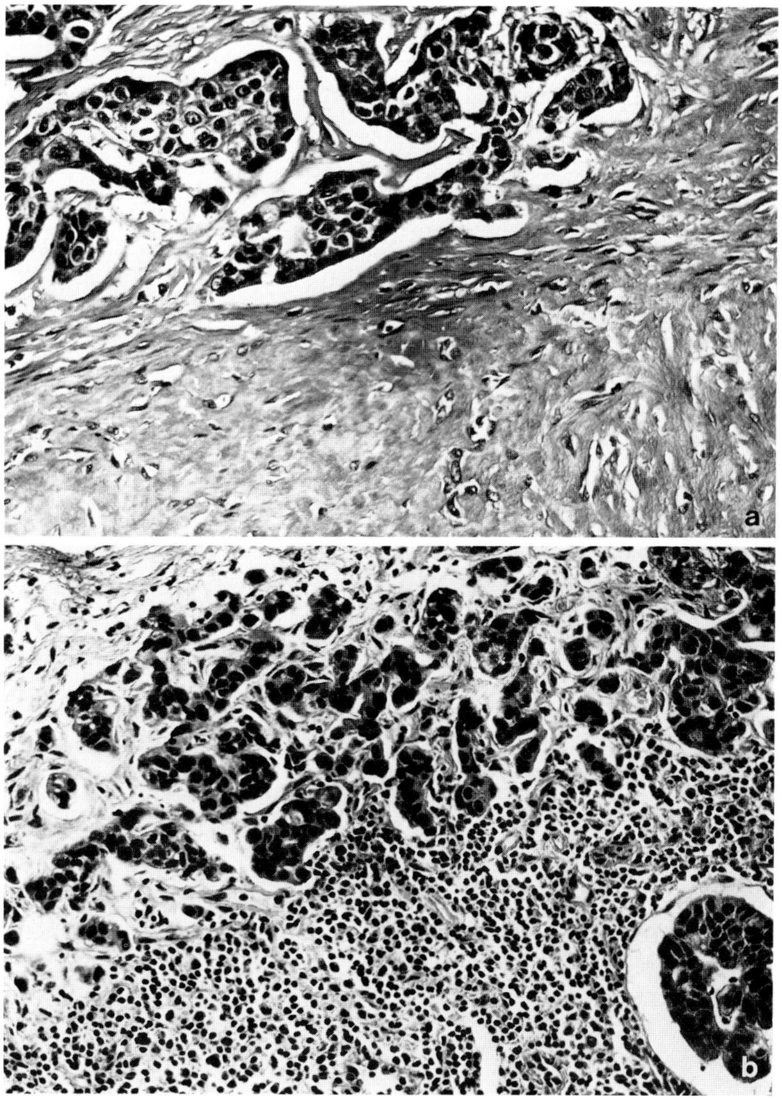

Figure 15.**121** Poorly differentiated squamous cell carcinoma in a pleomorphic parotid adenoma: **a** Tumor nests surrounded by remnants of the stroma of the pleomorphic adenoma. **b** Lymph node metastases of the same tumor. H & E. **a**, **b** 160×.

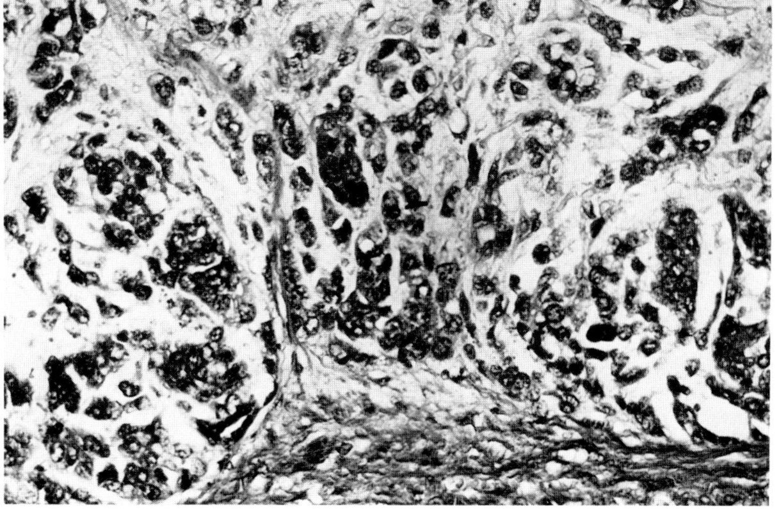

Figure 15.**122** Metastasizing undifferentiated carcinoma in a pleomorphic parotid adenoma: primary tumor with solid cell nests. H & E, 160×.

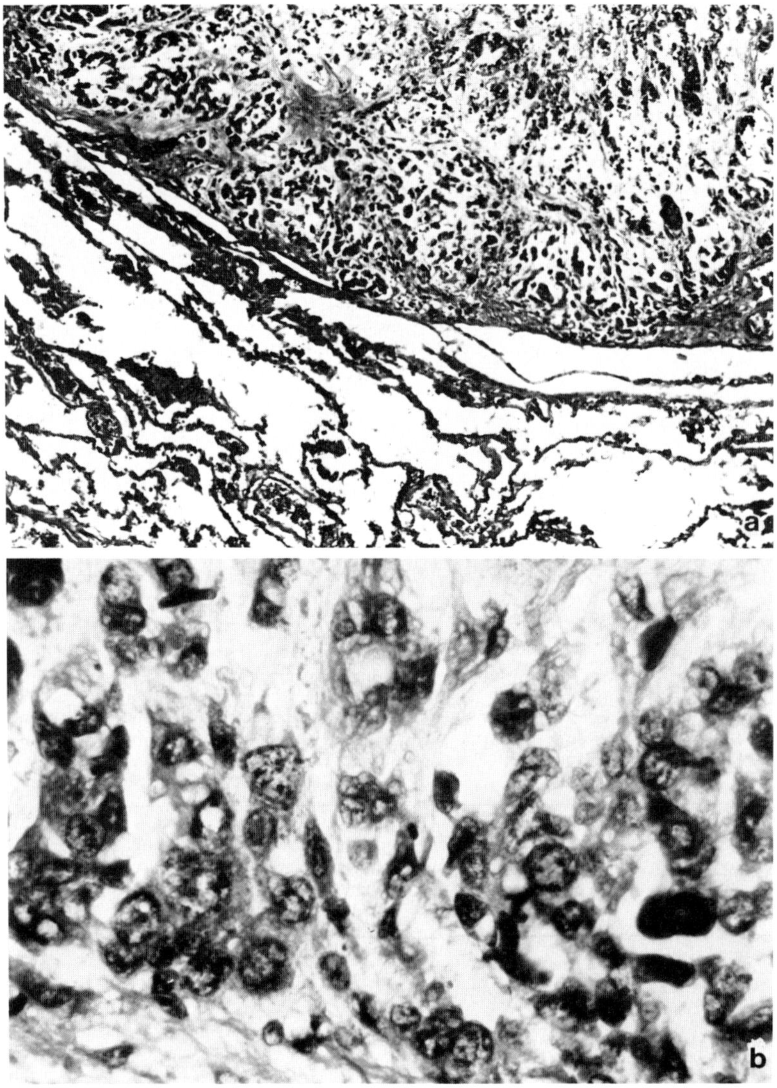

Figure 15.**123** Lung metastasis in the same patient shown in Figure 15.**122**: **a** Tumor focus bounded by lung tissue below. **b** Section from the metastasis. H & E. **a** 63×, **b** 400×.

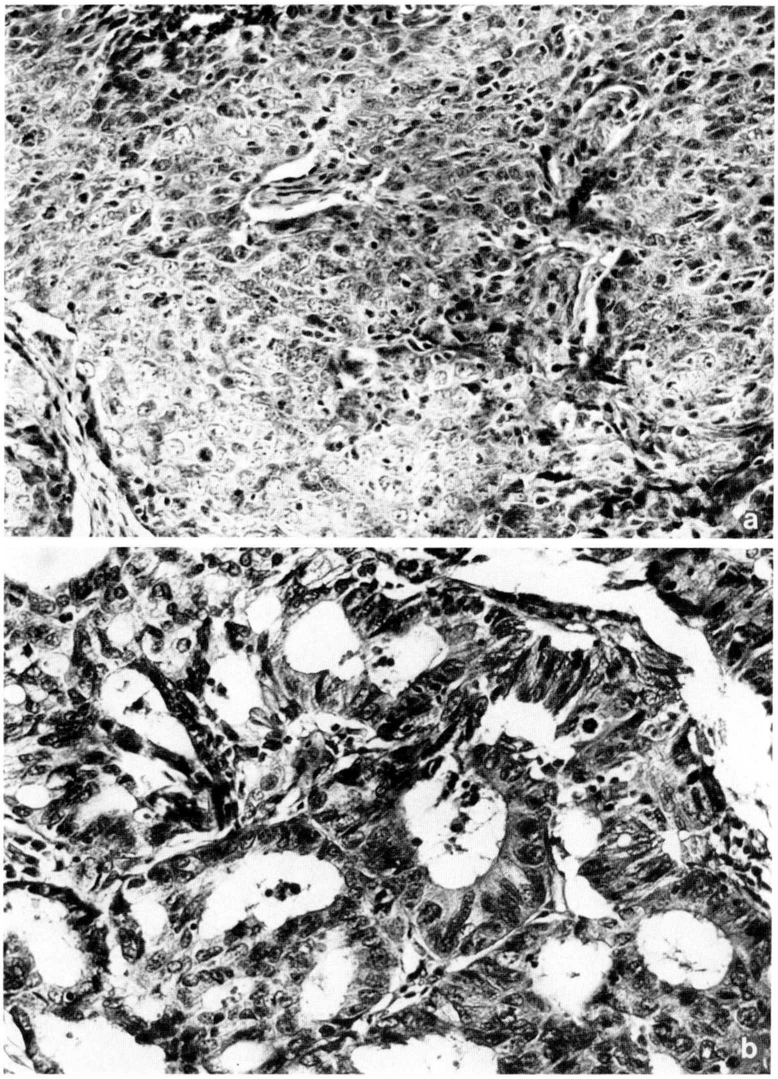

Figure 15.**124** Biphasic differentiation of a carcinoma in a pleomorphic parotid adenoma: **a** Differentiation to nonkeratinizing squamous cell carcinoma. **b** Differentiation to adenocarcinoma. H & E. **a**, **b** 160×.

Duct Carcinoma

The duct carcinomas form a small group of salivary tumors first described by Kleinsasser (Kleinsasser et al 1968, Hübner et al 1969) that are not included in the WHO classification (Thackray & Sobin 1972). These tumors affect the elderly: In our series, most of the patients were women in the seventh decade. Lymph node metastases are more common than blood-borne.

Clinical Aspects. Clinical aspects and course are not uniform: some tumors may grow extremely slowly, be well encapsulated, and mobile (Fig. 15.**68**), suggesting a diagnosis of a pleomorphic adenoma, whereas others grow quickly, are ill-defined, and of reduced mobility, with early lymph node metastases. The varying clinical course is probably ascribed to the fact that duct carcinomas resemble the mammary duct carcinoma (Kleinsasser et al 1968), consisting of several different histologic types.

In our series, the tumor was rare, forming 5% of the whole, with 80% of the tumors localized in the parotid gland, and a few in the submandibular and minor glands (Corio et al 1982, Seifert et al 1980, Jend-Rossmann 1980).

Histology. The organoid tumor architecture (Figs. 15.**125,** 15.**126a, b**) consists of two cell types (Kleinsasser et al 1968, Hübner et al 1969, Donath et al 1972, Fayemi & Toker 1974, Corio et al 1982). Dark cells lie on the internal surface of the duct structures, which resemble intercalated ducts, whereas clear glycogen-rich cells lie on the external surface. The tumor foci show a multinodular arrangement. Occasionally, clear papillary proliferations can be seen in the lumen of ductlike structures. Material resembling base-

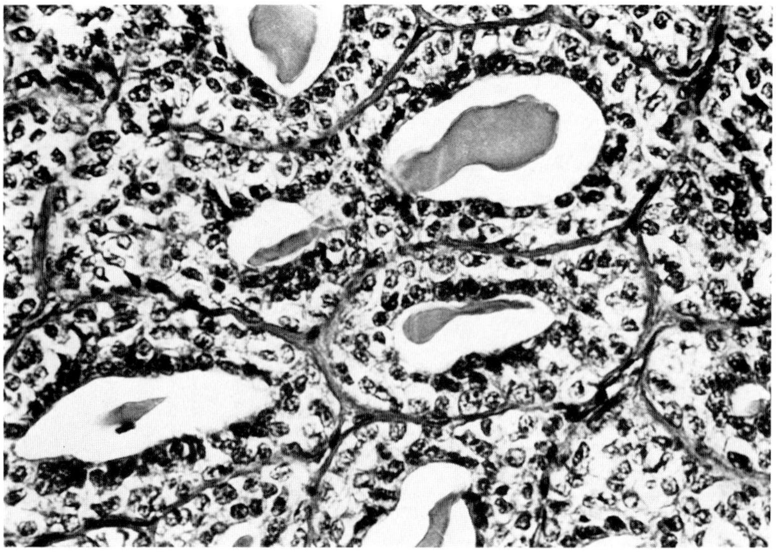

Figure 15.**125** Well-differentiated duct carcinoma of the parotid gland: dark narrow internal cell layer and external clear cell complexes of organoid architecture. H & E, 250×.

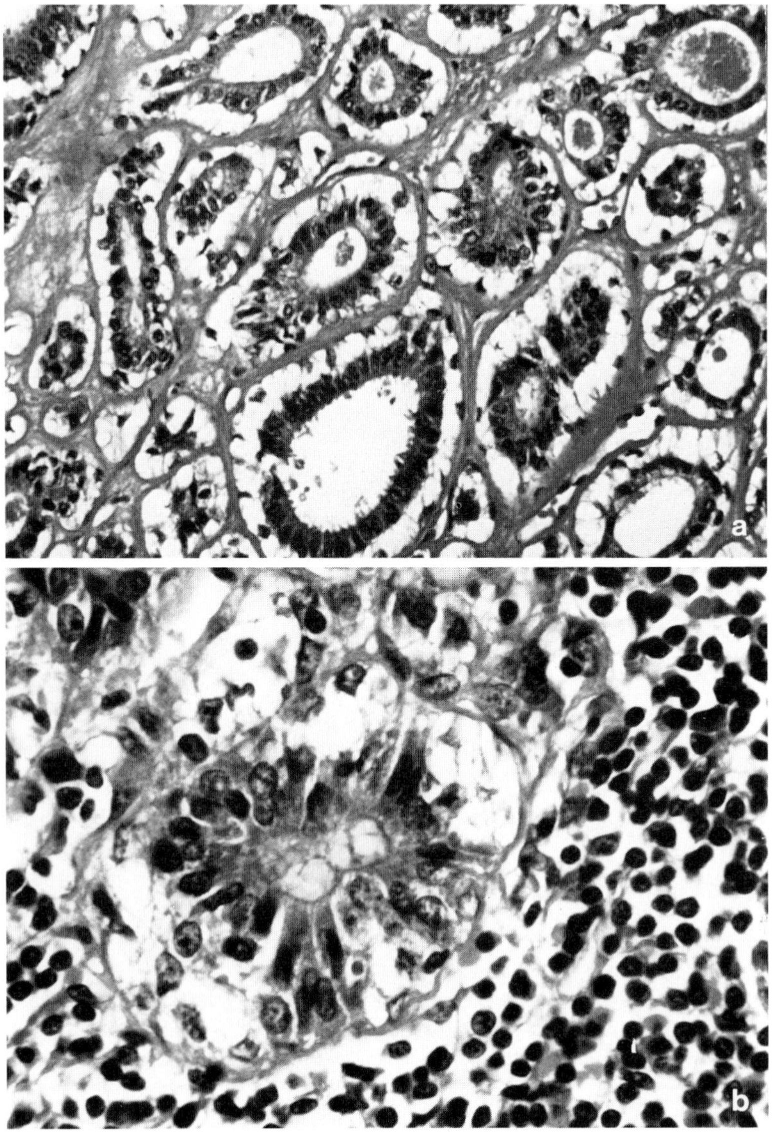

Figure 15.**126** Duct carcinoma of the parotid gland with lymph node metastases: **a** Primary tumor. **b** Lymph node metastasis. H & E. **a** 160×, **b** 400×.

ment membrane with hyaline transformation is laid down on the external surface of the clear cells. The proportion of clear and dark tumor cells within the tumor varies: at some points, the tumor may be composed purely of clear cells. Necrosis and pseudocystic transformations may be found in large foci of tumor. The margins of the tumor are not sharply demarcated. The duct carcinoma shows a positive reaction to CEA and lactoferrin in the tumor cells (Caselitz et al 1982, see also page 173f).

The *duct carcinoma of the comedo type* is a rare variant, comparable with the comedo tumor of the breast (Kleinsasser et al 1968). The tumor forms wide, sharply demarcated cell cords, with pseudocysts filled by cell debris within this cell complex. This creates a clear cribriform pattern. The tumor cells have a broad acidophilic cytoplasm of the striated duct cell type. Myoepithelial cells lie on the external surface of the cell walls (Hübner et al 1969). However, the dualism of the two cell forms of epithelial-myoepithelial duct carcinoma is absent. Increased cell atypia and mitoses are also characteristic of the comedo type.

Electron Microscopy. The dark ductal epithelium contains tonofilaments and desmosomes, and microvilli at some points on the luminal surface. The structure of the clear cells resembles the architecture of myoepithelial cells. Myofilaments, pinocytic vesicles, glycogen, and lipofuscin granules may be demonstrated in the cytoplasm. A multilayered basal membrane lies on the external surface (Brocheriou et al 1977).

Pathogenesis. The structure of this tumor resembles that of the intercalated duct system, and it may therefore also be termed an "epithelial-myoepithelial intercalated duct carcinoma" (Donath et al 1972). Synonyms include adenomyoepithelioma, tubular-solid adenoma, and glycogen-rich clear cell adenoma (Feyrter 1963, Bauer & Fox 1945, Saksela et al 1972). The abundant glycogen is in keeping with the fact that the forerunners of myoepithelial cells contain glycogen (Tandler 1965, Daley et al 1984).

Prognosis. Complete removal of the tumor secures a relatively favorable prognosis for the duct carcinoma. However, 30–40% of the tumors recur (Corio et al 1982), and in 10–20% regional lymph node metastases occur. The mortality is low, being less than 10%. Because of the small numbers, we have not divided the various duct carcinomas but include them all in prognostic group II (page 282), with a 5-year survival rate of 65%. The evolution of a duct carcinoma of the comedo type is more malignant than that of the tubular or papillary forms.

Treatment. The treatment of duct carcinoma consists of total parotidectomy, which may need to be combined with the resection of individual nerve fibers or the entire facial nerve, depending on the site of the tumor. The facial nerve may be reconstructed, if necessary. Since the patients are often already elderly, we often forego nerve reconstruction in favor of secondary cosmetic and functional procedures, such as tarsorraphy and masseteric transposition.

References

Bauer, W. H., R. A. Fox: Adenomyoepithelioma (cylindroma) of palate mucous glands. Arch. Path. (Chic.) 39 (1945) 96

Brocheriou, C., M. Auriol, F. Guilbert, F. Matar: Adenocarcinome canalaire à cellules claires de la parotide. Etude histologique et ultrastructurale d'un cas. Arch. Anat. Cytol. Path. 25 (1977) 201

Caselitz, J., M. Osborn, J. Wustrow, G. Seifert, K. Weber: The expression of different intermediate-sized filaments in human salivary glands and their tumours. Path. Res. Pract. 175 (1982) 266

Corio, R. L., J. J. Scuibba, R. B. Brannon, J. G. Batsakis: Epithelial-myoepithelial carcinoma of intercalated duct origin. A clinicopathologic and ultrastructural assessment of sixteen cases. Oral Surg. 53 (1982) 280

Daley, T. D., G. P. Wysocki, M. S. Smout, R. P. Slinger: Epithelialmyoepithelial carcinoma of salivary glands. Oral Surg. 57 (1984) 512

Donath, K., G. Seifert, R. Schmitz: Zur Diagnose und Ultrastruktur des tubulären Speichelgangkarzinoms: epithelial-myoepitheliales Schaltstückkarzinom. Virchows Arch. Path. Anat. 356 (1972) 16

Fayemi, A. O., C. Toker: Salivary duct carcinoma. Arch. Otolaryng. 99 (1974) 366

Feyrter, F.: Über das glykogenreiche retikulierte Adenom der Speicheldrüsen. Z. Krebsforsch. 65 (1963) 446

Hübner, G., O. Kleinsasser, H. J. Klein: Zur Feinstruktur der Speichelgangkarzinome. Ein Beitrag zur Rolle der Myoepithelzellen in Speicheldrüsengeschwülsten. Virchows Arch. Path. Anat. 346 (1969) 1

Jend-Rossmann, J.: Pathomorphologische Klassifikation von Tumoren der Submandibularis und Sublingualis. Analyse von 188 Fällen. Diss. Hamburg 1980

Kleinsasser, O., H. J. Klein, G. Hübner: Speichelgangcarcinome. Eine den Milchgangscarcinomen der Brustdrüse analoge Gruppe von Speicheldrüsentumoren. Arch. klin. exp. Ohr.-, Nas.- u. Kehlk.-Heilk. 192 (1968) 100

Saksela, E., J. Tarkkanen, J. Wartiovaara: Parotid clear-cell adenoma of possible myoepithelial origin. Cancer (Philad.) 30 (1972) 742

Seifert, G., H. Rieb, K. Donath: Klassifikation der Tumoren der kleinen Speicheldrüsen. Pathohistologische Analyse von 160 Tumoren. Z. Laryng. Rhinol. 59 (1980) 379

Tandler, B.: Ultrastructure of the human submaxillary gland. Z. Zellforsch. 68 (1965) 852

Thackray, A. C., L. H. Sobin: Histological Typing of Salivary Gland Tumours. World Health Organiziation, Genf 1972

Undifferentiated Carcinoma

Definition: Undifferentiated carcinomas cannot be placed in any specific tumor classification because of their primitive histologic and cytologic structure under light microscopy. Descriptions in the literature refer mainly to undifferentiated small cell duct carcinomas, whose tissue of origin is regarded as the duct cell system (Koss et al 1972, Blanck et al 1974, Wirman & Battifora

Tumor Type	Hamburg Salivary Gland Register (1965–1982) (663 tumors) %	Göttingen Series (1965–1975) (178 tumors) %
Acinic cell tumors	10.0	9.6
Mucoepidermoid tumors	19.5	11.2
Adenoid cystic carcinoma	16.5	18.0
Adenocarcinoma	10.0	11.9
Squamous cell carcinoma	7.5	7.3
Carcinoma ex pleomorphic adenoma	21.5	12.9
Other carcinomas	15.5	29.2
Duct carcinomas	3.5	3.9
Anaplastic carcinoma	5.5	21.9

Table 15.**10** Malignant Salivary Tumors: Frequency of Individual Tumors Related to the Total Number in the Göttingen Series (Chilla et al 1983) and in Hamburg Salivary Gland Register (Seifert & Donath 1976)

1976, Dubois et al 1977, Brocheriou et al 1977, Kumar et al 1979, Donath et al 1982).

Clinical Aspects. Undifferentiated carcinomas are difficult to distinguish from poorly differentiated adenocarcinoma and squamous cell carcinoma, so that data about the frequency of this tumor vary. In our own series, undifferentiated carcinomas formed 30% of all malignant salivary tumors (Table 15.**10**). The parotid gland is most frequently affected, as indeed it is with almost all malignant salivary tumors. The tumor affects men and women equally, with a peak age incidence in the sixth decade. The history is often short, because of the rapid growth, and the patient often presents for treatment in a late stage. In our series, undifferentiated tumors had the highest rate of facial nerve paralysis (60%), if the small group of solid adenoid cystic carcinomas is excluded. The frequency of lymph node metastases (64%) was only exceeded by squamous cell carcinoma, with 65%, and 20% developed distant metastases.

Histology. The tumor consists of poorly differentiated epithelial cell cords, usually arranged in a solid pattern. Adenoid structures may develop at some points. The polymorphic cell nuclei contain large nucleoli, demonstrate increased mitosis, and are surrounded by a narrow layer of cytoplasm. The stroma of the tumor may undergo hyaline transformation. Small cell and large cell types may be distinguished, depending on the size of the cell (Nagao et al 1982). Electron microscopy shows that small cell carcinomas have undifferentiated duct epithelium, also primitive neuroendocrine cells with hormone granules (Kraemer et al 1983; see also "Endocrine Carcinoma" later). Undifferentiated parotid carcinomas (Fig. 15.**127**)

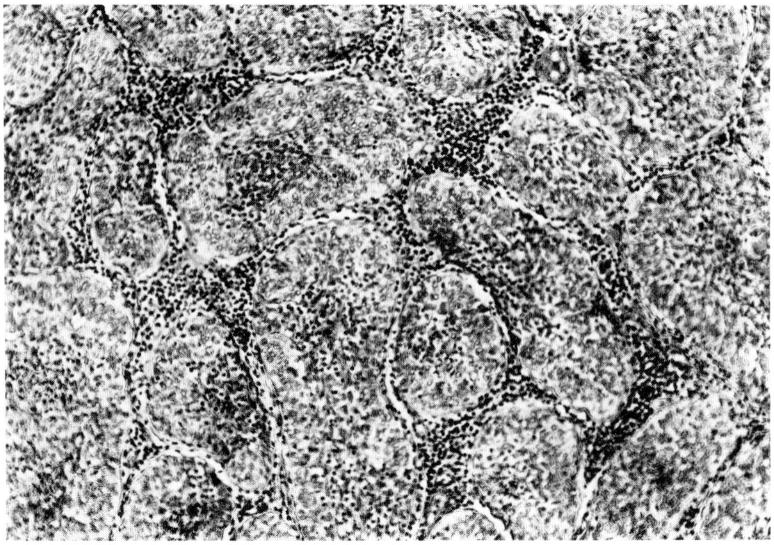

Figure 15.**127** Undifferentiated parotid gland carcinoma with a lymphoid stromal component. H & E, 160×.

with lymphoid stroma, whose architecture resembles nasopharyngeal carcinoma with lymphoid stroma, is a rare type (Wassef et al 1982, Nagao et al 1983). The differential diagnosis between a primary parotid carcinoma or the metastasis from a primary nasopharyngeal carcinoma may be very difficult (see also "Anaplastic Parotid Carcinoma later).

Electron Microscopy. Despite the cell polymorphism, cell types with organelles and secretory particles may be distinguished (Donath et al 1982, Yaku et al 1983). These include undifferentiated epithelial cells with clear cytoplasm that may contain glycogen granules and occasionally cilia. A further type of cell may be defined as a poorly differentiated duct cell. These cells contain primitive secretion products and a moderate number of cell organelles. Another cell type is characterized by microtubules, secretory granules, and a clear organelle content representing active secretory epithelial cells. Further types include epidermoid cells with desmosomes and tonofilaments (Nagao et al 1982) and myoepithelial cells with myofilaments and abundant organelles. The ultrastructural cytodifferentiation may be compared with that of the embryonal phase of development of the salivary gland (Donath et al 1978).

Pathogenesis. The tumor matrix of undifferentiated carcinoma originates from the primitive duct system. The basal reserve cells are pluripotent and can differentiate in several directions, including epidermoid cells (Regezi & Batsakis 1977). On the basis of electron microscopic findings, some undifferentiated carcinomas can thus be classified as poorly differentiated squamous cell carcinomas or duct carcinomas (Donath et al 1982). Acinar differentiation has not so far been observed, so that the term "embryonal carcinoma" (Vawter & Tefft 1966) should not be used, because one important characteristic of an embryonal tumor is absent, that is, the neoplastic proliferation of all cells of one organ anlage (Meister 1978, see page 276).

Because of their low 5-year survival rate of 25%, undifferentiated carcinomas are assigned to prognostic group IV (page 282), with the worst prognosis. A radical procedure combined with sacrifice of the facial nerve for tumors of the parotid gland, followed by radiation therapy, is the only potentially successful treatment (see page 278ff).

References

Blanck, C., A. Backstrom, C.-M. Eneroth, P. A. Jacobsson: Poorly differentiated solid parotid carcinoma. Acta Radiol. (Stockh.) 13 (1974) 17

Brocheriou, C., M. Auriol, F. Guilbert, A. Matar: Adenocarcinome canalaire à cellules claires de la parotide. Etude histologique et ultrastructurale d'un cas. Arch. Anat. Cytol. Pathol. 25 61977) 201

Donath, K., H. Dietrich, G. Seifert: Entwicklung und ultrastrukturelle Cytodifferenzierung der Parotis des Menschen. Virchow Arch. Path. Anat. 378 (1978) 297

Donath, K., G. Seifert, E. Sunder-Plassmann: Ultrastrukturelle Subklassifikation undifferenzierter Parotiscarcinoma. Analyse von 11 Fällen. J. Cancer Res. Clin. Oncol. 103 (1982) 75

Dubois, P. J., D. P. Orr, E. N. Meyers, L. E. Barnes: Undifferentiated parotid carcinoma with osteoblastic metastases. Amer. J. Roentgenol. 129 (1977) 744

Koss, L. G., R. H. Spiro, S. Hadju: Small cell (oat cell) carcinoma of the minor salivary gland origin. Cancer (Philad.) 30 (1972) 737

Kraemer, B. B., B. Mackay, J. G. Batsakis: Small cell carcinomas of the parotid gland. A clinicopathologic study of three cases. Cancer (Philad.) 52 (1983) 2115

Kumar, P. M., H. B. Marsden, A. H. Cameron, P. H. Morris-Jones, J. R. Mann: Carcinoma of the neck in young children: a light and electron microscopic study. J. Pathol. 128 (1979) 49

Meister, P.: Zur Pathologie der embryonalen Tumoren. Verh. Dtsch. Krebsges. 1 (1978) 275

Nagao, K., O. Matsuzaki, H. Saiga, I. Sugano, H. Shigematsu, T. Kaneko, T. Katoh, T. Kitamura: Histopathologic studies of undifferentiated carcinoma of the parotid gland. Cancer (Philad.) 50 (1982) 1572

Nagao, K., O. Matsuzaki, H. Saiga, B. Akikusa, I. Sugano, H. Shigematsu, T. Kaneko, T. Katoh, T. Kitamura, Y. Asano, M. Okamoto: A histopathologic study of benign and malignant lymphoepithelial lesions of the parotid gland. Cancer (Philad.) 52 (1983) 1044

Regezi, J. A., J. G. Batsakis: Histogenesis of salivary gland neoplasms. Otolaryng. Clin. North Amer. 10 (1977) 297

Vawter, G. F., M. Tefft: Congenital tumors of the parotid gland. Arch. Pathol. (Chic.) 82 (1966) 242

Wassef, M., Y. Le Charpentier, J. P. Monteil, K. Le Tien, A. Galian: Carcinome indifferencié a stroma lymphoide de la parotide (carcinome indifferencié de type nasopharynge?). Etude en microscopie optique, electronique et en immunofluorescence. Bull. Cancer (Philad.) 69 (1982) 11

Wirman, J. A., H. A. Battifora: Small cell undifferentiated carcinoma of the salivary gland origin. An ultrastructural study. Cancer (Philad.) 37 (1976) 1840

Yaku, Y., T. Kanda, T. Yoshihara, T. Kaneko, K. Nagao: Undifferentiated carcinoma of the parotid gland. Case report with electron microscopic findings. Virchows Arch. Path. Anat. 401 (1983) 89

Other Carcinomas

The group of other tumors embraces the rare but clearly defined types, such as sebaceous carcinoma, and those tumors whose classification is still a matter of dispute. Some of the following tumors possibly represent variants of already known types of carcinoma, so that they may in future be classified in one of the defined forms.

Sebaceous Carcinomas

Carcinomas arising in sebaceous cells are very rare and arise almost exclusively within the parotid gland (Silver & Goldstein 1966, Kleinsasser et al 1970, Batsakis et al 1972, Zechner & Albegger 1973, Shulman et al 1973, Akhtar et al 1973, Gnepp & Brannon 1984). The tumors consist of solid acinar or cystic epithelial cords with lipid droplets in the cytoplasm. Electron microscopy demonstrates microvilli and desmosomes but no tonofilaments. The tumors manifest local infiltration and metastasis. Sebaceous metaplasia

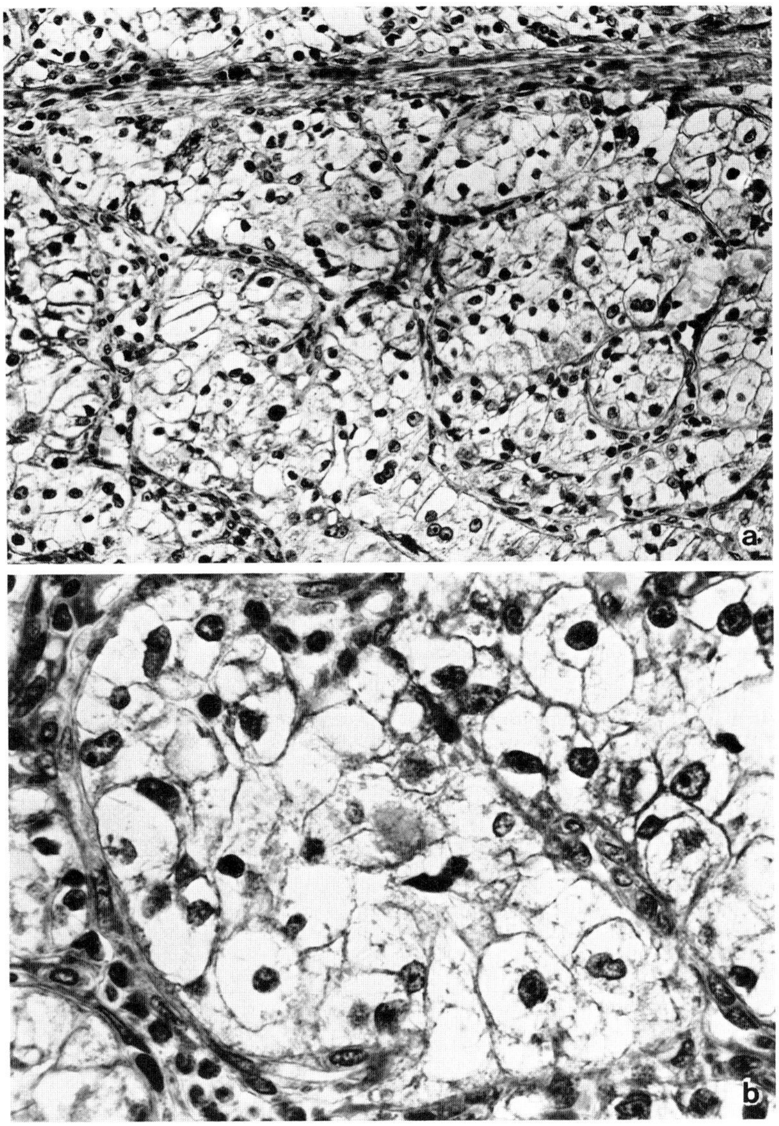

Figure 15.**128** Clear cell carcinoma of the palatal glands: trabecular and acinar clear cell tumor structures and vacuolated cytoplasm. Masson-Goldner. **a** 160×, **b** 400×.

is described on page 106 and sebaceous adenoma on page 215.

Clear Cell Carcinoma

This tumor arises mainly in the parotid and palatal glands. Cytochemical analysis or electron microscopy shows that this term embraces several tumors of different origin (Seifert & Donath 1978), as has already been indicated in the discussion of clear cell adenoma (page 216). The clear cytoplasm of the tumor seen under the light microscope (Fig. 15.**128a, b**) may be determined by low cell differentiation with a paucity of organelles. It can also be due to cytplasmic deposits of glycogen, mucus, lipid droplets, and clear secretory granules that are partially dissolved out of the tumor tissue by the fixation process and paraffin embedding. Numerous cell forms are to be considered as the tumor matrix, depending on the electron microscopic findings, including undifferentiated duct cells of the reserve cell type that possess only few cell organelles and desmosomes, and duct cells or primitive myoepithelial cells with glycogen granules in the cytoplasm and primitive epidermoid cells with tonofilaments in the cytoplasm and desmosomal links to the neighboring tumor cells. Thus, in clear cell carcinomas, immature duct carcinomas, adenocarcinomas, myoepithelial carcinomas, and immature nonkeratinizing squamous cell carcinomas may occur, with the corresponding ultrastructural differentiation (Mohamed 1976, Mohamed & Cherrick 1975, Echevarria 1967, Seifert & Donath 1978, Donath et al 1982, Gianola 1969, Stromeyer et al 1975, Stene & Koppang 1981, Chen 1983). Clear cell tumor foci in duct carcinoma have already

Batsakis, J. G., B. Kraemer, J. J. Sciubba: The pathology of head and neck tumors: The myoepithelial cell and its participation in salivary gland neoplasia. Head Neck Surg. (N. Y.) 5 (1983) 222

Beck, J. O.: The BW 1081 mouse salivary gland tumor. J. dent. Res. 39 (1959) 577

Belsky, J. L., N. Takeichi, T. Yamamoto, R. W. Cihak, F. Hirose, H. Ezaki, S. Inoue, W. J. Blot: Salivary gland neoplasms following atomic radiation: additional cases and reanalysis of combined data in fixed population, 1957–1970. Cancer (Philad.) 35 (1975) 555

Belsky, J. L., K. Tachikawa, R. W. Cihak, T. Yamamoto: Salivary gland tumors in atomic bomb survivors. J. Amer. med. Ass. 219 (1972) 864

Benjamin, E., D. H. Wright: Adenocarcinoma of the pancreas of childhood: A report of two cases. Histopathology 4 (1980) 87

Berg, J. W., R. V. P. Hutter, F. W. Foote jr.: The unique association between salivary gland cancer and breast cancer. J. Amer. med. Ass. 204 (1968) 771

Biggar, R. J., R. E. Curtis, D. A. Hoffman, J. T. Flannery: Second primary malignancies following salivary gland cancers. Brit. J. Cancer 47 (1983) 383

Borochovitz, D., W. K. Kam, M. Nolte, S. Graner, J. Kiss: Adenocarcinoma of the palate associated with nephrotic syndrome and epimembranous carcinoembryonic antigen deposition. Cancer (Philad.) 49 (1982) 2097

Brown, A. M.: A comparative assay of the in-vitro and in-vivo behavior of three chemically induced neoplasms of the rat submandibular glands. J. oral Path. 2 (1973) 33

Caputo, A., L. Orci: Morphological studies of a new transplantable salivary gland tumor in C3H mice. Z. Krebsforsch. 73 (1969) 46

Caselitz, J., A. Sendler, P. Schmiegelow, A. Salfelder: Morphologisches Reaktionsmuster von transplantiertem normalen Speicheldrüsengewebe in thymusaplastischen Mäusen. Verh. Dtsch. Ges. Path. 66 (1982) 615

Castelli, L., M. Marcante, A. Caputo: Further investigations on the behaviour of cultivated salivary gland adenocarcinoma of the mouse. Z. Krebsforsch. 79 (1973) 224

Cataldo, E., A. E. Reif: An explanation for the proportion of carcinomas and sarcomas seen in chemically induced murine submaxillary gland tumors. Cancer (Philad.) 50 (1982) 531

Donath, K. G. Seifert, J. Lentrodt: The embryonal carcinoma of the parotid gland. A rare example of an embryonal tumour. Virchows Arch. Path. Anat. 403 (1984) 425

El-Asfahani, A., G. I. Higashi, M. A. Ahmed: Chemical carcinogenesis of submandibular salivary gland in BALB/c mice and syngenetic passage of the tumor. Oral Surg. 48 (1979) 47

Emmelin, N., J. R. Garrett, P. Ohlin: Secretory activity and the myoepithelial cells of salivary glands after duct ligation in cats. Arch. oral Biol. 19 (1974) 275

Eversole, L. R.: Histogenic classification of salivary tumors. Arch. Path. (Chic.) 92 (1971) 434

Fasske, E., H. Themann: Stromamastocytose in virogenen transplantierbaren Speicheldrüsencarcinomen der Ratte. Z. Krebsforsch. 73 (1969) 75

Friborsky, V.: Induction of adenoid cystic carcinomas in the submaxillary gland in mice. Pathol. Microbiol. 28 (1963) 413

Janower, M. L., O. S. Miettinen: Neoplasms after childhood irradiation of the thymus gland. J. Amer. med. Ass. 215 (1971) 753

Ju, D. M. C.: Salivary gland tumors occurring after radiation of the head and neck area. Amer. J. Surg. 116 (1968) 518

Kleinsasser, O.: Einteilung, Morphologie und Verhalten der epithelialen Speicheldrüsentumoren. HNO (Berl.) 17 (1969) 197

Lamey, P.-J., M. M. Ferguson: Salivary gland viral oncogenesis in mice. J. dent. Res. 60 B (1981) 1117

Lamey, J.-P., J. P. Waterhouse, M. M. Ferguson: Pleomorphic salivary adenoma. Virally induced pleomorphic salivary adenoma in the CFLP mouse. Amer. J. Path. 109 (1982) 129

Manusco, T. F., M. J. Brennan: Epidemiological considerations of cancer of the gallbladder, bile ducts and salivary glands in the rubber industry. J. Occup. Med. 12 (1970) 333

Mark, J., R. Dahlenfors, C. Ekedahl: Chromosomal deviations and their specificity in human mixed salivary gland tumors. Anticancer Res. 1 (1981) 49

Mark, J., R. Dahlenfors, C. Ekedahl: Specificity and implications of ring chromosomes and dicentrics in benign mixed salivary gland tumours. Acta path. microbiol. immunol. scand. A 91 (1983a) 397

Mark, J., R. Dahlenfors, C. Ekedahl: Cytogenetics of the human benign mixed salivary gland tumor. Hereditas 99 (1983b) 115

Mori, M., Y. Takai, R. Naito, M. Hosaka, N. Murase: Immunohistochemical demonstration of epidermal growth factor and nerve growth factor in experimental carcinogenesis in the mouse submandibular gland. Virchows Arch. (Cell Pathol.) 45 (1984) 431

Newman, A. N., T. C. Calcaterra, S. Bhuta: Familial carcinoma of the submandibular gland. A case report and epidemiologic review. Arch. Otolaryng. (Chic.) 107 (1981) 169

Noyek, A. M., K. P. H. Pritzker, N. D. Greyson, M. Blackstein, J. S. Chapnik, B. J. Shapiro: Familial Warthin's tumor. I. Its synchronous occurrence in mother and son. II. Its association with cystic oncocytic metaplasia of the larynx. J. Otolaryng. 9 (1980) 90

Prior, P., J. A. H. Waterhouse: Secondary primary cancers in patients with tumors of the salivary glands. Cancer (Philad.) 36 (1977) 362

Rodendo, C., A. Garcia, F. Vazquez: Malignant lymphoepithelial lesion of the parotid gland: Poorly differentiated squamous cell carcinoma with lymphoid stroma. Cancer (Philad.) 48 (1981) 289

Saemundsen, A. K., H. Albeck, J. P. H. Hansen, N. H. Nielsen, M. Anvret, G. Henle, H. Henle, K. A. Thomsen, H. K. Kristensen, G. Klein: Epstein-Barr virus in nasopharyngeal and salivary gland carcinomas of Greenland eskimoes. Brit. J. Cancer 46 (1982) 721

Schneider, A. B., M. J. Favus, M. E. Stachura, M. J. Arnold, L. A. Frohman: Salivary gland neoplasms as a late consequence of head and neck irradiation. Ann. intern. Med. 87 (1977) 160

Schuster, G. S., T. R. Dirksen, B. Singh, D. H. Pashley: Altered enzyme release by virus infected mouse salivary glands. J. oral Pathol. 6 (1977) 203

Seifert, G.: Die epithelialen Speicheldrüsentumoren. In Schuchardt, K.: Fortschritte der Kiefer- und Gesichtschirurgie, Bd. XIV. Thieme, Stuttgart 1972 (S. 2).

Shafer, W. G.: Experimental salivary gland tumor genesis. J. dent. Res. 41 (1962) 117

Sheehan, R., G. Shklar: The effect of cyclophosphamide on experimental salivary gland neoplasia. Cancer Res. 32 (1972) 420

Shore-Freedman, E., C. Abrahams, W. Recant, A. B. Schneider: Neurilemmomas and salivary gland tumors of the head and neck following childhood irradiation. Cancer (Philad.) 51 (1983) 2159

Smith, J. A., M. J. Warhol, G. L. Brodsky: An immunohistochemical study of a carcinoma of the parotid gland exhibiting both ductal and acinic cell differentation. Oral Surg. 55 (1983) 267

Standish, S. M.: Early histologic changes in induced tumors of the submaxillary salivary glands of the rat. Amer. J. Path. 33 (1957) 671

Steinhardt, G.: 45 Jahre bestehendes Thorotrastom der Parotis. Dtsch. Z. Mund-Kiefer-Gesichts-Chir. 3 (1979) 189

Stenman, G., J. Mark: Specifity of the involvement of chromosomes 8 and 12 in human mixed salivary-gland tumours. J. oral Path. 12 (1983) 446

Stenman, G., J. Mark: Loss of the Y-chromosome in a cultured human salivary-gland adenocarcinoma. J. oral Path. 12 (1983) 458

Stenman, G., R. Dahlenfors, J. Mark, N. Sandberg: Adenoid cystic carcinoma: A third type of human salivary gland neoplasm characterized cytogenetically by reciprocal translocations. Anticancer Res. 2 (1982) 11

Takeichi, N., F. Hirose, H. Yamamoto, H. Ezaki, T. Fujikura: Salivary gland tumors in atomic bomb survivors in Hiroshima, Japan. II. Pathologic study and supplementary epidemiologic observations. Cancer (Philad.) 52 (1983) 377

Walker, M. J., P. K. Chaudhuri, D. C. Wood, T. K. Das Gupta: Radiation-induced parotid cancer. Arch. Surg. 116 (1981) 329

Wallace, A. C., J. T. MacDougall, J. Hildes, J. Lederman: Salivary gland tumors in Canadian eskimoes. Cancer (Philad.) 16 (1963) 1338

Wells jr., S. A., A. S. Rabson, R. A. Mahngren, A. S. Ketcham: In vitro neoplastic transformation of newborn hamster salivary gland tissue by oncogenic DNA viruses. Cancer (Philad.) 19 (1966) 1411

Wigley, C. B., J. Amos, P. Brookes: Different tumours induced by benzo(a)pyrene and its 7,8 dihydrodiol injected into adult mouse salivary gland. Brit. J. Cancer 37 (1978) 657

Treatment of Salivary Gland Tumors

Tumors of the salivary glands are characterized by a particularly wide histologic spectrum. Classification into histologic types and subtypes is not just a matter of nomenclature, but is of decisive significance for successful treatment. Close cooperation with a histopathologist is essential for several reasons: the place of aspiration cytology in the final decision, the problem of a biopsy to confirm the diagnosis, frozen section, and finally the examination of the tumor specimen after removal for final assessment with respect to postoperative radiotherapy, for confirmation of clearance around the tumor, and last but not least, to allow documentation for later analysis.

Operative Treatment

Surgery is the mainstay of treatment of salivary gland tumors. Radiation therapy is, with a few exceptions, restricted to a supportive role as postoperative radiotherapy for certain tumor groups, whereas chemotherapy has not yet made a significant contribution to the treatment of salivary gland malignancy. Surgery of the parotid gland places great demands on the skill of the surgeon because of the extratemporal segment of the facial nerve (page 329). The course of the nerve through the parotid gland generates certain problems: the operation must be radical enough, but with full regard for the nerve. The radicality of the procedure must not be compromized at the price of preservation of the facial nerve, but must rather be determined by the histologic nature of the tumor.

We have developed a concept for the treatment of salivary gland tumors (Haubrich & Miehlke 1978, Miehlke et al 1981) based on the histologic type: the surgery is divided into four categories (Table 15.**11**). In the course of the last 15 years, we have been able to adhere to this therapeutic concept based on the following principles:

- Preservation of the facial nerve in benign group I tumors and preservation of as much as possible of this nerve in the less malignant group II tumors (Table 15.**11**).
- Reconstructive procedures on the facial nerve, if it must be resected partially or completely for groups II and III tumors (Table 15.**11**), but not for group IV tumors or patients with a facial paralysis before operation.
- A radical neck dissection should not be carried out as a routine operation for all malignant tumors, but only for those with lymph node metastases or with advanced tumors extending beyond the organ of origin.

This treatment scheme must be modified on the basis of the results of a retrospective study of our patients treated for malignant tumors (Chilla et al 1980, 1981, 1983a, 1983b) and on the basis of the advanced techniques for reconstruction of the facial nerve (Miehlke et al 1981, Stennert et al 1982):

1. A radical procedure for all adenoid cystic carcinomas has almost never prevented recurrence of this tumor and has not improved the long-term prognosis. We feel that a radical procedure, for example sacrifice of a still-functioning facial nerve, is not always justified (see Chapter 22), but must be determined by the differentiation of the tumor into the histologic types of prognostic significance, that is tubular, cribriform, and solid subtypes (Chilla et al 1981).

2. We have become more willing to reconstruct the facial nerve even for the more malignant tumors as techniques have advanced and improved. The basic premise of these procedures is that the quality of the patient's remaining life can be improved, despite the generally poor long-term prognosis, without compromising the radicality of the tumor surgery. The prognosis of an individual patient is often very difficult to estimate. But considerable difficulties are encountered if a decision is made to reconstruct the nerve several years after the primary procedure.

Figure 15.**133** summarizes the established and more recent concepts of the treatment of malignant salivary tumors. The concept rests on division into four histologic prognostic groups, I–IV, which are not to be confused with the treatment concepts 1–4 given in Table 15.**11**. Adenoid cystic carcinoma belongs in the prognostic groups I and II on the basis of its 5-year survival rate, but it clearly has a worse long-term prognosis than the other tumors in these groups and is therefore placed in a category of higher surgical radicality, to emphasize that treatment can scarcely be carried out in accordance with a protocol (Chilla et al 1981).

Overlap between the various methods of treatment for the individual prognostic groups indicates that it is only possible to give recommendations about treatment depending on the general condition of the patient and on the site and extent of the tumor: the radicality of the surgery and the place of reconstruction of the facial nerve must be tailored for the individual patient.

Radiotherapy

Reports about the radiosensitivity of individual malignant salivary tumors vary widely (Butler 1972, Fletcher et al 1975, Jakobsson & Eneroth

Table 15.**11** Surgical Concept for Parotid Tumors (Haubrich & Miehlke 1978, Miehlke et al 1981)

Group 1	Group 2	Group 3	Group 4
Superficial or total parotidectomy with preservation of the facial nerve	Superficial or total parotidectomy with preservation of the facial nerve or partial resection and reconstruction by direct or indirect anastomosis (Conley's "big-little" operation)	Total parotidectomy with preservation of the facial nerve or total parotidectomy with radical neck dissection, resection, and reconstruction of the facial nerve by autologous nerve graft or combined nerve grafts	Total parotidectomy and radical neck dissection and if necessary resection of the mandible and mastoid with sacrifice of the facial nerve without reconstruction of the nerve (Conley's "big-big" operation)
No radiotherapy	No radiotherapy	Radiotherapy	Radiotherapy
Monomorphic adenoma (oncocytoma, basal cell adenoma)	Acinic cell tumor (Well differentiated forms)	Acinic cell tumor (poorly differentiated forms or recurrence)	Adenoid cystic carcinoma
Pleomorphic adenoma	Low grade mucoepidermoid tumor	Carcinoma ex pleomorphic adenoma	Carcinoma ex pleomorphic adenoma in advanced stages
Cystadenolymphoma		High grade mucoepidermoid tumor in locally limited stage	High grade mucoepidermoid tumor in advanced stage
Lymphangioma			
Neurinoma of the facial nerve (as access to the tumor the facial nerve can only be preserved in a few cases, and must then be reconstructed)		Local limited adenocarcinoma	Squamous cell carcinoma and undifferentiated carcinoma
		Duct carcinoma	Infiltrative adenocarcinoma
			All tumors causing facial paralysis or extensive infiltrating recurrent tumors

1970, Stewart et al 1968). The major gain from radiation therapy is a reduction and delay in the appearance of recurrences of tumor by postoperative radiotherapy (Elkons et al 1978, Fu et al 1977), which is the main indication for radiation therapy (Fig. 15.**133**). We have only used radiation therapy for inoperable patients or as a purely palliative measure. Orthovoltage therapy has now been almost completely replaced by telecobalt. In recent years, fast neutrons have also been used for the treatment of salivary malignancy. The results are controversial. (Catteral 1981, Geraci 1980, Henry et al 1979, Kaul & Hendrickson 1981). The dose of radiation used for postoperative treatment of malignant tumors is usually about 60 Gy.

Radiation therapy is not indicated for the treatment of benign salivary tumors. The previous frequent use of postoperative radiation therapy for a pleomorphic adenoma rested on the false concept that this tumor was thought to be semimalignant. Inadequate surgery, such as enucleation of a pleomorphic adenoma, followed by radiotherapy, as has been proposed again recently (Armitstead et al 1979), is to be condemned. This concept embraces two incorrect forms of treatment: firstly, enucleation of the tumor, which carries a high risk of local recurrence; secondly, irradiation of a nonmalignant tumor, which carries the risk of inducing a malignant one. Thus, an increased incidence of benign and malignant salivary tumors can be demonstrated after a latent interval of about two decades after irradiation of the parotid region for various reasons, such as hyperplastic tonsils (Maxon et al 1981, Walker et al 1981). The place of postoperative radiotherapy of individual malignant tumors has also not been agreed on. Adenoid cystic carcinomas are said not

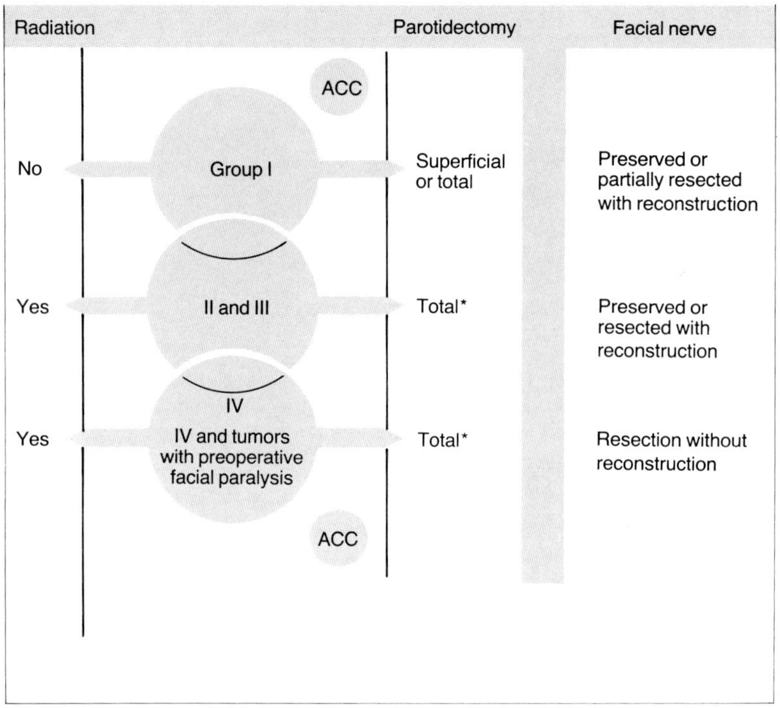

Figure 15.**133** Therapeutic concepts of malignant salivary gland tumors. ACC = adenoid cystic carcinoma. The group numbers relate to the prognostic groups I to IV determined by histology (see page 282, Figure 15.**135**). Group I includes well-differentiated acinic and mucoepidermoid tumors and tubular adenoid cystic carcinomas. Group II includes poorly differentiated acinic cell tumors, duct carcinomas, and cribriform and solid adenoid cystic carcinomas. Group III includes adenocarcinomas, poorly differentiated mucoepidermoid tumors, and squamous cell carcinomas. Group IV includes carcinoma ex pleomorphic adenoma and undifferentiated carcinoma.

to be radiocurable, but radiosensitive (Berdal et al 1970, Conley & Dingman 1974, Eneroth 1977, Grahne et al 1977, Leafstedt et al 1971, Moran et al 1961, Scherer et al 1972). This supposed radiosensitivity of adenoid cystic carcinomas has had no influence on the survival rate in our experience (Chilla et al 1981). The results of postoperative radiotherapy for patients with poorly differentiated acinic cell tumors were similar (Chilla et al 1983a). Radiotherapy is the treatment of choice for malignant lymphomas localized in the parotid region. The only place for surgery of such a tumor is to confirm the diagnosis and possibly to reduce the bulk of the tumor. There is no justification for sacrificing the facial nerve in such a patient.

Chemotherapy

Little is so far known about chemotherapy of malignant salivary tumors, with the exception of malignant lymphomas in the parotid area, which may be treated by irradiation therapy or chemotherapy, depending on their stage and histologic type (Rentschler et al 1977, Suen & Johns 1982). We have also treated a few patients with advanced malignancy, but with no effect on the course of the disease. This is also true of adenoid cystic carcinoma. However, there are conflicting reports of the response of this tumor to chemotherapy (Scheel & Kastenbauer 1981, Skibba et al 1981). It is extremely difficult to assess the efficacy of intra-arterial chemotherapy and the influence of the newer drugs on these slowly growing tumors, particularly the adenoid cystic carcinoma.

References

Armitstead, P. R., F. G. Smidey, H. G. Frank: Simple enucleation and radiotherapy in the treatment of the pleomorphic salivary adenoma of the parotid gland. Brit. J. Surg. 66 (1979) 716
Berdal, P., A. De Besche, E. Mylius: Cylindroma of salivary glands. Acta Otolaryng. (Stockh.) 263 (1970) 170
Butler, C.: Salivary gland tumours. J. Laryng. Otol. 86 (1972) 775
Catteral, M.: The treatment of malignant salivary gland tumors with fast neutrons. Int. J. Rad. Oncol. Biol. Phys. 7 (1981) 1737
Chilla, R., R. Casjens, U. Eysholdt, M. Droese: Maligne Speicheldrüsentumoren – Früherkennung. Nachsorge und Therapie. Arch. Oto-Rhino-Laryng. 237 (1983a) 227
Chilla, R., R. Casjens, U. Eysholdt, M. Droese: Maligne Speicheldrüsentumoren – Der Einfluß von Histologie und Lokalisation auf die Prognose. HNO 31 (1983b) 286
Chilla, R., R. Schrot, U. Eysholdt, M. Droese: Adenoidcystic carcinoma of the head and neck. ORL 42 (1980) 346
Chilla, R., R. Schrot, U. Eysholdt, M. Droese: Über die therapeutische Beeinflußbarkeit adenoid-zystischer Karzinome im Parotisbereich. HNO 29 (1981) 118
Conley, J., D. L. Dingman: Adenoid cystic carcinoma in the head and neck (cylindroma). Arch. Otolaryngol. 100 (1974) 81
Elkons, D., M. Colman, F. R. Hendrickson: Radiation therapy in the treatment of malignant salivary gland tumors. Amer. Cancer Soc. 41 (1978) 502
Eneroth, C. M.: Frequenz, Prognose und Behandlung der Speicheldrüsentumoren. HNO-Praxis 2 (1977) 159
Fletcher, E. H., N. V. Tapley, M. B. Patricio: Irradiation – radiotherapist's concept. In Conley, J.: Salivary Glands and the Facial Nerve. Thieme, Stuttgart 1975
Fu, K. K., S. A. Leibel, M. L. Levine, L. M. Friedlander, R. Boles, T. L. Phillips: Carcinoma of the major and minor salivary glands. Cancer (Philad.) 40 (1977) 2882
Geraci, J. P.: Neutron radiation therapy of parotid gland tumors. Acta radiol. Oncol. 19 (1980) 91

Grahne, B., C. Laurén, L. Holsti: Carcinoma adenoides cysticum im Kopf- und Halsbereich. HNO-Praxis 2 (1977) 181
Haubrich, J., A. Miehlke: Zur Therapie von Parotistumoren. Chirurg 49 (1978) 114
Henry, L. W., J. C. Blasko, T. W. Griffin, R. G. Parker: Evaluation of fast neutron teletherapy for advanced carcinomas of the major salivary glands. Cancer 44 (1979) 814
Jakobsson, P. A., C.-M. Eneroth: Variations in radiosensitivity of various types of malignant salivary gland tumors. Acta Otolaryng. 263 (1970) 186
Kaul, R., F. Hendrickson: Fast neutrons in the treatment of salivary gland tumors. Int. J. Radiat. Oncol. Biol. Phys. 7 (1981) 1667
Leafstedt, S. W., J. F. Gaeta, K. Sako, F. C. Marchetta, D. P. Shedd: Adenoid cystic carcinoma of major and minor salivary glands. Amer. J. Surg. 122 (1971) 756
Maxon, H. R., E. L. Saenger, S. R. Thomas, M. L. Shafer, C. R. Buncher, J. G. Kereiakes, C. A. McLaughlin: Radiation-associated carcinoma of the salivary glands. Ann. Otol. 90 (1981) 107
Miehlke, A., E. Stennert, R. Arold, R. Chilla, H. Penzholz, A. Kühner, V. Sturm, J. Haubrich: Chirurgie der Nerven im HNO-Bereich. Arch. Otorhinolaryng. 231 (1981) 89
Moran, J. J., S. M. Becker, L. W. Brady, V. B. Rambo: Adenoid cystic carcinoma – a clinicopathological study. Cancer (Philad.) 14 (1961) 1235
Rentschler, R., M. A. Burgess, R. Byers: Chemotherapy of malignant major salivary gland neoplasms. Cancer 40 (1977) 619
Scheel, J. V., E. R. Kastenbauer: Intraarterielle Cisplatin-Therapie beim adenoidzystischen Karzinom. HNO 29 (1981) 308
Scherer, E., G. Lehmann, M. John: Beitrag zur Strahlentherapie der Zylindrome im Kopf- und Halsbereich. Strahlentherapie 143 (1972) 361
Skibba, J. L., J. D. Hurley, H. V. Ravelo: Complete response of a metastatic adenoid cystic carcinoma of the parotid gland to chemotherapy. Cancer (Philad.) 47 (1981) 2543
Stenner, E., A. Miehlke, M. Schröder: Combined approach in extratemporal facial reconstruction. In Graham, M. D., W. F. House: Disorders of the Facial Nerve. Raven Press, New York 1982
Stewart, J. G., A. W. Jackson, M. K. Chew: The role of radiotherapy in the management of malignant tumors of the salivary glands. Amer. J. Roentgenol. 102 (1968) 100
Suen, J. Y., M. E. Johns: Chemotherapy for salivary gland cancer. Laryngoscope 92 (1982) 235
Walker, M. J., P. K. Chaudhuri, C. Wood, T. Gupta: Radiation induced parotid cancer. Arch. Surg. 116 (1981) 329

Prognosis of Malignant Salivary Gland Tumors

Of the factors that influence the prognosis of malignant salivary gland tumors, *histology* of the tumor has a preeminent place (Chilla et al 1983). If the patients are divided by histologic differentiation (typing) and subdifferentiation (grading), the survival rate varies widely (Fig. 15.**134**). The determinate survival rate (that is, the survival rate after correction for patients lost to follow-up or dying of intercurrent disease) after 5 years shows a wide variation from 23% for undifferentiated carcinoma to 100% for well-differentiated acinic cell tumors. Malignant salivary gland tumors can be divided into four prognostic groups (I–IV), based on this 5-year survival. The first group with a survival of 100% includes the well-differentiated acinic cell tumor, mucoepidermoid tumors, and tubular adenoid cystic carcinomas. The second group has a survival of 65% and includes the solid and cribriform adenoid cystic carcinomas and poorly differentiated acinic cell tumors and duct carcinomas. The third group with a 40% survival includes adenocarcinoma, poorly differentiated mucoepidermoid carcinoma, and squamous cell carcinoma. The fourth group with a 5-year survival of 25% includes carcinoma ex pleomorphic adenoma and the undifferentiated carcinomas (Fig. 15.**135**).

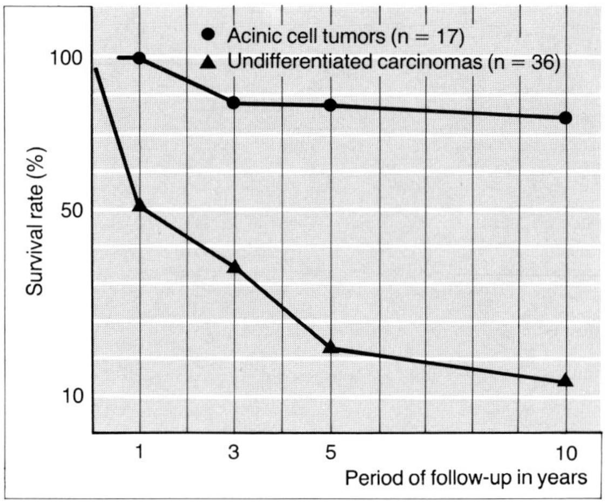

Figure 15.**134** Prognosis of acinic cell and undifferentiated carcinoma.

The histologic subtypes never fall in the same prognostic group. This divergence is particularly marked in the mucoepidermoid tumors: the highly differentiated forms are in group I, whereas the poorly differentiated forms are in group III.

In general, the 10-year survival is 10% worse than the 5-year survival, and the curves parallel each other with two exceptions: cribriform and solid adenoid cystic carcinomas, which change from group II into group IV. Highly differentiated mucoepidermoid tumors also change into group II rather than group I.

Our results accord largely with those of Eneroth (1977) and Fu et al (1977). Others (Levitt et al 1981, Spiro et al 1975) have found a considerably better prognosis for carcinoma ex pleomorphic adenoma and for acinic cell tumors, but in our experience, patients with a carcinoma ex pleomorphic adenoma are very unlikely to be cured. Boles et al (1980) also report a remarkable relatively unfavorable prognosis for acinic cell tumor, which was worse than that of adenoid cystic carcinoma, adenocarcinoma, and squamous cell carcinoma. However, the grade of differentiation of the acinic cell tumors was not reported, so that this series may have contained an unusually large proportion of poorly differentiated tumors.

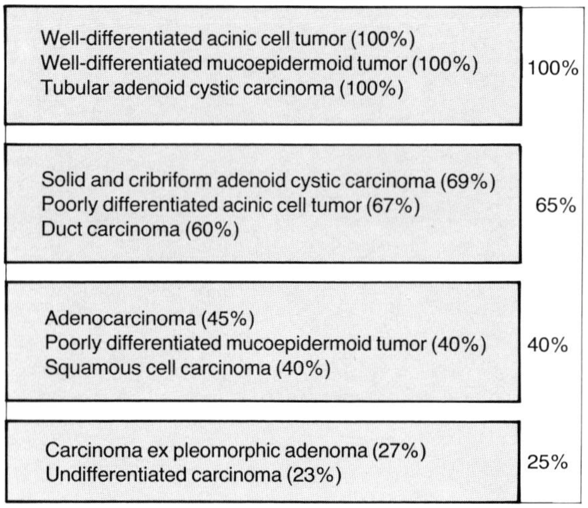

Figure 15.**135** Five-year survival of prognostic groups I to IV, based on 207 patients with malignant salivary tumors seen in the Göttingen Clinic between 1965 and 1975.

The extent of a malignant tumor, local recurrence, and lymph or blood-borne metastases obviously have a great influence on the prognosis. A *facial nerve paralysis* is a particularly unfavorable sign (Eneroth 1977). In our experience the 5-year survival is about 20%, and the 10-year survival is 15% (Fig. 15.**136**). Thus, patients with a face paralysis due to tumor should be included in the highest T stage (Levitt et al 1981, Spiro et al 1975).

Local recurrences, particularly repeated recurrences, are typical of the evolution of a salivary tumor. The rate of multiple recurrences in adenoid cystic carcinoma, acinic cell tumor, and the poorly differentiated mucoepidermoid tumor exceeds 50% (Fig. 15.**71**). The behavior of recurrent malignant salivary tumors varies widely. Thus, a disease-free interval lasting for years is common in adenoid cystic carcinoma, whereas all recurrences of squamous cell carcinoma are manifested in the first 2 years after operation (Figure 15.**138** and Table 15.**12**). The site of the recurrence depends on the direction of extension of the salivary malignancy (Fig. 15.**139**). The parotid

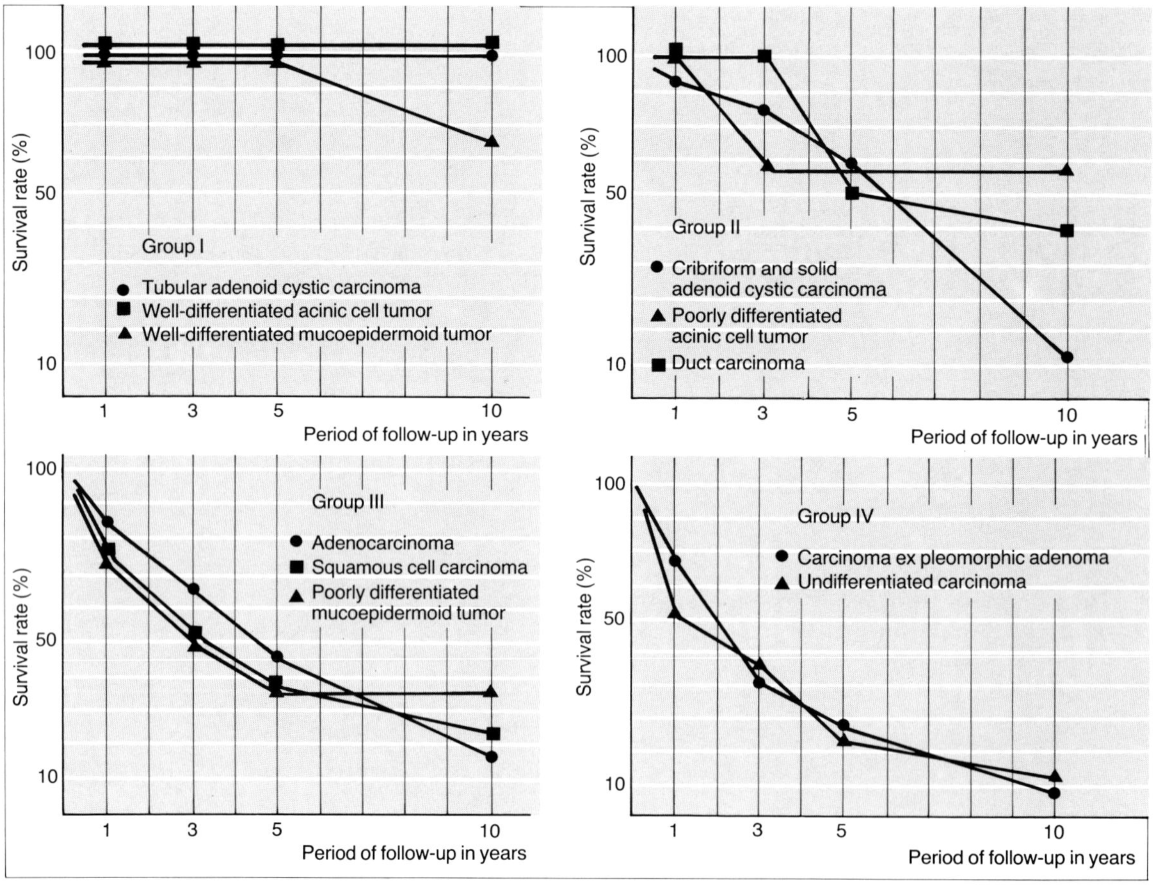

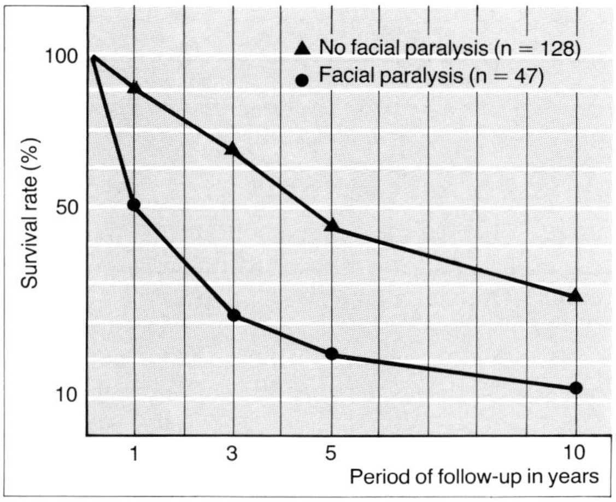

Figure 15.**136** Paralysis of the facial nerve and prognosis of patients with salivary tumors.

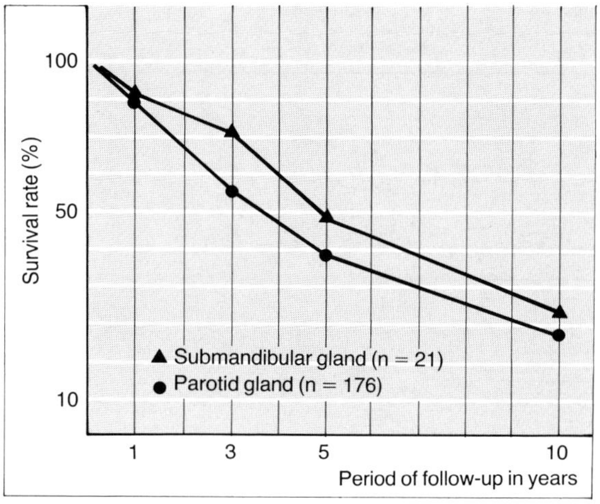

Figure 15.**137** Site and prognosis in malignant salivary tumors.

gland is not as easy to demarcate from the surrounding tissue as is the submandibular gland, and because of its anatomic relationships, it is difficult to assess. Follow-up is therefore difficult. Parotid malignancies often tend to spread along vessels and nerves. Adenoid cystic carcinoma is an impressive example of this growth tendency, but it also applies to recurrences of other tumors. Thus, concealed recurrences along the course of the maxillary artery into the pterygopalatine fossa are common. Tumors grow inferiorly, but more commonly superiorly in the carotid sheath to reach the base of the skull. They also extend along the external auditory meatus (Fig. 15.**140**) into the infratemporal fossa and extend along the facial nerve into the mastoid. Thus, a recurrence is often neither palpable nor visible and is only detected because of paralysis of a cranial nerve,

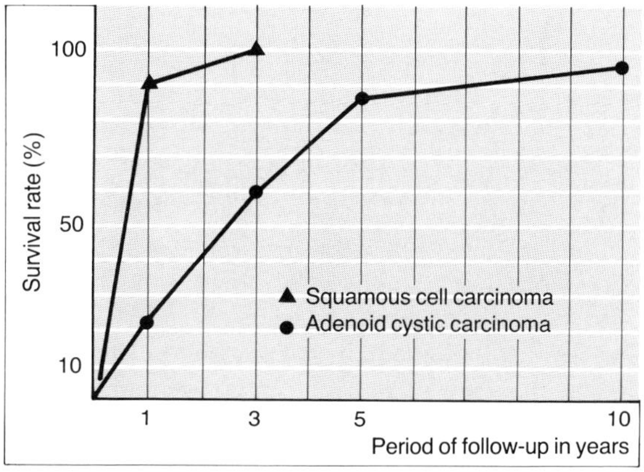

Figure 15.**138** Pattern of local tumor recurrence after the primary operation. The proportions relate to all patients who developed a recurrence during the course of their illness.

Table 15.**12** Recurrence-free Interval after Primary Treatment (Göttingen Series 1965–1975). The Percentage Figures Relate to the Total Number of Patients with Recurrence

Type of Tumor	Recurrence-free Interval		
	Less than 1 year %	3–5 year %	More than 5 years %
Acinic cell tumor	25	33	0
Adenocarcinoma	25	17	0
Adenoid cystic carcinoma	23	28	13
Carcinoma ex pleomorphic adenoma	50	14	7
Mucoepidermoid tumor	45	9	9
Squamous cell carcinoma	80	0	0
Duct carcinoma	20	0	0
Undifferentiated carcinoma	47	11	0

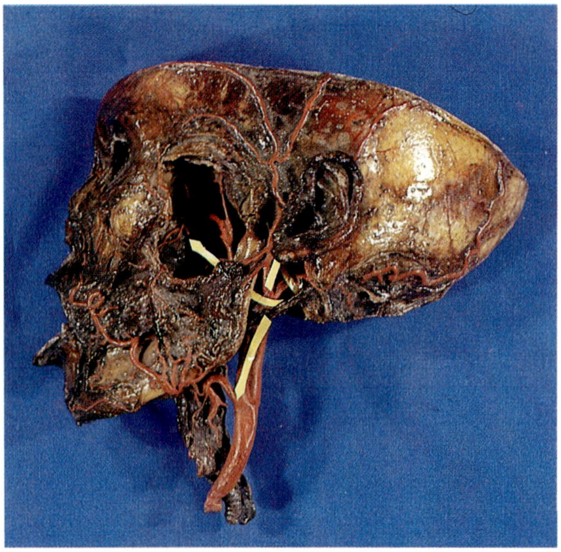

Figure 15.**139** Typical directions of spread of malignant salivary tumors and their recurrences, shown by an arrow. The coronoid process of the mandible has been removed.

for example, a swallowing disorder, or a vocal cord paralysis due to a lesion of the vagus nerve.

Lymph node and blood-borne *metastases* of salivary carcinomas also parallel the temporal course of local recurrence. At the time of presentation, 20% of our patients had a metastasis in the lymph nodes and 2% had a distant metastasis. However, these figures increased to 40% and 30%, respectively, during the evolution of the tumor. The lung is the site of predilection for distant metastases; metastases to the skeletal system and the liver are much less common. The timing of metastases is correlated with the appearance of local recurrence. A typical example is the adenoid cystic carcinoma whose blood-borne metastases almost always appear several years after primary treatment, and then are always associated with a late recurrence. These facts are impressive evidence of the decisive significance of the treatment of a primary tumor on the further progress of a patient with a malignant salivary tumor.

The *site* is said to be important in the prognosis of salivary tumors (Eneroth 1970). Tumors of the minor salivary glands have the most favorable prognosis, followed by parotid tumors and finally those of the submandibular gland. We have been unable to confirm these findings, particularly the prognosis of submandibular tumors (see Fig. 15.**137**) (Chilla et al 1983).

The histologic structure and site of a salivary tumor have a considerable influence on prognosis but are not capable of being influenced by the surgeon. We must attempt to influence the course of the highly malignant salivary tumors by taking advantage of the factors that can be influenced, such as treatment, early recognition, and aftercare.

References

Boles, R., J. Raines, M. Lebovits, K. K. Fu: Malignant tumors of salivary glands. A university experience. Laryngoscope 90 (1980) 729

Chilla, R., R. Casjens, U. Eysholdt, M. Droese: Maligne Speicheldrüsentumoren – Der Einfluß von Histologie und Lokalisation auf die Prognose. HNO 31 (1983) 286

Eneroth, C.-M.: Incidence and prognosis of salivary-gland tumours at different sites. Acta Otolaryng. 263 (1970) 174

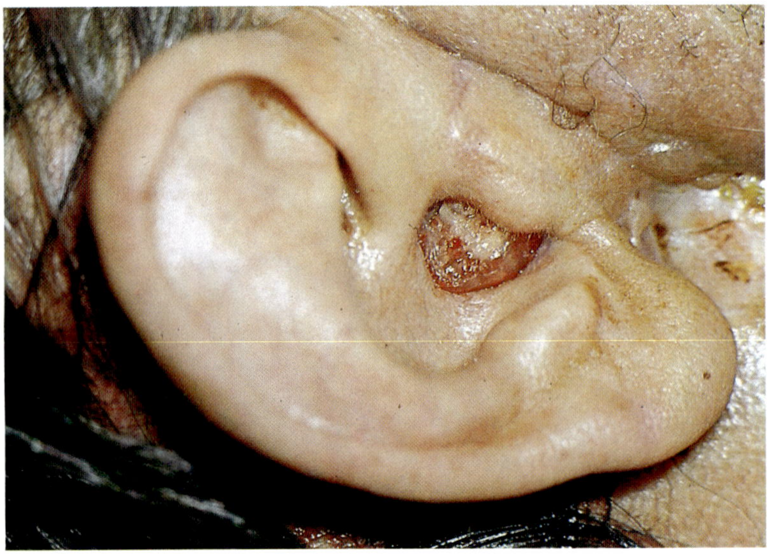

Figure 15.**140** Recurrence of a squamous cell carcinoma of the parotid gland breaking through into the external auditory meatus.

Eneroth, C.-M.: Frequenz, Prognose und Behandlung der Speicheldrüsentumoren. HNO-Praxis 2 (1977) 159
Eneroth, C.-M.: Facial nerve paralysis. A criterion of malignancy in parotid tumors. Arch. Otolaryng. 95 (1972) 300
Fu, K. K., S. A. Leibel, M. L. Levine, L. M. Friedlander, R. Boles, T. L. Phillips: Carcinoma of the major and minor salivary glands. Cancer 40 (1977) 2882
Levitt, S. H., R. B. McHugh, O. Gómez-Marin, V. J. Hyams, E. H. Soule, E. W. Strong, A. H. Sellers, J. E. Woods, O. M. Guillamondegui: Clinical staging system for cancer of the salivary gland: a retrospective study. Cancer 47 (1981) 2712
Spiro, R. H., A. G. Huvos, E. W. Strong: Cancer of the parotid gland. A clinico-pathologic study of 288 primary cases. Amer. J. Surg. 130 (1975) 452

16. Nonepithelial Salivary Tumors

The nonepithelial tumors of the salivary gland arise from local mesenchymal tissues, including the blood and lymphatic vessels, the neural structures, the connective and fatty tissue, and the neighboring muscle. They can spread within the gland or invade the periglandular tissue. Tumors of the intra- and periglandular lymph nodes, including malignant lymphomas and metastases, are discussed in Chapter 17, and extraglandular tumors are discussed in Chapter 18 because of their significance in differential diagnosis.

One hundred and twenty patients with nonepithelial tumors (excluding lymph node tumors and extraglandular tumors) were recorded in the Salivary Gland Register at the Pathology Department of the University of Hamburg in the years 1965–1981. These patients represent 4.5% of the 2700 patients with salivary gland tumors registered in the same period, and 52.5% were angiomas (Table 16.**1**), 18.5% lipomas, 17.5% neural tumors, and 4% other benign mesenchymal tumors, such as fibromas, osteochondromas and granular cell tumors. Thus, more than 90% of this group are benign, and only 7.5% are represented by sarcomas of varying degrees of differentiation.

The nonepithelial salivary gland tumors demand individual consideration because of their differential diagnosis and treatment. Thus, neurinomas of the extratemporal course of the facial nerve are often misdiagnosed as pleomorphic adenoma or a cystadenolymphoma and subjected to an operation that can cause facial paralysis. Almost 90% of nonepithelial tumors are localized to the parotid gland, the rest are in the submandibular gland. This difference is due to the fact that the parotid gland is more richly permeated by vascular and neural tissue than the submandibular gland, and it is not separated from the neighboring tissue by a well-developed capsule, as is the submandibular gland.

Table 16.**1** Classification of 120 Nonepithelial Salivary Gland Tumors in the Salivary Register 1965–1981

Type of Tumor	Men	Women	Total	%
Angioma	31	32	63	52.5
Pure hemangioma	17	22	39	
Mixed hemangioma and lymphangioma	4	3	7	
Pure lymphangioma	9	5	14	
Hemangiopericytoma	1	2	3	
Lipoma	20	2	22	18.5
Neural tumors	11	10	21	17.5
Neurinoma	3	6	9	
Neurofibroma	6	3	9	
Neurofibromatosis	2	1	3	
Other benign tumors	3	2	5	4.5
Fibromas	1	–	1	
Osteochondromas	1	1	2	
Granular cell tumors	1	1	2	
Sarcomas	6	3	9	7.5
Malignant histiocytoma	3	1	4	
Malignant schwannoma	1	1	2	
Rhabdomyosarcoma	1	1	2	
Malignant hemangioendothelioma	1	–	1	
Total	71	49	120	100.0

Table 16.**2** Age Distribution of 120 Nonepithelial Salivary Gland Tumors in the Salivary Gland Tumor Register, 1965–1981

Age (yr)	Heman-giomas*	Lymph-angiomas	Lipoma	Neural Tumors	Other Benign Tumors	Sar-comas
0–10	22**	6	–	3	1	–
11–20	10	2	–	–	–	–
21–30	3	2	3	2	1	–
31–40	5	3	4	4	–	1
41–50	–	–	5	4	1	1
51–60	4**	1	5	3	1	2
61–70	4**	–	5	4	–	1
71–80	–	–	–	1	–	3
Over 80	1	–	–	–	1	1
Total	49	14	22	21	5	9

* Includes mixed hemangiomas and lymphangiomas.
** Includes one hemangiopericytoma.

The age distribution (Table 16.**2**) demonstrates further differences among the nonepithelial tumors. Almost two thirds of all tumors develop in the first three decades of life. This is especially true of hemangioma and lymphangioma, which arise primarily in the first decade. Also 25% of all hemangiomas arise in the first decade. The significance of the age factor in diagnosis and treatment of tumors is discussed further in Chapter 19. Neural tumors and lipomas usually occur after the fourth decade and then affect each decade equally up to the seventh.

Angioma

Vascular tumors are the most frequent salivary tumors of children. A summary of the literature shows that about 40% of all tumors in the first decade of life are angiomas (Schuller & McCabe 1977, Nussbaum et al 1976). The following types of angioma may be distinguished by their architecture.

Hemangioma

Parotid hemangiomas occur most commonly in infants and more often in girls than boys (Schröder 1965, Helpap 1966, Brands & Menges 1968, Lopes-Tello & Krämer 1971). Many parotid hemangiomas are present at birth and resolve spontaneously toward the end of the first year of life. Parotid hemangiomas mainly arise in the superficial lobe and endow the thin overlying infantile skin with a blue transluscent color. The soft well-vascularized tumor invades the body of the gland like a sponge (Fig. 16.**1**). Secondary inflammation or circulatory disorders cause partial sclerosis and vascular thrombosis. Phleboliths of various sizes are thus caused by calcification (Hébert et al 1975). Periglandular hemangiomas arising in the masseter muscle can masquerade as a painful parotid tumor (Chilla 1983).

Hemangiomas may be classified as capillary or cavernous, depending on the width of the lumen (Seifert 1965). The lumen is lined by a single layer of epithelium and contains a varying quantity of erythrocytes. Cavernous hemangiomas usually arise from primary capillary hemangiomas. Capillary hemangiomas were found in about 30% of the material in the Salivary Gland Register, and about 60% were cavernous hemangiomas, and 10% were mixed hemangiomas and lymphangiomas; 40% of the hemangiomas were localized in the parotid gland, whereas in the remaining 60%, angiomatous proliferation had developed in periglandular soft tissue. The gland tissue, particularly the end pieces, disappears due to proliferation of the blood vessels, whereas the ducts remain recognizable for a relatively long period within the vascular tumor (Fig. 16.**2a**, **b**, 16.**3a**, **b**). The marked cellularity of proliferative capillary hemangiomas and the apparent invasive spread can mimic a malignant vascular tumor of the angiosarcomatous type. This is especialy true of congenital capillary hemangiomas, which may also be termed benign infantile hemangioendothelioma (Nagao et al 1980). In this type of tumor, the endothelial cells are arranged occasionally in several layers with a solid arrangement, but on the whole are uniformly differentiated (Seifert 1965).

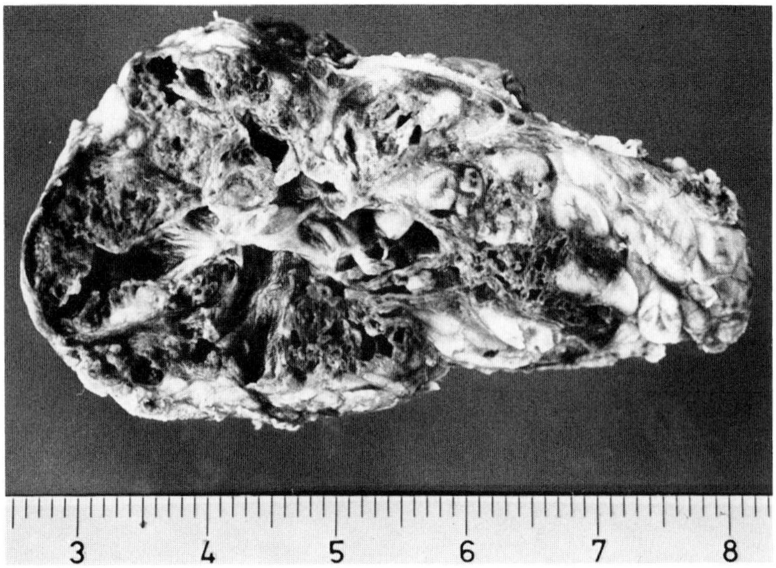

Figure 16.**1** Cavernous hemangioma of the parotid gland: spongelike permeation of the gland by hollow blood spaces.

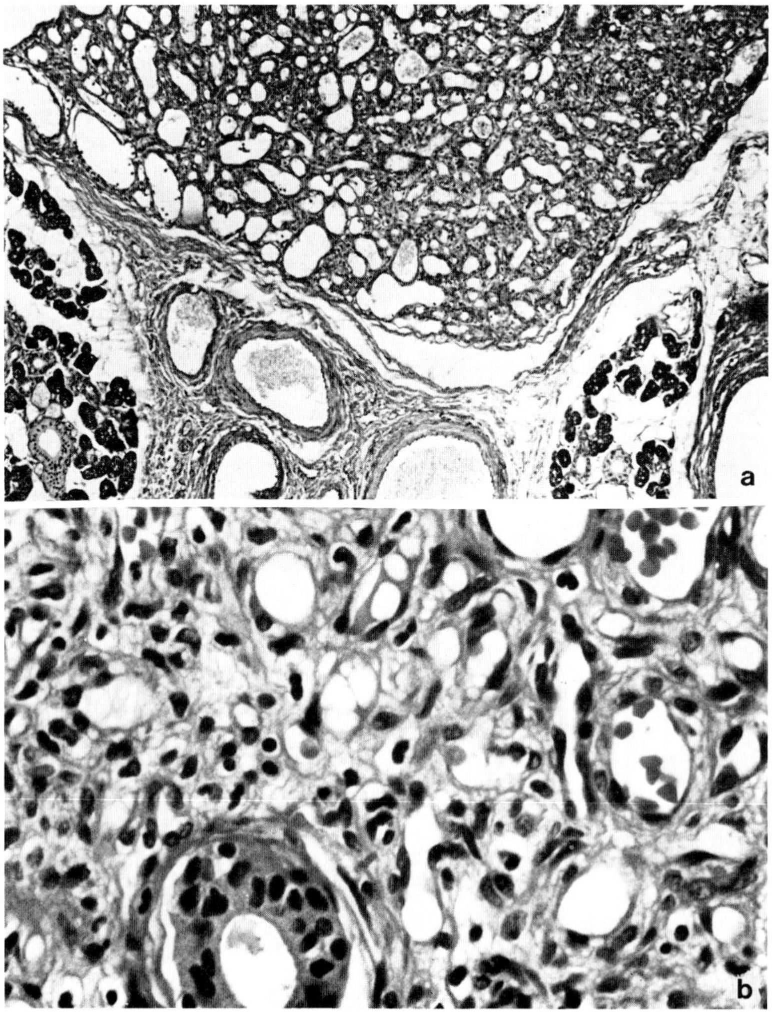

Figure 16.**2** Cavernous hemangioma of the parotid gland:
a Cavernous dilated thin-walled blood spaces with endothelial lining, and marginal rests of parenchyma. **b** Segment of the tumor with inclusion of a striated duct.
H & E. **a** 63×, **b** 160×.

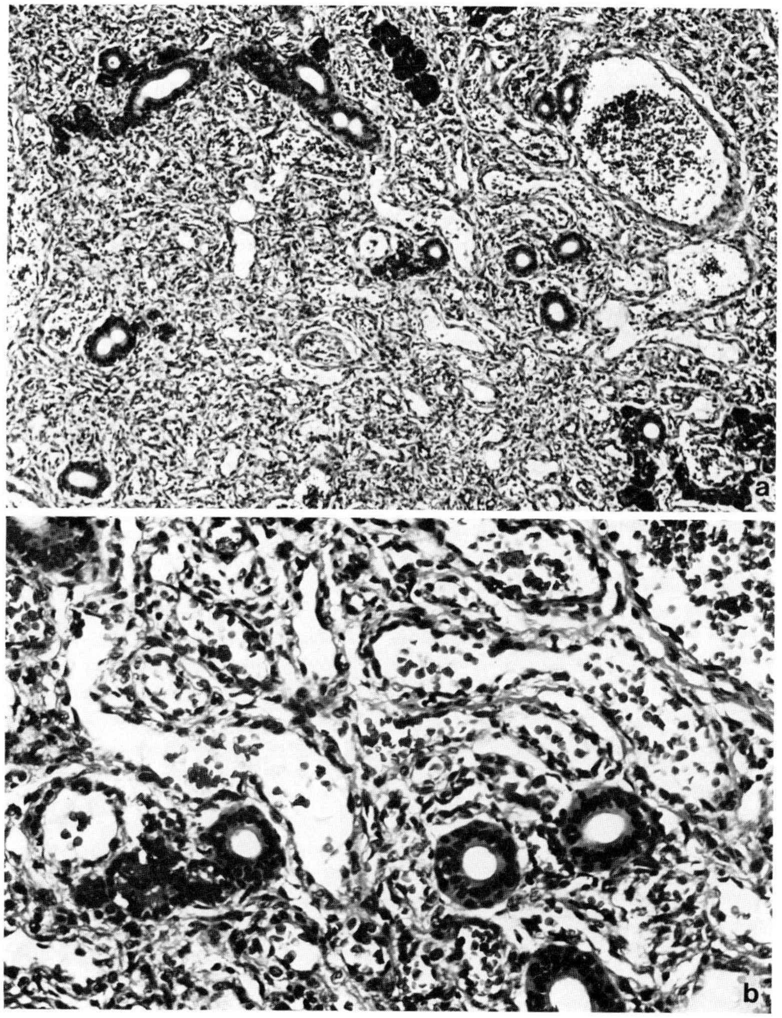

Figure 16.**3** Capillary hemangioma of the parotid gland: **a** Displacement of the gland parenchyma by strongly proliferating capillaries with remnants of the duct system in between. **b** Thin-walled capillaries with regular endothelial boundaries. H & E. **a** 63×, **b** 160×.

Lymphangioma

Lymphangiomas are considerably rarer than hemangiomas, and in our material were more common in boys than girls (Seifert 1965). The relatively soft gelatinous tumor spreads mainly in the periglandular fatty tissue, especially of the spaces inferior to the parotid or submandibular gland and less within the actual gland parenchyma. The lumen of the vessels contains cell-free lymph, which does not occur with hemangiomas. Cystic lymphangioma with its flat epithelial lining is characteristic (Fig. 16.**4a, b**). Sclerosis and obliteration of the lymph vessels can occur due to degenerative changes. Macroscopically, these tumors may be recognized by their compressibility. They can be emptied and they will refill when the patient puts his head between his knees.

Hemangiopericytoma

Primary benign hemangiopericytomas of the salivary glands are very rare (Pellegrini et al 1967, Cernea et al 1969, Hubert et al 1970, Neal & Starke 1973, Massarelli et al 1980). This tumor is characterized by spindle-shaped cell proliferation arising from the pericytes of the external capillary wall with an intact endothelium (Fig. 16.**5**). The basement membrane of the capillary wall is preserved. In addition, reticular fibers are developed between the proliferation of pericytes. Atypical mitoses and other forms of cell atypia are absent. The stroma can show degenerative hyaline changes.

Treatment of Angiomas

Angiomas can regress spontaneously from the sixth month of life after formation of a vessel lumen. In infants, removal should therefore be avoided if at all possible, because the anatomic

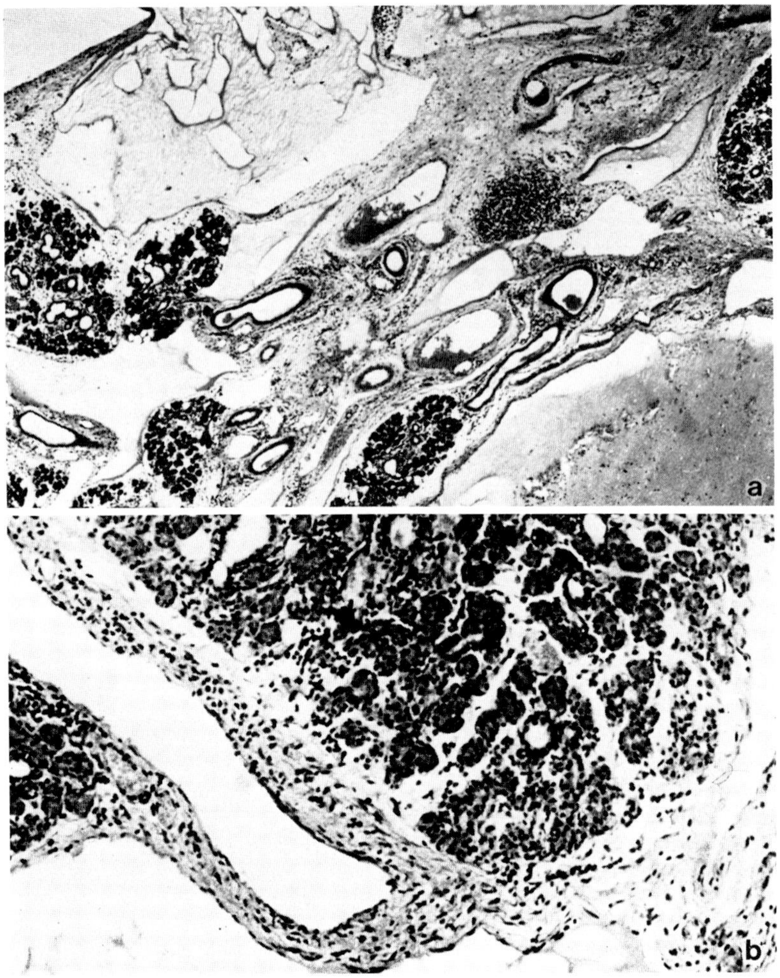

Figure 16.**4** Cystic lymphangioma of the parotid gland: displacement of the gland tissue by thin-walled dilated lymph vessels with cell-free lymph in the lumen. H & E. **a** 25×, **b** 160×.

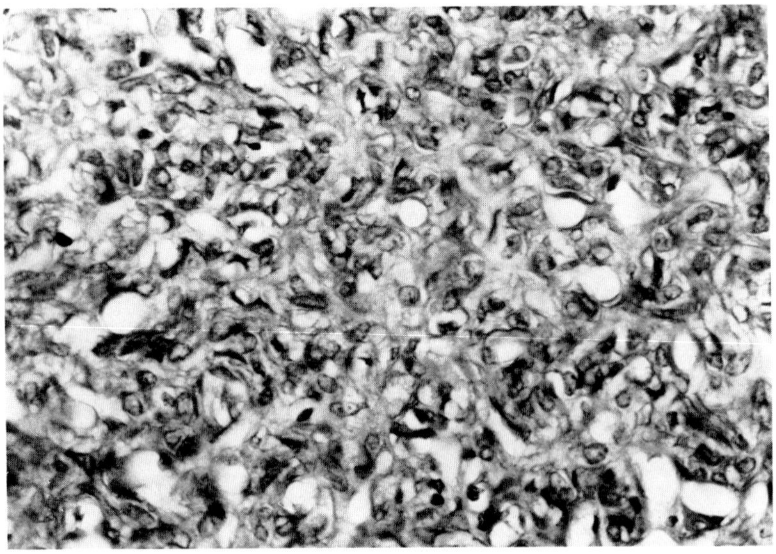

Figure 16.**5** Hemangiopericytoma of the parotid gland: pericytic proliferation and intact capillaries with regular endothelium between them. H & E, 400×.

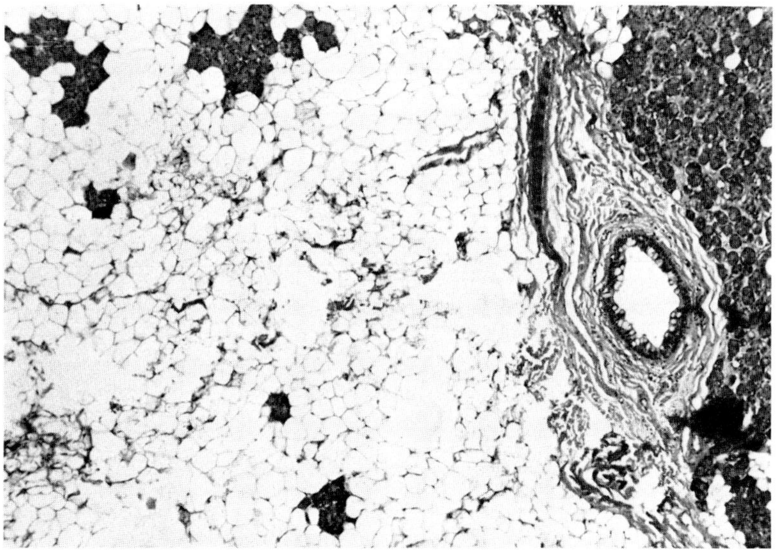

Figure 16.**6** Intraglandular lipoma of the parotid gland: replacement of the gland tissue by fat. A remnant of the gland with a duct is shown on the right. H & E, 160×.

structures are so small and because of the delicacy of the facial nerve. Radiation therapy causes both types of tumor to regress, but this treatment carries the danger of atrophy of the skin and, even worse, the risk of a radiation-induced carcinoma many years later. The best policy therefore is to wait until the child has reached school age: it is then possible to remove the angioma and preserve the facial nerve because the structures are by now much larger (Denecke 1969, Miehlke 1960, 1973). The operation demands considerable experience, because the cavernous spaces surround the delicate peripheral branches of the facial nerve and must be freed from the branches of the nerve a millimeter at at time. The rubber band technique (see page 329ff) is particularly valuable for these patients. Further details of tumors in children are discussed in Chapter 19.

Lipoma

Of all lipomas, 95% arise in the parotid gland and only 5% in the submandibular gland. In our own material, more than 90% occurred in men. Lipomas demonstrate both intraglandular and periglandular extension, but are distinguished from lipomatosis by the formation of a capsule. Macroscopically, lipomas are soft and yellow in color, so that they can be confused with a cystadenolymphoma before the operation, and the true nature of the tumor becomes apparent only after it has been exposed. The removal of a lipoma presents no particular operative difficulties provided that the trunk of the facial nerve and its branches are exposed. The technique is described on page 329ff. Lipomas consist histologically of uniform fat cells arranged in lobules between which narrow connective tissue septa with blood vessels are developed (Baker et al 1981, Janecka et al 1977, Walts & Perzik 1976, Peiro-Escriva et al 1982). The tumors grow by expansion and displace the parenchyma (Fig. 16.**6**), but the atrophy that they produce is not pronounced, as in an angioma. Intraglandular lipomas of the parotid must be distinguished from the subaponeurotic form and also from diffuse lipomatosis (Adams et al 1982) (see also page 168).

Neural Tumors

Neural tumors appear in middle life. In our material, 85% originated in the parotid and 15% in the submandibular gland. The histologic structure of neural tumors of the salivary glands does not differ from that of similar tumors of other organs, so that they can be classified by the general classification of tumors of the nervous system (Harkin & Reed 1968).

Solitary Schwannoma (Neurinoma, Neurilemmoma)

This group contains 40% of all neural tumors. Most extratemporal facial nerve schwannomas are benign: they cause symptoms by pressure on the surrounding structures. The fascicles of the facial nerve are strangulated in the stylomastoid canal by the increase in size of the tumor within the canal.

Schwannomas are encapsulated, gray in color, and have a cystic surface. The histologic picture

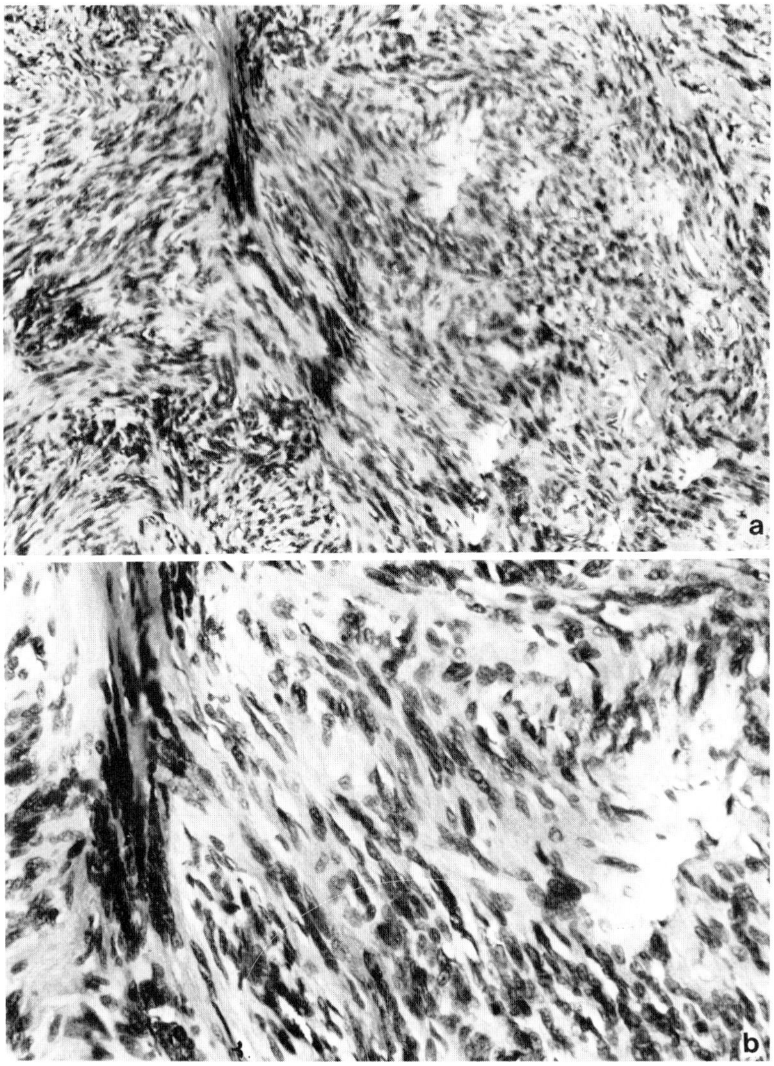

Figure 16.**7** Solitary schwannoma of the parotid gland: spindle cell masses of Schwann cells with fascicular arrangement and palisading of the cell nuclei (Antoni type A). H & E. **a** 160×, **b** 400×.

(Fig. 16.**7a, b**) is characterized by spindle cell growths of the perineural Schwann cells, which demonstrate a fascicular or palisade arrangement. A collagen matrix develops between these fiber bundles (Aston & Sparks 1975, Avery & Sprinkle 1972, Conley & Janecka 1974, Kavanagh & Panje 1982, Shore-Freedman et al 1983, Helidonis et al 1978).

The palisade arrangement of the tumor cells is typical of the Antoni type A of Schwannoma. Under the electron microscope, the Schwann cells possess notched cell nuclei and a rich provision of organelles in the cytoplasm (lysosomes, Golgi apparatus, mitochondria, and granular endoplasmic reticulum). The fibroblasts lying between the Schwann cells contain no "long-spacing collagen" (Kessoku et al 1980). The Antoni type B of schwannoma is characterized by an abundant edematous translucent matrix, numerous vessels, thin cell cords, and a tendency to cystic degeneration. The rich cellularity of the schwannoma and the palisade arrangement of the tumor cells can simulate a sarcoma. The differential diagnosis of malignant schwannoma is discussed on page 298.

Solitary Neurofibroma

This tumor is roughly as common as the solitary schwannoma. It presents as a circumscribed nodule but, unlike the schwannoma, does not have a capsule (Figs. 16.**8**, 16.**9**). Neurofibromas arise from the nerve fibers and can also include Schwann cells. A collagen matrix lies between the cells with inclusion of mucoid or myxomatous structures that usually contain acid mucopolysaccharides and demonstrate a positive staining with alcian blue, in contrast to schwannomas of Antoni-type B, which usually do not stain with alcian

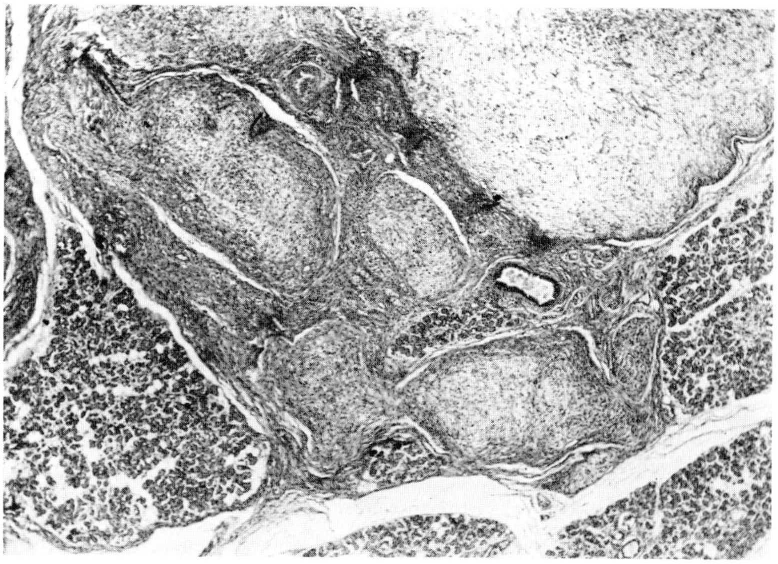

Figure 16.**8** Solitary neurofibroma of the parotid gland: multiple poorly demarcated nodular formations within the gland. H & E, 25×.

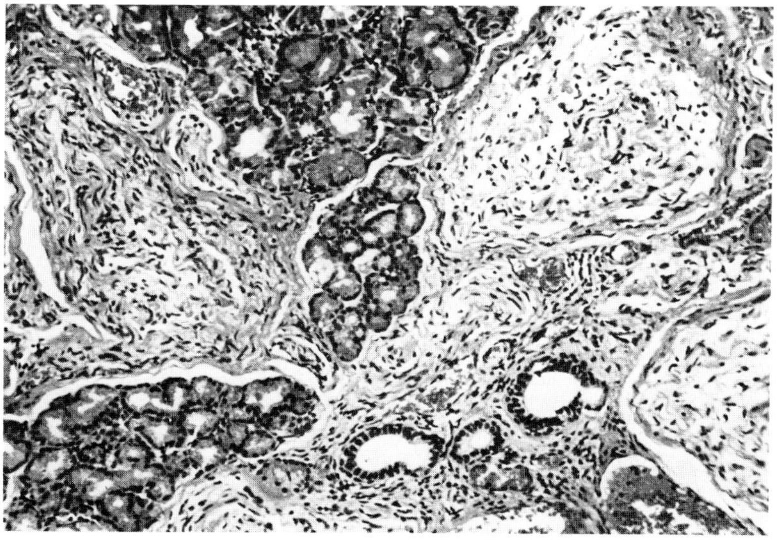

Figure 16.**9** Plexiform neurofibroma of the parotid gland showing neural fiber bundles permeated by myxomatous tissue, and collagenous fiber structures. H & E, 160×.

blue. The neurofibromas form plexiform or fusiform structures (Weitzner 1980, Martin et al 1981).

Neurofibromatosis (Von Recklinghausen's Disease)

Multiple nodules appear, often presenting for the first time in childhood. Important clinical signs include cutaneous manifestations (café-au-lait spots and nevoid telangiectasia), pigmented lesions of the buccal mucosa, lesions of the central nervous system, such as tuberous sclerosis, and signs of the Sturge-Weber syndrome, such as nevus flammeus of the face, particularly in the area of distribution of the first branch of the trigeminal nerve, congenital glaucoma, and a tendency to paroxysmal attacks of epilepsy. An autosomal dominant inheritance may be demonstrated in many cases (Schätzle & Haubrich 1975). Ten percent of these tumors undergo sarcomatous degeneration (Haguenau 1948, Kreyberg 1954, Redon 1955). Histologic examination demonstrates the structures of a plexiform neurofibroma and also of a cystic schwannoma, mostly of Antoni type B, within the nodes (Brasfield and Das Gupta 1972). The cells are arranged in whirls and may have Schwann cell inclusions. A myxoid matrix may be observed in addition to fascicles of collagen fibers. Hypertrophic nerve fibers and also degenerative changes may be observed.

Treatment of Neural Tumors

Before treating a *facial nerve schwannoma*, it is vital to establish if it is benign or malignant by a careful open biopsy. The extratemporal course of the nerve is exposed by the technique described on page 329ff.

If histologic examination demonstrates the tumor to be one of the very rare malignant schwannomas, the treatment should be the radical removal of the tumor with a wide margin of normal tissue followed by a full dose of radiotherapy. A benign schwannoma of the intratemporal segment of the facial nerve should usually be resected and the continuity of the nerve restored by an autologous nerve graft at the same procedure.

The treatment of a *schwannoma of the extratemporal course of the facial nerve* follows the same principles as that of a tumor of the intratemporal course. If a facial paralysis is present before the operation, the diseased nerve segment is removed with a wide margin and the defect is bridged by a free autologous nerve graft. If the tumor arises from a branch of the facial nerve distal to the bifurcation, the resection of the entire facial branch will have no undesirable sequelae because function will be restored by the abundant anastomotic network. In individual cases, it may be necessary to restore the continuity of the facial nerve by direct or indirect anastomosis using an autologous nerve graft. If the tumor takes origin from the facial nerve trunk but has not caused a paralysis, a considerable problem arises. It will usually be necessary to resect the involved segment of the nerve and to restore anatomic continuity by a free autologous nerve graft. Although this procedure is logical and oncologically sound, the patient has a complete facial paralysis that lasts about a year.

It is difficult for the surgeon faced with a histologically benign tumor to make a conscious decision to resect the facial nerve, thus causing a facial nerve paralysis, particularly since these patients are usually in the middle years of life and in an active period of their lives.

This decision requires a careful assessment of the patient's emotional and social status. It may be justifiable to take a calculated risk, if the tumor is proved to be benign, and to adopt a conservative policy with close follow-up. A long personal experience of this tumor has shown this policy to be justifiable. We also believe that other surgeons, such as Conley and Lundgreen share this view, since both have reported cases in which they have removed the tumor either by an incision along the nerve sheath (Conley 1975) or by removal of the tumor down to its points of origin from the facial nerve (Lundgreen 1947), thus taking great care to preserve the function of the facial nerve. Recurrences are seldom seen after subtotal removal (Roos et al 1956). The decision to adopt a conservative policy in these cases is certainly more difficult than that of complete removal and reconstruction. Surgery in these cases should be tailored to the individual patient, and careful follow-up is essential after any conservative procedure to detect the occasional malignant transformation.

Treatment of neurofibromatosis in von Recklinghausen's disease is particularly difficult. Removal of tumors in the parotid area requires attention to the following points: numerous neurofibromas should only be removed if they are causing a severe cosmetic deformity. A prerequisite is that *all nodules* must be removed. Sarcomatous degeneration of untreated neurofibromas is much more common than spontaneous malignancy. Since the disease is usually generalized, neurofibromas causing only moderate swelling of the lateral part of the face and not causing a facial paralysis should not be removed.

Other Benign Tumors

The tumors in this heterogenous group are entirely localized in the parotid gland.

Fibromas

Pure fibromas are very rare. Typically, they are firm in consistency, and their histologic characteristics are a collagenous network of fiber structure (Fig. 16.**10a, b**). They must be distinguished from pleomorphic adenoma with a stroma rich in fascicles (page 184), and from tumors such as desmoids (Fig. 16.**11**) arising from adjacent tissue (Majmudar & Winiarski 1978). Xanthofibromas of the parotid are extremely rare (Cancura 1969).

Osteochondroma

This tumor is extremely rare in the parotid area (Fig. 16.**12a, b**), and as with fibromas must be distinguished from unilateral degenerative changes in a pleomorphic adenoma. Chondromas or osteomas in early childhood may indicate a dysgenetic origin from remnants of the branchial arches.

Granular Cell Tumor

This tumor mainly affects the tongue and the larynx, and the salivary glands only rarely (Seifert et al 1977). In our two cases, the tumors arose in the parotid gland, had reached a size of 1.5 cm, were fully mobile, encapsulated, and at operation

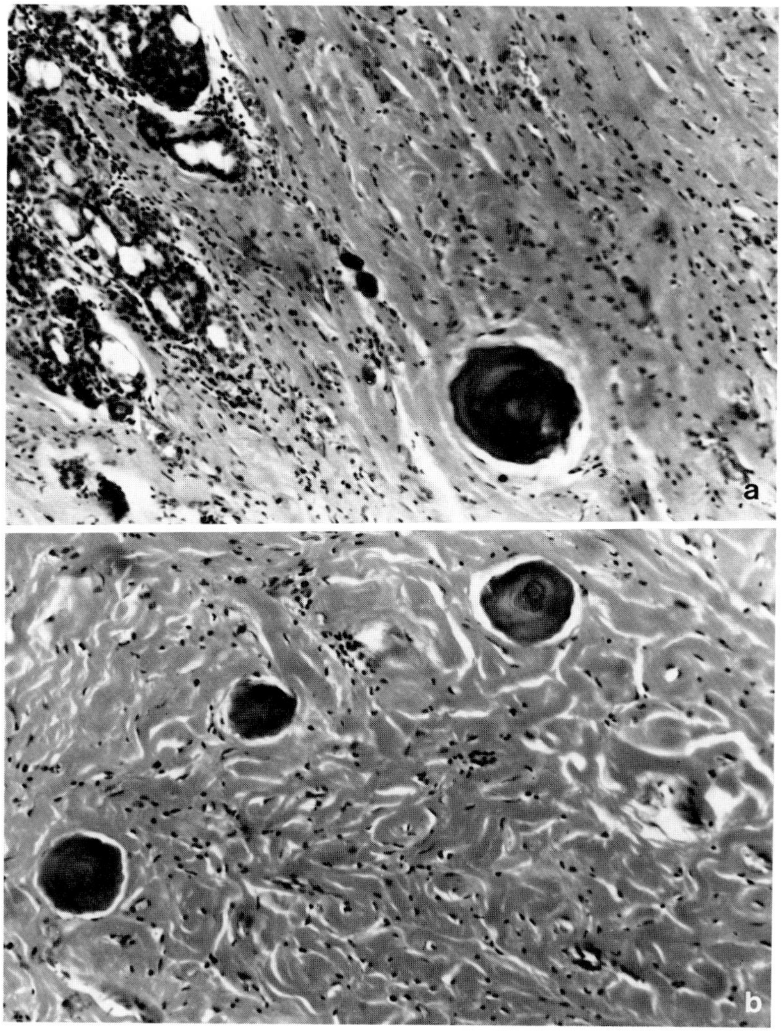

Figure 16.**10** Fibroma of the parotid gland with calcification. H & E. **a, b** 63×

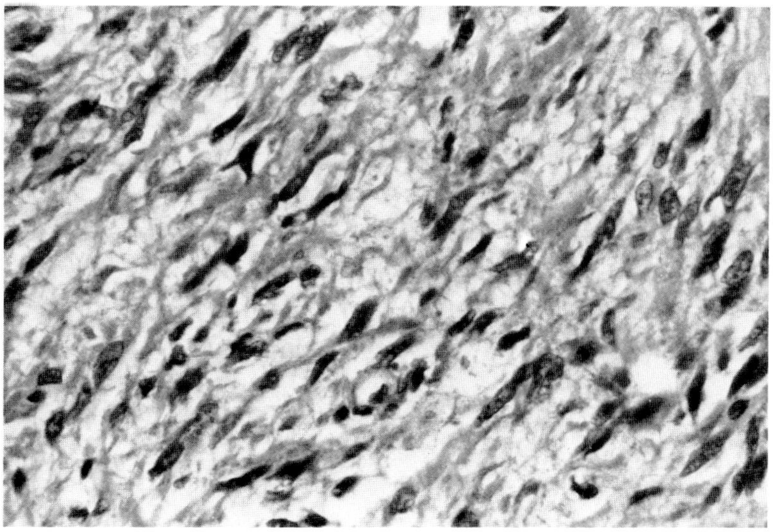

Figure 16.**11** Desmoid with infiltration of the parotid gland: collagenous fiber bundles with inclusion of spindle-shaped fibroblasts. H & E, 400×.

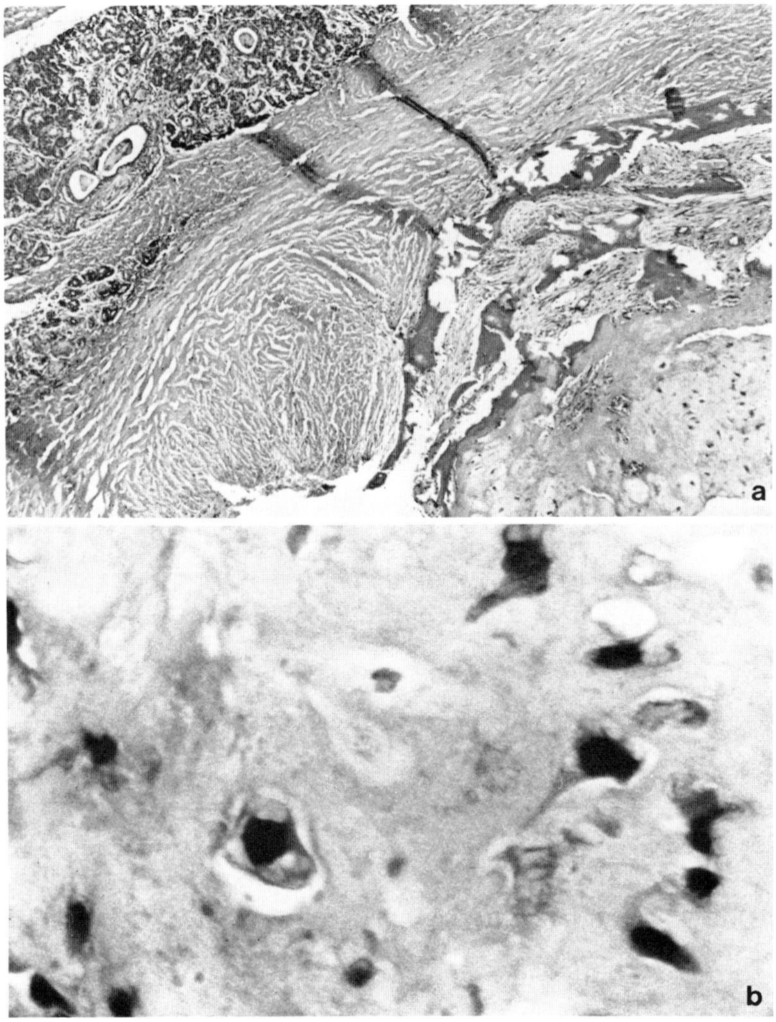

Figure 16.**12** Osteochondroma of the parotid gland: **a** Cartilage and bone tissue permeating the parotid gland. **b** Section of the tumor with cartilaginous cells. H & E. **a** 25×, **b** 400×.

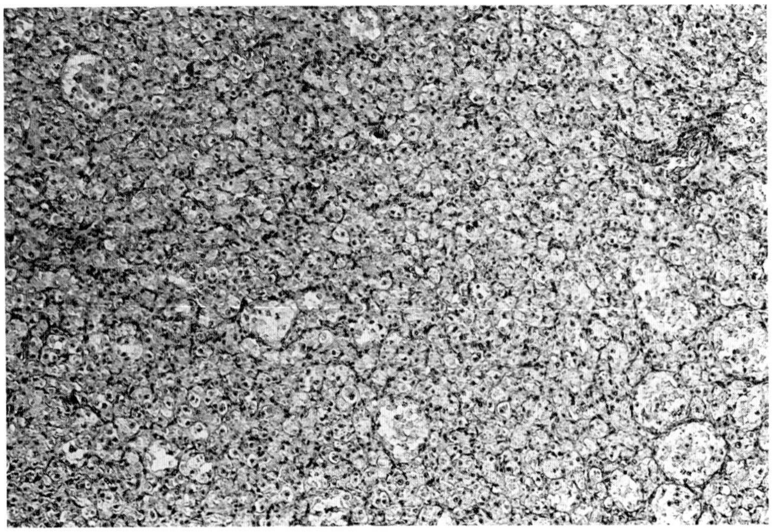

Figure 16.**13** Granular cell tumor of the parotid gland: alveolar-lobular arrangement of tumor cell cords. Masson-Goldner, 63×.

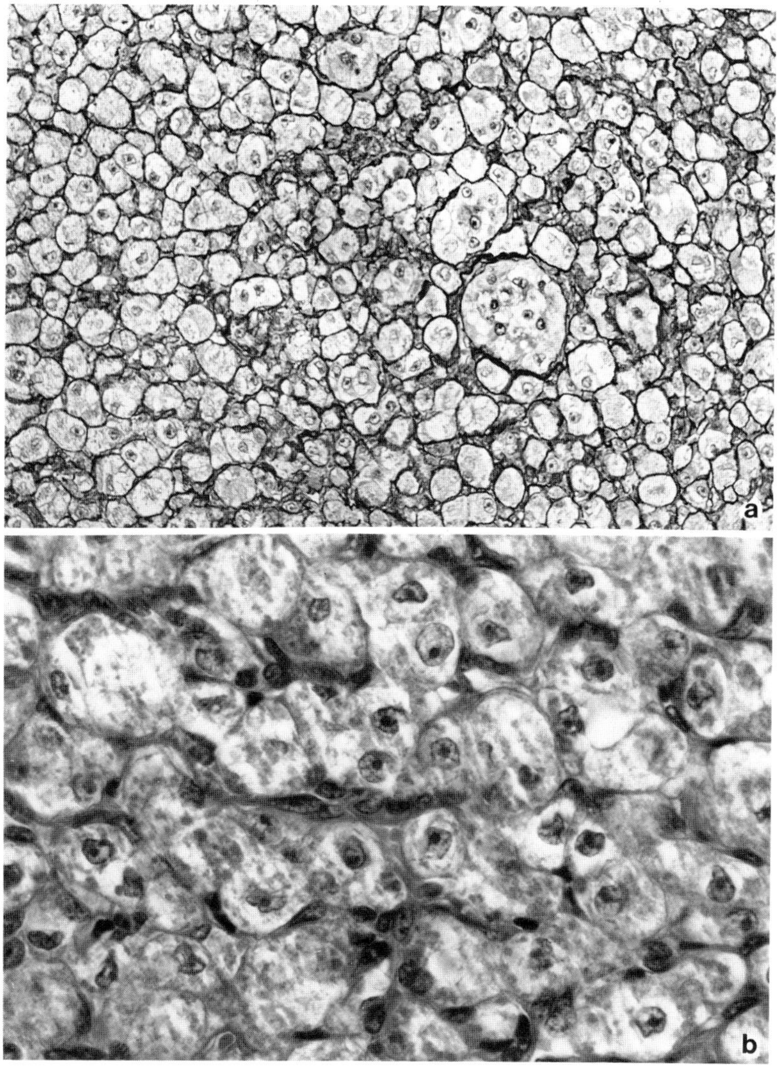

Figure 16.**14** Granular cell tumor of the parotid gland: **a** Reticular arrangement with sheaths of alveolar cell complexes. Gomori, 160×. **b** Section showing tumor cells rich in cytoplasm and granular cell transformation of the cytoplasm. H & E, 400×. (Seifert et al 1977.)

were closely related to the facial nerve. The histologic characteristics (Figs. 16.**13**, 16.**14a, b**) are solid, alveolar cell structures with broad acidophilic granular cytoplasm. The granules are PAS positive and also contain mucopolysaccharides. A fine network develops from basement membrane substances that lie between the cells. The granular cell tumor must be distinguished from alveolar soft part sarcoma, acinic cell tumor, and paraganglioma.

Pseudotumorous Granulomas

Odd cases of eosinophilic lymphofollicular granuloma (Kimura's disease) (Miyamoto & Tani 1977) and a lymphomatoid granulomatosis (Jensen et al 1982) localized in the parotid gland have been recorded.

Sarcoma

Only tumors arising primarily from the mesenchyme of the salivary gland should be assigned to this category (Volpe & Mazabraud 1981). Malignant tumors arising from the external auditory meatus, the mandible, the base of the skull, or the middle ear that invade the parotid and simulate a salivary gland tumor will not be considered here (see Chapter 19).

Malignant Fibrous Histiocytoma

This tumor has occasionally been described in the parotid gland (Sphapshay et al 1979, Benjamin et al 1982). We have seen four patients with this disease. The criteria of malignancy include infiltration and polymorphic architecture consisting of immature histiocytes with giant cell nuclei, mul-

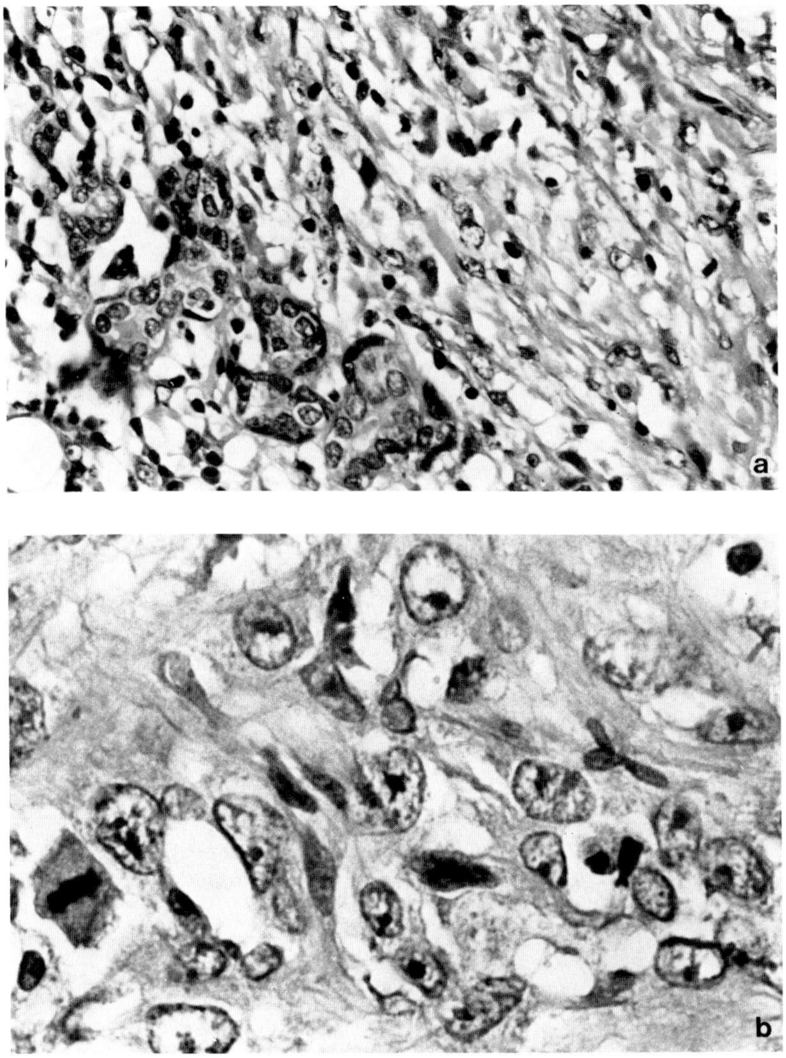

Figure 16.**15** Malignant histiocytoma of the parotid gland: pleomorphic architecture with infiltration of the parotid (**a**) and increased mitoses. H & E. **a** 400×, **b** 1000×.

tinucleated giant cells, mitoses, and whorls of fibers (Fig. 16.**15a, b**).

Malignant Schwannoma

This tumor is distinguished histologically from benign schwannomas by plump spindle cells, an increased frequency of mitoses, and syncytial fascicles. The cellular abundance and the aggressive growth pattern are important characteristics that distinguish this tumor from the benign schwannoma (Figs. 16.**16**, 16.**17**).

Rhabdomyosarcoma

Embryonal rhabdomyosarcomas arise in children and adolescents particularly (Stobbe & Dargeon 1950). The characteristics are polymorphous tumor cells with distended nuclei and spindle-shaped solid cytoplasm. Cross-striation of the tumor cells may be absent. Myoglobin or desmin may be demonstrated in the tumor cells by immunocytochemistry of unfixed material (Fig. 16.**18**).

Angiosarcoma

This group includes especially the malignant hemangioendothelioma (Tomec et al 1979) and hemangiopericytoma. A hemangioendothelioma consists of a malignant proliferation of endothelial cells with a luminal and pericapillary extension (Fig. 16.**19a, b**), whereas a hemangiopericytoma consists of malignant transformation of pericytes with intact endothelial cells. Unlike the benign hemangioma or hemangiopericytoma, the malignant tumors have abundant mitoses and abnormal cell forms with bulky nuclear structures. Treatment is along usual oncologic lines, depending on the stage of the tumor.

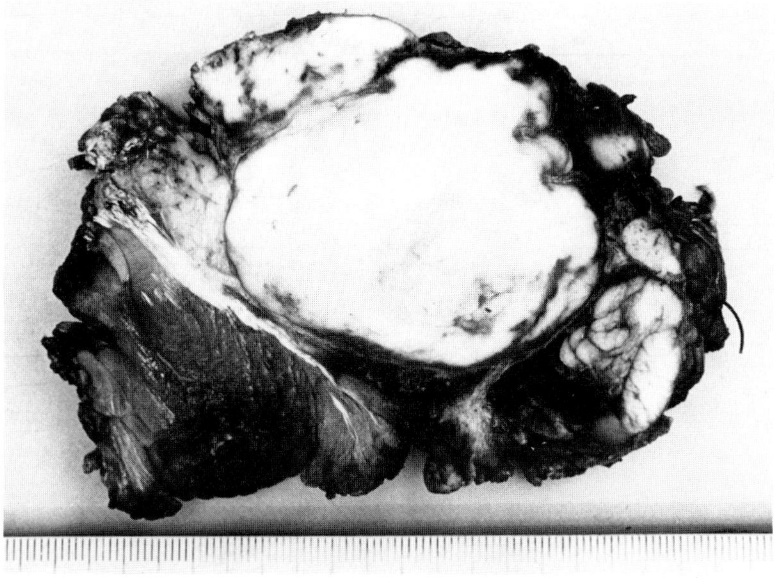

Figure 16.**16** Malignant schwannoma of the parotid gland: cut surface of the specimen with infiltration of the body of the gland.

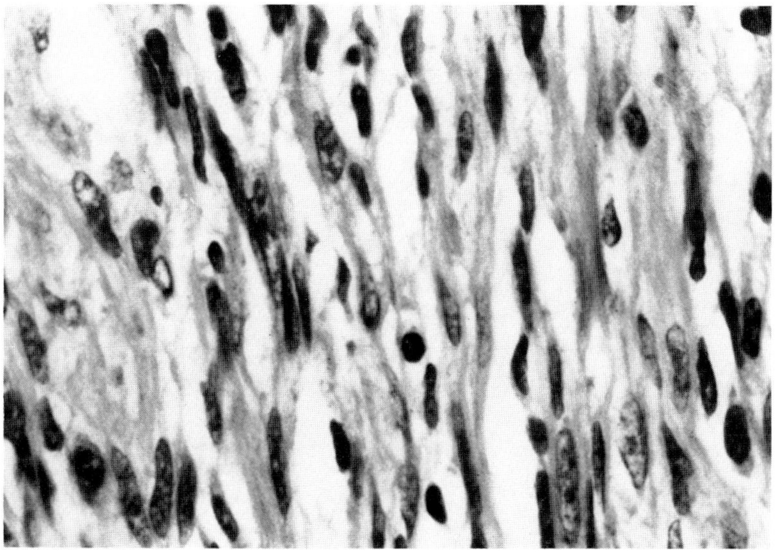

Figure 16.**17** Malignant schwannoma of the parotid gland: spindle-shaped tumor cells with nuclear polymorphism and mitoses. H & E, 700×.

References

Adams, G., M. V. Goycoolea, C. Foster, L. Dehner, R. D. Anderson: Parotid lipomatosis in a 2-month-old child. Otolaryngol. Head Neck Surg. 89 (1982) 402

Aston, S. J., F. C. Sparks: Intraparotid neurilemmoma of the facial nerve. Arch. Surg. 110 (1975) 757

Avery, A. P., P. M. Sprinkle: Benign intraparotid schwannomas. Laryngoscope 82 (1972) 199

Baker, St. E., J. L. Jensen, R. W. Corell: Lipomas of the parotid gland. Oral Surg. 52 (1981) 167

Benjamin, E., S. Wells, H. Fox, N. L. Reeve, F. Knox: Malignant fibrous histiocytomas of salivary glands. J. clin. Pathol. 35 (1982) 946

Brands, Th., G. Menges: Das Hämangiom der Glandula parotis. Zbl. Chirurg. 93 (1968) 557

Brasfield, R. D., T. K. Das Gupta: Von Recklinghausen's Disease. A clinicopathological study. Ann. Surg. 175 (1972) 86

Cancura, W.: Ein Fall eines Xanthofibroms in der Ohrspeicheldrüse. Mschr. Ohrenheilk. 103 (1969) 554

Cernea, P., D. Debry, P. Laudenbach, R. Moreau, C. Brocheriou, M. Cathelin, J. M. Vaillant, P. Guilbert, J. M. Soubiran, C. Chevallier, G. Hosxe, G. Peri: Hémangiopéricytome de la parotide. Rev. Stomat. (Paris) 70 (1969) 132

Chilla, R.: Kavernöses Hämangiom im M. Masseter. Ein Beitrag zur Differentialdiagnose des schmerzhaften Parotistumors. HNO (Berl.) 31 (1983) 88

Conley, J.: Salivary Glands and the Facial Nerve. Thieme, Stuttgart 1975

Conley, J., I. Janecka: Neurilemmoma of the facial nerve. Plast. Reconstr. Surg. 52 (1973) 55

Denecke, H. J.: Zur Chirurgie des N. facialis im Bereiche der Parotis und der Schädelbasis. Wien. klin. Wschr. 71 (1959) 180

Haguenau, M., Med. Diss. Paris 1948; Zit. nach Rauch, G.: Die Speicheldrüsen des Menschen, Thieme, Stuttgart 1959

Harkin, J. C., R. J. Reed: Tumors of the Peripheral Nervous System. Armed Forces Institute of Pathology, Washington 1968

Hébert, G., D. Quimet-Oliva, J. Ladouceur: Vascular tumors of the salivary glands in children. Amer. J. Roentgen. 123 (1975) 815

Helidonis, E., G. Dokianakis, P. Pantazopoulos: A schwannoma of the parotid gland. Report of a case. J. Laryngol. Otol. 92 (1978) 833

Helpap, B.: Hämangiome der Parotis und Tumoren der

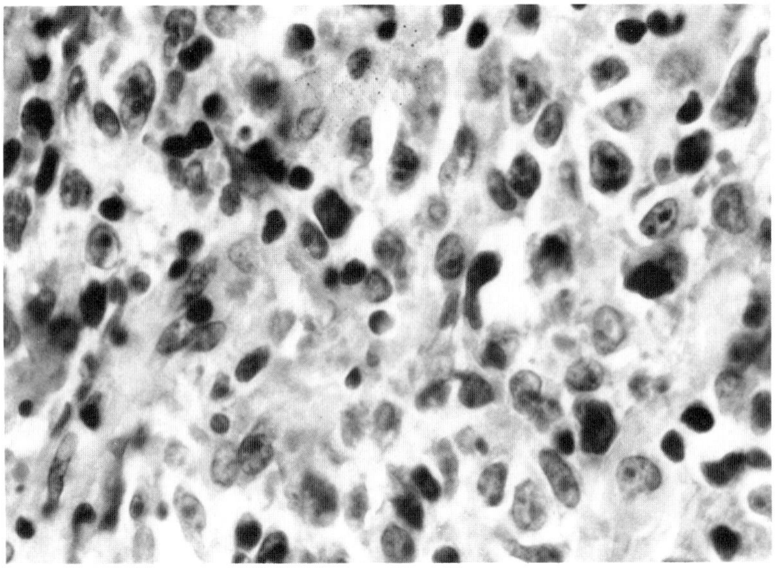

Figure 16.**18** Rhabdomyosarcoma of the parotid gland: polymorphous tumor architecture with some broad cytoplasmic borders, myoglobin, and numerous mitoses. H & E, 700×.

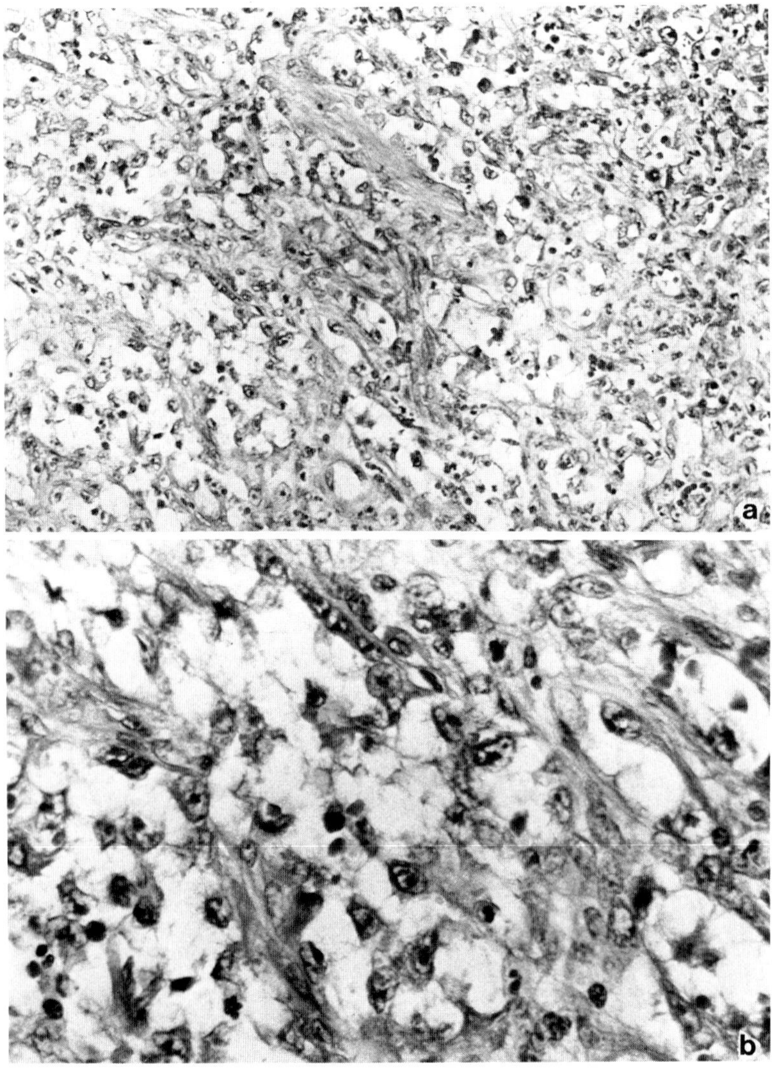

Figure 16.**19** Malignant hemangioendothelioma of the submandibular gland: **a** Vascular neoformation with irregular arrangement of cells. **b** Polymorphic endothelial cells with atypical mitoses. H & E. **a** 160×, **b** 400×.

nichtchromaffinen Paraganglien im Kiefer-Wangen-Bereich bei Kindern – eine differentialdiagnostische Betrachtung. Z. Laryng. Rhinol. 45 (1966) 444

Hubert, J. C., D. Drevet, R. Gay: A propos d'un cas d'hémangiopéricytome parotidien. J. Franc. Otorhinolaryng. 19 (1970) 659

Janecka, I. P., J. Conley, K. H. Perzin, G. Pitman: Lipomas presenting as parotid tumors. Laryngoscope 87 (1977) 1007

Jensen, J. K., C. Lund, J. Schlichting: Lymphomatoid granulomatosis presenting primarily in a parotid gland. J. Laryngol. Otol. 96 (1982) 961

Kavanagh, K. T., W. R. Panje: Neurogenic neoplasms of the seventh cranial nerve presenting as a parotid mass. Amer. J. Otolaryng. 3 (1982) 53

Kessoku, A., T. Kitamura, T. Kaneko, T. Kanda, H. Suzuki: Zur Ultrastruktur des Neurinoms des Nervus facialis. Z. Laryng. Rhinol. 59 (1980) 288

Kreyberg, H., zit. nach Redon, H.: Chirurgie des glandes salivaires. Masson, Paris 1955

Lopez-Tello, C. S., D. Krämer: Parotishämangiome im Kindesalter. Arch. Kinderheilk. 182 (1971) 258

Lundgreen, N.: Neurinoma of N. facialis. Acta Oto-laryng. 35 (1947) 535

Majmudar, B., N. Winiarski: Desmoid tumor presenting as a parotid mass. J. Amer. Med. Ass. 239 (1978) 337

Martin, C., R. Kohler, J. P. Laydevant, H. Martin: Un nouveau cas de neurofibrome parotidien. J. Franc. Otorhinolaryng. 30 (1981) 41

Massarelli, G. F. Tanda, V. Fois, L. Oppia: Hemangiopericytoma of the parotid gland. Report of a case and review of the literature. Virchows Arch. Path. Anat. 386 (1980) 81

Miehlke, A.: Chirurgie des N. facialis. Urban & Schwarzenberg, München 1960

Miehlke, A.: Surgery of the Facial Nerve. Urban & Schwarzenberg, München; Saunders, Philadelphia 1973

Miyamoto, Y., T. Tani: Eosinophilic lymphofollicular granuloma in parotid gland (Kimura's disease): A report of two cases. Kawasaki Med. J. 3 (1977) 15

Nagao, K., O. Matsuzaki, H. Shigematsu, T. Kaneko, T. Katoh, T. Kitamura: Histopathologic studies of benign infantile hemangioendothelioma of the parotid gland. Cancer 46 (1980) 2250

Neal, T. F., W. R. Starke: Hemangiopericytoma of the parotid gland: a case report with autopsy. Laryngoscope 83 (1973) 1953

Nussbaum, M., S. Tan. M. S. Som: Hemangiomas of the salivary gland. Laryngoscope 86 (1976) 1015

Peiro-Escriva, J., J. Palao-Esteve, J. Bonet-Marco, H. Morera-Faet: Lipoma de la glandula parotida. Rev. Mex. Radiol. 36 (1982) 113

Pellegrini, G., S. Verdaguer, F. Boyre, J. L. de Firmas, F. Philip: Hémangiopéricytome parotidien. Rev. Laryng. 28 (1967) 421

Redon, H.: Chirurgie des glandes salivaires. Masson, Paris 1955

Roos, D. B., L. T. Byars, L. V. Ackerman: Neurilemmomas of the facial nerve presenting as parotid gland tumors. Ann. Surg. 144 (1956) 258

Schätzle, W., J. Haubrich: Pathologie des Ohres. Springer, Berlin 1975

Schröder, H. J.: Beitrag zur Pathogenese und Klinik des Parotishämangioms. Z. Laryng. Rhinol. 44 (1965) 594

Schuller, D. E., B. F. McCabe: Salivary gland neoplasms in children. Otolaryng. Clin. North Amer. 10 (1977) 399

Seifert, G.: Die Speicheldrüsengeschwülste im Kindesalter. Zschr. Kinderchir. 2 (1965) 285

Seifert, G., M. Heckmayr, K. Donath: Der Granularzelltumor der Parotis. Differentialdiagnostische Kriterien. Z. Laryng. Rhinol. 56 (1977) 695

Shore-Freedman, E., C. Abrahams, W. Recant, A. B. Schneider: Neurilemomas and salivary gland tumors of the head and neck following childhood irradiation. Cancer (Philad.) 51 (1983) 2159

Sphapshay, S. M., R. H. Wingert, J. S. Davis: Fibrous histiocytoma of the parotid gland. Laryngoscope 89 (1979) 1808

Stobbe, G. D., H. W. Dargeon: Embryonal rhabdomyosarcoma of head and neck in children and adolescents. Cancer 3 (1950) 826

Tomec, R., L. Ahmad, Y. S. Fu, S. Jaffe: Malignant hemangioendothelioma (angiosarcoma) of the salivary gland. An ultrastructural study. Cancer (Philad.) 43 (1979) 1664

Volpe, R., A. Mazabraud: Primary sarcomas of the parotid gland. A clinicopathologic report of two cases. Pathologica 73 (1981) 541

Walts, A. E., S. L. Perzik: Lipomatous lesions of the parotid gland. Arch. Oto-Laryng. 102 (1976) 230

Weitzner, S.: Plexiform neurofibroma of major salivary glands in children. Oral Surg. 50 (1980) 53

17. Lymph Node Diseases of the Salivary Gland

Clinical Data

The parotid and submandibular glands have close contact with lymph nodes and contain lymph nodes completely surrounded by parenchyma. The *parotid lymph nodes* (Figure 17.**1**) consist of a para- and an intraglandular group, the former being closely related to the parotid capsule and lying mainly in front of the tragus. Other lymph nodes lie on the lateral surface of the parotid gland, on the anterior and lower pole of the parotid, and between the parotid gland and the sternocleidomastoid muscle. About 20 to 30 lymph nodes lie within the parotid parenchyma (Conley 1975). The para- and intraglandular lymph node groups are united by lymph vessels,

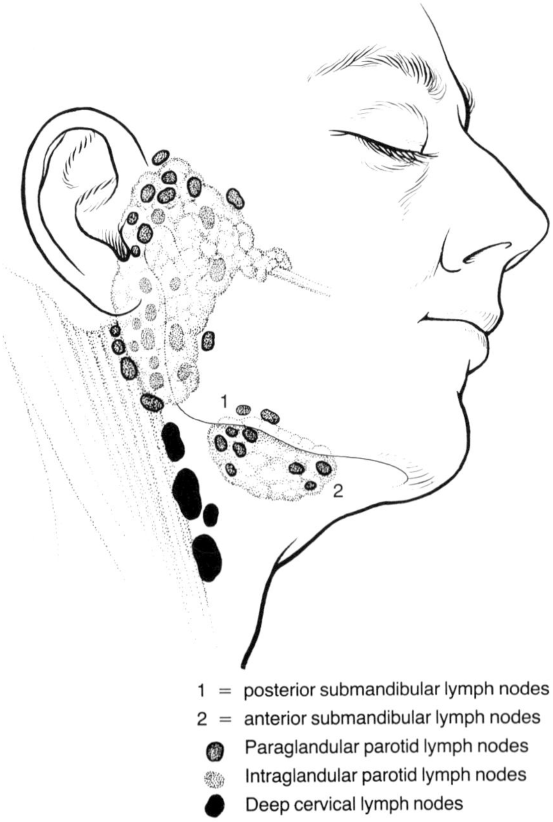

Figure 17.**1** Lymph nodes of the parotid and submandibular glands.

but also drain lymph directly from their own territory, which includes the skin of the temporal, frontal, and parotid regions and the anterior surface of the auricle (see also page 1 and page 310ff).

Several lymph node groups are also enclosed within the submandibular space. These paraglandular submandibular lymph nodes (Fig. 17.**1**) can be divided into an anterior, a middle, and a posterior group (Pernkopf 1957). The afferent lymph vessels arise from the anterior part of the tongue, the floor of the mouth, the teeth of the lower jaw, the skin of the nose, and from the anterior part of the cheek.

Swelling of the salivary glands may be produced not only by diseases of the gland tissue, but also by the regional lymph nodes (Seifert 1979). Circumscribed enlargement of the regional lymph nodes may mimic a salivary gland tumor. The differential diagnosis therefore plays an important role in further treatment. In 8070 cases of salivary gland disease in the Salivary Gland Register (1965–1982), 399 patients had lymph node disease in the parotid or submandibular glands, that is, 5% of the entire series. The distribution of the diseases can be seen in Table 17.**1**: 55% were due to various forms of lymphadenitis, including sarcoidosis (13%), tuberculosis (12%), and toxoplasmosis (4%), 35% were malignant lymphomas, and 10% were metastases. The classification of the lymph node lesions was carried out in cooperation with the Lymph Node Register at the Pathology Institute of the University of Kiel, using the Kiel classification of malignant lymphomas (Lennert et al 1978).

Lymphadenitis

Nonspecific inflammation of the para- and intraglandular parotid lymph nodes is usually due to infection in the drainage area of these lymph nodes, but in many cases it is no longer possible to obtain a history of the primary infection. The inflammation causes a unilateral swelling in the parotid region, which, unlike sialadenitis, does not usually involve the gland parenchyma. If the inflammation extends to the parenchyma, which it

Table 17.**3** Frequency and Classification of 139 Malignant Lymphomas in the Salivary Gland Register 1965–1982

Type of Lymphoma	No.	%	
Non-Hodgkin's lymphoma	118		85
Well-differentiated lymphoma	88		63
chronic lymphatic leukemia		2	
Immunocytoma		22	
Centrocytic-centroblastic lymphoma		39	
Poorly differentiated lymphoma	30		22
Centroblastic lymphoma		3	
Lymphoblastic lymphoma		4	
Hodgkin's lymphoma	21		15
Lymphocyte predominant		4	
Nodular-sclerosing form		4	
Mixed type		5	
Lymphocyte depleted		2	
Total	139		100

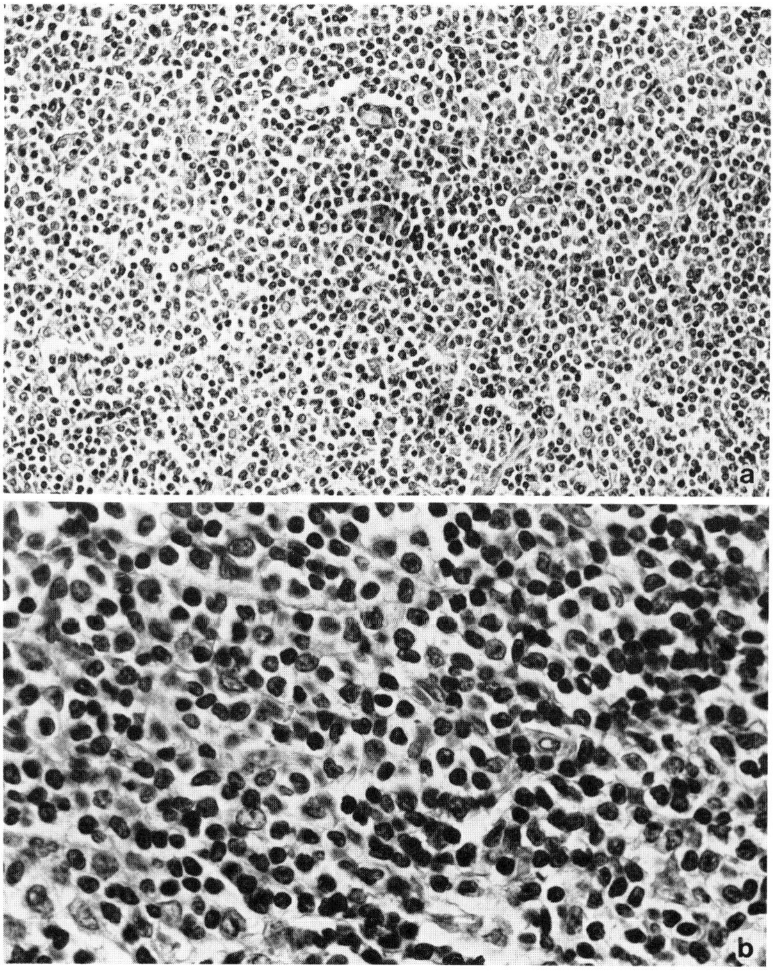

Figure 17.**5** Highly differentiated malignant immunocytoma of the parotid gland: **a** Diffuse infiltration. **b** Architecture consisting of lymphoid and plasmacytoid cells. PAS. **a** 160×, **b** 400×.

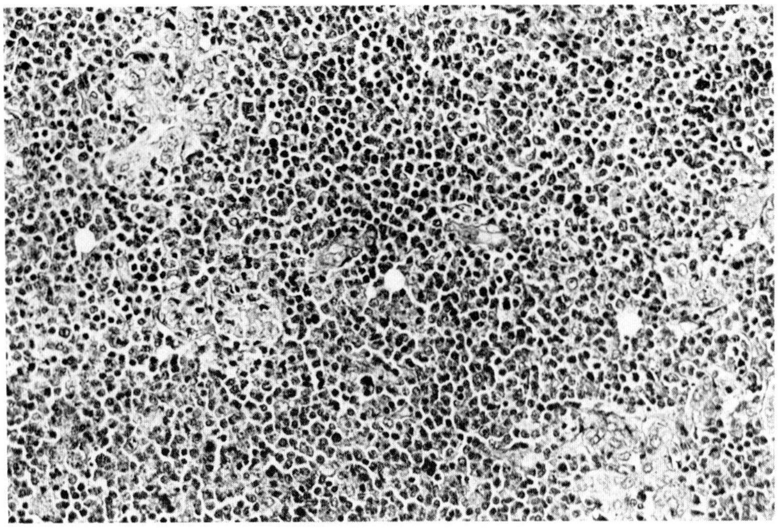

Figure 17.**6** Poorly differentiated malignant immunoblastic lymphoma with a high degree of malignancy. Diffuse infiltration of the gland. PAS, 160×.

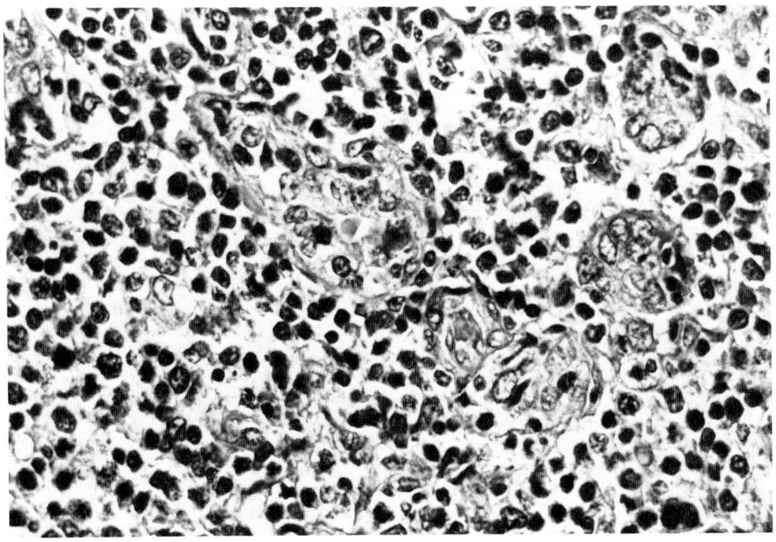

Figure 17.**7** Immunoblastic lymphoma (same case as in Figure 17.**6**): remnants of duct structures between the lymphomatous infiltrate. H & E, 400×.

tomas arising in the parotid gland are rare (Ferlito et al 1980). The immunoblastic lymphoma dominates the poorly differentiated lymphomas (Figure 17.**6** & 17.**7**). However, secondary malignant lymphomas arising in myoepithelial immune sialadenitis are more likely to be well differentiated (Table 17.**2**): 90% are well-differentiated malignant lymphomas, mainly immunocytomas, and only 10% are poorly differentiated immunoblastic lymphomas (Figs. 17.**8**–17.**10**). Similar findings regarding the frequency of malignant lymphomas are given by Schmid et al (1982b). Of 26 malignant lymphomas associated with Sjögren's syndrome, 23 were immunocytomas and three were transitional forms with immunoblastic lymphoma. In contrast, the centrocytic-centroblastic lymphoma is the dominant type in primary malignant lymphomas in patients without Sjögren's syndrome: 15 of 21 cases in Schmid's series were of this type, whereas only two were polymorphic cell immunocytomas, and there were two each of poorly differentiated centroblastic or immunoblastic lymphomas (Schmid et al 1982a).

The *occurrence of non-Hodgkin's lymphoma in myoepithelial sialadenitis* (Sjögren's syndrome) has been investigated by immunocytochemistry. In myoepithelial immune sialadenitis, there is an increase of immunoglobulin G (IgG)-containing plasma cells and a slight increase of IgM-containing plasma cells in the area surrounding the myoepithelial islands (von Gumberz & Seifert 1980).

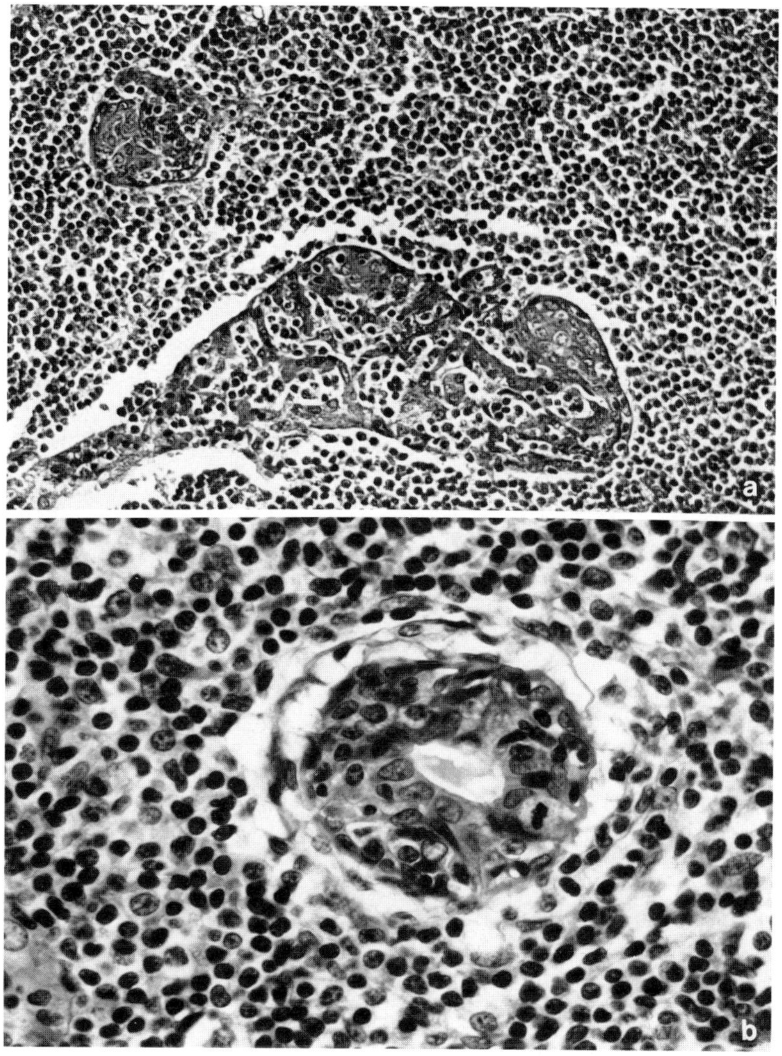

Figure 17.**8** Immunocytoma of the parotid gland with myoepithelial parotitis: **a** Diffuse lymphoid cell infiltration with inclusion of myoepithelial cell islands. **b** Section from the lymphomatous infiltrate with remnants of a cell island. H & E. **a** 160×, **b** 400×.

A polyclonal plasma cell population is present overall. Monoclonal IgM infiltrations, mainly of kappa type, may be defined as early or prelymphomas (Lennert et al 1979, Schmid et al 1982b). These infiltrates present as small circumscribed proliferative zones that finally may become confluent to form a larger focus of lymphoma. In some cases, this neoplastic process is accompanied by a focal epithelioid cell proliferation. A disorder of T cell function, in particular the T suppressor cells, leading to an increased T cell proliferation, has been discussed in the genesis of malignant lymphomas arising in a patient with immune sialadenitis (see also page 154).

Hodgkin's lymphomas are considerably more uncommon than B cell lymphomas and only constitute 15% of malignant lymphomas of the salivary glands. The lymphocyte-predominant and nodular-sclerosing forms with a better prognosis are more common than lymphocyte-depleted forms with a worse prognosis. Mixed forms have an intermediate position.

Diagnosis and Treatment

A biopsy excision must be carried out to confirm the diagnosis and to allow further classification of the tumor. A parotidectomy has the advantage of providing the pathologist with an abundance of material and furthermore is the appropriate treatment if the tumor is not malignant.

If further investigation, including tumor staging, indicates that the disease is confined to a salivary gland and the neighboring lymph nodes, the treatment for virtually all patients is radiation therapy. In all other cases radiation therapy is combined with chemotherapy, depending on the type and stage of the lymphoma. In our material, the 5-year determinate survival rate for patients with well-differentiated salivary gland lymphomas of

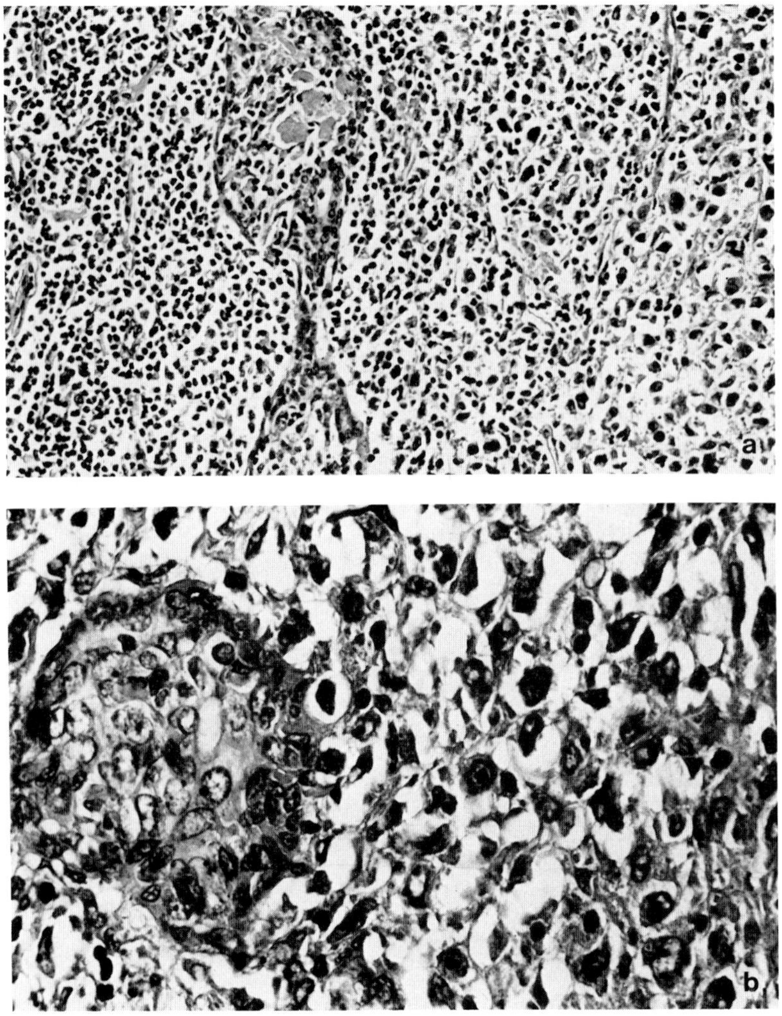

Figure 17.**9** Immunoblastic lymphoma of the parotid gland arising in myoepithelial parotitis. Infiltration by polymorphic immunoblasts with remnants of myoepithelial cell islands. H & E. **a** 160×, **b** 400×.

Hodgkin's type was 80%, whereas it was only 40% for the more highly malignant types. Patients with myoepithelial sialadenitis require continuous follow-up, because they are at risk of developing a malignant lymphoma (see before and page 154).

Leukemia

Infiltrates of the salivary glands are occasionally observed in patients with advanced leukemia or chronic lymphatic leukemia. Usually, it has already been known for a long time that the patient has the disease, and there is rarely a question of differential diagnosis from other salivary tumors. The term "Mikulicz syndrome" should now be consigned to history: an explanation of this term follows in an attempt to clear up the confusion caused by it. The symmetrical swelling of both parotid and salivary glands that characterizes Mikulicz syndrome may have several causes. The cause in the first patient described was possibly a Sjögren's syndrome (see page 146), but the term has since been used for benign and malignant tumors, leukemic infiltrates, and malignant lymphomas of this site. Since all the diseases embraced by the term "Mikulicz syndrome" are now well defined, this term should be allowed to disappear from the literature.

Metastases

Distant metastases to the salivary glands are rare, although occasional cases have been reported, usually of widespread metastases from an advanced carcinoma. A wide variety of tumors have been reported, including leiomyosarcoma of the uterus (Vollrath et al 1981), a small cell bronchial carcinoma (Albahany et al 1972), a hypernephroma (Gandon et al 1977), a colonic carcinoma (Nussbaum 1976), and a personal case of a breast carcinoma. Yarrington (1982) found a distant metastasis to be the indication for operative treat-

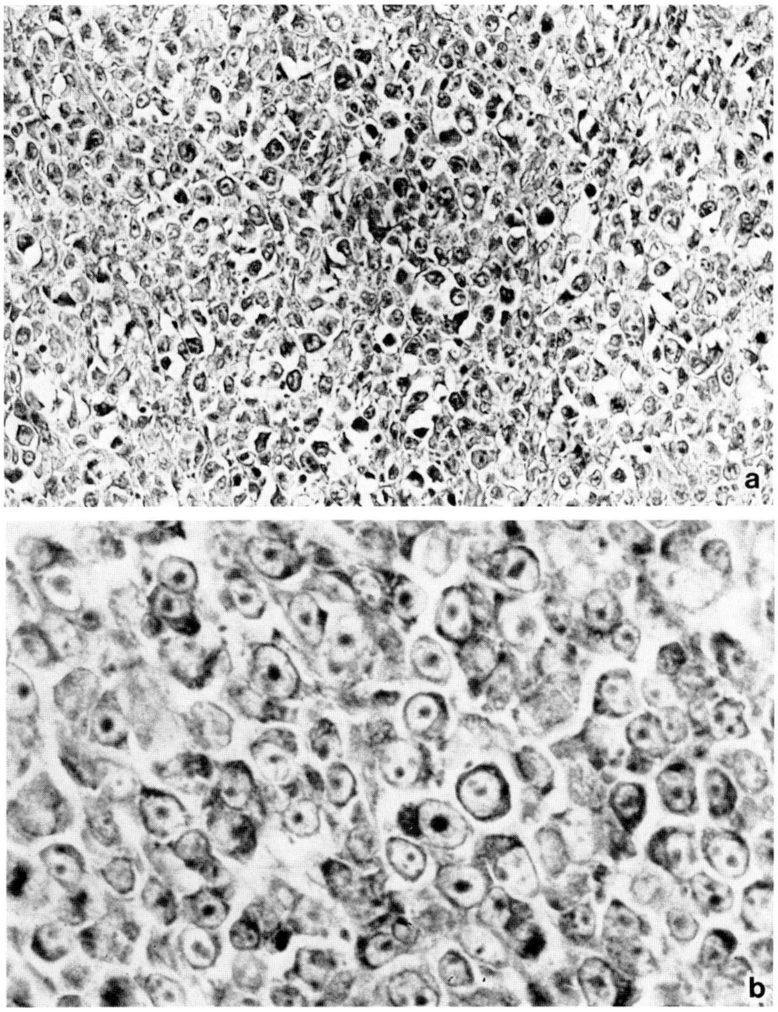

Figure 17.**10** Immunoblastic lymphoma of the parotid gland: immunoblasts with large clear nuclei and distinct nucleoles. Giemsa. **a** 160×, **b** 400×.

ment of a parotid swelling in 4% of his 250 parotidectomies; carcinoma of the lung was the most common primary tumor.

Para- or intraglandular metastases in the parotid of tumors of the skin of the head and neck should be taken into account in planning diagnosis and treatment. The skin areas that drain initially into the parotid lymph nodes (Fig. 17.**11**) include:

- The parotid region, consisting of the preauricular skin and the skin of the posterior part of the cheek
- The anterior surface of the auricle (Fig. 17.**12**)
- The temporal region
- The forehead (Fig. 17.**13a, b**).

Other regions that may also need to be considered include:

- The skin of the eyelids and the conjunctiva
- The upper lip
- The nose
- The anterior part of the cheek
- The posterior surface of the auricle and the retroauricular region

Lymph node metastases of malignant skin tumors to the parotid lymph nodes have been reported both in retrospective studies (Conley & Arena 1963, Jackson & Ballantyne 1981, Nichols et al 1980) and also in prospective studies (Storm et al 1977). The principal primary tumors responsible were melanomas, followed by squamous cell carcinomas. In 81 patients with parotid metastases, the primary tumor in 45% was a malignant melanoma and a squamous cell carcinoma in 38% (Conley & Arena 1963).

The *treatment* of clinically manifest para- or intraparotid lymph node metastases must follow the concepts that we have already laid down for primary squamous cell carcinoma of the parotid gland (see page 253). Squamous cell carcinoma metastatic to the parotid gland often lies in a more

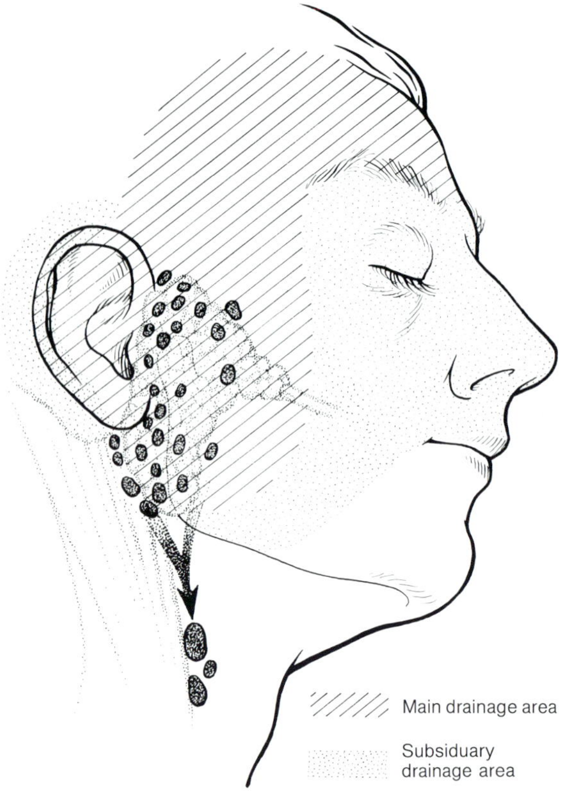

Figure 17.**11** Drainage area of the para- and intraglandular lymph nodes of the parotid gland.

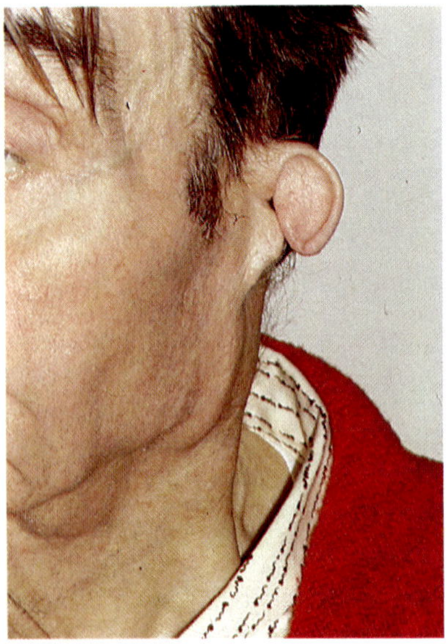

Figure 17.**12** Metastases of an auricular carcinoma to the parotid lymph nodes. The auricle had been excised previously.

favorable position than primary carcinoma of the gland, since metastases of a skin carcinoma almost always invades solely the paraglandular lymph nodes or the lymph nodes within the superficial lobe of the parotid (Fig. 17.**13a, b**). Resection of the facial nerve is therefore seldom needed. Parotidectomy, combined if necessary with resection of the primary tumor, is the treatment of choice for all operable tumors. Radiation therapy is reserved for postoperative treatment and for the treatment of inoperable patients.

If in addition the patient has lymph node metastases in the neck, the parotidectomy is combined with a radical neck dissection. If lymph nodes are not palpable in the neck before the operation, the jugular chain should be inspected during the procedure through an extended parotidectomy incision. If a frozen section shows evidence of metastasis, a radical neck dissection should be carried out.

We do not consider it justifiable to carry out superficial parotidectomy with prophylactic radical neck dissection for a skin carcinoma lying in the drainage region of the parotid without palpable lymph nodes (Storm et al 1977). The vast majority of skin carcinomas arising in elderly subjects due to exposure to the weather seldom metastasize (Jackson & Ballantyne 1981). However, an elective neck dissection may be justifiable in malignant melanomas, even in the absence of palpable lymph nodes, depending on its type and the depth of infiltration. The decision requires careful cooperation with the pathologist and the dermatologist. This policy applies to *malignant lymphoepithelial lesions* also (Ferlito & Donati 1977, Redondo et al 1981). This matter has already been discussed on pages 267 and 273. The epidermoid nature of the tumor cells is shown by demonstration of desmosomes and intracytoplasmatic tonofilaments with the electron microscope. The similarity of the tumor architecture to an undifferentiated nasopharyngeal carcinoma must be considered carefully in the differential diagnosis.

The *submandibular gland* is much less often the site of a metastasis, and distant metastases within this gland are rare. The submandibular lymph nodes that have close contact with the submandibular gland are indeed often the first metastatic site of carcinomas of the tongue and floor of the mouth, carcinomas of the submandibular gland itself, and malignant skin tumors in the area of drainage of these lymph nodes (see before). The submandibular gland and the adjacent lymph nodes are therefore removed in continuity with a classic radical neck dissection and also with a suprahyoid dissection.

Figure 17.**13** Metastases of a skin carcinoma to the left parotid: **a** Scar due to resection of a squamous cell carcinoma of the skin of the lateral part of the forehead. **b** Metastases arising 3 years after the initial operation on the skin. **c** Intraoperative view showing removal of the metastasis of the superficial lobe, by total parotidectomy with preservation of the facial nerve. A sling is shown around the temporofacial segment. **d** Operative specimen showing relatively well-demarcated metastasis.

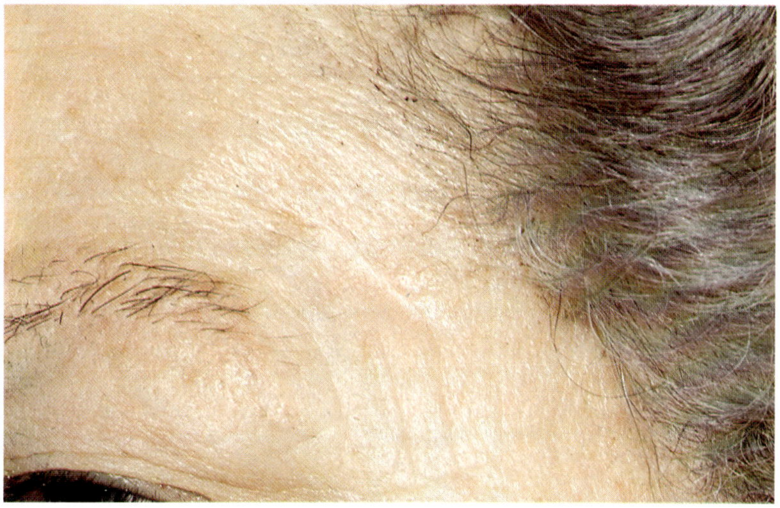

a

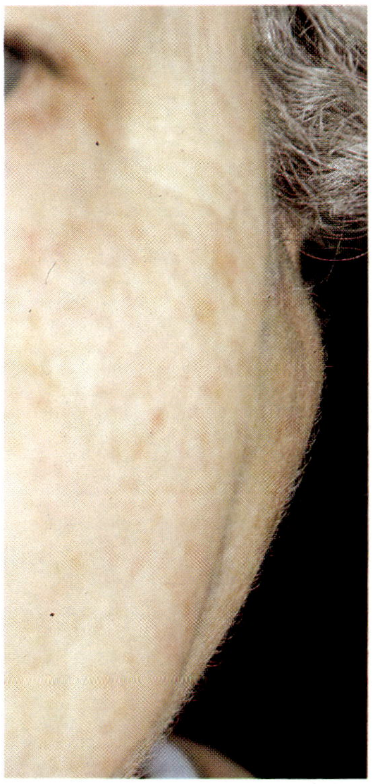

b

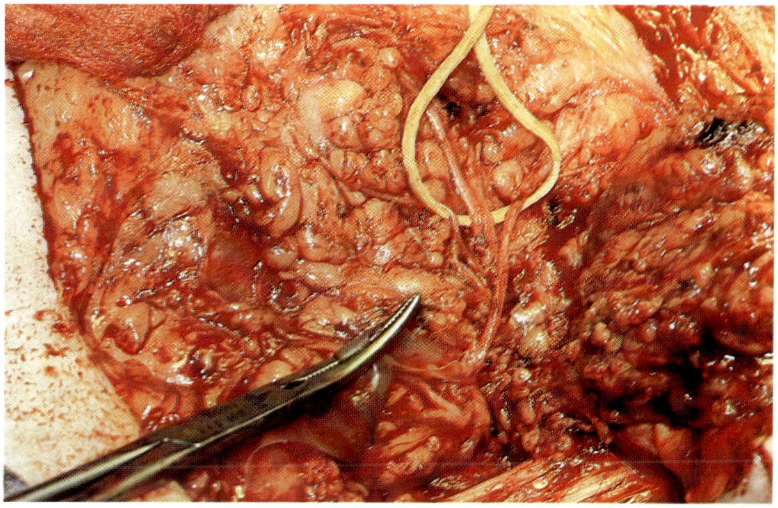

c

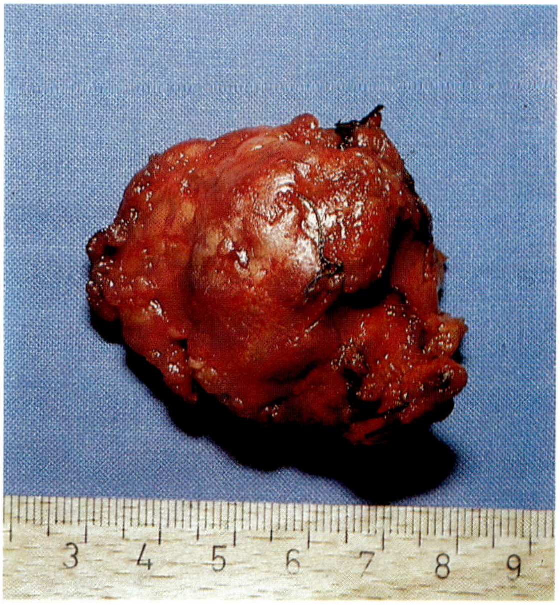

d

References

Albahany, A., J. Rigault, L. Roisin, J. E. Fleury: Métastase intraparotidienne bilatérale d'un épithélioma bronchique à petites cellules. Rev. Stomat. (Paris) 73 (1972) 229

Azzopardi, J. G., D. J. Evans: Malignant lymphoma of parotid associated with Mikulicz's disease (benign lymphoepithelial lesion). J. clin. Path. 24 (1971) 744

Bathard-Smith, P. J., H. S. Coonar, A. F. Markus: Hodgkin's disease presenting intra-orally. Brit. J. Oral Surg. 16 (1978/79) 64

Batsakis, J. G., E. G. Bernacki, D. H. Rice, M. E. Stebler: Malignancy and the benign lymphoepithelial lesions. Laryngoscope 85 (1975) 389

Blok, P., L. van Delden, I. van der Waal: Non-Hodgkin's lymphoma of the hard palate. Oral Surg. 47 (1979) 445

Bolognini, G., G. Riva: Lymphoproliferative Erkrankungen und Paraproteinämien beim Sjögren-Syndrom. Schweiz. med. Wschr. 105 (1975) 1493

Chilla, R., H.-O. Meyfarth, C. Arglebe: Über die operative Behandlung der chronischen Ohrspeicheldrüsenentzündung. Arch. Otorhinolaryng. 234 (1982) 53

Colby, T. V., R. F. Dorfman: Malignant lymphomas involving the salivary glands. Path. Ann. 14 (1979) 307

Conley, J.: Salivary Glands and the Facial Nerve. Thieme, Stuttgart 1975

Conley, J., S. Arena: Parotid gland as a focus of metastases. Arch. Surg. 87 (1963) 757

Ferlito, A., L. F. Donati: Malignant lymphoepithelial lesions. Undifferentiated ductal carcinomas of the parotid gland. J. Laryng. 91 (1977) 869

Ferlito, A., F. Polidoro, G. Recher: Extramedullary plasmacytoma of the parotid gland. Laryngoscope 90 (1980) 486

Freeman, C., J. W. Beng, S. J. Cutter: Occurrence and prognosis of extranodal lymphomas. Cancer 29 (1972) 252

Gandon, J., J. Trotoux, P. Marandas, Y. Calmette: Les métastases des cancers du sein au niveau des glandes salivaires. A propos d'un cas de métastase intraparotidienne. Ann. Oto-Laryng. (Paris) 94 (1977) 485

Gumberz, Chr. von, G. Seifert: Immunoglobulin-containing plasma cells in chronic parotitis and malignant lymphomas of the parotid gland. Comparing immunocytochemical observations of frequency and localization. Virchows Arch. Path. Anat. 389 (1980) 79

Hashimoto, N., K. Kurihara: Pathological characteristics of oral lymphomas. J. oral Path. 11 (1982) 214

Heckmayr, M., G. Seifert, K. Donath: Maligne Lymphome und Immunsialadenitis. Z. Laryng. Rhinol. 55 (1976) 593

Hyman, G. A., M. Wolff: Malignant lymphomas of the salivary glands. Review of the literature and report of 33 new cases, including four cases associated with the lymphoepithelial lesion. Amer. J. clin. Path. 65 (1976) 421

Jackson, G. L., A. J. Ballantyne: Role of parotidectomy for skin cancer of the head and neck. Amer. J. Surg. 142 (1981) 464

Karcher, D. S., D. J. Perry, M. A. Hurwitz, B. Detrick-Hooks: T-cell lymphoma occurring in the oropharynx. Cancer 50 (1982) 1155

Kassan, S. S., T. L. Thomas, H. M. Moutsopoulos, R. Hoover, R. P. Kimberly, D. R. Budman, J. Costa, I. G. Decker, T. M. Chused: Increased risk of lymphoma in Sicca syndrome. Ann. Inter. Med. 89 (1978) 888

Lapes, M., K. Antoniades, W. Gartner jr., R. Vivacqua: Conversion of a benign lymphoepithelial salivary gland lesion to lymphocytic lymphoma during dilantin therapy. Correlation with dilantin-induced lymphocyte transformation in vitro. Cancer 38 (1976) 1318

Lehrer, St., B. Roswit, Qu. Federman: The presentation of malignant lymphoma in the oral cavity and pharynx. Oral Surg. 41 (1976) 441

Lennert, K., H. Knecht, M. Burkert: Vorstadien maligner Lymphome. Verh. Dtsch. Ges. Path. 63 (1979) 170

Lennert, K., N. Mohri, H. Stein, E. Kaiserling: The histopathology of malignant lymphoma. Brit. J. Haemat. 31 (1975) Suppl. 193

Lennert, K., N. Mohri, H. Stein, E. Kaiserling, H. K. Müller-Hermelink: Malignant Lymphomas other than Hodgkin's Disease. Springer, Berlin 1978

Macht, S. D., S. D. Pett, N. T. Tsangaris: Non-Hodgkin lymphoma of the parotid gland: diagnosis, evaluation and treatment. Ann. Plast. Surg. 2 (1979) 37

Miller, R., E. T. Yanagihara, A. A. Dubrow, R. J. Lukes: Malignant lymphoma in a Warthin's tumor. Report of a case. Cancer 50 (1982) 2948

Nichols, R. D., L. A. Pinnock, R. T. Szymanowski: Metastases to parotid nodes. Laryngoscope 90 (1980) 1324

Nichols, R. D., J. W. Rebuck, J. C. Sullivan: Lymphoma of the parotid gland. Laryngoscope 92 (1982) 365

Nime, F. A., H. S. Cooper, C. Eggleston: Primary malignant lymphomas of the salivary glands. Cancer 37 (1976) 906

Nussbaum, M., H. T. Cho, M. L. Som: Parotid space tumors of non-salivary origin. Ann. Surg. 183 (1976) 10

Pernkopf, E.: Topographische Anatomie, 4. Bd., 1. Hälfte. Urban & Schwarzenberg, München 1957

Podoshin, L., Y. Talmon, A. Grischkan, M. Fradis: Primary lymphoma of the parotid gland. J. Laryng. 93 (1979) 417

Redondo, C., A. Garcia, F. Vazquez: Malignant lymphoepithelial lesion of the parotid gland: Poorly differentiated squamous cell carcinoma with lymphoid stroma. Cancer 48 (1981) 289

Ree, H. J., V. B. Rege, R. E. Knisley, W. R. Thayer, R. P. D'Amico, J. Y. Song, J. P. Crowley: Malignant lymphoma of Waldeyer's ring following gastrointestinal lymphoma. Cancer 46 (1980) 1528

Schmid, U., D. Helbron, K. Lennert: Primary malignant lymphomas localized in salivary glands. Histopathology 6 (1982a) 673

Schmid, U., D. Helbron, K. Lennert: Development of malignant lymphoma in myoepithelial sialadenitis (Sjögren-syndrome). Virchows Arch. Path. Anat. 395 (1982b) 11

Schwarze, E.-W., B. Mrowietz, G. van Ackeren: Maligne Lymphome im Oropharynx – unter besonderer Berücksichtigung der Non-Hodgkin-Lymphome. Verh. Dtsch. Krebs-Ges. 4 (1983) 267

Schubert, J., U. Wagner: Klinische Erstmanifestationen von malignen Lymphomen im Kiefer-Gesichtsbereich. Dtsch. Z. Mund-Kiefer-Gesichts-Chir. 3 (1979) 144

Seifert, G.: Wangenschwellungen bei Speicheldrüsenentzündungen. HNO 27 (1979) 119

Seifert, G.: Lymphoid lesions of the oral cavity. Path. Res. Pract. 167 (1980) 179

Seligman, B. R., F. Rosner, J. Davenport: Primary lymphosarcoma of the parotid gland. Cancer 33 (1974) 239

Storm, F. K., F. R. Eilber, F. C. Sparks, D. L. Morton: A prospective study of parotid metastases from head and neck cancer. Amer. J. Surg. 134 (1977) 115

Talal, N., L. Sokoloff, W. Barth: Extrasalivary lymphoid abnormalities in Sjögren's syndrome (reticulum cell sarcoma, "pseudolymphoma", macroglobulinemia). Amer. J. Med. 43 (1967) 50

Tomich, Ch. E., W. G. Shafer: Lymphoproliferative disease of the hard palate: A clinicopathologic entity. Oral Surg. 39 (1975) 754

Türk, R., F. Horak: Nicht-Hodgkin-Lymphome im Hals-, Nasen-, Ohrenbereich, Z. Laryng. Rhinol. 61 (1982) 516

Tyzak, Th.: Maligne Lymphome der Kopfspeicheldrüsen. – Eine morphologische Analyse von 108 Fällen nach der Kiel-Klassifikation. Diss., Hamburg 1982

Vinceneux, P.: Assosiation d'un lymphome malin des glandes salivaires et d'un Syndrome de Sjögren. Nouv. Presse Med. 5 (1976) 1719

Vollrath, M., M. Droese, B. Hinney: Die Parotis als Zielorgan von Nah- und Fernmetastasen. Z. Laryng. Rhinol. 60 (1981) 39

Yarington, C. T.: Metastatic malignant disease to the parotid gland. Laryngoscope 91 (1981) 517

Zulman, J., R. Jaffe, N. Talal: Evidence that the malignant lymphoma of Sjögren's syndrome is a monoclonal B-cell neoplasm. New Engl. J. Med. 299 (1978) 1215

18. Periglandular Tumors

Tumors arising from organs adjacent to the salivary glands can invade the gland or displace it in such a way that they mimic a salivary tumor. Benign and malignant tumors, pseudotumors, and congenital anomalies may all simulate salivary tumors. The parotid gland is much more at risk than the submandibular gland because of its position, its larger surface, and its relationship to several other structures. The penalty of failing to diagnose a periglandular tumor includes an unnecessary operation (for a masseteric hypertrophy, for example) or exposure of the patient to unnecessary risk. A typical example of the latter is a sebaceous cyst, an operation usually assigned to very junior members of the staff. A sebaceous cyst in the lateral part of the face can infiltrate the parotid gland, so that the operation requires the surgeon to have mastered the technique of parotid gland and facial nerve surgery. We have on several occassions seen injuries to the facial nerve arising from operations for a sebaceous cyst.

The *skin* of the parotid region is much less commonly the site of a basal cell carcinoma or a squamous cell carcinoma than the rest of the skin of the face, but more commonly than the skin of the trunk and the limbs. *Basal cell carcinoma* is usually restricted to the skin layer, and infiltration of the parotid parenchyma is only seen in recurrences. In contrast, *squamous cell carcinoma* of the parotid region can reach a considerable size (Fig. 18.**1**) and invade deeply into the parenchyma of the gland. Tumors of this type should be treated like parotid malignancies, that is, by resection of the skin, total parotidectomy, and, if necessary, partial or complete resection of the facial nerve. Reconstruction of the facial nerve is justified. We regularly use postoperative radiation therapy for large squamous cell carcinomas. Since the intraparotid lymph nodes are the first station for the preauricular skin region, parotidectomy may be required for tumors of this area. We do not consider an elective neck dissection to be justifiable.

Lipomas (page 74) may also present as tumors in the parotid or submandibular region. They usually arise from subcutaneous fatty tissue, and are often multiple, in which case the diagnosis is easy. However, an isolated lipoma of the parotid region can cause difficulties in diagnosis, so that large tumors should be treated by a parotidectomy with exposure of the facial nerve. This is also true of *sebaceous cysts,* if it is suspected that the tumor extends deeply in the anterior or posterior part of the cheek (Fig. 18.**2**).

Cysts, adamantinomas, and malignant bone tumors of the *mandible* (Fig. 18.**3**) can invade or displace the parotid gland (Fig. 18.**4**). Radiology of the mandible is therefore always advisable to elucidate the cause of a parotid tumor, if this is not absolutely clear. Arthritis of the *temporomandibular joint* causing swelling of the joint may also present as a parotid tumor, but the reverse situation is more common. Patients with a deep adenoid cystic carcinoma often have a history of temporomandibular joint disorders and several of our patients had already been submitted to operations on the joint before the diagnosis of adenoid cystic carcinoma of the parotid gland was finally made. Tumors of the joint are rare (Hölscher et al 1978), but must be included in the differential diagnosis of a parotid tumor.

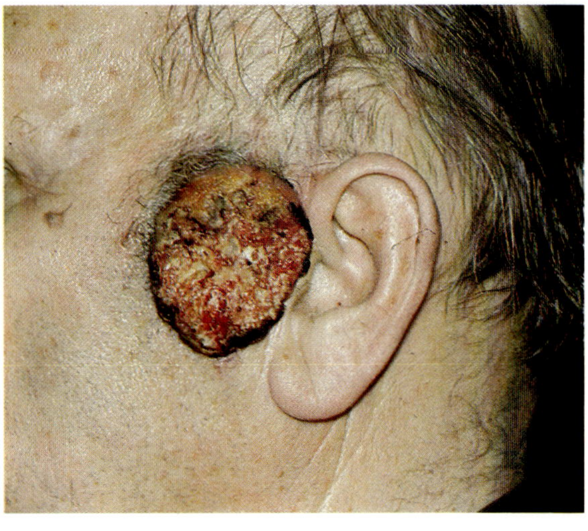

Figure 18.**1** Exophytic skin carcinoma of the parotid region.

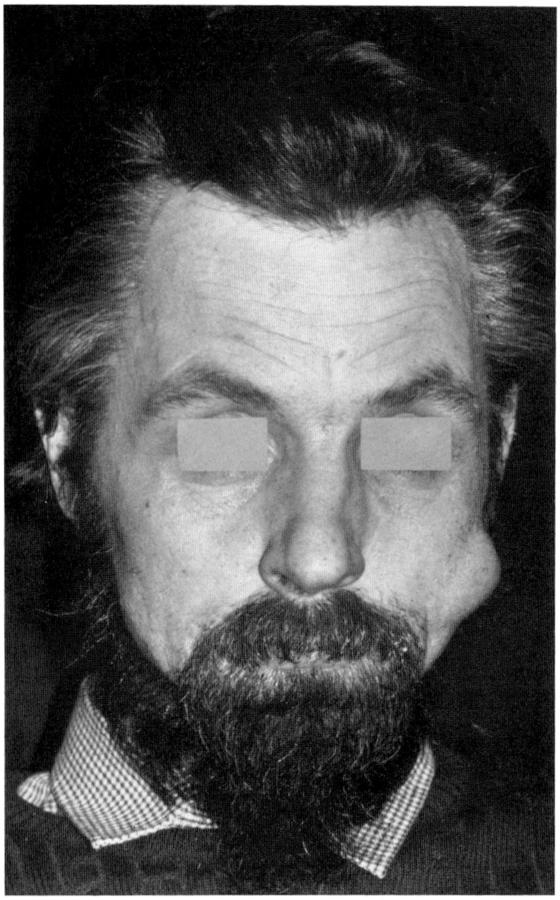

Figure 18.**2** Sebaceous cyst of the anterior part of the cheek.

Tumors of the *masseteric muscle,* such as *hemangioma* (Fig. 18.**5**), can mimic a parotid tumor, but hypertrophy of this muscle is more common and is usually due to incorrect function of the masticatory apparatus. A *masseteric hypertrophy* can reach a considerable size (Fig. 18.**6**). The diagnosis can usually be established rapidly by the variation in size on palpation with the muscle relaxed and under tension.

Branchial cleft fistulas occasionally pass through the parotid region (page 164) and are then closely related to the facial nerve (Chilla & Miehlke 1984). The diagnosis is easy to make if the fistula opens into the external auditory meatus (Fig. 18.**7**), in the posteroinferior part of the face, or on the neck. However, branchial cleft fistulas (duplicate meatus) may have no visible opening, and they then mimic a parotid tumor (Fig. 18.**8**). The diagnosis is only made when the tumor is removed.

References

Chilla, R., A. Miehlke: Zur Klinik und Topographie des "doppelten Gehörgangs". Z. Laryng. Rhinol. 63 (1984) 229

Hölscher, A. H., G. Rahlf, E. Stennert, A. Schauer: Riesenzelltumor der Sehnenscheide mit Synovialchondrom. Z. Laryng. Rhinol. 57 (1978) 904

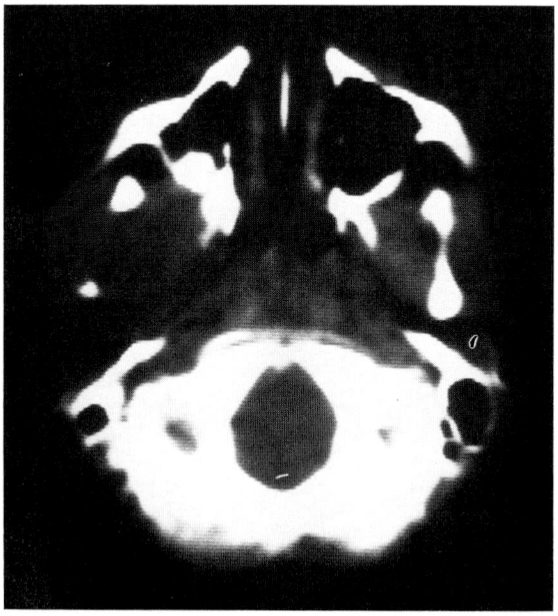

Figure 18.**3** Aggressive fibromatosis of the left infratemporal fossa (Computed tomography scan). The disease has destroyed the ascending ramus of the mandible widely and mimics a parotid tumor (see also Fig. 18.**4**).

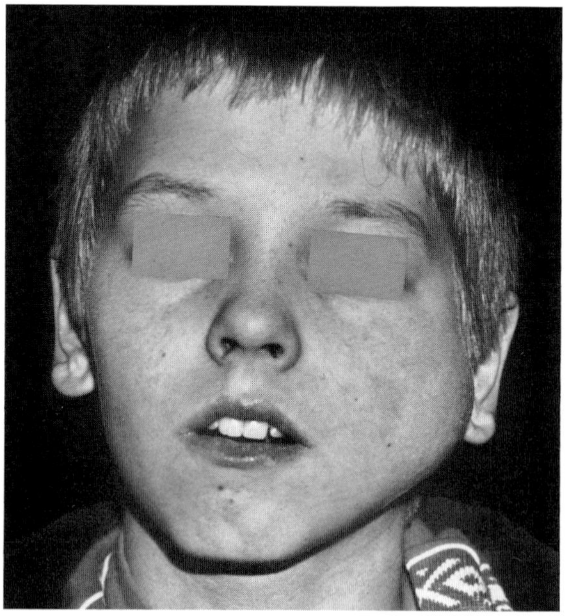

Figure 18.**4** Aggressive fibromatosis of the left infratemporal fossa.

ma simplex can often be completely removed, a cavernous lymphangioma often recurs.

Opinions differ about the relative frequency of benign epithelial tumors in childhood. According to Kauffman and Stout (1963), the pleomorphic adenoma is not the most frequent benign tumor, as it is in the adult, whereas Jacques et al (1976) stated that the pleomorphic adenoma was indeed the most common benign epithelial tumor in patients less than the age of 18 years. Further large studies have been able to confirm these views: 17 of 23 patients with epithelial tumors had pleomorphic adenomas in one series (Byars et al 1957) and 10 of 12 in another series (Bianchi & Cudmore 1978).

Malignant tumors of the salivary glands in childhood are very rare and are mainly seen in older children, although they can occur in newborn infants and in the first year of life (Danziger 1964, Hendrick 1964, Vawter & Tefft 1966, Eneroth 1976, Jacques et al 1976, Schuller & McCabe 1977). Opinions vary about the frequency of malignant salivary gland tumors in childhood. Whereas in adulthood, 15–25% of salivary gland tumors are malignant, several investigators have observed that half of all nonangiomatous tumors in childhood are malignant (Castro et al 1972, Chong et al 1975, Schuller & McCabe 1977, Blanck et al 1979). The data in the literature are difficult to interpret, because the age groups, the sites of the tumor, and the histologic classifications all vary.

Mucoepidermoid tumor appears to be the most common malignant tumor of childhood (Foote & Frazell 1954, Schuller & McCabe 1977, Blanck et al 1979, Dahlquist & Östberg 1982) followed by acinic cell tumor. Adenoid cystic carcinoma, adenocarcinoma, and undifferentiated carcinoma also occur.

Diagnosis and treatment follow the guidelines laid down for adults, that is, early removal of the tumor by subtotal parotidectomy, and preservation of the facial nerve, if possible. Postoperative radiation therapy is advisable for many tumors, such as high-grade mucoepidermoid tumors, undifferentiated carcinomas, and many adenoid cystic carcinomas.

It is difficult to make a definite statement about prognosis because of the small number of malignant tumors arising in childhood. The impression is, however, that mucoepidermoid and acinic cell tumors have a good prognosis if treated by surgery.

References

Barnhart, R. A., A. K. Brown jr.: Cystic hygroma of the neck. Report of a case. Arch. Otolaryng. 86 (1967) 74

Bianchi, A., R. E. Cudmore: Salivary gland tumours in children. J. Ped. Surg. 13 (1978) 6

Blanck, C., C.-M. Eneroth, P. Jakobsson: Malignant tumours of the parotid gland in the first two decades. Opuscul. Med. 24 (1979) 143

Byars, L. T., L. V. Ackermann, E. Peacock: Tumours of salivary gland origin in children. Ann. Surg. 14 (1957) 40

Castro, E. B., A. G. Huvos, E. W. Strong, F. W. Foote: Tumours of the major salivary glands in children. Cancer 29 (1972) 312

Catania, V. C., F. Bozetti, A. Santangelo, B. Salvadori: Parotid gland tumours in infants and children. Tumori 63 (1977) 195

Chong, G. C., O. H. Beahrs, M. L. C. Chen, A. B. Hayles: Management of parotid gland tumours in infants and children. Mayo Clin. Proc. 50 (1975) 279

Conley, J.: Salivary Glands and the Facial Nerve. Thieme, Stuttgart 1975

Dahlquist, A., Y. Östberg: Malignant salivary gland tumours in children. Acta Otolaryngol. 94 (1982) 175

Danziger, H.: Adenoid cystic carcinoma of the submaxillary gland in an 8-month-old infant. Can. Med. Ass. J. 91 (1964) 759

Eneroth, C.-M.: Die Klinik der Kopfspeicheldrüsentumoren. Arch. Oto-Rhino-Laryng. 213 (1976) 61

Foote, F. W., E. L. Frazell: Tumours of the major salivary glands. In: Atlas of Tumour Pathology. Sect. IV, Fasc. 11. Armed Forces Institute of Pathology, Washington/D. C. 1954

Hendrick, J. W.: Mucoepidermoid cancer of the parotid gland in a one year old child. Amer. J. Surg. 108 (1964) 907

Hoffmann, K., M. A. Block: Tumours of major salivary glands in children. Mich. Med. 67 (1968) 1461

Jaques, D. A., O. S. Kroll, R. G. Chambers: Parotid tumours in children. Amer. J. Surg. 132 (1976) 469

Kauffman, S. L., A. P. Stout: Tumours of the major salivary glands in children. Cancer 16 (1963) 1317

Rauch, S.: Zur Klinik der gut- u. bösartigen mesenchymalen Speicheldrüsentumoren. In Schuchardt K.: Fortschr. Kiefer- u. Gesichtschirurgie, Bd. XIV. Thieme, Stuttgart 1970

Rauch, S.: Sialadenome des Säuglings. In Schuchardt, K.: Fortschr. Kiefer- u. Gesichtschirurgie, Bd. XV. Thieme, Stuttgart 1972

Schuller, D. E., B. F. McCabe: Salivary gland neoplasms in children. Otolaryng. Clin. North Amer. 13 (1977) 399

Seifert, G.: Die Speicheldrüsengeschwülste im Kindesalter. Z. Kinderchir. 2 (1965) 285

Vawter, G. F., M. Tefft: Congenital tumours of the parotid gland. Arch. Path. 82 (1966) 242

Watson, W., W. D. McCarthy: Blood and lymph vessel tumours; a report of 1056 cases. Surg. Gynec. Obstet. 71 (1940) 569

Woodring, A. J.: Cervical cystic hygroma: a review of the literature and report of an unusual case. Ann. Otol. 77 (1968) 978

20. Differential Diagnosis of Salivary Swellings

The differential diagnosis of chronic parotid swellings may be difficult, whereas acute inflammation of bacterial or viral origin causing typical symptoms and signs are usually easy to diagnose.

True tumors must be distinguished from nonneoplastic salivary diseases to enable logical treatment decisions to be made. A careful history, palpation, and assessment of the function of the facial nerve are the basic steps. A bilateral, soft, painless swelling of the parotid gland, fluctuating in size, indicates a sialadenosis or a chronic myoepithelial sialadenitis. Further evidence of a sialadenosis is given by the presence of metabolic diseases, such as diabetes mellitus, hyperthyroidism, gonadal dysfunction, pituitary insufficiency, or disorders of the autonomic nervous system. If the sialadenosis has been present for a long time, a sialogram demonstrates a typical pattern of very thin fine ducts without terminal dilation. Whereas some investigators have been able to demonstrate reduced or absent secretion by sialometry, we have been unable to demonstrate a change in the flow rate in patients with sialadenosis confirmed by histopathology. Similarly, the values for protein and amylase secretion do not differ from those of control subjects (see Chapter 8). Sialochemistry may show that the potassium content of saliva is increased and sodium is reduced compared with normal. A radioisotope scan provides little definite evidence of a sialadenosis. The most certain method of proving the diagnosis is by an open biopsy or aspiration cytology.

The diagnosis of chronic myoepithelial sialadenitis (page 146ff) rests on the demonstration of the often concomitant Sjögren's syndrome with a simultaneous rheumatoid manifestation, such as positive rheumatoid factor, C-reactive protein, an increased erythrocyte sedimentation rate, a protein shift with an increase of gamma globulins, lupus erythematosus cells, and antinuclear factors. Chronic myoepithelial sialadenitis, like sialadenosis, is almost always bilateral, but unlike sialadenosis occurs for the first time in the older age groups: the peak age incidence is in the fifth to sixth decades, and most patients are women. The sialogram shows similar changes to those of chronic recurrent parotitis. In the advanced stage of the disease the sialogram shows a typical picture of parenchymatous atrophy. The most certain way of establishing the diagnosis is by biopsy.

Chronic recurrent parotitis (page 115) is distinguished from sialadenosis and chronic myoepithelial sialadenitis by the fact that it is often unilateral, painful, and firm in consistency and the saliva is often purulent. A further characteristic is the symptomfree interval that almost all patients with chronic recurrent parotitis demonstrate. Even though tension pain may occasionally occur in chronic myoepithelial sialadenitis, it is not so frequent as in chronic recurrent parotitis. Finally, the acute episodes of chronic recurrent parotitis usually respond to antibiotics, whereas sialadenosis and chronic myoepithelial sialadenitis do not.

Inflammation of the temporomandibular joint may express itself as a parotid swelling. The pain on opening the mouth and the ache localized in the temporomandibular joint in the presence of an otherwise unremarkable salivary gland indicate the correct diagnosis. Special radiographic views of the temporomandibular joint may be of diagnostic value.

Intra- and periglandular tuberculous lymph nodes in the absence of radiologic evidence of calcification are usually mistaken for tumors and removed. Their true nature is then revealed on histologic examination. Schätzle (1970) describes a patient with stage III syphilitic infection of the parotid gland, which was also confused with a tumor. Serologic investigation established the diagnosis.

Salivary gland tumors present little difficulty in differential diagnosis. A unilateral, clearly demarcated tumor that is painless and that in the patient's opinion has recently increased in size is almost certainly benign. Cystadenolymphoma has the same diagnostic criteria, but is often bilateral.

Pain, incomplete or complete peripheral paralysis of the facial nerve, indistinct tumor margins, and enlarged regional lymph nodes are certain signs of malignancy. Unlike an idiopathic facial paralysis, a paralysis due to a malignant tumor usually develops slowly. Sialography and radioisotope imaging usually play a subordinate role in the diagnostic spectrum. The diagnosis is confirmed by aspiration cytology or by postoperative histologic examination.

Occasionally, mandibular tumors are confused with parotid tumors, but this can be resolved by radiologic examination.

Lesions arising from the epidermis, such as dermoid or epidermoid cysts lying over the gland, can mimic a parotid gland tumor. The superficial position of the lesion usually indicates that it is not a salivary gland tumor.

Metastases to the intra- and paraglandular lymph nodes are extremely important. Melanomas of the skin of the head metastasize with remarkable frequency to the parotid lymph nodes, and they can often be diagnosed by their bluish color seen through the overlying skin (Fig. 20.**1**). A very nodular tumor should suggest a metastasis.

The salivary tissue, particularly that of the parotid gland, may be affected relatively uncommonly by systemic disorders of the lymphatic system, for example, Hodgkin's lymphoma and other malignant lymphomas. A sudden increase in size of the parotid gland in a patient with chronic myoepithelial sialadenitis should be suspected as being due to malignant transformation and should be verified by hematologic and histologic investigations.

Sarcoidosis of the intra- or paraglandular lymph nodes usually declares itself by a nodular swelling, often combined with an incomplete facial paralysis. The diagnosis is confirmed by the presence of parahilar lymph nodes on a chest radiograph, a positive Kveim test, reduced tuberculin sensitivity, and increased gamma globulin levels. Histologic verification is also very valuable.

Tumors of the ascending ramus of the mandible or odontogenic tumors must be distinguished from parotid tumors by radiographs (Ganz & Niemeyer 1967, Schätzle et al 1970). The most common lesions are cysts or cystic adamantinomas.

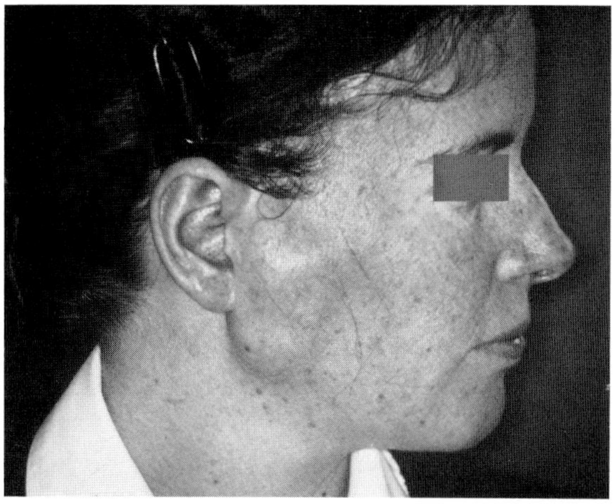

Figure 20.**1** Intraparotid metastasis of a melanoma. The primary tumor lay on the skin of the head.

Cysts and fistulas arising from the ear and branchial cysts and fistulas are often confused with parotid lesions. Minnigerode and Haubrich (1965) describe a congenital duplication of the external auditory meatus that was discovered during a parotidectomy.

Lastly, hypertrophy of the masseter muscle must be mentioned, since this can be confused with a salivary lesion. The soft salivary tissue can then be distinguished from hard muscular tissue under tension by bimanual palpation.

References

Ganz, H., W. Niemeyer: Unterkieferhantelcyste. Ein Beitrag zur Differentialdiagnose der Parotistumoren. Arch. klin. exp. Ohr-, Nas.- u. Kehlk.-Heilk. 188 (1967) 515

Minnigerode, B., J. Haubrich: Angeborene echte Gehörgangsverdoppelung, eine seltene embryogenetische Überschußbildung. Z. Laryng. Rhinol. 44 (1965) 706

Schätzle, W.: Zur Fehldiagnose "Parotistumor". HNO 18 (1970) 11

21. Neural Diseases of the Salivary Glands

Motor, sensory, and nervous elements are all represented in the salivary glands. *Motor nerve fibers* constitute the greater part of the extratemporal course of the facial nerve. Preservation of function of this nerve is the most important factor in every operation in this region, particularly parotidectomy (page 333ff). It is important to preserve the marginal mandibular branch of the facial nerve and the hypoglossal nerve lying deep in the submandibular triangle in removal of the submandibular gland. Malignant tumors of the parotid gland can infiltrate the facial nerve, causing paralysis of the facial musculature. Adenoid cystic carcinoma in particular tends to spread along the nerve sheaths (page 239). A facial nerve paralysis of a deep, invisible, and often impalpable parotid tumor is often the first symptom that takes the patient to the doctor. An idiopathic facial paralysis is then commonly diagnosed, because this is much the most common cause of such a paralysis, but this diagnosis must only be made after the exclusion of other causes. The correct diagnosis is established by the history of a slowly progressive paralysis and functional examination of the facial nerve; the diagnosis is confirmed by surgery.

The parotid region receives *sensory nerve fibers* from the trigeminal nerve (the auriculotemporal nerve) and the great auricular nerve arising from the cervical plexus. The great auricular nerve can usually not be preserved at parotidectomy. Its trunk reaches the posterior part of the parotid and there breaks up into individual branches that pass through the parotid capsule to the auricle. The auriculotemporal nerve enters the parotid region at the level of the temporomandibular joint and there lies in close relationship with the temporal vessels. This nerve is usually not demonstrated at parotidectomy, but it is certainly often ligated with the branches of the temporal vessels. The resulting loss of sensation of the posterior part of the cheek and the auricle gradually recovers within about a year.

The *autonomic nerve fibers* supply the sweat glands of the skin, the vessels, and cells of the salivary parenchyma, including the myoepithelial cells of the parotid and submandibular glands. Sympathetic and parasympathetic nerve fibers contribute to this innervation to a varying extent. Denervation or aberrant reinnervation are complications of surgery, which are also used sometimes for treatment of salivary disorder.

Denervated Salivary Gland

If the autonomic nerve supply to the acinar cells is interrupted, a series of processes is set in motion that show a certain regularity (Stefano and Perec 1981). Neurogenic transmitters (norepinephrine in the case of the sympathetic nerves) stored in these fibers are released after division of the autonomic fibers. The acinar cells are thus stimulated and produce a *degeneration secretion* (Emmelin & Trendelenburg 1972). This degeneration secretion begins some hours after denervation and only ceases a few days later when the stores of the nerve fibers are completely discharged (see Chapter 8).

If the sensitivity of acinar cells to various sympathomimetic agents is tested later, sensitivity to norepinephrine, that is, the natural neurogenic transmitter, is increased after sympathetic denervation *(prejunctional supersensitivity)*.

This prejunctional supersensitivity is due to the fact that the storage mechanism for norepinephrine in the nerve fibers is eliminated, so that a similar dose of norepinephrine results in a higher concentration on the adrenergic receptors of the acinar cells. True postjunctional supersensitivity of the acinar cells develops gradually and can only be demonstrated several weeks later. It is demonstrated against all sympathomimetic agents that can activate the adrenergic receptors of the acinar cells and probably rests on the simultaneous increase of adrenergic receptors in the membranes of the acinar cells (Arnett & Davis 1979, Chilla et al 1981, Pointon & Banerjee 1979).

The changes of secretion of the salivary glands after denervation of the parenchyma in the experimental animal have been studied by Emmelin especially (Emmelin 1968, Emmelin & Strömblad 1958, Emmelin & Trendelenburg 1972). Similar lesions are found after denervation of human salivary glands. Whereas the immediate effects of denervation of salivary tissue have been well investigated, knowledge about the long-term effects of autonomic denervation is scant.

Parasympathetic denervation of the submandibular gland by chorda tympani neurectomy is used for the treatment of sialorrhea (page 75). Its disadvantages are partial loss of taste. The chorda tympani may also be destroyed in chronic middle ear disease (Griffith 1977), although injury to the nerve is more commonly due to middle ear operations (Chilla et al 1979). If the chorda tympani is completely divided, the secretory capacity of the submandibular gland is reduced to a minimal resting secretion for many years (Chilla et al 1982), whereas complete recovery usually occurs after extension of the nerve.

Parasympathetic denervation of the parotid gland is used in the treatment of chronic recurrent parotitis, sialadenosis, and salivary fistula. Division of the auriculotemporal nerve (the postganglionic parasympathetic denervation) or division of the tympanic plexus (the preganglionic parasympathetic denervation) obviously does not have the permanent inhibitory influence on the secretion of the parotid gland of chorda tympani neurectomy on the secretion of the submandibular gland. The success of parasympathetic parotid denervation for these diseases is thus in general modest (Chilla 1981). To what extent this is due to remaining sympathetic innervation of the gland, to unaffected pathways of parasympathetic innervation, or the high regenerative capacity of the autonomic nervous system has not yet been determined.

Frey's Syndrome

Sweating and redness of the skin often associated with burning and pilomotion of the skin (Herxheimer 1958, Laage-Hellman 1957) of the cheek after stimulation by chewing or taste were first described by Duphenix (1757) after incision of a parotid abscess. A more accurate description was given by Lucie Frey (1923) after a shotgun injury of the parotid gland complicated by infection. Frey's syndrome (gustatory sweating or auriculotemporal syndrome) affects not only the territory of the auriculotemporal nerve, but also that supplied by the great auricular nerve (Laage-Hellman 1957). It may be caused by a forceps delivery (Dey 1953, Haxton 1948b), central nervous system lesions (Forbes & Doy 1963), cervical sympathectomy (Ashby 1960, Haxton 1948a, 1948b, Herxheimer 1958, Tankel 1951), and radical neck dissection (Myers & Conley 1970, Spiro & Martin 1965).

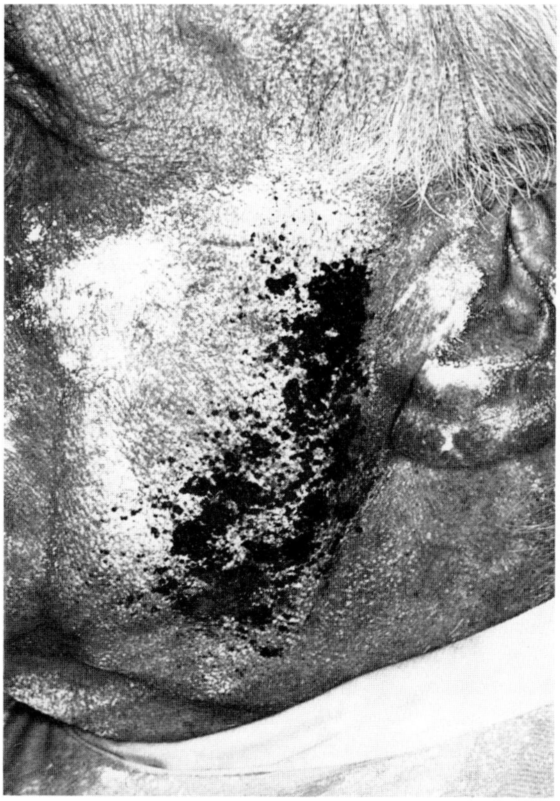

Figure 21.**1** Frey's syndrome after superficial parotidectomy showing the starch-iodine reaction caused by discharge of sweat in the parotid region after a gustatory stimulus. The patient had been submitted to parotidectomy 18 months previously (the dark area is the area that stains blue).

The most common causes are injuries to or operation on the parotid gland or the surrounding area (Chisa et al 1964, Hogemann 1951, Kaplan & Spring 1960, Laage-Hellman 1957). Indeed Frey's syndrome is an unavoidable result of parotid surgery, since it can be demonstrated objectively after almost 100% of all parotidectomies (Laage-Hellman 1957) by the starch-iodine method described by Minor (1928) (Fig. 21.**1**). Usually, however, the disease is not clinically manifested. Only about 20–30% of patients notice the symptom themselves and far fewer are distressed by it.

The explanation of Frey's syndrome is probably the inappropriate regeneration of injured autonomic nerve fibers (Ford & Woodhall 1938). Both cholinergic sympathetic fibers to the sweat glands and also the cholinergic parasympathetic nerve fibers for the parotid acinar cells are divided at parotidectomy (Fig. 21.**2a–c**). They run partially with sensory nerve fibers (the auriculotemporal nerve includes trigeminal fibers, sympathetic fibers, and parasympathetic secretory fibers; the

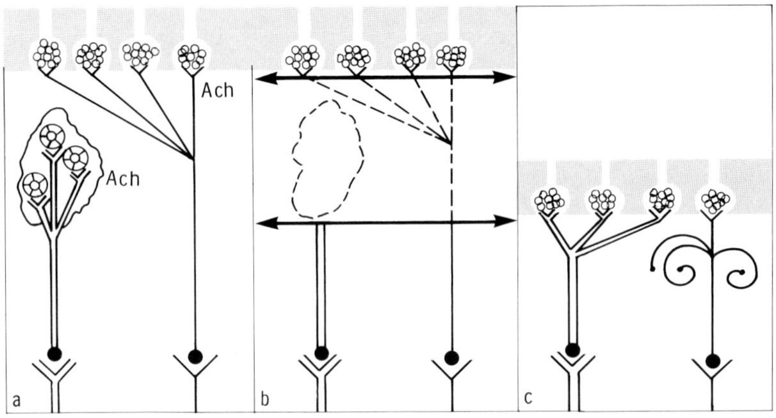

Figure 21.**2** Pathogenesis of Frey's syndrome (according to Laage-Hellmann). **a** Normal sympathetic-cholinergic innervation of the sweat glands and parasympathetic-cholinergic innervation of the parotid gland. **b** Division of the sympathetic and parasympathetic nerve fibers by parotidectomy. **c** Reinnervation of the sweat glands by parasympathetic-secretory and sympathetic nerve fibers.

great auricular nerve includes fibers from the cervical plexus and sympathetic fibers). The new sprouting axons of the postganglionic parasympathetic nerve cells reach the sweat glands of the skin in addition to any remaining acinar cells. Since the afferent limb of the reflex arc remains unchanged, taste stimulates the secretion of sweat rather than saliva. This is accompanied by reddening of the skin due to the parasympathetic vascular effect, that is, an absence of parasympathetic secretory nerve fibers to the skin vessels. The syndrome is usually confined to the territory of the auriculotemporal and great auricular nerves that supply the skin of the parotid region.

Gustatory sweating after lesions of the sympathetic nervous system also affects other parts of the body (Haxton 1948a and 1948b). This obviously cannot be described as an auriculotemporal syndrome. Lesions of the parasympathetic secretory parotid innervation are not to be expected in lesions of the cervical sympathetic nervous system, so that inappropriate regeneration, as already described, cannot be the cause. Nonetheless gustatory sweating after sympathetic lesions can be explained by inappropriate nerve regeneration, if it is recalled that all salivary gland tissue is supplied by postganglionic adrenergic sympathetic nerve fibers. If the preganglionic sympathetic fibers in the sympathetic trunk are injured, nerve fibers destined for the salivary glands may connect up with the sweat gland innervation (Hogemann 1951). It is thus easy to understand that gustatory sweating after a sympathetic lesion can be relieved by stellate ganglion block. This is not true of the typical auriculotemporal syndrome after a parotid operation (Haxton 1948a, 1948b, Hogemann 1951).

The theory of inappropriate neural regeneration is now generally accepted. Other theories postulate that gustatory sweating may be due to irritation of the auriculotemporal nerve by scar tissue (Frey 1923, Gray 1959), by hypersensitivity of the denervated sweat glands to neurogenic transmitters (Cannon & Rosenblueth 1949), or by transaxonal excitation (Chorobski 1951) between parasympathetic and sympathetic nerve fibers in the presence of normal reinnervation of the sweat glands.

The theory of inappropriate neural regeneration is supported by the latency of appearance of Frey's syndrome (Laage-Hellman 1957), Laage-Hellman's experiments (1958b), and the stimulation experiments on the tympanic plexus in patients with known gustatory sweating carried out by Ross (1970).

Attempts to prevent Frey's syndrome by modifications of the technique of parotidectomy have been unsuccessful. These include resection of the auriculotemporal nerve (Kidd 1955) and turning in a muscle flap from the sternocleidomastoid muscle under the skin of the parotid (Jost et al 1960, Kornblut et al 1974).

The basis of all proposed **therapeutic procedures** is either to eliminate the parenchyma of the sweat gland or to prevent its function:

1. *Elimination of the sweat gland parenchyma*
   a) Skin excision (Langenskiöld 1946)
   b) Radiotherapy (Morfit & Kramish 1961, Needles 1936, Rumball 1964)
2. *Inhibition of sweat gland function*
   a) Pharmacologic methods:
   - Systemic anticholinergics agents (Shelley & Horvath 1951)
   - Injection of anticholinergic agents into the parotid region (Herxheimer 1958)
   - Local application of anticholinergic ointments, for example 1–3% scopolamine ointment (Laage-Hennman 1958a)
   - Glycopyrrolate (Hays 1978)

- Local anesthesia of the tympanic plexus or the otic ganglion (Glaister et al 1958)

b) Surgical procedures

- A fascia lata underlay of the skin (Wallis & Gibson 1977)
- Excision of the auriculotemporal nerve (Coldwater 1954, Hunt et al 1966)
- Division of the glossopharyngeal nerve (Gardner & McCubbin 1956)
- Tympanic neurectomy (see later)

Of the many treatments described, anticholinergic ointment and denervation of the inappropriately innervated sweat glands have proved to be the most useful.

Radiation therapy is not justifiable because of the high dose required to destroy the sweat glands. The systemic use of anticholinergic agents has many side effects. Repeated local anesthesia of the otic ganglion or the tympanic plexus is scarcely practicable, and excision of the skin is not very effective.

Systemic side effects of scopolamine such as occur on local application may be observed: one third of the patients complain of dryness of the mouth (Laage-Hellman 1958a, 1958b, 1958c). If the ointment is put in the eyes, the patient may complain of an uncomfortable disturbance of accomodation or vision, and there is also the danger of narrow angle glaucoma. These side effects are said to be less if glycopyrrolate is used, since this substance is less well absorbed and does not pass the blood-brain barrier (Hays 1978).

Methods of treatment designed to disrupt the reflex of gustatory sweating by destroying autonomic nerve fibers aim to achieve long-term success.

Excision of auriculotemporal nerve has not had the effect that was hoped for (Coldwater 1954, Hunt et al 1966, Laage-Hellman 1958a). Furthermore it is often difficult to carry out in a previously operated area, and carries the danger of injury to the facial nerve (Edison 1974).

The otic ganglion lying at the base of the skull is difficult to reach, and intracranial division of the glossopharyngeal nerve is inadequate for this relatively harmless condition.

Tympanic neurectomy was proposed by Hemenway (1960) for elimination of the gustatory-sudomotor reflex. Observations that Frey's syndrome disappears after anesthesia of the tympanic plexus (Van Dishoeck 1968) and that it can be produced by stimulation of the plexus (Ross 1970) had encouraged many investigators to use tympanic neurectomy for long-term treatment of gustatory sweating (Blumenfeld & Friedman 1967, Van Dishoeck 1978, Edison 1964, Golding-Wood 1962, Hunt et al 1966, Laage-Hellman 1958b, Parisier et al 1978).

Hays (1978) has summarized the results of 73 patients reported in the literature: tympanic neurectomy had an excellent result in 56% of cases, a satisfactory result in 26%, and no effect in 16%. Thus, a satisfactory outcome can be achieved in 82% of cases, and this result was maintained in the long term. Tympanic neurectomy is therefore a valuable alternative to local anticholineric agents; furthermore, it has the advantage of good long-term results after only one relatively simple microsurgical procedure on the ear.

References

Arnett, C. D., J. N. Davis: Denervation-induced changes in alpha and beta adrenergic receptors of the rat submandibular gland. J. Pharmacol. exp. Therap. 211 (1979) 394

Ashby, W. B.: Gustatory sweating and pilomotor changes. Brit. J. Surg. 47 (1960) 406

Blumenfeld, R. J., J. E. Friedman: Intratympanic surgical treatment of Frey's syndrome. Arch. Otolaryng. 86 (1967) 2

Cannon, W. B., A. Rosenblueth: The Supersensitivity of Denervated Structures. Macmillan, New York 1949

Chilla, R.: Chirurgie der Nerven im HNO-Bereich: Vegetative Hirnstrukturen. Arch. Oto-Rhino-Laryng. 231 (1981) 353

Chilla, R., M. Brüner, C. Arglebe: Function of submaxillary gland following iatrogenic damage to chorda tympani nerve. Acta Otolaryng. 87 (1979) 152

Chilla, R., H. Nicklatsch, C. Arglebe: Late sequelae of iatrogenic damage to chorda tympani nerve. Acta Otolaryng. 94 (1982) 461

Chisa, N., C. G. Medelson, J. D. Damley: Auriculotemporal syndrome. Arch. Derm. 90 (1964) 457

Chorobski, J.: A syndrome of crocodile tears. Arch. Neurol. Neurosurg. Psychiat. 65 (1951) 299

Coldwater, K. B.: Surgical treatment of the auriculotemporal syndrome. Arch. Surg. 69 (1954) 54

Dey, D. L.: A variant of auriculotemporal syndrome. Aust. N. Z. J. Surg. 22 (1953) 310

van Dishoeck, H. A. E.: The auriculo-temporal or Frey syndrome and tympanic neurectomy. Laryngoscope 78 (1968) 122

Duphenix, M.: Observations sur les fistules du canal salivaire de Stenon. I. Sur une playe compliquée à la joue où le canal salivaire fut déchiré. Mem. Acad. Royal Chir. 3 (1757) 431

Edison, B. D.: Frey's syndrome, diagnosis and treatment. E. N. T. Month. 53 (1974) 50

Emmelin, N.: Degeneration secretion from parotid glands after section of the auriculotemporal nerves at different levels. J. Physiol. 195 (1968) 407

Emmelin, N., B. C. R. Strömblad: A "paroxysmal" secretion of saliva following parasympathetic denervation of the parotid gland. J. Physiol. 143 (1958) 506

Emmelin, N., U. Trendelenburg: Degeneration activity after parasympathetic or sympathetic denervation. Rev. Physiol. 66 (1972) 147

Forbes, J., R. Doy: Unilateral gustatory sweating. Cent. Afr. J. Med. 9 (1963) 398

Ford, F. R., B. Woodhall: Phenomena due to misdirection of regenerating fibers of cranial, spinal and autonomic nerves. Arch. Surg. 36 (1938) 480

Frey, L.: Le syndrome du nerf auriculo-temporal. Rev. Neurol. 2 (1923) 97

Gardner, W. J., J. W. McCubbin: Auriculotemporal syndrome; gustatory sweating due to misdirection of regenerated nerve fibers. J. Amer. med. Ass. 160 (1956) 272

Glaister, D. H., J. R. Haennshaw, P. F. Heeron, A. W. Peck, D. H. Patey: The mechanism of postparotidectomy gustatory sweating (the auriculo-temporal syndrome). Brit. Med. J. 1958/II, 942

Golding-Wood, P. H.: Tympanic neurectomy. J. Laryngol. Otol. 76 (1962) 683

Gray, H.: Anatomy of the Human Body, ed. 27. Lea & Febinger, Philadelphia 1959

Griffith, I. P.: Observations on the pathology of chorda tympani nerve in temporal bone sections. J. Laryng. Otol. 91 (1977) 151

Haxton, H. A.: Treatment of hyperhidrosis. Brit. Med. J. 1948a/I. 636

Haxton, H. A.: Gustatory sweating. Brain 71 (1948b) 16

Hays, C. L. L.: The Frey syndrome: a review and double blind evaluation of the topical use of a new anticholinergic agent. Laryngoscope 88 (1978) 1796

Hemenway, W. G.: Gustatory sweating and flushing (the auriculotemporal syndrome – Frey's syndrome). Laryngoscope 70 (1960) 84

Herxheimer, A.: Gustatory sweating and pilomotion. Brit. Med. J. 1958/I, 688

Hogemann, K.-E.: Surgical-orthopaedic correction of mandibular protrusion. Acta Chir. Scand. (Suppl.) 159 (1951) 94

Hunt, W., D. Joseph, R. Newell, H. H. Hanna: Gustatory sweating: report of a case treated by tympanic neurectomy. Arch. Otolaryng. 83 (1966) 260

Jost, G., F. Legent, S. Baupelot: Le comblement des dépressions résiduelles après parotidectomie par un lambeau du sterno-cléidomastodien. Utilisation de l'incision de Lotte. Ann. Otolaryng. (Paris) 85 (1960) 367

Kaplan, H., P. N. Spring: Gustatory hyperhidrosis associated with subcondylar osteotomy. J. Oral Surg. 8 (1960) 50

Kidd, H. A.: Total parotidectomy with preservation of facial nerve. A review of 47 cases. Brit. Med. J. 1955/II, 1309

Kornblut, A. D., P. Westphal, A. Miehlke: The effectiveness of a sternomastoid muscle flap of preventing post-parotidectomy occurence of the Frey syndrome. Acta Otolaryng. (Stockh.) 77 (1974) 368

Laage-Hellman, J.-E.: Gustatory sweating and flushing after conservative parotidectomy. Acta Otolaryng. (Stockh.) 48 (1957) 234

Laage-Hellman, J.-E.: Treatment of gustatory sweating and flushing. Acta Otolaryng. (Stockh.) 49 (1958a) 132

Laage-Hellman, J.-E.: Gustatory sweating and flushing – aetiological implications of response of sweat glands to various stimuli. Acta Otolaryng. (Stockh.) 49 (1958b) 363–374

Laage-Hellman, J.-E.: Gustatory sweating and flushing – aetiological implications of latent period and mode of development after parotidectomy. Acta Otolaryng. (Stockh.) 49 (1958c) 306

Langenskiöld, A.: Gustatory local hyperhidrosis following injuries in the parotid region. Acta Chir. Scand. 93 (1946) 293

Minor, V.: Ein neues Verfahren zur klinischen Untersuchung Untersuchung der Schweißabsonderung. Dtsch. Z. Nervenheilk. 101 (1928) 302

Morfit, H. M., D. Kramish: Auriculotemporal syndrome (Frey syndrome) following surgery of parotid tumors. Amer. J. Surg. 102 (1961) 777

Myers, E. N., J. Conley: Gustatory sweating after neck dissection. Arch. Otolaryng. 91 (1970) 534

Needles, W.: The auriculotemporal syndrome with suggestion regarding therapy. Arch. Neurol. Neurosurg. Psychiat. 35 (1936) 357

Parisier, S. C., W. J. Binder, A. Blitzer, W. H. Friedman, W. F. Marovitz: Evaluation of tympanic neurectomy and chorda tympanectomy for gustatory sweating and benign salivary gland disease. Ear Nose Throat J. 57 (1978) 213

Pointon, S. E., S. P. Banerjee: Alpha- and beta-adrenergic receptors of the rat salivary gland. Elevation after chemical sympathectomy. Biochim. Biophys. Acta 584 (1979) 231

Ross, J. A. T.: The function of the tympanic plexus as related to Frey's syndrome. Laryngoscope 80 (1970) 1816

Rumball, W. G.: The Frey syndrome, and intratympanic procedure for its control. Proc. Canad. Otol. Laryng. Soc. 18 (1964) 92

Shelley, W. B., P. N. Horvath: Comparative study on the effect of anticholinergic compounds on sweating. J. Invest. Dermatol. 16. (1951) 267

Spiro, R. H., H. Martin: Gustatory sweating following parotid surgery and radical neck dissection. Ann. Surg. 165 (1965) 118

Stefano, F. J. E., C. J. Perec: Denervation supersensitivity in salivary glands. Trends Pharmacol. Sciences 2 (1981) 107

Tankel, H.: Case of gustatory sweating. J. Neurol. Neurosurg. Psychiat. 14 (1951) 129

Wallis, K. A., T. Gibson: Gustatory sweating following parotidectomy: Correction by a fascia lata graft. Brit. J. Plast. Surg. 31 (1978) 68

22. Surgery of the Salivary Glands

Surgery of the Parotid Gland; Extratemporal Facial Nerve Surgery

Any operation on the parotid gland is to be regarded as an operation on the facial nerve. This principle also applies to surgery of the submandibular gland in which the hypoglossal and the lingual nerves require particular care. A spectrum of surgical procedures will be described, ranging from exposure of the trunk of the facial nerve and its branches to various reconstructive procedures on the extratemporal segment of the facial nerve. The surgery of the submandibular and sublingual glands will be discussed in a later section.

Exposure of the Extratemporal Trunk of the Facial Nerve

Two basic methods are available:

1. Exposure of the branches of the facial nerve at the periphery followed by retrograde disssection toward the trunk.
2. Exposure of the trunk of the facial nerve before its exit from the stylomastoid foramen followed by dissection in a peripheral direction.

Retrograde Dissection. If the parotid gland is regarded as a triangle standing on its apex, access to the nerve may be chosen from each of the three sides and each angle. Sistrunk (1921), Kidd (1950), Arson & Ott (1923), Byars (1952), and Pollack (1957) used exposure of the marginal mandibular ramus of the facial nerve at the inferior pole of the gland. This was then used to lead dissection to the nerve trunk. Exposure of the nerve may be facilitated by first demonstrating the facial vein (Fig. 22.**1**), since this runs under the marginal mandibular ramus in a vertical direction anterior to the angle of the jaw.

Moser (1954) exposed the branches to the frontal belly of the occipitofrontal muscle and the orbicularis oculi muscle. Dissection was thereafter carried in a retrograde direction toward the bifurcation. One of these branches can be found by blunt dissection with two Freer dissectors between the wall of the orbit and the tragus.

Bailey (1947) began dissection at the anterior edge of the parotid gland using the parotid duct as a landmark. The buccal ramus is in an immediate relationship running in the same direction. Retrograde dissection can also be carried along this nerve to the bifurcation of the trunk. Various incisions are available for each of these methods.

Antegrade Dissection. The Canadian surgeon Janes advocated a new direct approach to the trunk of the nerve in 1940. He maintained that exposure of the trunk of the nerve was relatively easy with some experience. This operation is the basis of the present technique of many surgeons. The facial nerve trunk is exposed anterior to the stylomastoid foramen during its course through the retromandibular fossa by partially dividing the insertion of the sternocleidomastoid muscle to the mastoid process, thus exposing the posterior belly of the digastric muscle. The facial nerve lies directly medial to and above the latter structure.

This technique can be used with some modifications, if a radical neck dissection is first carried out for a malignant tumor and a parotidectomy in continuity then follows. In this case, the sternocleidomastoid muscle is resected completely, exposing the digastric muscle. The trunk of the facial nerve can be exposed rapidly and safely by one more small step. We call this "surgical access."

The incision for the radical neck dissection is extended superiorly behind the angle of the jaw and abuts the lobule of the ear in a Y shape. The knife is carried down to the periosteum of the lower part of the mastoid process to expose the mastoid apex and the anterior surface of the mastoid process. The posterior belly of the digastric muscle is followed to its point of origin on the medial surface of the mastoid process: the facial nerve trunk lies 1–1.5 cm deep and medial to this point. The following maneuver has been described for identification of the trunk (Perzik 1958): the anterior surface of the index finger is pushed beneath the posterior belly of the digastric to its origin. The fingernail then lies directly on

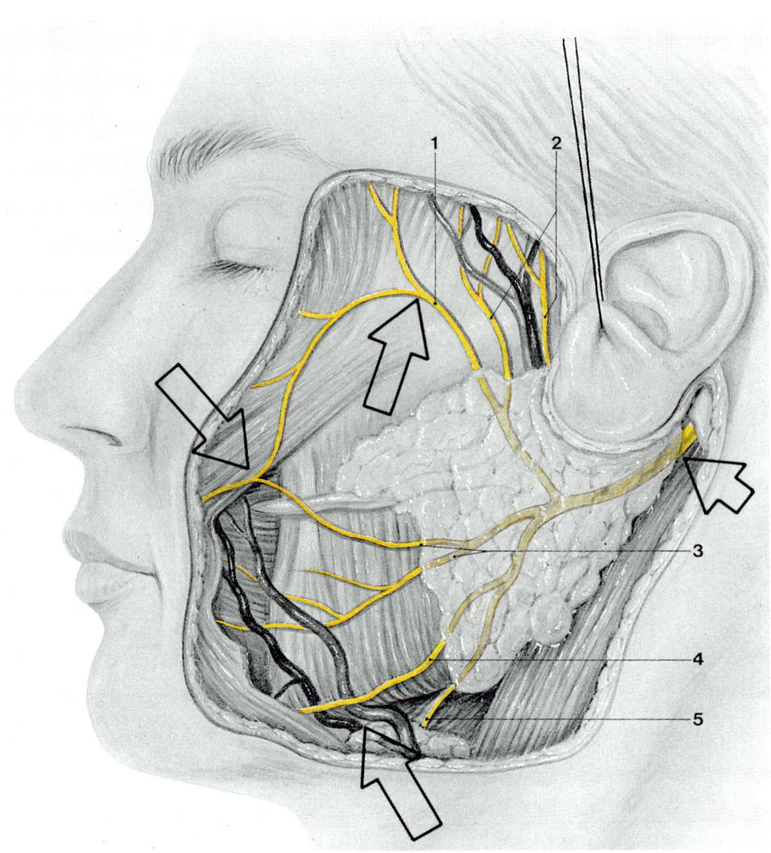

Figure 22.**1** Demonstration of surgical access to the trunk of the facial nerve and its peripheral branches:
1 = zygomatic ramus
2 = temporal ramus
3 = buccal ramus
4 = marginal mandibular ramus
5 = cervical ramus

the trunk of the nerve (Fig. 22.**2**). The facial nerve is now exposed using a Freer's semiblunt raspatory curved on the flat. The capsule of the posterior part of the parotid gland is displaced anteriorly, and dissection is carried along it on the trunk of the facial nerve, which is protected by the index finger. The nerve then appears as a white gleaming structure that cannot be missed, embedded in fatty tissue. At this point, its diameter is 3–4 mm. It is the only structure of this color and thickness running across this space. The bifurcation of the facial nerve often lies very close to the stylomastoid foramen. The main cervicofacial branch may then be the first part of the nerve encountered in the dissection. The bifurcation is then found by retrograde dissection. Figure 22.**2** shows the typical position of the finger over the posteriorly displaced posterior belly of the digastric muscle. The facial nerve trunk can be seen lying on the fingernail.

The situation is different if the facial nerve must be exposed for the removal of a *benign* parotid tumor or for other indications, such as a severe deep injury of the parotid gland. Unneccessary incisions on the neck should then be avoided for cosmetic reasons, and in these cases we prefer an "otologic" incision using the anatomic landmarks familiar to the otologist.

Hogg and Kratz (1958) showed that the tympanomastoid fissure is an excellent landmark for the direct exposure of the facial nerve trunk at its exit from the stylomastoid foramen. The facial nerves lies 6–8 mm medial to the end point of the tympanomastoid fissure.

The procedure begins with a retroauricular incisions, such as is familiar to every otologist. This incision is extended toward the angle of the jaw and then carried around the lobule of the ear in a Y shape (Fig. 22.**3**). The suprameatal spine is exposed by displacing the membranous meatus anteriorly. The tympanomastoid fissure lies immediately distal to the suprameatal spine. The meatus is displaced with the elevator until the entire extent of the tympanomastoid fissure is visible.

The parotid gland is exposed anterior and inferior to the ear by sharp dissection of the subcutaneous tissue until its anterior border is almost reached. The knife is used in such a way that it is turned away from the parotid gland and cuts lightly against the subcutaneous tissue. The branches of

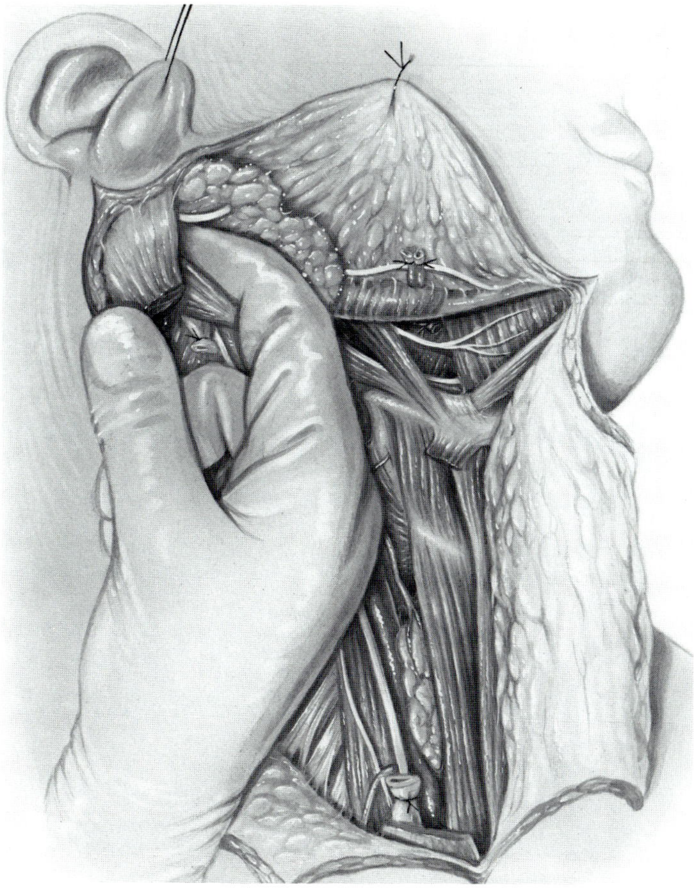

Figure 22.**2** Surgical access to the trunk of the facial nerve in the retromandibular fossa with simultaneous radical neck dissection. The marginal mandibular ramus has been protected by retraction with a sling of the facial artery and vein.

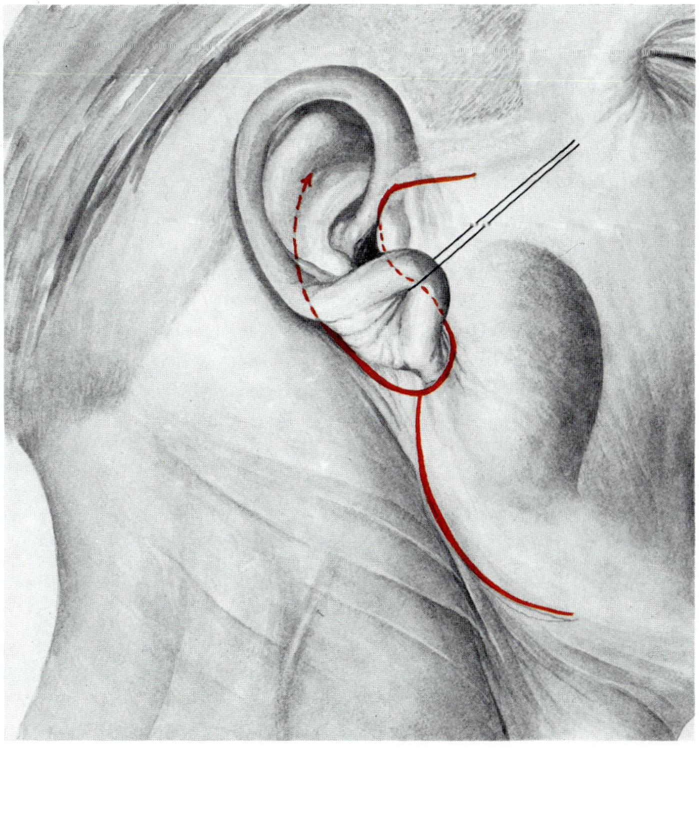

Figure 22.**3** Y-shaped incision.

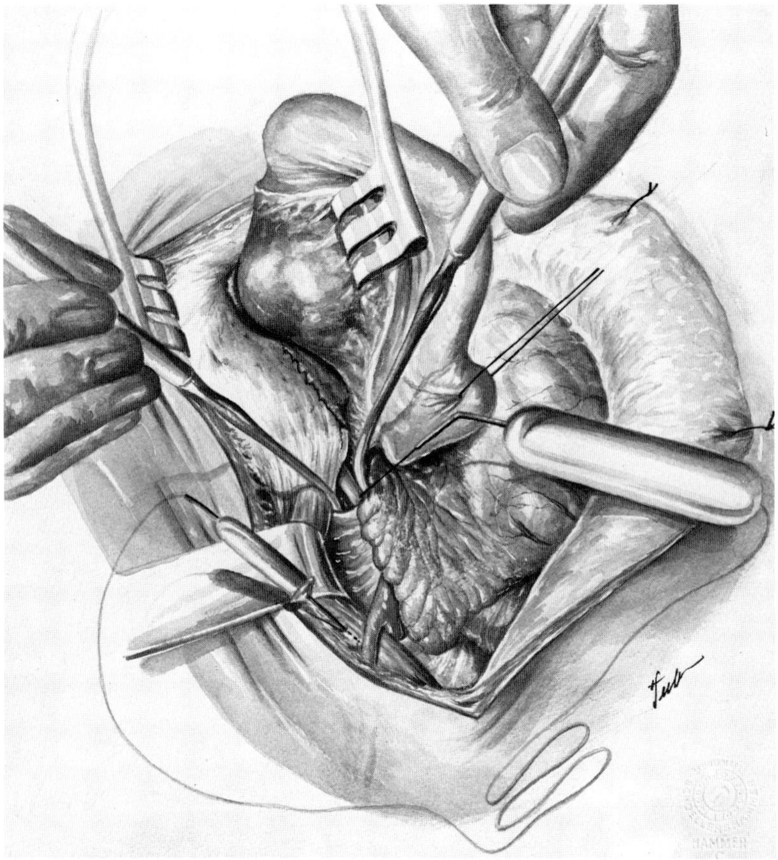

Figure 22.**4** The trunk of the facial nerve exposed in the retromandibular fossa. In this case the stimulator is being used to identify the nerve.

the facial nerve at the anterior edge of the parotid gland lie fairly superficial in the fascia over the masseter muscle: the skin must therefore not be elevated as far as this point. The skin flap that has been developed is fixed to the towels with silk sutures.

The lobule of the ear is now retracted anteriorly using a nylon suture and the incision running toward the angle of the jaw is deepened by freeing the posterior edge of the parotid gland without opening the capsule and displacing it anteriorly with an elevator. The great auricular nerve is often encountered during this step. We always put a black silk suture round this nerve, which is now divided to free the posteroinferior quadrant of the parotid gland. The anterior surface of the sternocleidomastoid muscle can now be exposed by sharp dissection. The resulting space is opened up by using the two index fingers to displace the posterior part of the parotid anteriorly and the sternocleidomastoid muscle and the posterior belly of the digastric muscle posteriorly.

The high point of the operation has now been reached, that is, the search for the facial nerve trunk in the retromandibular fossa. This is achieved by first exposing the tympanomastoid fissure and following it to its end. It must be emphasized again that the trunk lies 6–8 mm deep to the end of the tympanomastoid fissure, although the stylomastoid foramen lies 1 cm medial to this point. Since the trunk of the nerve runs laterally toward the surgeon immediately after its exit from the stylomastoid foramen, it appears to lie more superficial.

A 10 ml hyaluronidase solution is now injected with a fine needle immediately distal to the end of the tympanomastoid fissure to expand the tissue planes. At this point, the surgeon should put on a loupe with 2.5× magnification. Two Freer's elevators are then pushed into the depth of the retromandibular fossa at the end of the tympanomastoid fissure while the capsule of the posterior part of the parotid gland is pulled anteriorly with a wide periosteal elevator or a Schönborn hook. The facial nerve trunk will be found at a depth of 6–8 mm embedded in loose fatty tissue, running diagonally across the retromandibular fossa like a silver-white gleaming cable having the thickness of a knitting needle. Figure 22.**4** shows the trunk being looked for using a stimulator. This instrument is only used if the surgeon is in any doubt.

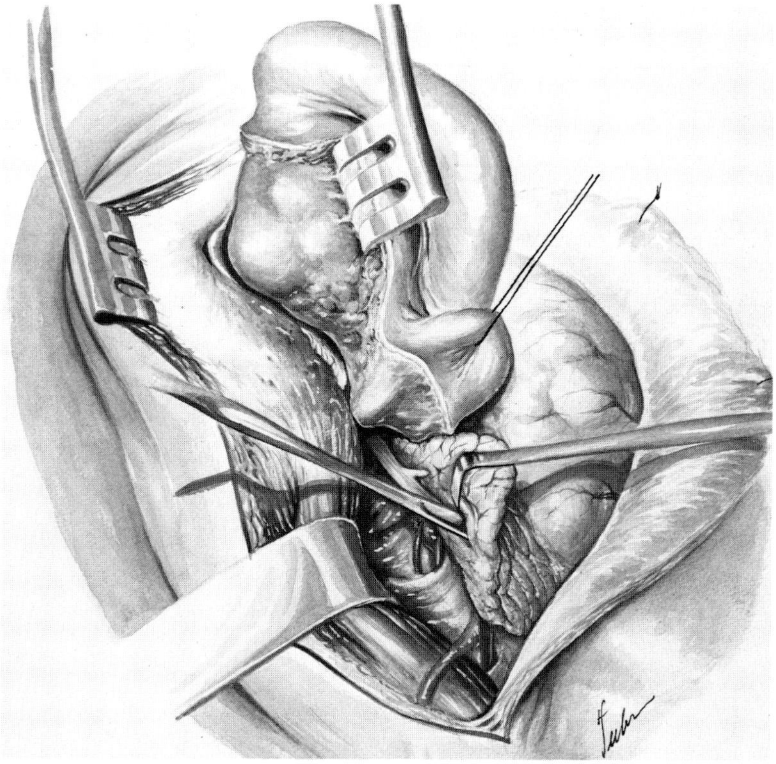

Figure 22.**5** Exposure of the cervicofacial branches of the facial nerve.

It must be emphasized yet again that the nerve trunk can be expected to be found 6–8 mm deep to the end of the tympanomastoid fissure, although the stylomastoid foramen lies 1 cm medial to this point. The facial nerve as it rises from the depth of the retromandibular fossa is often covered by 1 or 2 tributaries of the retromandibular vein. These vessels must be dealt with by bipolar coagulation forceps (using a current of 3–4 mA) and then divided.

The trunk of the nerve is often not found at the first attempt, but this is no cause for alarm. A Lahey swab soaked in epinephrine solution is placed in the fossa, and left in place for 2–3 minutes.

After waiting 2–3 minutes, the operation then proceeds using the two elevators as described previously. The field is widened by an assistant retracting the mandible anteriorly. The nerve can often be suspected and felt before it comes into view. We therefore regard it as an advantage to use a loupe in this phase of the operation, rather than the operating microscope. The operating microscope does not provide the required overview of the surrounding tissue. As soon as the trunk of the nerve has been exposed, a sling cut from a rubber glove is placed around it.

It is of dubious value and possibly dangerous to use the styloid process as a landmark for finding the nerve trunk, as is often recommended. In a third of all patients, the styloid process is absent, and in many others it is not palpable. The facial nerve runs lateral to the styloid process, so that the nerve can be damaged in a search for the styloid process, which lies medial to the nerve.

The *stimulator can be useful for identification of the facial nerve,* particularly in an operation for a deep lobe tumor that displaces the trunk laterally and that can then look like a strand of connective tissue. We do not usually use the stimulator to look for the trunk, but there is no doubt that this apparatus is very helpful in operations for a recurrent tumor. The stimulator is indispensible when dissecting the peripheral parts of the nerve to determine the territory of individual nerve fibers. This point will be discussed again later.

Superficial Parotidectomy

Once the trunk of the nerve has been exposed, the next phase begins, that is, peripheral dissection by retraction of the lateral lobe using a periosteal elevator or a Schönborn hook until the bifurcation of the nerve is clearly visible. The surgeon should now take a short rest and insert a gauze swab soaked in epinephrine into the wound.

Dissection of the branches of the facial nerve to expose the parotid plexus completely now fol-

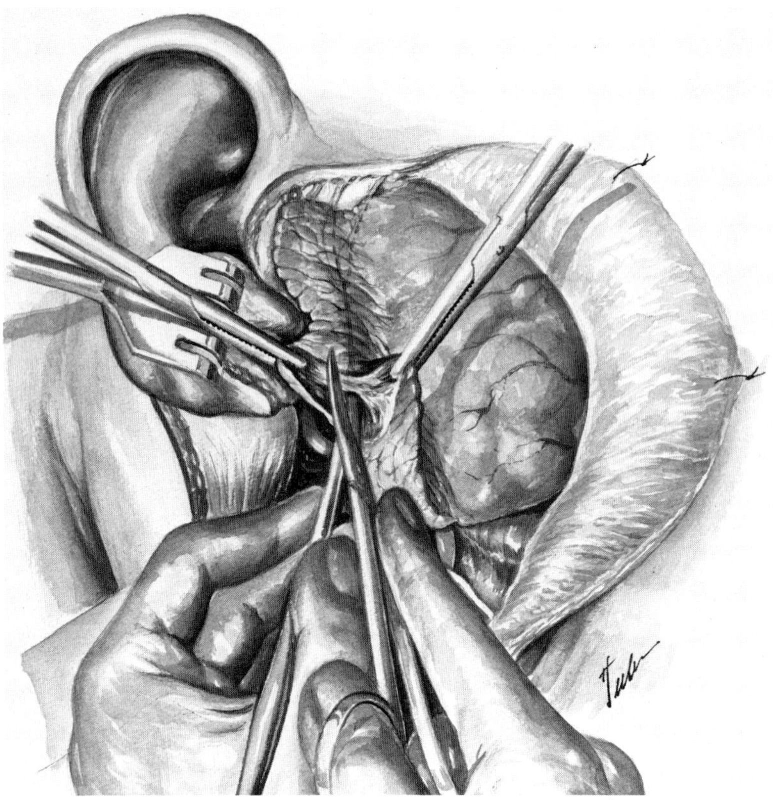

Figure 22.**6** Exposure of the temporofacial branches after splitting of the superficial lobe of the parotid gland.

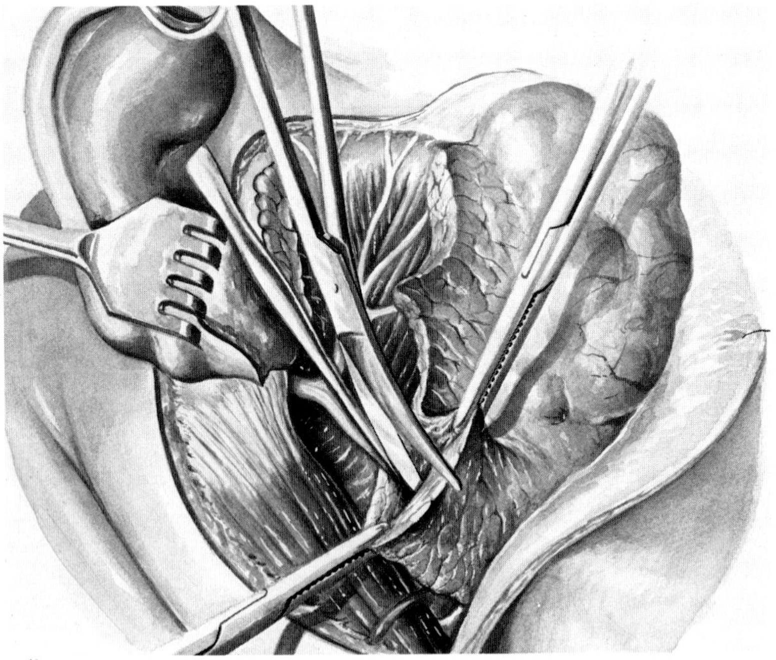

Figure 22.**7** The superficial lobe of the parotid gland has been split for further exposure of the facial branches.

lows. We use the tunnel technique, whose principle rests on the division of the lateral lobe into sectors: a Freer's elevator is pushed peripherally directly over the branches of the facial nerve (Fig. 22.**5**). With the elevator thus riding on the nerve, narrow scissors are inserted into the tunnel over the instrument and the overlying parotid tissue is divided (Figs. 22.**6**, 22.**7**). Dissection is thus carried step by step toward the periphery of the facial nerve branches, as the mass of the lateral lobe

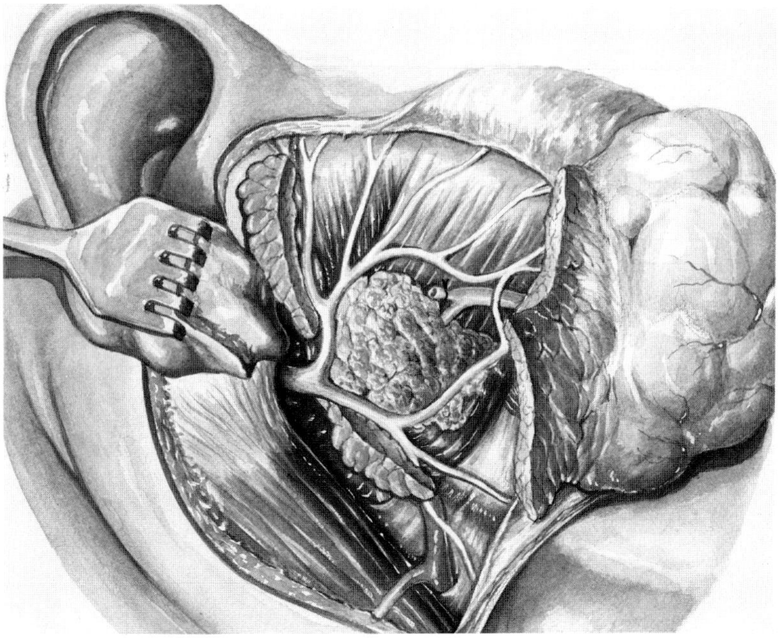

Figure 22.**8** The superficial lobe has been removed, and the entire facial nerve plexus has been exposed. The isthmus and the deep lobe of the parotid gland can be seen. The parotid duct leading from the superficial lobe has been ligated.

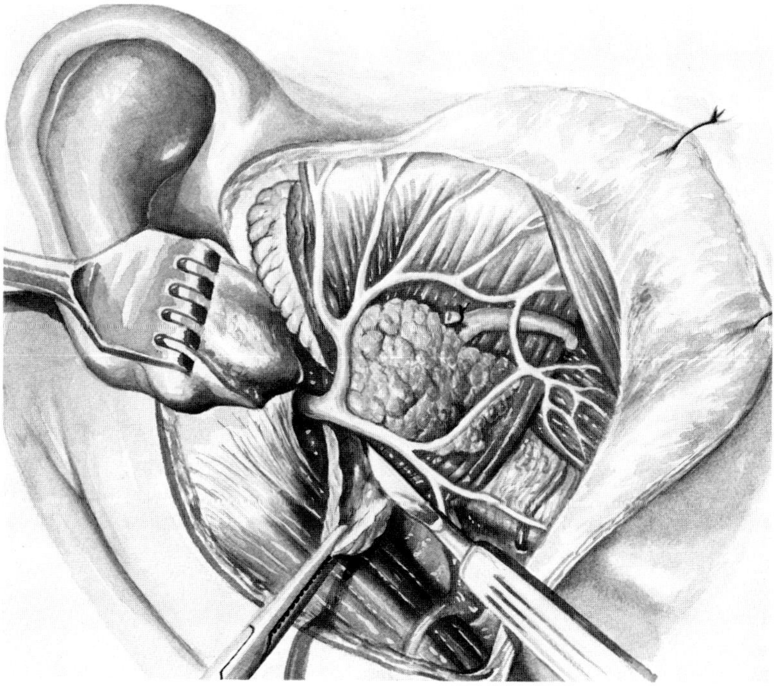

Figure 22.**9** The posteroinferior quadrant of the superficial lobe being removed.

becomes thinner and thinner. Finally, the exposed peripheral branches of the facial nerve turn deeply to reach the muscles. Dissection ends at this point. The superficial lobe of the parotid gland is divided into several sectors by dissecting the individual nerve fibers in this manner (Fig. 22.**7**). Since the surgeon works under vision at all times, the individual segments of the gland can be removed without danger of injury to the nerve (Fig. 22.**8**).

The dissection is carried well clear of the tumor to ensure that the tumor and the surrounding tissue are removed. This usually succeeds in benign tumors, since the nerve runs away from the tumor. Other techniques to be described later are used for malignant tumors.

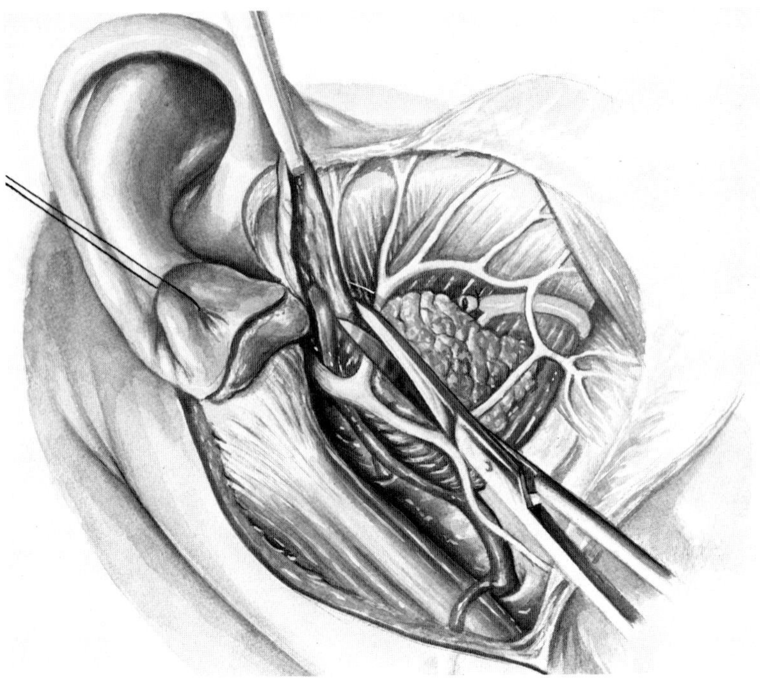

Figure 22.**10** The postero-superior quadrant of the superficial lobe being removed.

Occasionally, the parotid duct may be exposed during dissection of the buccal ramus, which often has several parallel branches. It should be divided to allow complete mobilization of the parotid gland (Fig. 22.**8**). The peripheral stump of the duct is ligated with chromic catgut to prevent reflux of saliva from the mouth into the wound. All small bleeding points are either ligated or dealt with by bipolar coagulation. In chronically infected glands, the vessels are ligated with normal catgut, and in noninfected cases by synthetic catgut.

Figure 22.**9** shows removal of the remaining posteroinferior quadrant of the parotid gland using the knife. The last step of a superficial parotidectomy is removal of the remaining posterosuperior quadrant of the gland (Fig. 22.**10**) remembering that the superficial temporal artery and vein are in an immediate relationship. It is usually necessary to doubly ligate and divide them to prevent brisk hemorrhage. The posterosuperior quadrant turns anterior to the tragus and behind one of the vertical branches of the facial nerve into the depth of the wound. This part of the parotid gland is freed by dissection along the tragal cartilage with blunt narrow scissors or a knife, until the triangular part of the cartilaginous meatus (named the pointer by Conley) is reached.

This pointer was used by Conley (1955, 1957) and Rankow (1968) as a landmark for identification of the trunk of the facial nerve. Its apex points directly to the facial nerve trunk in the depths of the retromandibular fossa.

The deep groove formed behind the ascending ramus of the mandible can be improved cosmetically by filling it with a muscular transposition flap from the sternocleidomastoid muscle, spread out over the main branches of the facial nerve and sutured into position with catgut (Fig. 22.**11**). It is also claimed that covering the facial branches by muscle tissue prevents the auriculotemporal syndrome (see page 325) (Jost et al 1978), but a trial on 70 patients, half of whom had the transposed muscle flap and half did not, showed that the flap did not prevent the appearance of Frey's syndrome (Kornblut et al 1974).

A suction drain is now introduced and the wound is closed in layers with subcutaneous and skin sutures (Fig. 22.**12**).

Total Parotidectomy with Preservation of the Facial Nerve

A total parotidectomy with preservation of the facial nerve is indicated for a benign tumor in the isthmus, or in the deep lobe or a recurrent tumor. The facial nerve must be elevated clear of the deep lobe before it can be removed. Small rubber bands are placed carefully around the individual branches of the facial nerve, and the deep lobe is dissected off the medial surface of the nerve using fine curved neurologic scissors. The nerve

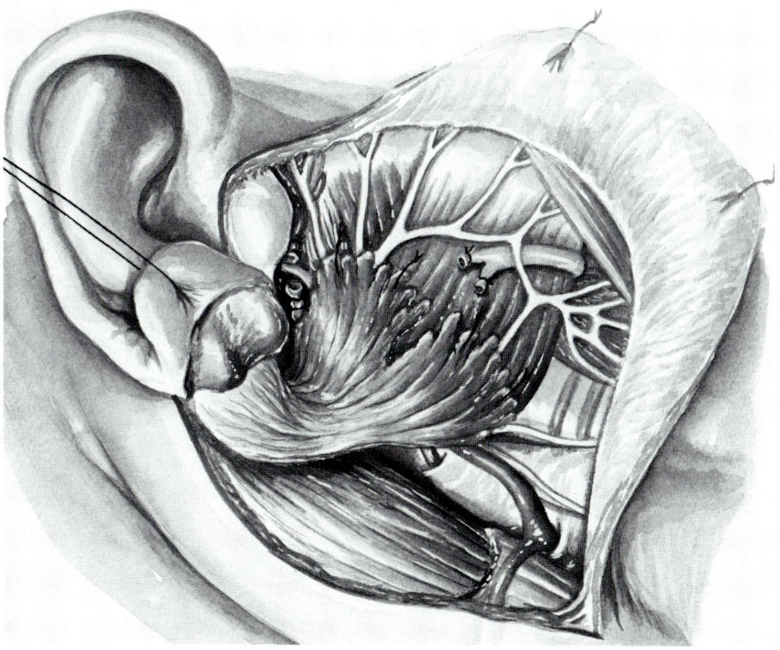

Figure 22.**11** A flap taken from the sternocleidomastoid muscle to fill out the operative defect.

branches that are not being worked on are covered temporarily with small swabs soaked in Ringer's solution. Isolation of the deep lobe now follows: it is adherent to the temporomandibular joint, the mandible, and the surrounding muscles, such as the stylohyoid, the styloglossus, and the digastric. This part of the gland is also closely related to the external carotid and maxillary arteries, so that double ligature of the external carotid artery is often indicated. Finally, the branches of the facial nerve are separated gently, and the deep lobe is delivered between them and is removed (Fig. 22.**13**).

A total parotidectomy is occasionally followed by a facial paralysis, but this is usually only a neurapraxia and at worst a mild form of axonotmesis. The paralysis resolves spontaneously within days or weeks.

Removal of Dumbbell Tumors

The removal of tumors lying deep in the retromandibular portion or the parapharyngeal part of the parotid gland presents greater difficulty (Fig. 22.**14**). These tumors are also called dumbbell tumors. Many of them are only recognized late because of their concealed site. The characteristic pain on pressure in front of the mastoid process that they cause must be emphasized (Denecke 1959). These tumors often present as a swelling of the pharyngeal wall or the tonsillar region (Fig. 22.**15**). They are difficult to remove because of their extent and because they are clamped between the styloid process and the stylomandibular ligament.

The stylomandibular ligament is divided and the ascending ramus of the mandible is retracted as

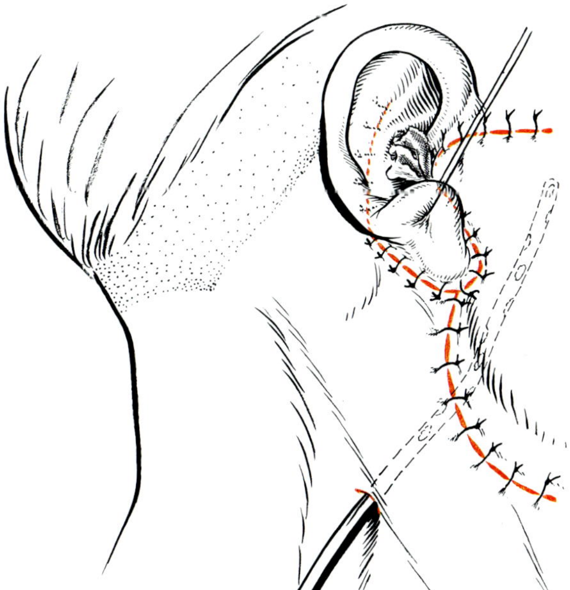

Figure 22.**12** Closure of the wound with suction drainage.

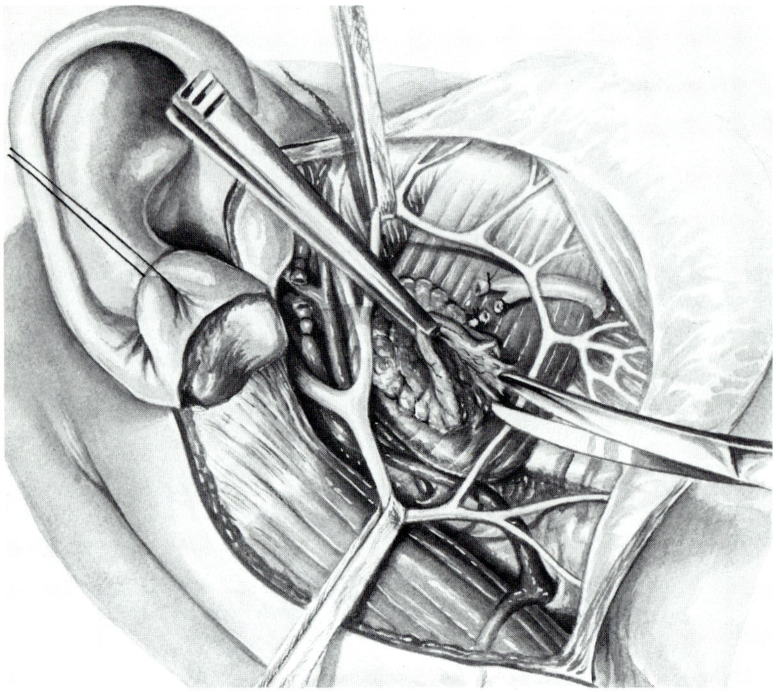

Figure 22.**13** Removal of the deep lobe of the parotid gland using the rubber sling technique.

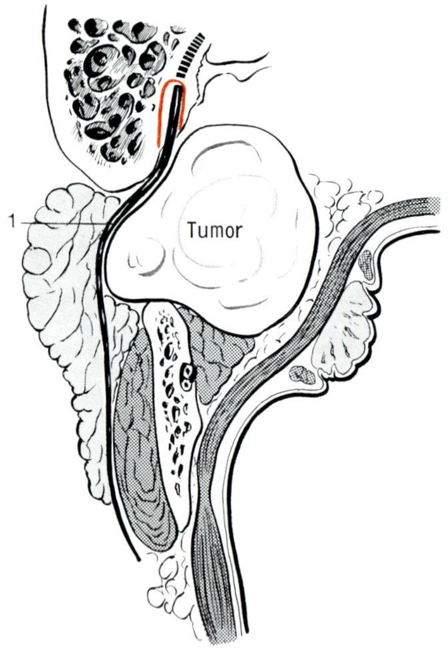

Figure 22.**14** Semidiagrammatic appearance of a dumbbell tumor. 1 = the facial nerve.

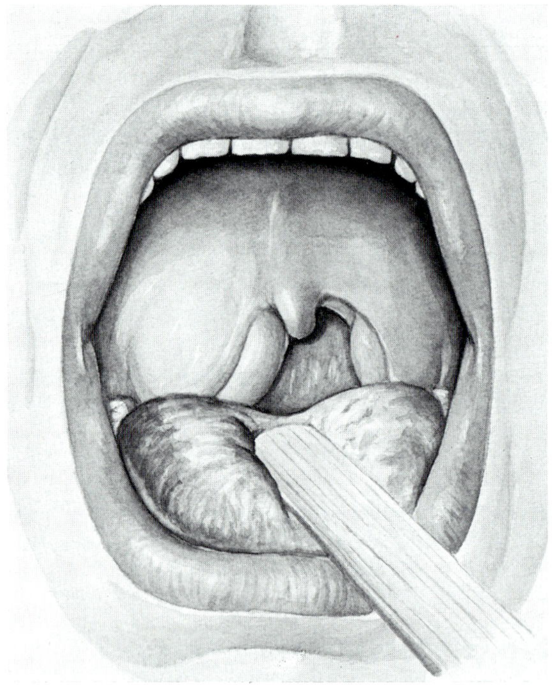

Figure 22.**15** Oral view of a dumbbell tumor.

far anteriorly as possible to open up the operative field. It is appropriate to divided the external carotid artery, the maxillary artery, or the superficial temporal artery and the corresponding veins. The facial nerve trunk is first exposed as previously described, and the superficial lobe is removed. Removal of the mastoid tip and of the posterior part of the ascending ramus of the mandible, using a chisel or drill, and resection of the styloid process provide further space.

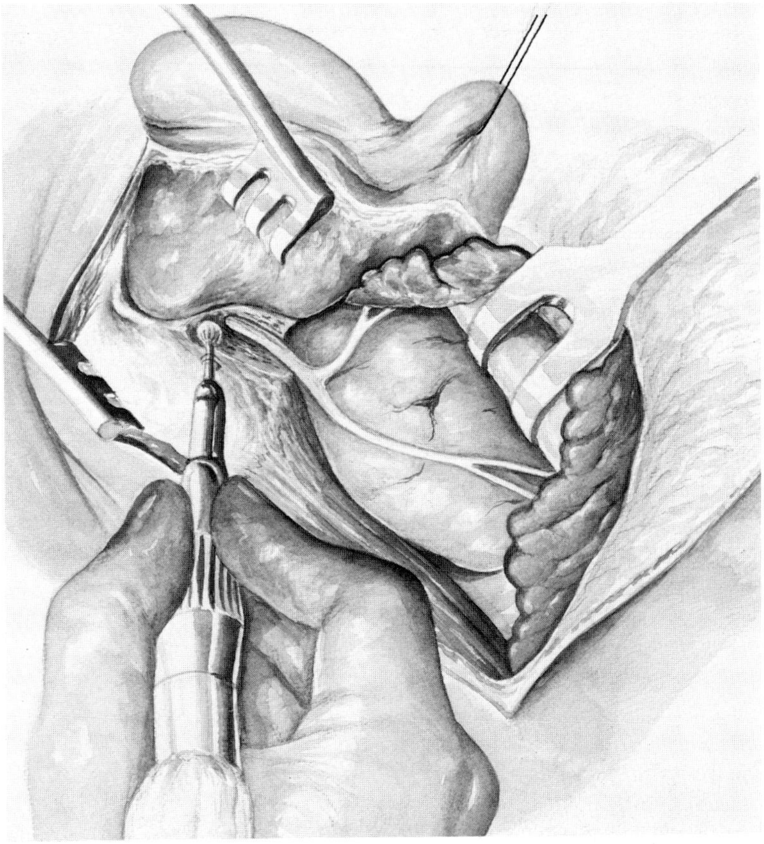

Figure 22.**16** The stylomastoid canal being drilled to mobilize the trunk of the facial nerve.

Sometimes, temporary division of the ascending ramus of the mandible is indicated. After the tumor has been removed, the bone ends are carefully readapted and fixed by wire or by compression plates.

The tumor is now mobilized using an elevator. If delivery of the tumor from the depths of the retromandibular fossa carries the risk of overstretching of the facial nerve, it may be appropriate to open up the stylomastoid canal and to lift the mastoid segment of the facial nerve out of it. This prevents overstretching of the trunk. Figure 22.**16** shows exposure of the nerve in the stylomastoid canal, and the surface of the tumor under the nerve.

Once the tumor has been mobilized, it is then relatively easy to retract the trunk of the facial nerve above or below the tumor, which is then removed without further stretching of the nerve. A muscle transposition graft should always be used after removal of a dumbbell tumor to reduce the size of the operative defect. Introduction of a suction drain and wound closure now follows.

Special Procedures for Recurrent Tumors

In clinics that are particularly interested in parotid gland surgery, the problem of the patient with a recurrent tumor presents itself relatively often. These recurrences are due to unsatisfactory resections of malignant tumors, and incorrect primary operations (particularly enucleation) for pleomorphic adenomas.

The typical picture of a recurrent pleomorphic adenoma is that the entire operative field is seeded by small miliary masses of recurrent tumors about 1 cm in size. The cause of this widespread recurrence is rupture of the capsule of the pleomorphic adenoma at the first operation, scattering microscopic pieces of tumor over the operative field. Scar tissue forms in the retromandibular fossa and makes identification of the facial nerve trunk difficult or impossible.

We always use the stimulator to facilitate identification of the facial nerve trunk embedded in scar tissue. The anesthetist must be warned before the operation not to use relaxants.

It is often necessary to abandon the search for the trunk of the facial nerve, since this may be too dangerous. The facial nerve is then exposed by its peripheral branches. These branches are sought at typical sites and are then used to lead dissection backward to the bifurcation and the facial nerve trunk.

Dissection using these individual nerve trunks has already been mentioned briefly on page 329ff. Their identification using appropriate landmarks must now be discussed.

We begin with the "superior operation" (Fig. 22.**1**): that branch of the temporofacial ramus running to the orbicularis oculi muscle and to the frontal part of the occipitofrontal muscle is looked for within the gland, using a loupe. This branch can be found by blunt dissection halfway between the edge of the orbit and the tragus using a Freer's elevator. One of the fine silvery strands is found running in the expected direction after retracting the gland.

If the first attempt fails, further dissection must be abandoned because of the danger to the fine nerve fibers.

Attention now turns to the marginal mandibular ramus (Fig. 22.**1**) of which there are often two. Finding this nerve can often be facilitated by first finding the facial artery and vein running vertically under the marginal mandibular ramus anterior to the angle of the jaw. They are found just below the mandible and followed superiorly to expose the nerve branches in the loose connective tissue below the parotid gland.

If this approach to the facial nerve fails, the final method that can be tried is to find the parotid duct at the anterior border of the parotid gland and to dissect here to find the buccal branch above or below it. Occasionally, there are two rami.

Once the fibers of the facial nerve have been found by one of these methods, it is easy to dissect in a retrograde direction, using the tunnel technique, a millimeter at a time, until the bifurcation is reached. Dissection is then continued in a peripheral direction along the cervicofacial or temporofacial rami (page 329ff), once more splitting the superficial lobe into segments. Depending on the site of the recurrence, it may be necessary to follow the trunk into the retromandibular fossa. This is not very difficult once the bifurcation of the facial nerve trunk has been reached.

Total Parotidectomy with Sacrifice of the Facial Nerve

If the histopathologic type of the tumor and its extent demands the use of the most radical form of parotid surgery, then a total parotidectomy in continuity with a radical neck dissection is carried out with sacrifice of as much as necessary of the facial nerve. Total parotidectomy and radical neck dissection, planned as a monobloc operation, also often demand resection of the masseter muscle and of the ascending ramus of the mandible.

After such an operation, the patient has a grotesque deformity of the face that results from complete paralysis of the facial nerve for the rest of his life. The work of Lathrop (1963, 1964), Maxwell (1954a), Maxwell et al (1953) and Conley (1955, 1957, 1970, 1975) to develop methods of bridging the defect in the nerve are among the greatest advances of facial surgery of our time. The astonishing results that may be achieved with these nerve reconstructions have freed surgery of the facial nerve from inappropriate and life-threatening compromises. Since the overriding consideration must be radical removal of the tumor, the operation is usually combined with a radical neck dissection, as mentioned previously. Reconstruction of the facial nerve can be carried out at the same time, or up to a few weeks later.

We have often found it more suitable to carry out the operation in two stages a few weeks apart to give the pathologist and the surgeon the opportunity to assess the histopathologic findings and to discuss the next procedure.

If reconstruction is to be carried out at a second stage, the individual branches and the trunk are marked with silver clips immediately distal or proximal to the resection site. The clips are embedded in silicon tubes and are then sutured to the underlying tissue. This step facilitates the finding of the trunk and the branches when the wound is opened again. Screening is occasionally helpful in finding the clips later.

Radical Neck Dissection as part of a Monobloc Procedure

Some remarks about the anatomy of the cervical lymph node system must be made to help understand the monobloc operation, which is often necessary for malignant tumors of the parotid. Three chains of lymph nodes may be distinguished in the neck running in a superoinferior direction (Leicher et al 1956). They are interconnected by numerous vertical and horizontal lymph vessels (see also Figs. 22.**17**, 22.**18**).

The common carotid artery and the jugular vein are accompanied by the main jugular lymphatic trunk and chain of jugular lymph nodes.

A second important pathway is the chain of lymph nodes running under the sternocleidomastoid muscle near its posterior border. These lymph nodes lie in the fatty tissue that surrounds the accessory nerve and that fills the space between the sternocleidomastoid, trapezius, and scalenus muscles.

A prelaryngeal and paratracheal series of nodes running in an inferior direction in the center of the neck forms a third chain.

These lymphatic pathways of the neck receive the lymph, not only from immediately adjacent organs and tissues, but also lymph that has been previously filtered by regional lymph nodes draining circumscribed territories.

The upper deep cervical nodes thus collect all the lymph of the head, not directly, but rather as the second or third station draining the regional lymph nodes of the individual territories of the head. Thus, lymph is filtered in the upper deep cervical node after it has run through the parotid and preauricular lymph nodes (Fig. 22.**17**). This lymph originates from the external ear and middle ear, the parotid gland, the lateral part of the face, the parotid and forehead region, including the orbital cavity, and the lip.

The lower deep cervical nodes are the last station for the lymph arising in the head, which has already been filtered by the superior jugular nodes, before it finally reaches the bloodstream (Lanz & Wachsmuth 1955). The superficial cervical lymph nodes in the occipital triangle embedded in fatty tissue along the accessory nerve are the first regional filters of the lymph from the skin and the muscles of the back of the neck and from the skin of the head, especially that of the occipital region. The occipital nodes usually communicate with this group. Also, some of the lymph from the retroauricular lymph nodes drains into the superficial cervical lymph nodes as a secondary station (Fig. 22.**18**).

The site of predilection for metastases of malignant tumors of the parotid gland is the upper deep cervical nodes, particularly those in the angle of the facial vein (marked 1 in Fig. 22.**19**), and the carotid bifurcation (marked 2 in Fig. 22.**19**). The lymph drains from here along the internal jugular vein into the lower deep cervical nodes (marked 3 in Fig. 22.**19**).

The management of malignant tumors of the parotid gland thus often embraces two areas that are closely connected by the protective chain of lymph nodes. Cure is only possible if all regional lymph node metastases are removed as well as the primary tumor.

A radical neck dissection in continuity with the primary tumor of the parotid gland is often indi-

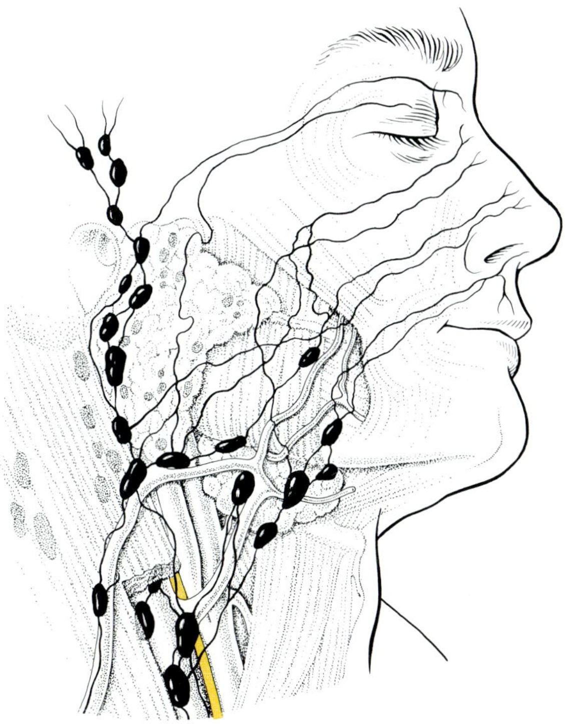

Figure 22.**17** The lymph nodes of the face and neck.

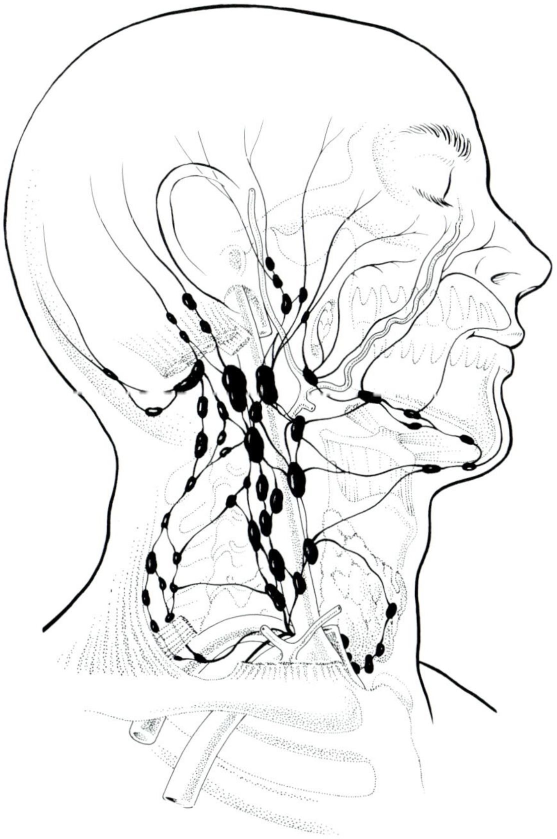

Figure 22.**18** The lymph nodes of the lateral part of the neck. The drainage area and lymphatics of the upper deep cervical nodes. (von Lanz and Wachsmuth.)

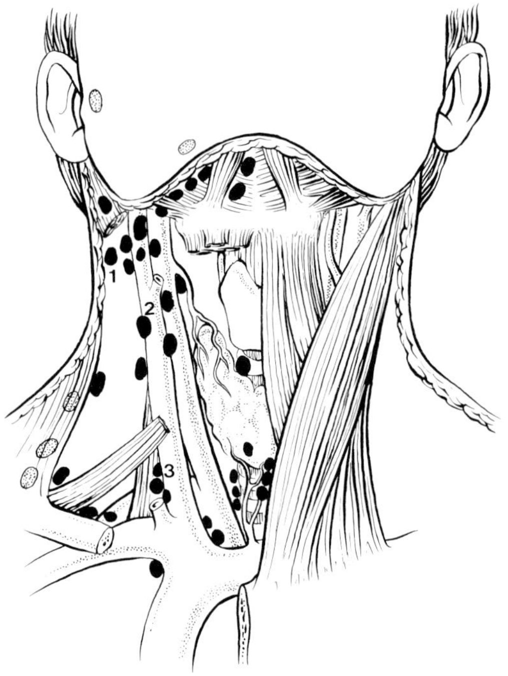

Figure 22.**19** Semidiagrammatic illustration of the most important lymph nodes, adapted from a diagram of the Columbia-Presbyterian Medical Center, New York.
1 and 2 = the upper deep cervical lymph nodes:
1 = the group around the insertion of the sternocleidomastoid muscle, 2 = the group around the jugular vein, 3 = the lower deep cervical nodes.

cated. The following structures must be removed as a routine: the sternocleidomastoid muscle, the omohyoid muscle, the anterior border of the trapezius muscle, the internal and external jugular vein, the facial vein, the accessory nerve, the entire cervical plexus preserving the phrenic nerve, and the submandibular gland. All that remains is the carotid artery, the brachial plexus, and the phrenic, vagus, and hypoglossal nerves.

In individual cases, the surgeon must decide whether a functional neck dissection with preservation of the accessory nerve or the jugular vein (Pietrantoni & Agazzi 1961, Bocca 1972) is justified. We consider that preservation of the accessory nerve in all cases of high-grade cancer compromises the effectiveness of radical neck dissection and influences the prognosis (Conley 1970, 1975). The accessory nerve runs directly inferior to the base of the skull through fat and connective tissue in which the subdigastric lymph nodes of the jugular chain are embedded. It is exactly these lymph nodes and lymphatics which are mandatory to remove. We therefore feel that in such cases it is better to carry out a radical neck dissection with sacrifice of the accessory nerve and to replace the nerve with an autologous transplant using the sural nerve (Anderson & Flowers 1969, Harries & Dickey 1965, Fisch & Michael 1973, Samii 1980, Miehlke et al 1981). Deliberate sacrifice and reconstruction of the accessory nerve during radical neck dissection is in accordance with sound oncologic principles, that is:

1. Radical and complete removal of all potentially dangerous tissue with a wide margin of healthy tissue.
2. Reconstruction of important structures, in this case the accessory nerve by a free autologous nerve graft. Further details are discussed by Miehlke (1981).

Reconstruction of the Facial Nerve

In the last decade, it has become acknowledged that a very radical procedure is essential for the removal of parotid tumors. The operative procedure must be tailored to the biologic behavior of the tumor. The range of surgical procedures extends from parotidectomy with preservation of the facial nerve to total parotidectomy with sacrifice of the nerve en bloc with radical neck dissection and resection of the mandible, if necessary (Fig. 22.**20**; see also page 340). This has already been discussed.

Operations are now available that include reconstruction of the trunk and branches of the facial nerve.

Four techniques will now be described for reconstruction of the facial nerve, depending on the size and site of the defect:

1. Direct anastomosis
2. Indirect anastomosis
3. Autologous nerve graft
4. Combined graft (diversification technique)

Reconstruction of the facial nerve with one of these methods has now become established so that many patients have regained the use of their facial muscles with considerable improvement in their quality of life. Before the technique is discussed some facts must be highlighted that have led to modifications and improvements in microsurgical suturing technique.

Preliminary Remarks on Nerve Suture

Several well-developed procedures allow successful nerve regeneration. The prerequisites are growth of the axon cylinder from the central stump and wallerian degeneration of the

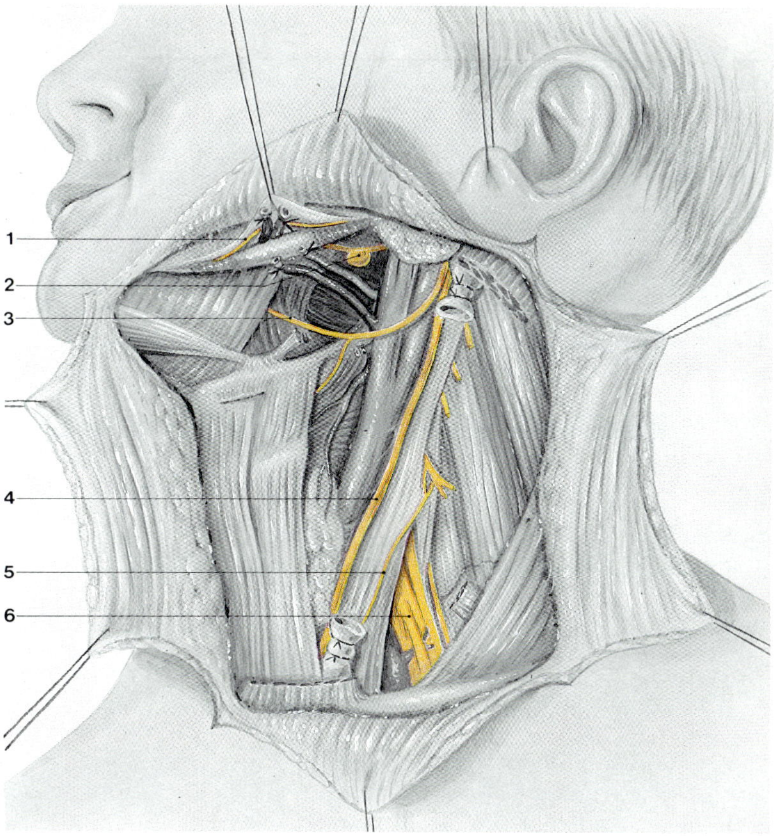

Figure 22.**20** Appearance after a radical neck dissection.
1 = marginal mandibular ramus.
2 = lingual nerve with submandibular ganglion.
3 = hypoglossal nerve.
4 = vagus nerve.
5 = phrenic nerve.
5 = brachial plexus.

peripheral part of the nerve. The outgrowth of axons begins in the first few days after the nerve is divided, that is, at the time at which the proliferation of the Schwann cells begins to form Büngner's bands in the peripheral stump. Büngner's band are protoplasmic bands formed from sheath cells in which the neurofibrils and neuroplasm of regenerating peripheral nerves lie embedded and grow. The degenerated stump serves to receive the axon cylinder growing out from the proximal stump. A fibrin membrane forms between the two stumps in the first 3 days. The fibrin is converted into cords that orient themselves in the direction of the axis of the nerve stumps. The Schwann cells arising from the central and peripheral stumps are conducted along this fibrin bridge toward each other until they finally unite.

It is known from the work of Weiss and Hiscoe (1948) that there is a stream of cytoplasm that moves in the axis cylinder of the nerve fibers in a peripheral direction at a speed of 1–5 mm/day. In addition to this slow axonal flow by which the main amount of the axoplasm is moved peripherally, there is also a much faster transport of 40–500 mm/day. These fast-flowing agents include lipoproteins, proteins, neurosecretory material, and catecholamines (Kreutzberg & Schubert 1971, Rieske & Kreitzberg 1978). The beginning of the outgrowth of the first newly formed axons can be seen 2 to 4 days after division of the nerve in the anastomosis. Delicate connective tissue can only be observed in the anastomosis from about the seventh day.

The proliferation of the connective tissue proceeds mainly from the epineurium of the nerve stump. (Figure 22.**21** should facilitate understanding of the following discussion). The investigations of Millesi et al (1972) and Millesi (1978) have shown that this connective tissue from around the anastomosis migrates between the two nerve stumps and thus lies between their fascicles if the anastomosis tends to retract. Furthermore, Millesi et al (1972) affirmed that the extent of the soft tissue proliferation at this site could be influenced by trauma during preparation of the nerve stumps for anastomosis, and by the suture itself.

Direct Anastomosis

The experiments just described carried out by Millesi and his colleagues have led to far-reaching changes in suturing technique:

1. The epineurium of the nerve stumps is resected for at least 3 mm to eliminate the site for

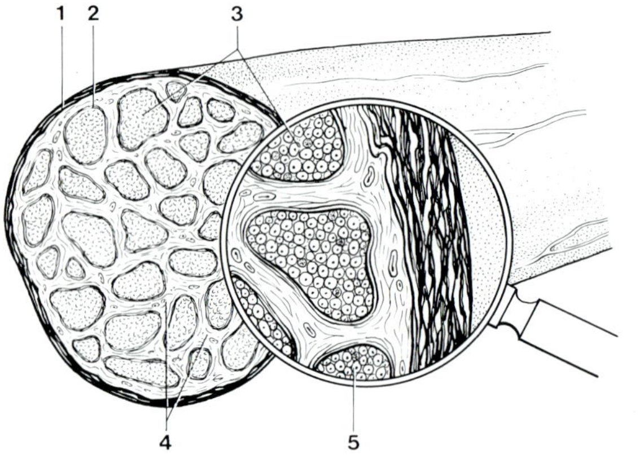

Figure 22.**21** Section of a nerve. 1 = epineurium, 2 = perineurium, 3 = fascicle, 4 = interfascicular epineurium, 5 = neurite.

connective tissue invasion into the anastomosis between the fascicles. Resection of the epineurium with a minimum of trauma using fine-pointed watchmakers forceps and neurectomy scissors should encompass the entire circumference of the nerve stumps.

2. The operative trauma of freshening and adapting the nerve stumps for anastomosis must be kept to a mimimum. The operating microscope is used for freshening the stumps, for resection of the epineurium, for identification of the fascicles, and for the suture itself to minimize the inevitable trauma to the nerve stumps.
3. The nerve stumps must be joined without tension at all costs. The previous view that slight tension was useful in an end-to-end suture to direct the fibrin membrane to form a guide is now no longer accepted because this tension favors the invasion of proliferating connective tissue.
4. The exposed fascicles of the two nerve stumps are joined at corresponding points where possible, by one or two fine sutures. The fascicles in the intra- and extratemporal course of the facial nerve can be identified as far as the bifurcation.
5. The use of sutures should be kept to a mimimum. The suture should be placed through the perineurium, if possible (Fig. 22.**22a, b**). In particular situations, epi- and perineural sutures should be used (Figure 22.**22c**), and wherever possible fibrin glue should be used rather than sutures. A 10–0 monofilament suture with an atraumatic needle is used for the fascicular suture. The suture is passed through the perineurium and tied just tightly enough to ensure that the nerve stumps lie snugly against each other. All compression is to be avoided. If a perineural suture is not possible because of the small size of the peripheral branches, an epineural suture is used. In this situation the epineurium is not removed. The suture is led through the epineurium and at the same time through the perineurium (Fig. 22.**22c**). A relatively exact approximation of the proximal and distal fascicles of even the finest peripheral branches can be obtained by this method.
Suture material is not used for anastomosis in the stylomastoid canal. The nerve stumps are approximated exactly in the gutter of the canal after resecting the epineurium. Cohesion between the freshened nerve stumps suffices, if the anastomosis is free from tension. Natural adhesion is achieved within 20 minutes.
Experiments have shown that a fibrin film unites the circumference of the cut ends with one another within 2 to 3 days, and a connective tissue bridge develops after 7 days.
6. Protection of the anastomosis had a secure place in the classic method of nerve suturing. A sheath of various tissues, such as serosa, amnion, collagen, and artificial materials, such as Milipore and silicone, was thought to prevent the ingrowth of connective tissue. It is now known that encasing the nerve does not prevent proliferation of connective tissue. This tissue arises mainly from the epineurium that

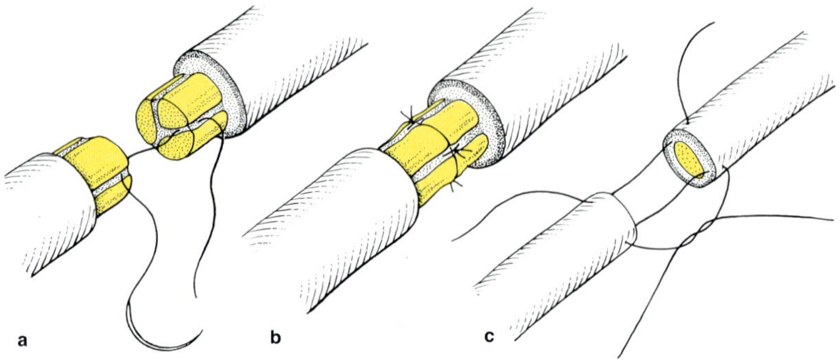

Figure 22.**22a–c** Microsurgical suture, perineural suture (**a**, **b**) and epineural and perineural suture (**c**).

remains within the sheath, so that the epineurium must be resected.

We now therefore seldom use protection of the suture site, although we still do so if it is necessary to support, protect, and immobilize the anastomosis, for example, in the lateral facial region to prevent distortion of the suture site by chewing.

Now we only use very well-tolerated artificial collagen prepared in fine tubes (Braun, Melsungen). A half-open cylinder is cut with a wide window. The cylinder is slit up one side so that it can be laid easily around the nerve. When the cylinder has been placed in position, the suture can be checked for optimal accuracy through the window. A drop of autologous plasma is then introduced through the window (Fig. 22.**23**) to stabilize the suture and to form a bridge for the newly sprouting Schwann cells. Finally, several further drops of fibrin glue are placed at the end of the collagen tube to ensure adhesion of the collagen cylinder to the nerve sheath and to provide the anastomosis with additional stability.

A fine sheet of serosa can be used instead of the collagen cylinder to wrap around an anastomosis of the extratemporal segment. Fibrin glue is again introduced on both ends of the sheet. The accuracy of the suture can be checked under the operating microscope through the fine transparent serosa. Amnion is also suitable for this purpose.

Indirect Anastomosis

It is conceivable that a wide resection of one of the important end branches of the facial nerve must be undertaken, whereas one of the other less important branches can be preserved. The remaining long segment of the latter can then be anastomosed to the more important branch (Fig. 22.**24**). The same technique is used as for direct anastomosis.

Free Autologous Nerve Graft

If the main trunk of the facial nerve or several peripheral branches must be sacrificed, the methods discussed so far are no longer practicable, and a free autologous nerve graft must be used.

Two nerves can be considered as donor sites:

a) The great auricular nerve.
b) The sural nerve.

The Great Auricular Nerve. The great auricular nerve is sought through a perpendicular incision running from the external auditory meatus to the first skin fold of the neck: it lies immediately

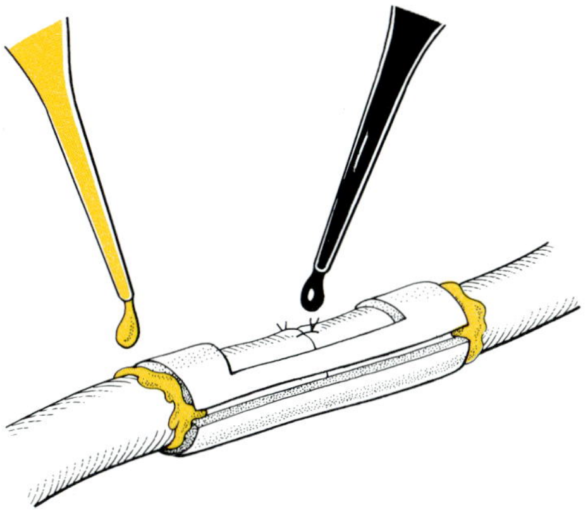

Figure 22.**23** Microsurgical nerve suture encased in a collagen cylinder. A drop of serum is introduced into the window in the cylinder, and the two ends of the window are stuck to the circumferance of the nerve with fibrin glue to provide better support for the anastomosis.

posterior to the external jugular vein running in the subcutaneous tissue (Fig. 22.**25**). A segment of the nerve is removed that must be considerably longer than the defect. Several branches may also be harvested on occasion.

If the entire nerve must be reconstructed, it is advisable to take a part of the cervical plexus in addition (Figs. 22.**26**, 22.**27**). If the nerve must be reconstructed after a tumor operation, the nerve

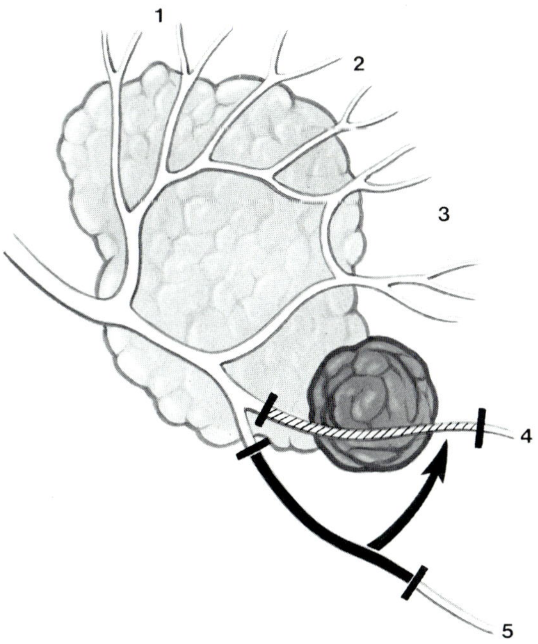

Figure 22.**24** Indirect anastomosis. 1 = temporal ramus, 2 = zygomatic ramus, 3 = buccal ramus, 4 = marginal mandibular ramus, 5 = cervical ramus.

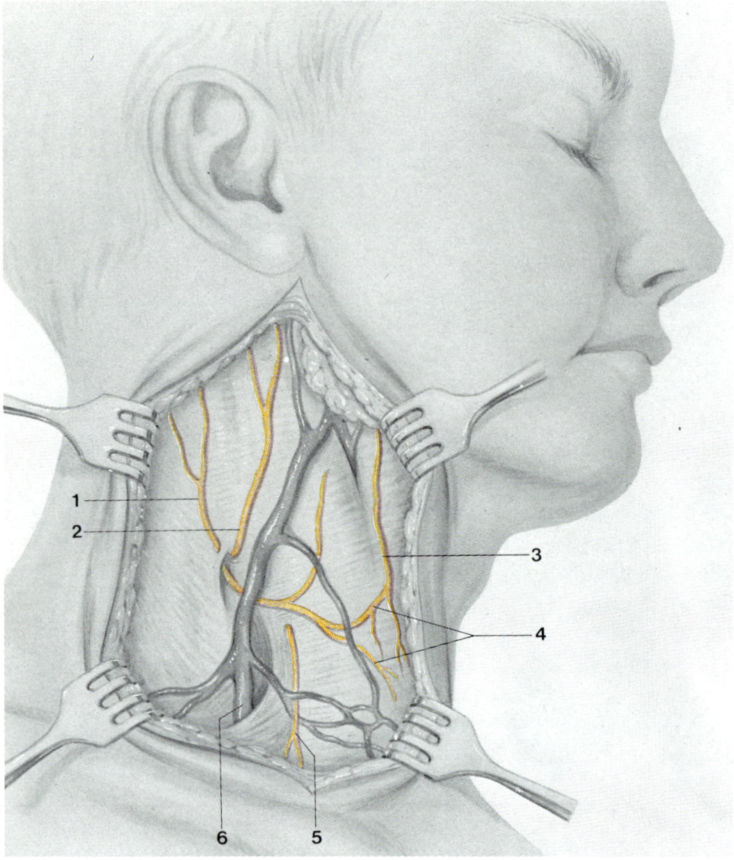

Figure 22.**25** Some of the important cervical nerves. 1 = lesser occipital nerve,
2 = great auricular nerve,
3 = the cervical ramus of the facial nerve,
4 = the transverse cervical nerve,
5 = supraclavicular nerve,
6 = external jugular vein.

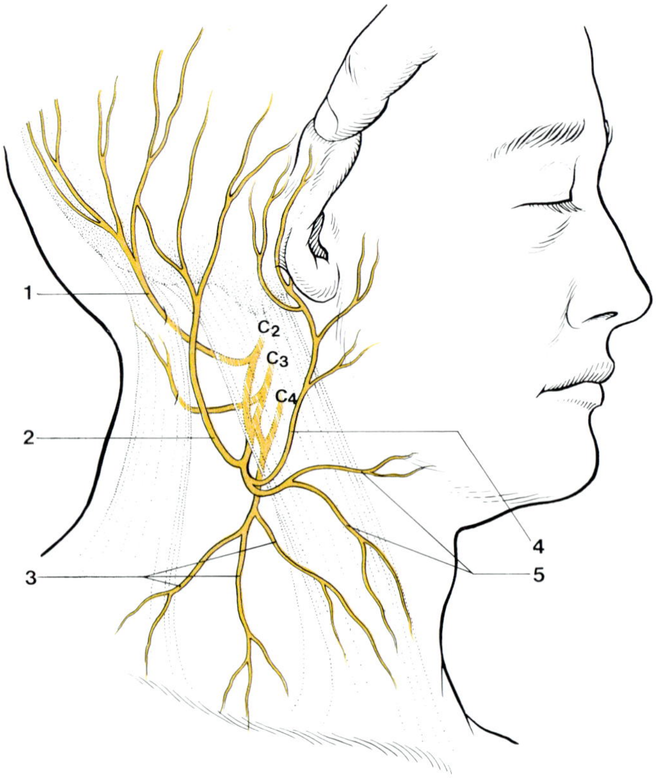

Figure 22.**26** The cervical plexus.
1 = Greater occipital nerve arising from C_1.
2 = Lesser occipital nerve arising from C_2.
3 = Supraclavicular nerve arising from C_3 and C_4.
4 = Great auricular nerve arising from C_2 and C_3.
5 = Transverse cervical nerve.

graft is taken from the opposite side of the neck, because of the possible danger of microscopic lymph node metastases on the same side.

The epineurium is resected as previously described, and the nerve graft is cut slightly longer than the defect.

The Sural Nerve. The sural nerve is usually harvested by a second operative team. Its proximal segment consists of several fascicles: peripherally, it supplies the skin of the posterolateral part of the ankle and of the lateral part of the dorsum of the foot with several branches (Fig. 22.**28**).

A vertical incision 2–3 cm long is made between the malleolus and the Achilles tendon. The sural nerve can be found in the subcutaneous fatty tissue at this point by retracting the saphenous vein laterally. The nerve is now mobilized as far distally as possible and its end branches are divided 3–5 cm distal to the site of incision. Several small horizontal incisions are made up to the level of the calf over the course of the nerve. The nerve is now removed by a ring-shaped stripper. The stripper is pushed proximally by careful rotating movements in the subcutaneous tissue with simultaneous tension on the nerve, until the calf is reached. The sural nerve is divided at this point and removed at the malleolus after releasing it from the surrounding subcutaneous fatty tissue through the several incisions.

The graft is now reduced in size to slightly more than that of the defect and the epineurium is resected as far as possible.

In recent years we have tried to place the site of the anastomosis in the bony gutter of the stylomastoid canal. It has proved to be unimportant whether the graft is a little too long or too short. It is much more important that the anastomosis produces an exact approximation of the fascicles and fixation in this position. The gutter of the stylomastoid canal presents the best conditions for this procedure.

The trunk of the facial nerve is divided with a fine knife or a razor blade just distal to the origin of the chorda tympani, provided that there is no reason for cutting it higher (Fig. 22.**29**). The distal stump is dissected from the bony canal. The transverse connective tissue fibers running over the stylomastoid foramen in the direction of the nerve must be divided and separated (Fig. 22.**30**).

A 3 mm section of the epineurium is now resected from the stump of the facial nerve within the mastoid process. A first trial is made of the graft for size. The individual fascicles of the facial nerve and the graft are approximated one at a

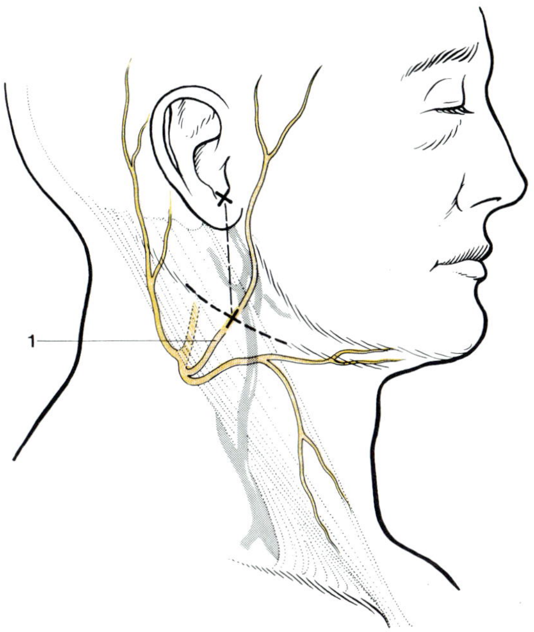

Figure 22.**27** The great auricular nerve (1).

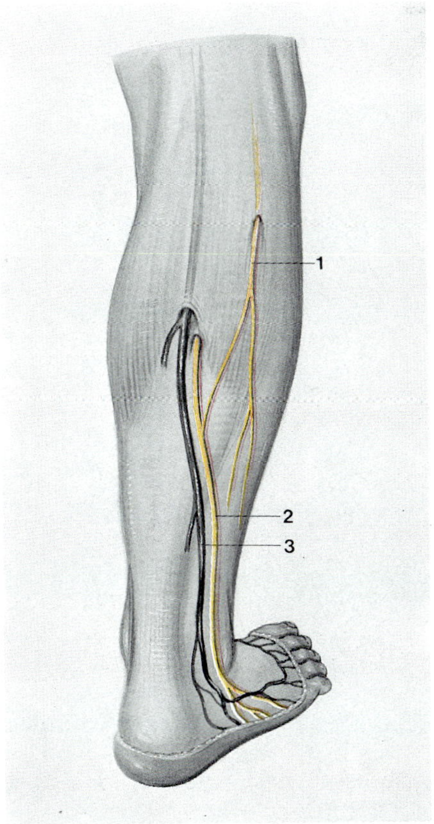

Figure 22.**28** The sural nerve, 1 = the fibular communicating ramus, 2 = the sural nerve, 3 = the lesser saphenous vein.

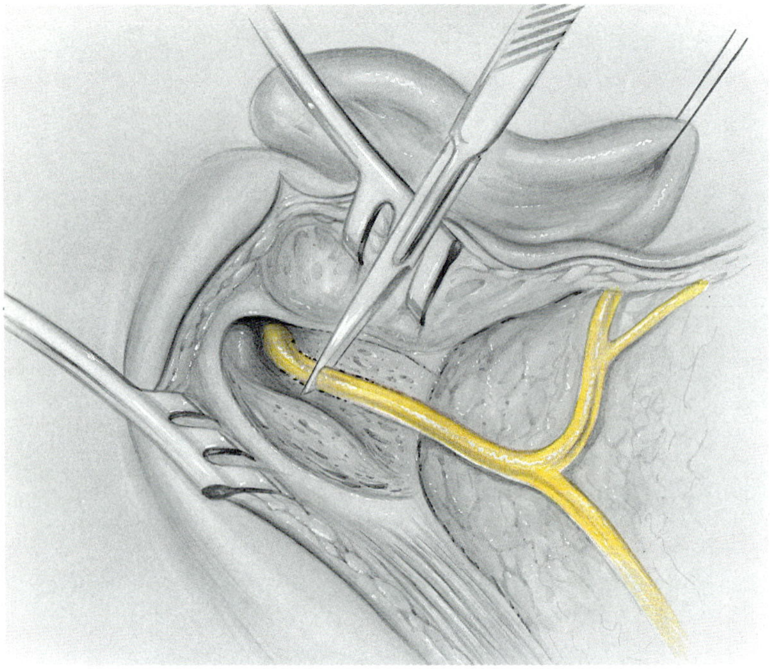

Figure 22.**29** Division of the trunk of the facial nerve in the stylomastoid canal.

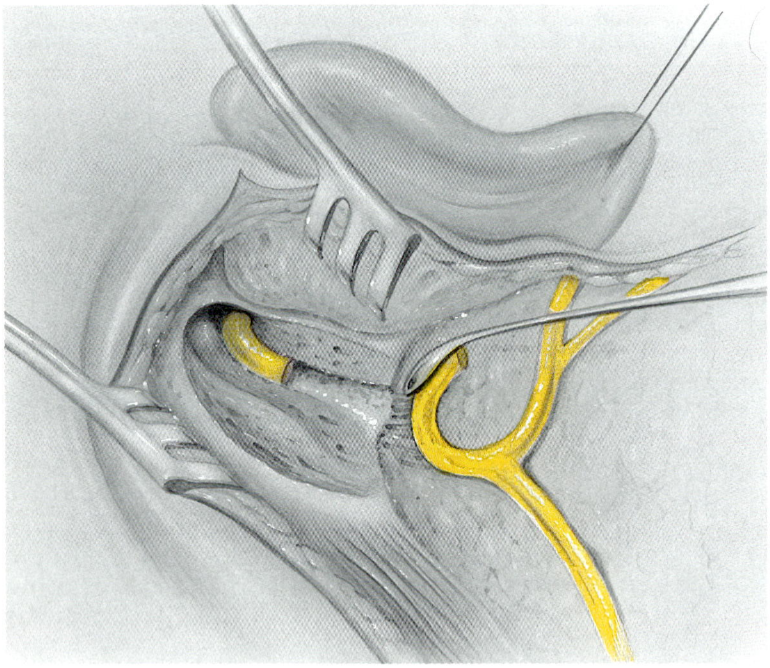

Figure 22.**30** Release of the trunk of the facial nerve from the stylomastoid canal.

time, if possible ensuring that the anastomosis is entirely free from tension. A drop of autologous plasma is placed over the anastomosis with a pipette (Fig. 22.**31**); covering with serous sheet or amnion may also be used.

This completes the proximal anastomosis of the facial nerve to the graft.

If the posterior wall of the stylomastoid canal has been destroyed so that there is no bed available for the graft, an artificial support can be constructed from fatty tissue, as proposed by Jongkees (personal communication 1972).

The peripheral stumps of the graft are approximated one at a time to the resected stumps of the

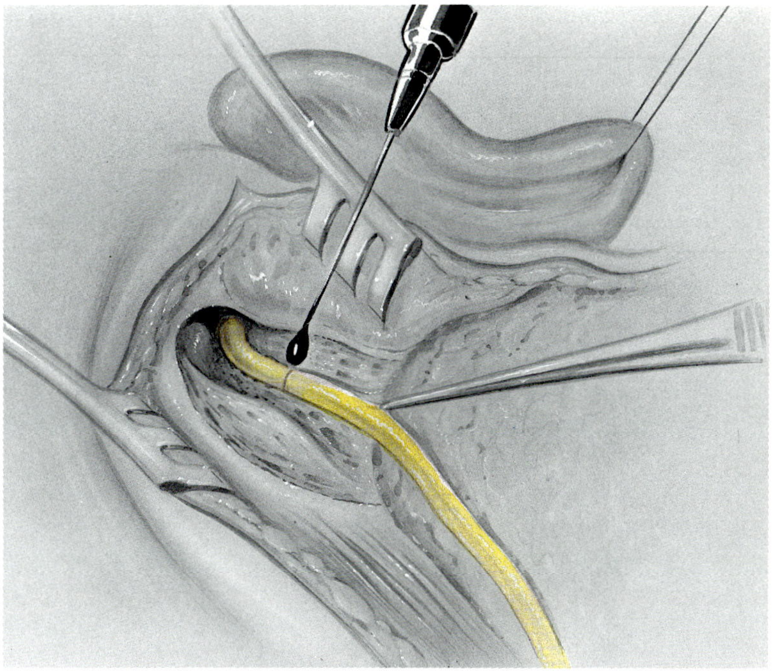

Figure 22.**31** Anastomosis of a free nerve graft from the great auricular nerve or sural nerve to the stump of the facial nerve in the stylomastoid canal.

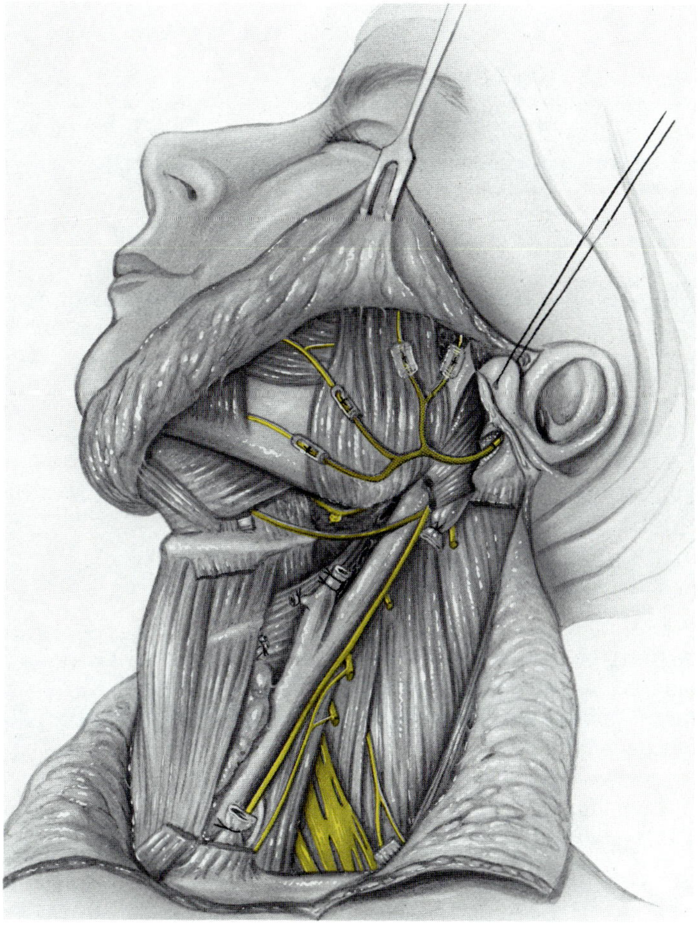

Figure 22.**32** Reconstruction of the facial nerve using a free branched autologous nerve graft from the great auricular nerve.

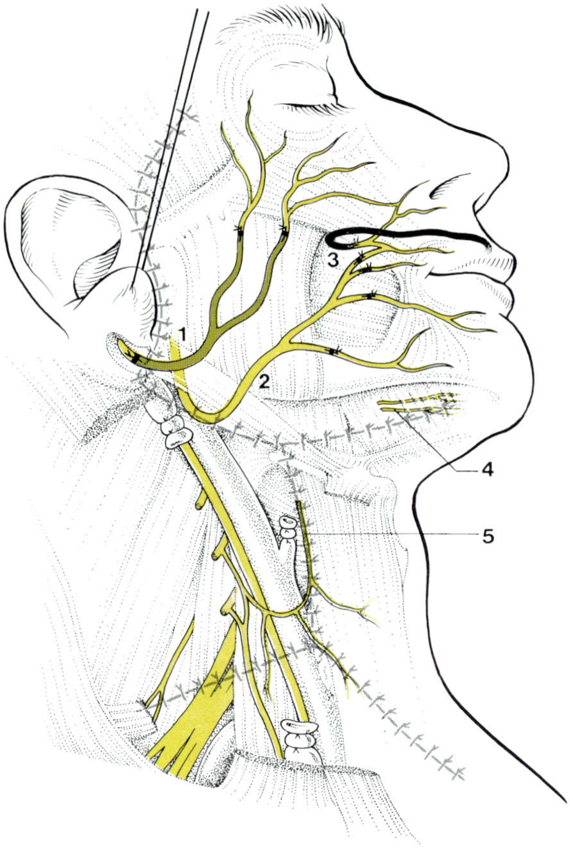

Figure 22.**33** Diversification technique.
1 = nerve interposed between the trunk of the facial nerve and its peripheral branches to the eye. 2 = the hypoglossal nerve transposed to the buccal perioral branches of the facial nerve, 3 = facio-facial anastomosis to the buccal rami. 4 = divided peripheral hypoglossal nerve branches. 5 = divided ansa cervicalis.

facial nerve and sutured with atraumatic 10–0 monofilament under the operating microscope using the perineural or epineural suture technique.

The peripheral anastomosis may be relieved of tension by fixing it to the surrounding soft tissue by a suture placed through the epineurium and pulled toward the anastomosis.

When adapting the graft (Fig. 22.**32**) to the remaining peripheral branches, on occasion there may be insufficient proximal branches to match the peripheral branches. In this situation, neighboring peripheral branches may be brought together by a perineural suture, after resection of the epineurium at the site of contact (Stennert 1982) (see color plate III, Fig. 4, page 359).

Combined Nerve Grafts

For many years, we used the well-established technique of hypoglossal-facial anastomosis as part of the rehabilitation program, but now we use the suture technique of Millesi et al (1972), previously described. The function of the *perioral musculature* recovers satisfactorily after hypoglossal-facial anastomosis, but recovery around the eye is less satisfactory. A detailed follow-up of a large number of patients undergoing intratemporal reconstruction of the facial nerve has shown that the fibers running to the orbicularis oculi muscle, particularly those intended for the blink reflex, demonstrate a marked ability to regenerate.

Finally, sympathetic movements always occur after resection and reconstruction of the facial nerve, by end-to-end suture or by autologous nerve graft.

There are several types of sympathetic movement. The most frequent, the most obvious, and the most disturbing is the simultaneous elevation of the angle of the mouth with closure of the eyelids.

We wondered therefore if it would no be possible to make use of the extensive recovery of function in the perioral musculature after hypoglossal-facial anastomosis, on the one hand, and the recovery of function in the eye region after a facial nerve graft, on the other hand.

We therefore attempted *diversification* using two donor nerves, firstly, the original facial nerve, and secondly, the hypoglossal nerve.

The original facial nerve is used exclusively for the temporofacial branches, whereas the hypoglossal nerve is used exclusively for the cervicofacial branch (Fig. 22.**33**). We thus achieve the following:

1. The motor impulses are conducted to the region of predilection of the two donor nerves.
2. The most frequent type of sympathetic movements, that is, simultaneous elevation of the mouth and closure of the lids, is kept to a mimimum.

If the lower part of the face is reinnervated by the hypoglossal nerve, one of the great advantages of modern reconstructive surgery of the nerve is lost, that is, recovery not only of voluntary movement, but also of emotional expression.

There are numerous anastomoses between the extratemporal branches of the facial nerve, which were described in Chapter 1. Connections between the cervicofacial and temporofacial territories are found in between 18% (Chilla 1979) and 67% (Davis et al 1956) of subjects, mainly running via the buccal ramus.

In all patients with these direct connections between the temporofacial and cervicofacial regions undergoing reconstruction with two separate anastomoses of the facial nerve with the facial nerve trunk and the hypoglossal nerve, emotional impulses may be conducted over the buccal connections from the upper to the lower parts of the distribution of the facial nerve.

Some patients do not achieve this secondary transmission of emotional impulses from the upper to the lower part of the face, because they do not possess these connections between the two main trunks of the facial nerve. In this situation, the cross-face anastamosis originally described by Scaramella (1971) and later by Anderl (1979) and Samii (1980) is used. An incision is made on the anterior edge of the parotid gland on the healthy side to expose one or two buccal branches. These are then joined to one or two peripheral branches on the diseased side using a sural nerve graft in a subcutaneous tunnel through the upper lip (Fig. 22.**34**). The cervicofacial fibers alone are reanastomosed so that this area is brought under adequate emotional influence from the opposite side.

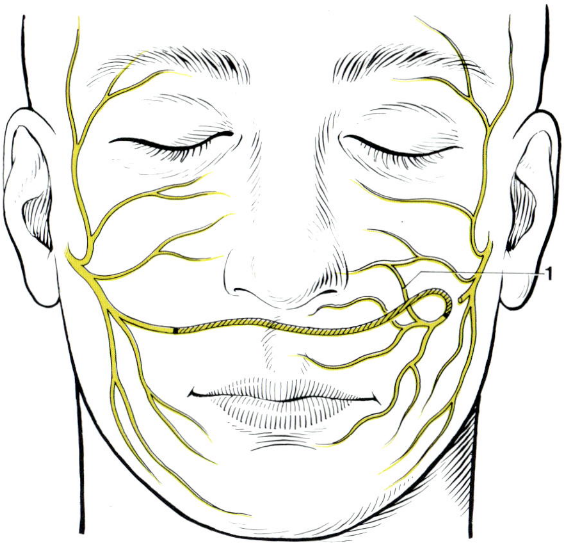

Figure 22.**34** Cross-face anastomosis using a sural graft (Samii's technique). 1 = a further branch.

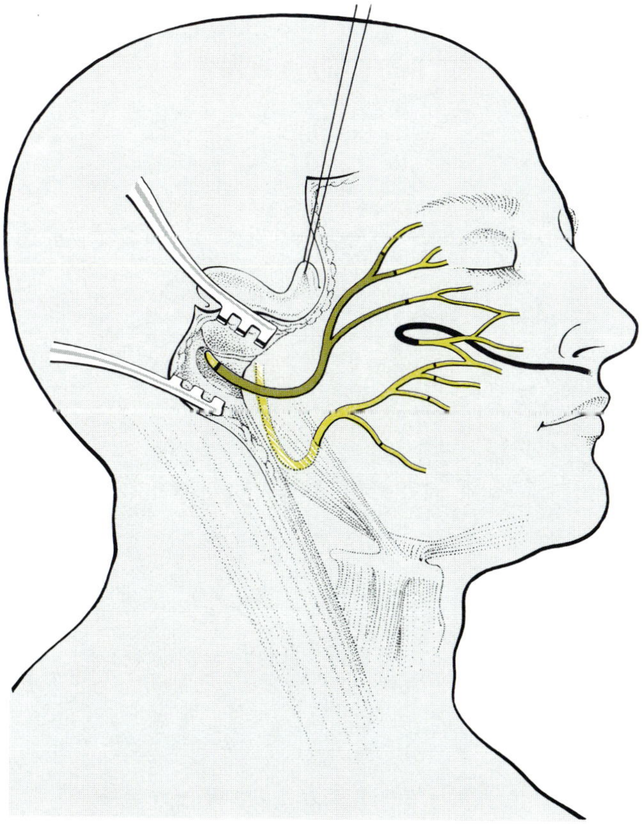

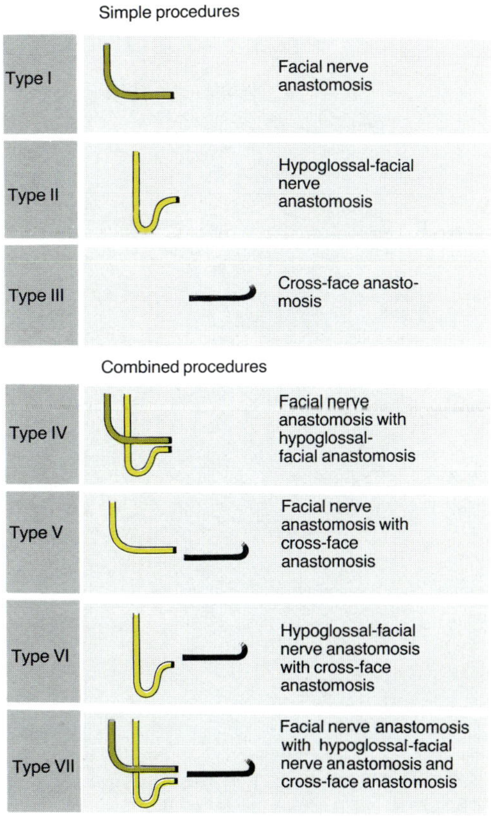

Figure 22.**35a** Diversification technique: the upper part of the facial nerve fibers are anastomosed to the original trunk of the facial nerve using a free nerve graft. The lower part of the facial nerve fibers are anastomosed to the hypoglossal nerve; in addition a cross-face anastomosis has been used. **b** The Göttingen scheme for extratemporal reconstruction of the facial nerve.

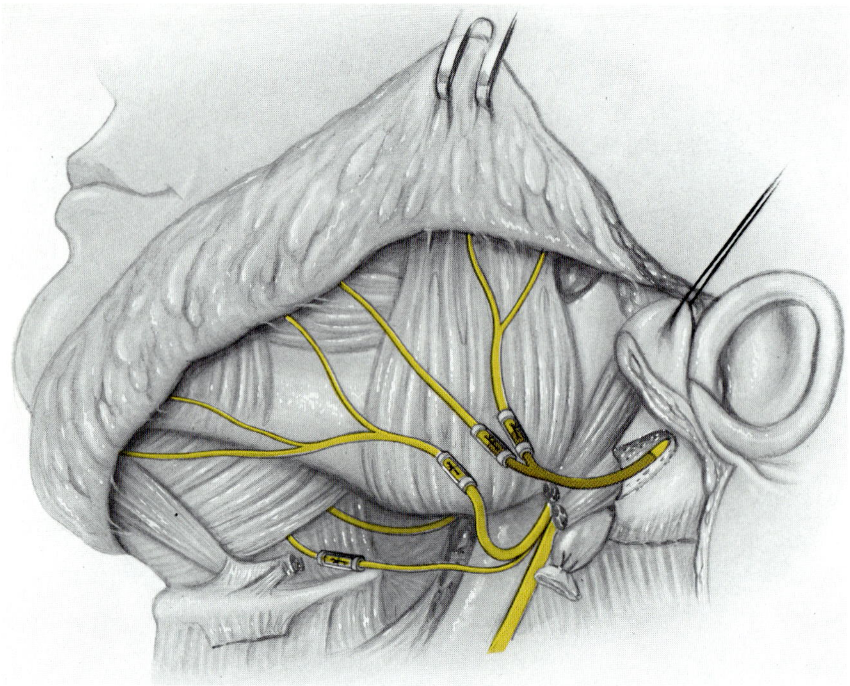

Figure 22.**36** The lower part of the facial nerve fibers reconstructed using the hypoglossal nerve.

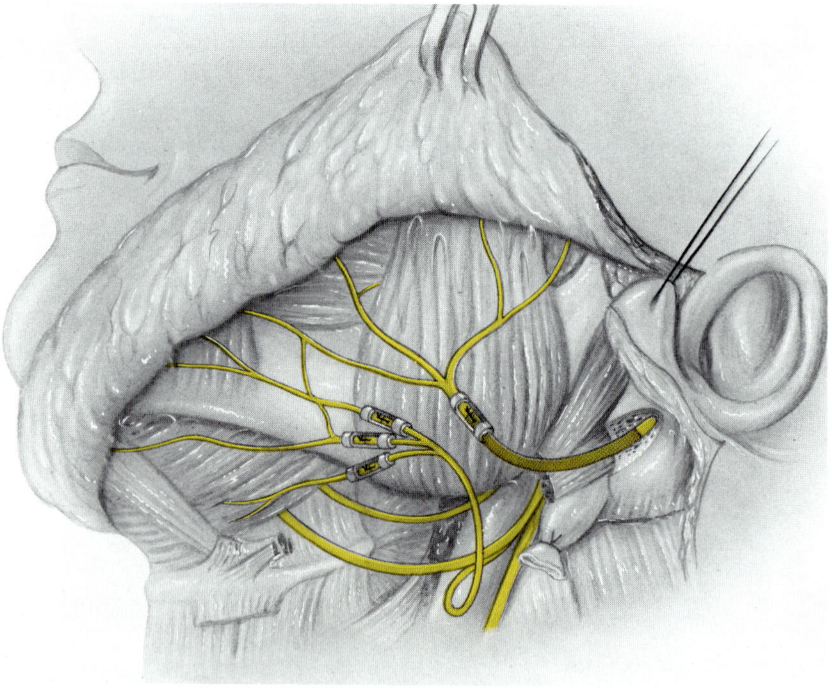

Figure 22.**37** Lower part of the facial nerve fibers reconstructed using the ansa cervicalis.

Several possibilities are thus available, some well known, some more recent, for reconstruction of the peripheral fibers of the facial nerve. Depending on the anatomic situation, the following classification was proposed by Stennert et al (1979) (Fig. 22.**35**):

Current techniques:

Type I: use of the ipsilateral facial nerve alone
Type II: use of the ipsilateral hypoglossal nerve alone
Type III: facio-facial anastamosis

Combination techniques:

Type IV: use of the ipsilateral facial nerve combined with the hypoglossal nerve

Type V: use of the ipsilateral facial nerve combined with facio-facial anastomosis

Type VI: use of the ipsilateral hypoglossal nerve combined with facio-facial anastomosis

Type VII: use of the ipsilateral facial nerve and hypoglossal nerve plus facio-facial anastomosis

Types IV and VII must be regarded as the ideal procedures from a functional point of view (Fig. 22.**35**).

The motor function of the tongue is deliberately sacrificed, if the hypoglossal nerve is used as a donor nerve for the lower part of the face. This must be explained to the patient beforehand. Many patients scarcely realize that they have lost the function of the tongue, and the remaining patients usually adapt to its loss within a few weeks. Nonetheless, we anastomose the motor branch of the ansa cervicalis to the hypoglossal nerve stump to minimize loss of function of the tongue (Fig. 22.**36**).

If the ansa cervicalis is well developed, it may be used for anastomosis to the lower facial nerve fibers in place of the hypoglossal nerve (Fig. 22.**37**). This is undoubtedly the most elegant solution, because mobility of the tongue is not lost.

Various possible techniques for reconstruction of the facial nerve are shown in Plates **I–IV**.

Plate 1

Figure **1** Preparation of a direct anastomosis using aluminium foil to provide a working surface. 1 = gelatine sponge, 2 = nerve trunk, 3 = graft, 4 = silicone.

Figure **2** Further preparation for a direct anastomosis showing epineurial resection of the nerve stumps.

Figure **3** Anastomosis being carried out with several atraumatic 9–0 sutures. The aluminium foil has now been removed.

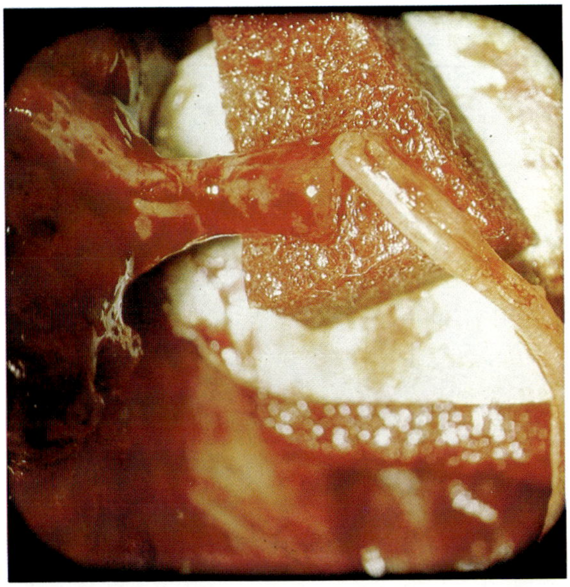

1

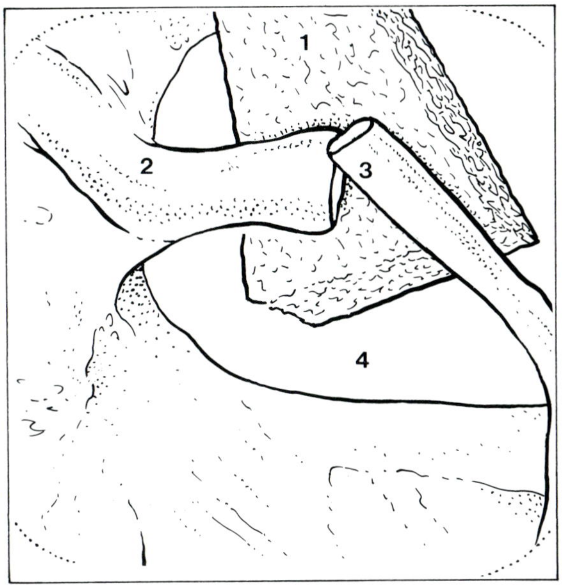

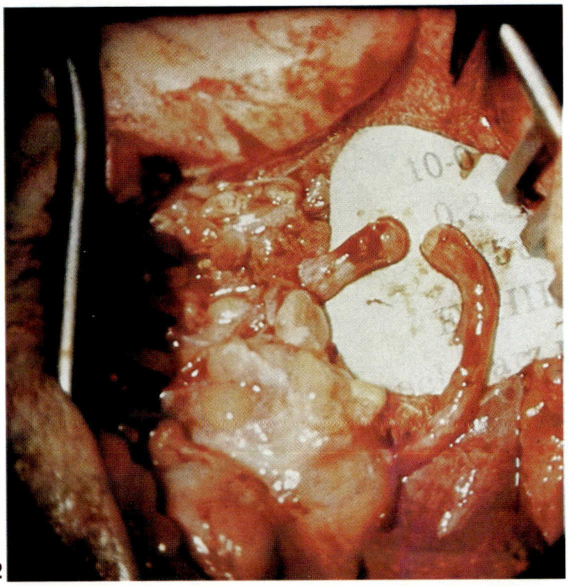

2

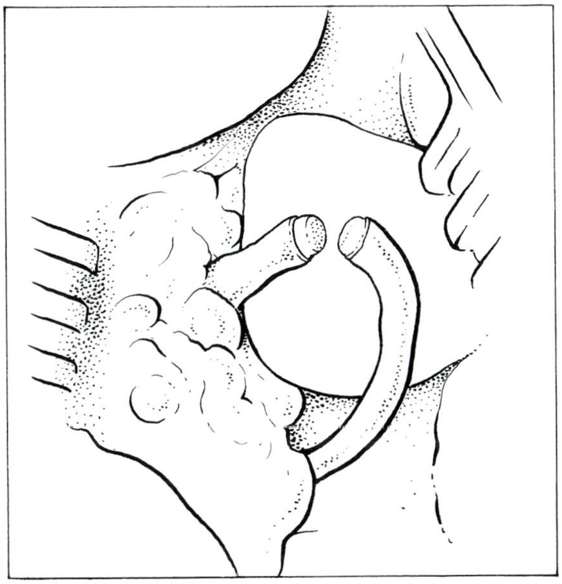

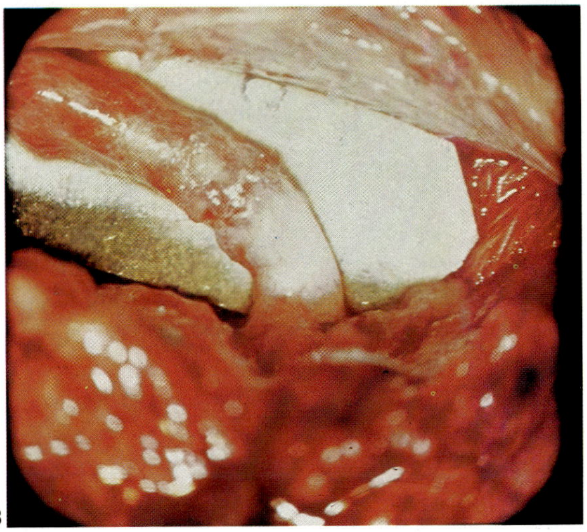

3

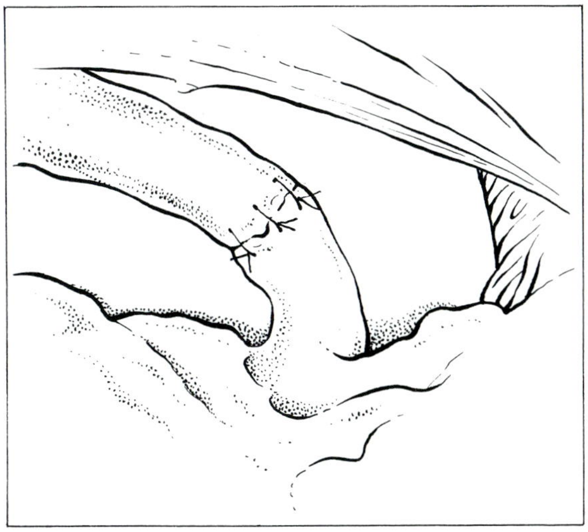

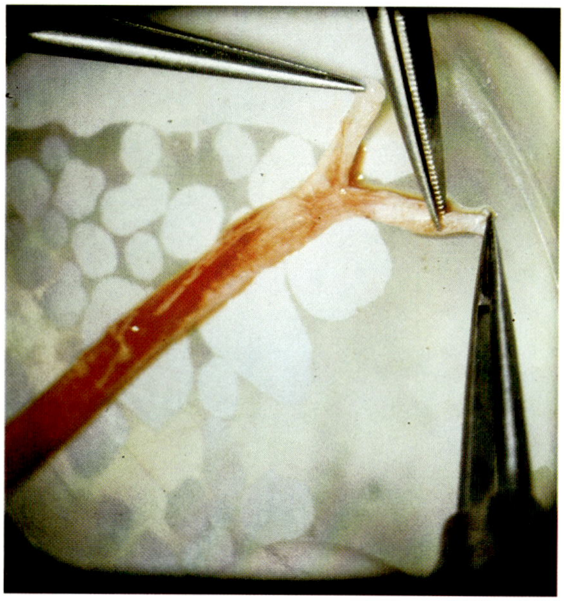

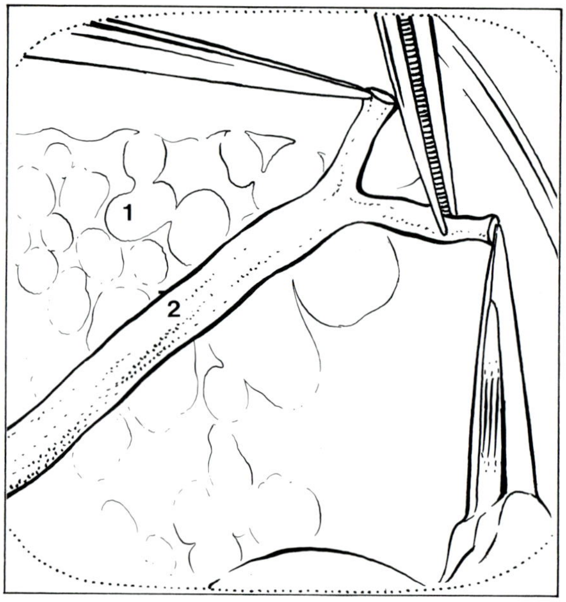

Figure **1** Preparation of a free autologous nerve graft. A relatively long graft with two branches is being prepared for grafting.

1 = Petri dish, 2 = split sural nerve.

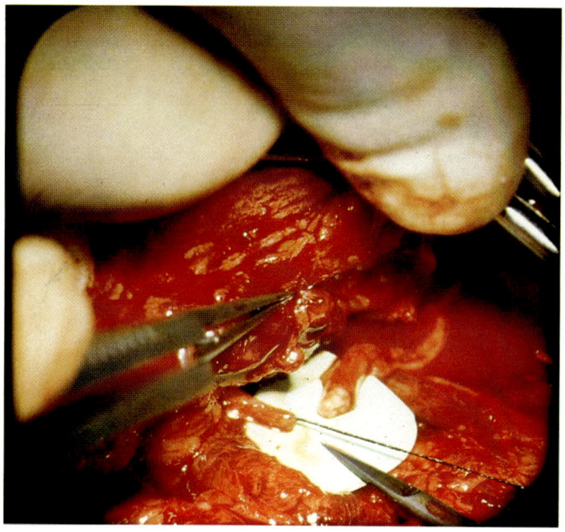

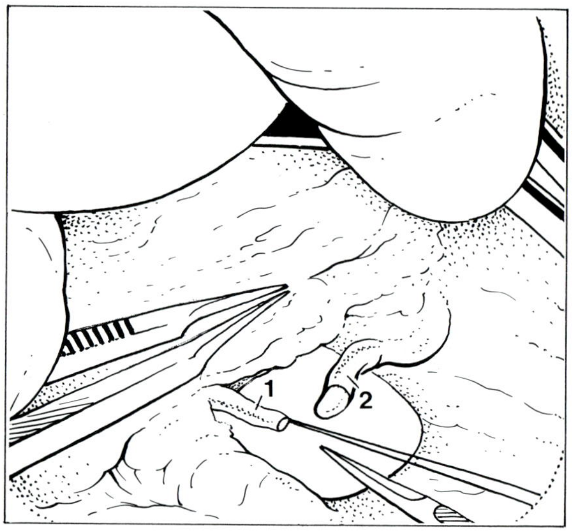

Figure **2** Preparation for anastomosis of two branches after epineural resection.

1 = end of the graft, 2 = peripheral branch.

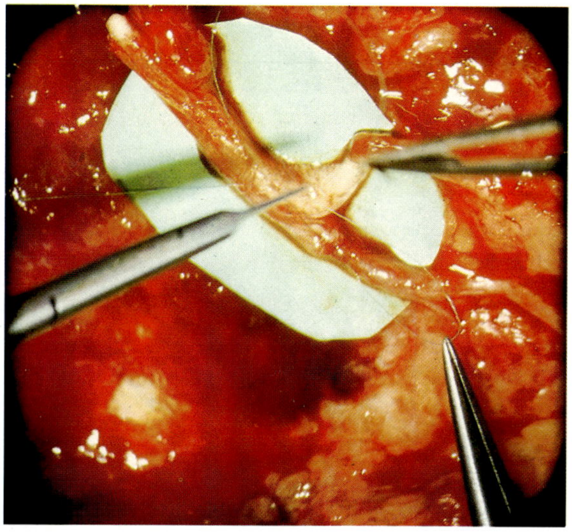

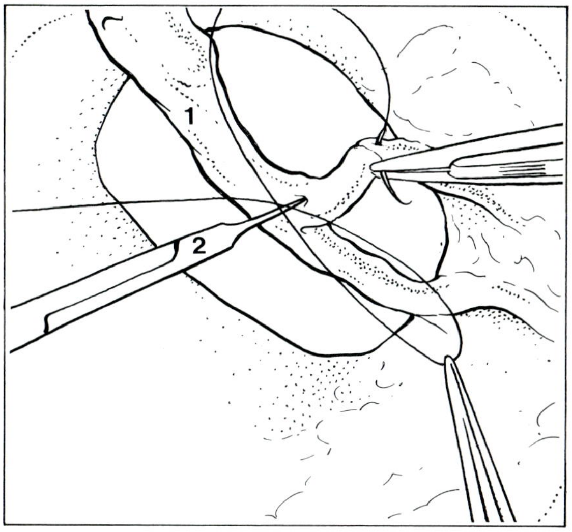

Figure **3** Anastomosis of both branches of the autologous nerve graft to the corresponding peripheral branches of the pes anserinus being carried out. 1 = the graft, 2 = graft being pushed toward the peripheral nerve.

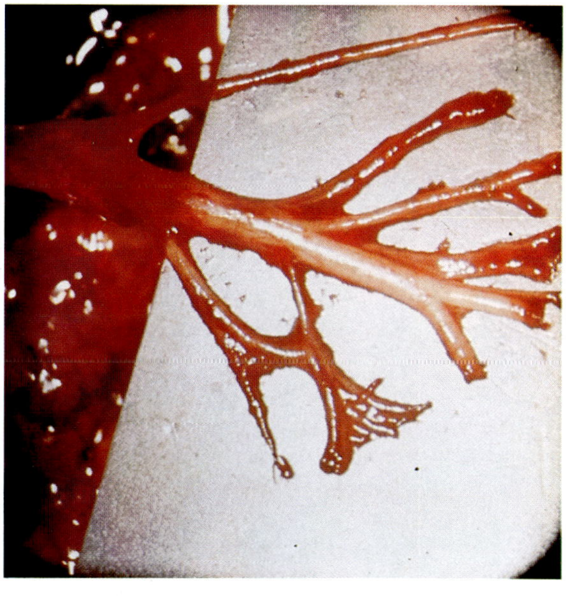

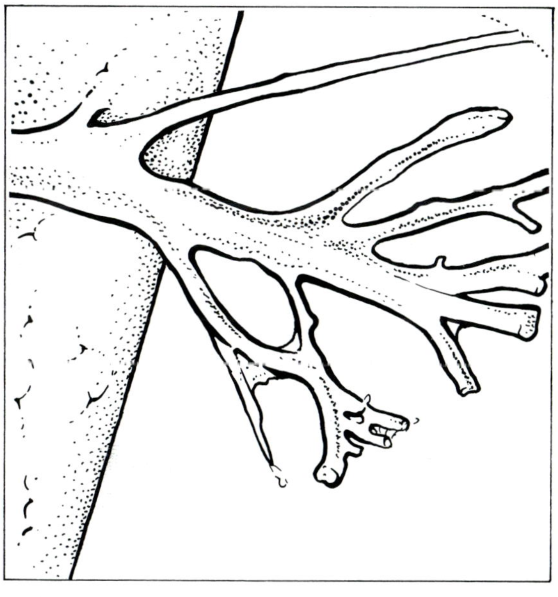

Figure **4** Autologous nerve graft from the sural nerve with numerous branches, which is very suitable for reconstruction of the facial nerve. A similar pattern of graft can be obtained from the great auricular nerve, even if it does not have so many branches.

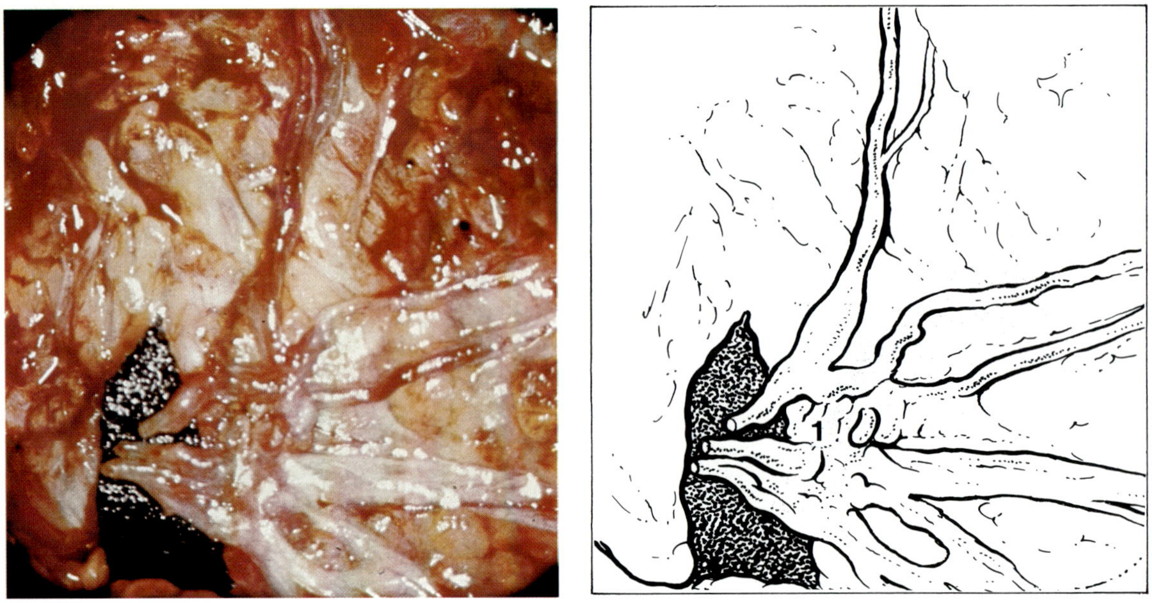

Figure **1** Maceration of the fibers of the facial nerve due to a traumatic salivary fistula. 1 = the degenerated, atrophic pes anserinus.

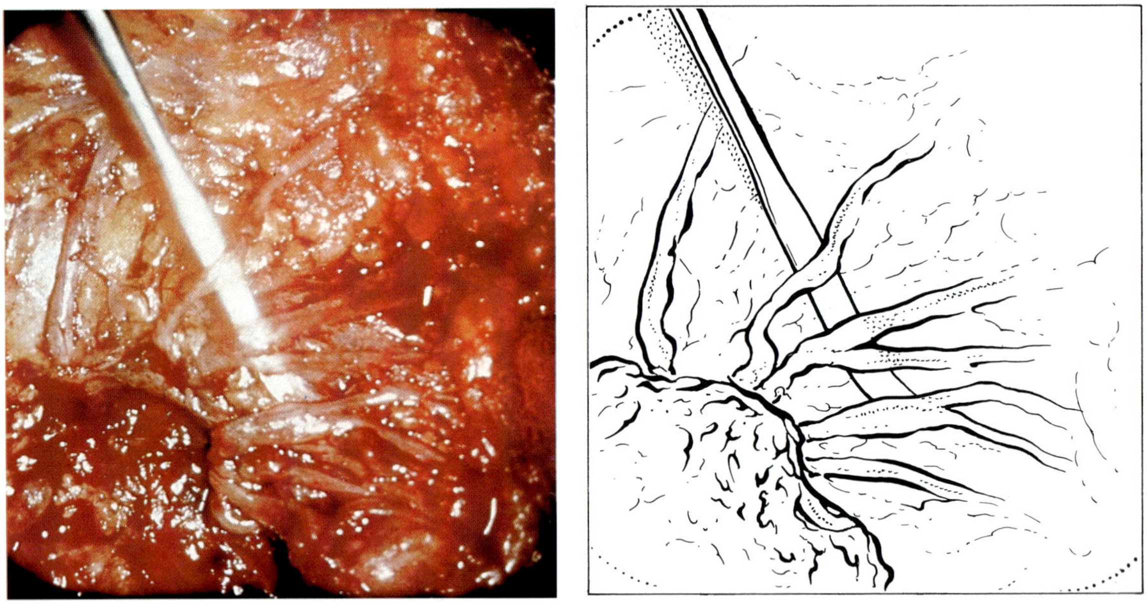

Figure **2** The individual peripheral branches of the facial nerve (temporofacial, buccal, cervicofacial, and more peripheral rami) displayed by an elevator. The degenerated pes anserinus has been resected.

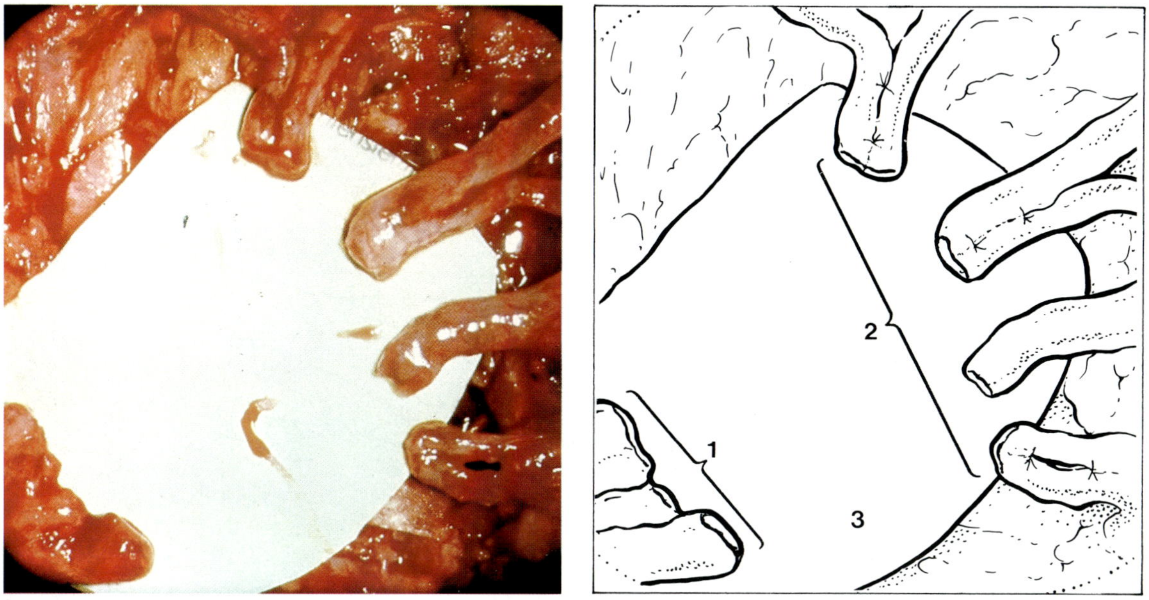

Figure **3** An extensive defect of the facial nerve is shown. Only three central stumps are available for a total of seven peripheral branches. The central stumps lie immediately to the bifurcation. The number of branches can be reduced by suturing neighboring branches after resection of the epineurium at points of contact using the finest epineurial suture (Fig. **4**). The defect can then be bridged by only three free grafts. 1 = the three central branches, 2 = the seven freshened stumps, 3 = the silicone plate.

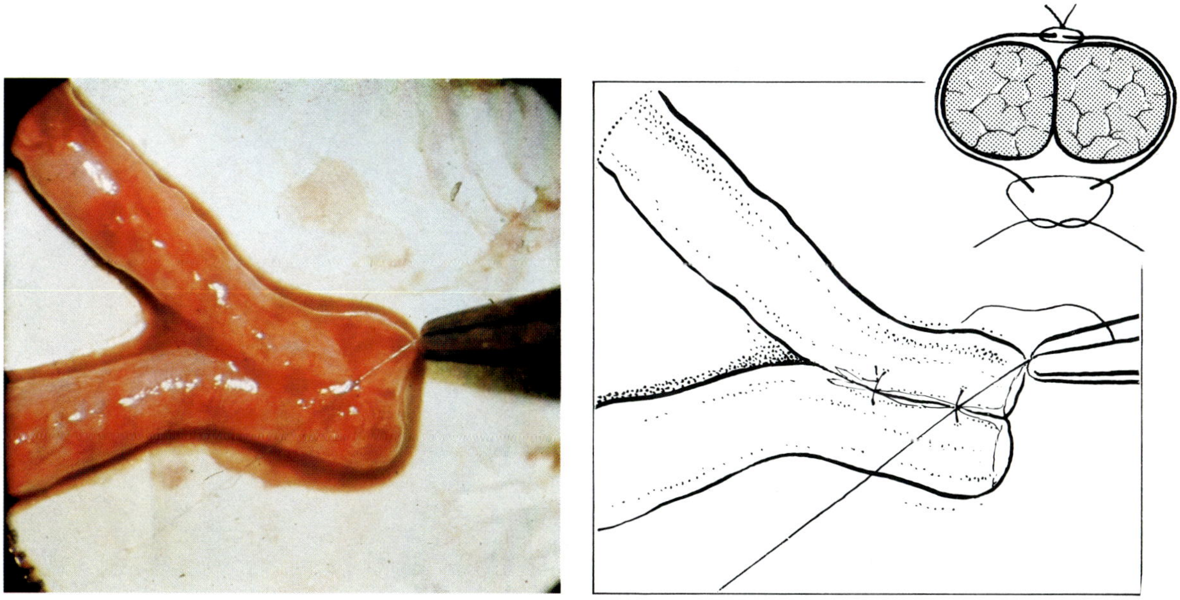

Figure **4** Approximation of neighboring facial branches, and resection of the epineurium at the point of contact so that the fascicles lie close to each other. An epineurial suture has been used.

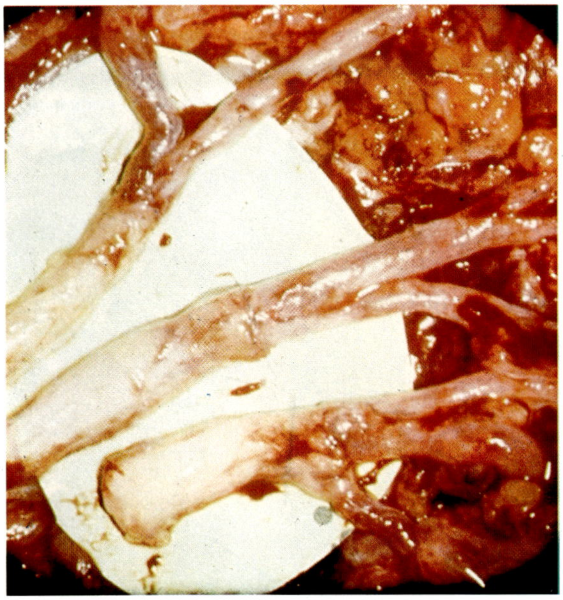

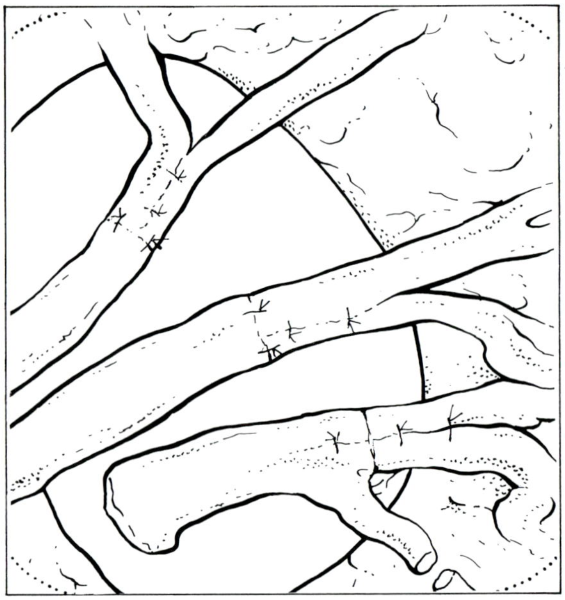

Figure **5** Bridging of a defect in the facial nerve using three relatively short grafts taken from a donor nerve.

Plate IV

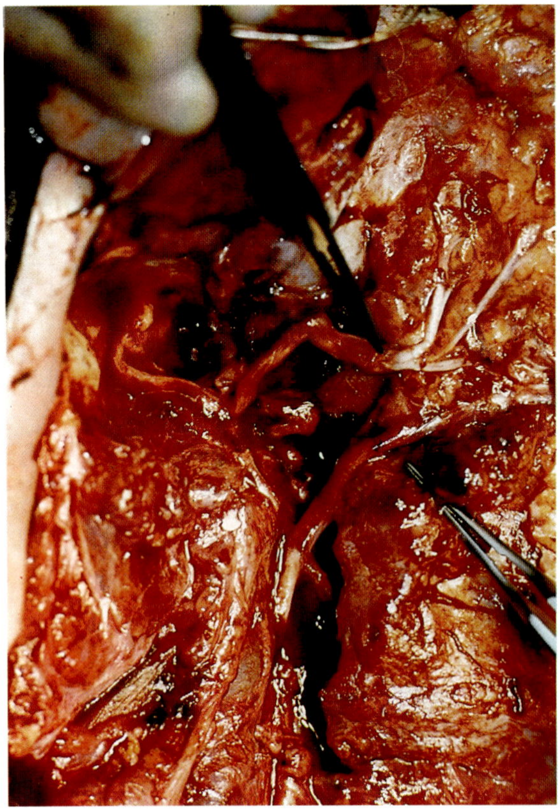

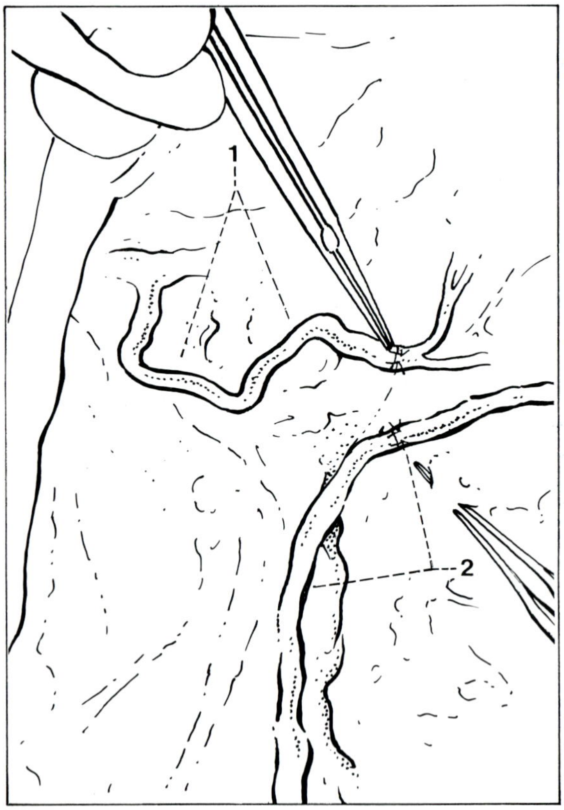

Figure **1** Diversification technique for reconstruction of one complete ramus of the facial nerve. A free facio-facial anastomosis is shown above (1), and a hypoglossal-facial anastomosis (2) below.

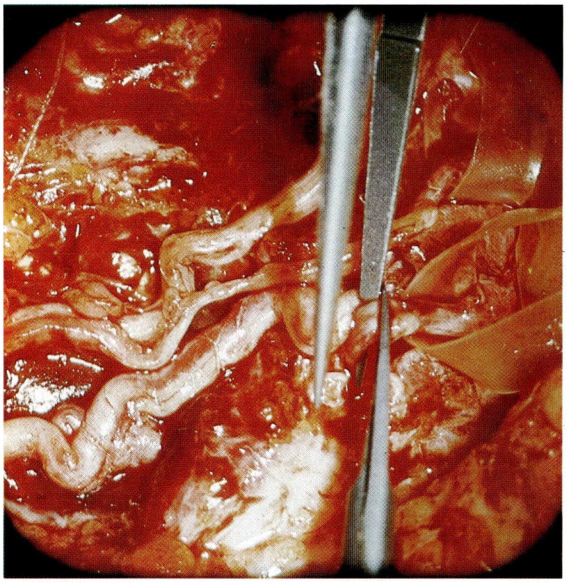

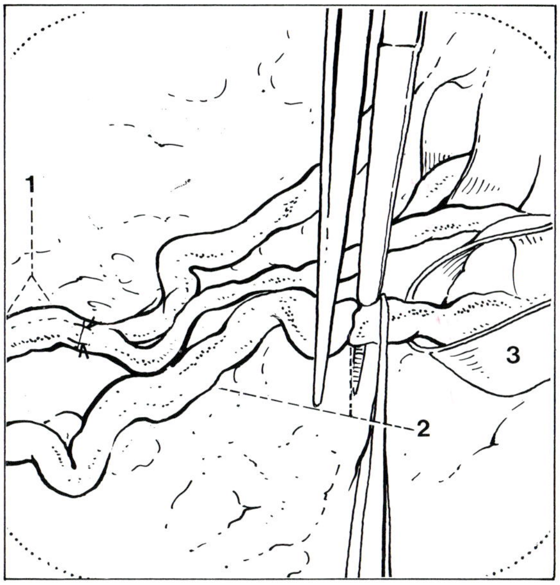

Figure **2** Another example of the diversification technique. An autologous facio-facial anastomosis is shown above (1), and a hypoglossal facial anastomosis below (2). 3 = a rubber band.

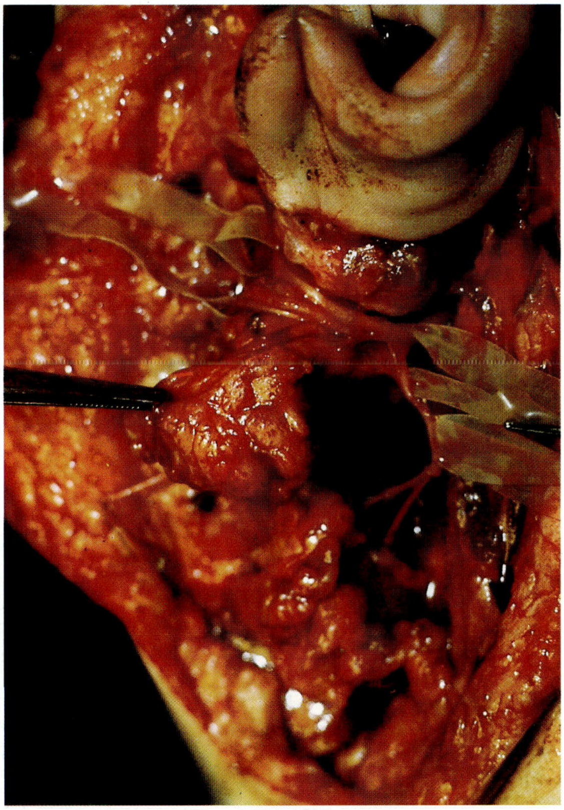

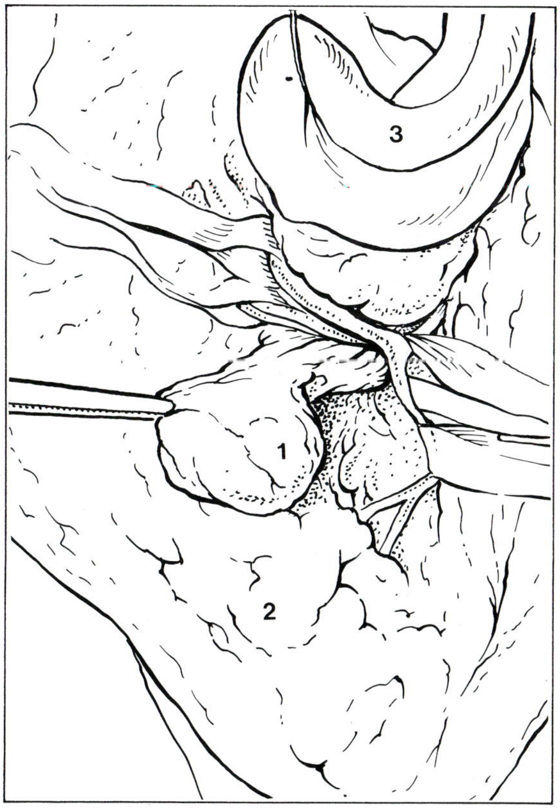

Figure **3** A branchial fistula (1) or duplicate external auditory meatus. The saccular structure passes beneath the bifurcation of the facial nerve. 2 = branchial fistula, 3 = the facial nerve retracted by several other bands.

Injuries of the Parotid Gland and the Facial Nerve

The increasingly severe injuries of the face in industrial and road traffic accidents are regrettable, but an inevitable part of our increasingly mechanized life style. Open facial wounds with destruction of the facial nerve will also continue to occur so long as men indulge in senseless wars. Facial nerve surgery has developed to deal with these serious injuries, and suitable operative techniques for each situation are now available.

We will deal first with injuries of the lateral part of the facial nerve, using as an example a road traffic accident resulting in deep lacerations of the parotid gland and a defect in the facial nerve. Recovery of function of the injured nerve depends on the initial method of treatment.

Various procedures may be considered for reconstruction of extensive defects of the trunk and branches of the nerve. Destruction of the parenchyma of the parotid gland exposes the neural tissue to lysis by saliva escaping into the wound. A parotidectomy should therefore usually be carried out, since preservation of the injured parenchyma often leads to a salivary fistula, even with the most careful apposition and suture technique. This fistula then later requires a parotidectomy. Time is thus lost, tissue is destroyed by the saliva, and the prospects of healing are worsened.

Our policy is thus as follows:

1. Probing of the parotid duct from the mouth to confirm whether the duct is damaged. A silver probe or fine polyethylene catheter are used as for sialography. In doubtful cases, methylene blue is introduced through the catheter to demonstrate a fistula.
2. If the parotid duct is intact and the parenchyma of the parotid gland is only slightly injured, the wound is sutured carefully with fine atraumatic sutures.
3. A superficial or total parotidectomy is carried out, depending on the site of the wound, for injuries of the parotid duct and deeper destruction of the gland parenchyma.
4. Optimal access to the trunk and branches of the facial nerve is achieved by this procedure. The nerve can be inspected and sutured, if it is injured.

Naturally, the best results are obtained if the facial nerve is repaired at the same time as the wound closure. Primary facial suture or primary nerve graft offer a better chance of success.

It is occasionally not possible to repair the facial nerve primarily, for several reasons, such as severe shock and absence of the appropriate instruments. In such situations focal inflammation often makes it difficult to find the facial nerve later. The surgeon who carries out the primary wound care must therefore ensure that the nerve stumps are marked with temporary sutures or silver clips. The ends of the nerves are freed for several millimeters, and the end of the nerve stump is marked with a silver clip. A silicone tube of appropriate diameter, about 5 mm in length, is split longitudinally and laid around the freed end of the nerve. A fine silk suture, if possible colored, is passed through the nerve stump immediately proximal to the silver clip, tied to the silicone cylinder, and at the same time fixed to the underlying tissue.

The silicone cylinder with the ends of the nerve and the silver clips can be easily found at the time of the secondary procedure.

If only simple primary care facilities are available, the widely damaged parotid gland itself should be irrigated with an antibiotic solution, and a rubber dam drain should be introduced to drain the saliva. Stennert (1982) has proposed that a silicone sheet cut to the appropriate shape and with many holes in it should be stitched to the wound surface to prevent the adhesions that occur within the wound. When the wound is reopened, the wound surfaces can be easily peeled apart, thus opening up the operative field quickly and in the correct layer without damage to the nerve endings.

If all these preparatory procedures have been carried out at the primary operation, a secondary suture may be undertaken in the third week, after resolution of the acute phase of the trauma. The prospects of success are as good as after primary suture, because in the third week, after division of the nerve the proliferation of the Schwann cells is at its most pronounced, and suturing is facilitated by swelling of the nerve stumps.

It must be remembered that the Büngner's bands in the distal stump degenerate slowly after about 3 weeks and are replaced by connective tissue. The loss of Schwann cells in the distal stump can be a disadvantage for conduction and maturation of the regenerating nerve fibers.

Even if neither primary suture nor early secondary suture procedures are carried out and no clear record is available of the original findings, there is certainly no reason to abandon the patient or even to adopt a hopeful "wait and see" policy, which in truth has no hope of success.

At this point, the time schedule drawn up by the neurologist Zülch (1961) must be discussed; the first signs of recovery of function appear within 2 to 3 weeks of *contusion of the nerve*. If the damage to the axis cylinder is so severe that recovery of function is only possible by *regeneration*, the first signs of recovery of function can only be expected after 3 to 4 months even in the most favorable cases. The facial muscles remain ready for reinnervation for about 1 year.

Exploration of the nerve is thus recommended, if the first signs of recovery of function do not appear within 4 to 5 months.

Despite these theoretical considerations, practice shows that in many cases reinnervation of the facial musculature can be achieved in many cases when it was no longer expected. Electrical investigations, particularly electromyography and electroneuronography (Esslen 1973), have proved to be of great clinical value in making this important decision. These tests can be supplemented by muscle biopsy and by the succinyl test (Nessel 1970).

So far, relatively few of these operations have been carried out (probably fewer than 1000 in all the world), so that it is not easy to describe the results of this type of reconstruction. However, it can be said that the results appear to be encouraging: Conley, who without doubt has the greatest experience, summarizes his results as follows:

- 46% achieve very good results
- 28% achieve less satisfactory results
- 26% are unsuccessful.

Our results of about 200 reconstructions of the facial nerve are similar.

However, it has been quite rightly remarked by Maxwell that even a poor result is better than that which can be achieved by a muscle graft or fascial implant. The injured facial nerve should therefore always be reconstructed if at all possible, using one of the methods described in this chapter.

Procedures Other than Reconstruction of the Facial Nerve

In some patients whose facial nerve must be sacrificed because of the degree of malignancy of the tumor or its spread, or because the facial nerve was already paralyzed, it may not be possible to reconstruct the facial nerve. The only recourse is then a procedure to improve the static appearance of the paralyzed face.

In 1916 Rosenthal developed the operation of muscular neurotization for reanimation of the paralyzed facial musculature. Animal experiments carried out by Erlacher (1914) had shown that nerve fibers grow from healthy into paralyzed muscles, which then recovered tone and some voluntary movement provided that the muscles adhere over a wide area. The masseter and temporalis muscles are used for implantation: both are innervated by the motor division of the trigeminal nerve. Muscle flaps are developed from the masseter or temporalis muscle respecting the site of entry and course of the branches of the trigeminal nerve within the muscle, and are then transported to the orbicularis oculi or orbicularis oris muscles. In many respects, Rosenthal's procedure resembles the muscle rotation flap developed by Lexer (1931) to elevate the paralyzed facial muscles, so that the procedure is now described as the Lexer-Rosenthal operation.

The temporalis muscle is freed through an incision, shown in Figure 22.**38**. A muscle flap about 1.5 cm wide based on the zygomatic arch is developed. The orbicularis oculi muscle is freed from the underlying tissue at the corner of the eye. The temporalis flap is transposed through a subcutaneous tunnel to the corner of the eye and stitched to the anterior edge of the orbicularis oculi muscle.

The masseter muscle is freed from the lower border of the mandible, and a muscle flap 1.5 cm wide based on the zygomatic arch is split off. The orbicularis oris muscle and the facial muscles radiating into it are dissected free around the angle of the mouth. The masseter muscle flap is fed through a subcutaneous tunnel and sutured to the orbicularis oris muscle over a wide area under marked tension. Chromic catgut sutures are placed in the same direction as the muscle fibers so as not to impede the required neurotization. Conley (1979) improved the masseter flap by shortening and limiting the incision in the masseter muscle so as not to disturb the radiating branches of the motor root of the trigeminal nerve. Furthermore, the transposed part of the masseter muscle is drawn as far as possible toward the middle of the upper or lower lip and is stitched over as wide an area as possible. Pronounced overcorrection is desirable, but this settles rapidly.

Pichler (1948) developed an anterior and posterior pedicled flap of the entire temporalis muscle (Fig. 22.**39**). This flap is turned down over the zygomatic arch (Fig. 22.**40**), drawn through a subcutaneous tunnel, and then fixed to the orbicularis oris muscle through small incisions at the center of the mandible and at the angle of the mouth. Gohrbandt (1972) refined the procedure by extending the temporalis graft to include fas-

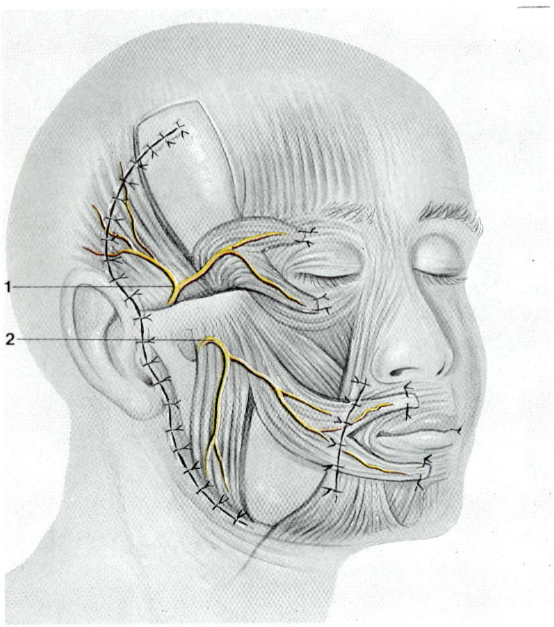

Figure 22.**38** Masseter and temporalis muscleplasty with careful preservation of the trigeminal nerve. 1 = the deep temporal nerve (V3), 2 = the masseteric nerve (V3).

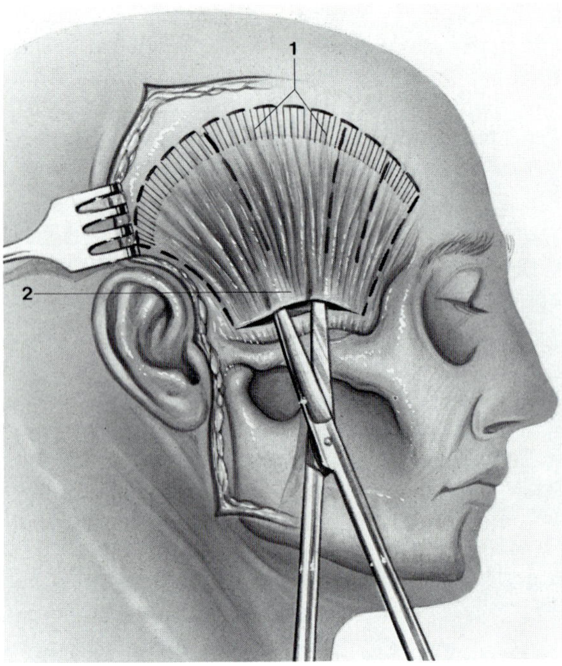

Figure 22.**39** Preparation for fascial transplantation with freeing of the galea aponeurotica. 1 = epicranium, 2 = freeing of the aponeurosis.

cial strips from the line of origin of the muscle from the galea aponeurotica. A certain degree of myoneurotization is possibly to be expected in this procedure also. One disadvantage is the swelling over the zygomatic arch formed by the temporalis muscle. This is thrown into greater relief, because the profile of the temple above the zygomatic arch appears to be even more sunken because the temporalis muscle has been removed. The defect can be filled by pieces of alloplastic material, such as Silastic or ceramics, or by homologous tissue, such as bone or cartilage, cut to the appropriate size (Fig. 22.**41**).

Doubt has lately been cast on the attractive theory of myoneurotization by the motor root of the trigeminal nerve. Electromyography on patients who had undergone a Rosenthal procedure (Struppler & Scheininger 1961) using simultaneous recording from synergistic facial or trigeminal musculature excluded an innervation of the facial muscles by motor trigeminal fibers.

However, even a slight degree of movement produced by the masseter or temporalis muscle and a certain degree of tone of the face, combined with improvement of the ability to chew and speak is very useful. Furthermore, a few of our patients were able to smile.

The muscle tranposition should be used in young persons who are prepared to undertake the self-training for transmission of the masseteric or temporal traction to the facial musculature. A simple fascial sling is also available to provide static improvement.

There are many modifications of the fascial sling originally described by Blair (1941) using the fascia lata of the thigh as the donor site (Stein 1913). The transplanted fascia is nourished by ingrowth of blood vessels at the receptor site. A loss of traction due to atrophy is not to be feared. The principle of the operation is to surround the orbicularis oris with a subcutaneous fascial sling suspended from a fixation point on the anterior part of the zygomatic arch. Gillies (1934) placed a further narrow fascial strip in a figure of eight around the paralyzed half of the mouth to improve elevation of the angle of the mouth.

Finally, muscleplasty and fascial slings may be combined (McLaughlin 1953) (Fig. 22.**42**). We will use this procedure as an example for the similar procedures described by Aschan (1956) and Ragnell (1958). The movement of the temporalis muscle is transmitted to the paralyzed half of the face by insertion of fascia lata strips. The tendon of the temporalis muscle is divided from the coronoid process and is fastened to a wide

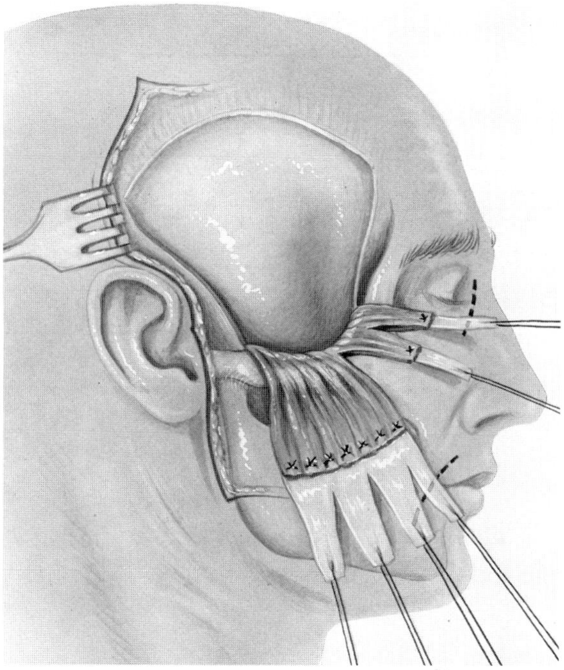

Figure 22.**40** Fascial graft before adjustment.

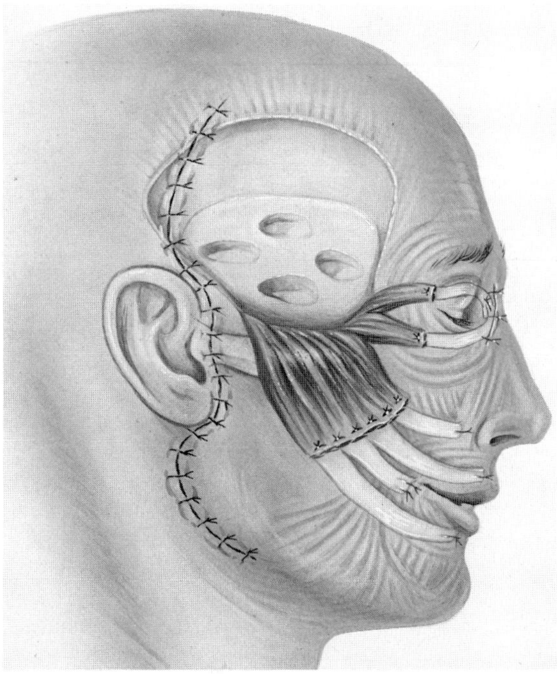

Figure 22.**41** Fascial transplantation completed, and filling of the defect in the temporal area with a plastic, such as Silastic or ceramics, or homologous tissue, such as cartilage or bone.

fascial sling by a short narrow fascial strip. The sling is drawn in a figure of eight around the paralyzed muscle.

We usually combine this procedure with a face lift carried out through an appropriately extended incision.

In many cases of facial paralysis, the facial asymmetry appears to be even more pronounced because of the apparent or real overaction of the nonparalyzed side. This situation is due to an unexplained muscle tone. A limited procedure to reduce the tone of the facial muscles on the contralateral side may then be valuable.

A selective neurectomy may be carried out on those nerve fibers that are mainly responsible for the pronounced facial distortion (Marino 1956). One of the two marginal mandibular branches of the facial nerve on the healthy side may be divided to correct asymmetry of the lower face. The marginal mandibular branch consists of two rami in only half the cases. The excessive function of the upper lip can be reduced in a similar manner by neurectomy of one of the two buccal rami. These operations should only be carried out after strict definition of the operative area using a stimulator and simultaneous intraoperative electromyographic recordings.

An alternative to neurectomy is a limited local excision of the facial muscles to suppress the contralateral facial muscles (Niklison 1965). For example, in pronounced distortion of the lower lip on laughing due to partial paralysis of the contralateral marginal mandibular ramus, the depressor anguli oris and the depressor labii inferioris muscles can be defined through a mucosal incision within the mouth on the sound side, and a piece of the muscle removed. A similar procedure may also be carried out on the upper lip, if the levator labii superioris and zygomatic muscles are responsible for distortion during speech and emotional movements. In such cases the muscles may be resected through a skin incision in the nasolabial fold.

These procedures for suppressing antagonistic muscle traction should only be carried out after a delay of several years because the contractures responsible for the facial asymmetry may occasionally relax spontaneously for reasons as yet unknown.

Face lifts and cutaneous and subcutaneous excisions in the nasolabial area to adjust the angle of the mouth and the philtrum (Kapovits 1961) have proved useful for making the nasolabial fold more animated (Fig. 22.**43**). Further improvements are

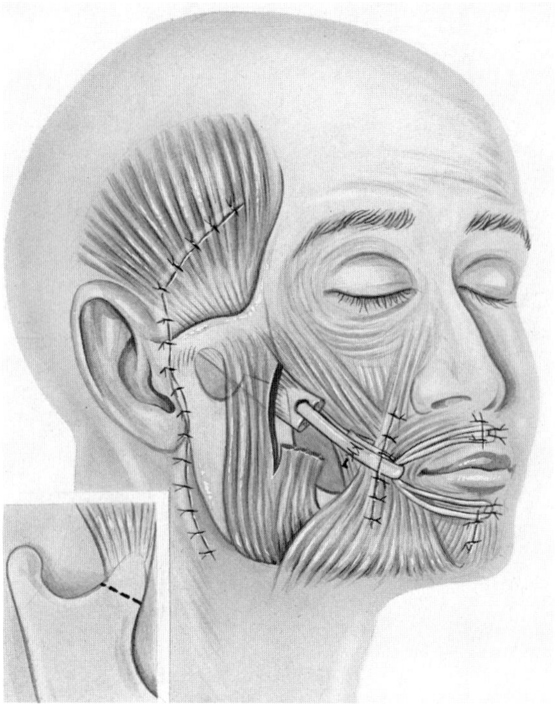

Figure 22.**42** Fascial graft using McLaughlin's technique.

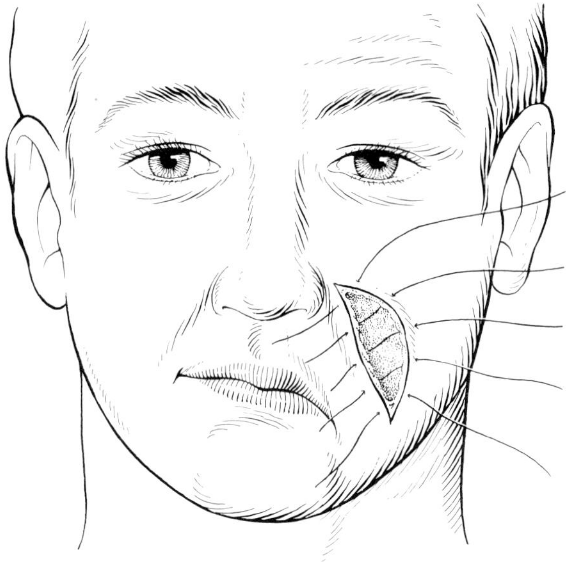

Figure 22.**43** Regional correction with formation of an artificial nasolabial fold using Kapovits' technique.

achieved by removal of unsightly swellings and overhanging parts of the skin.

Finally, the inability of the eyelids to close with the ever-present danger of drying of the conjunctiva presents a specific problem.

In ectropion of the lower lid due to loss of tone of the orbicularis oculi muscle, the lacrimal canaliculus is no longer bathed in tears, and normal drainage of tears is lost, leading to epiphora. The ectropion can be dealt with by partial excision and a transposition flap of the lower lid. In other cases, a tarsorrhaphy is advised, but this produces a noticeable cosmetic defect. The operation described by Egerton & Wolfort (1969) (Fig. 22.**44a, b**) of narrowing the palpebral fissure by subcutaneous traction produces better cosmetic results. The operative details can be seen in the diagram. It must be admitted that after some time the lower lid often prolapses again, but this can be easily corrected.

In addition to static methods for narrowing the palpebral fissure, there are procedures intended to restore some degree of movement.

The levator palpebrae superioris muscle innervated by the oculomotor nerve is the main muscle for retracting the upper lid. The orbicularis oculi muscle innervated by the facial nerve closes the lids. Lid movements are largely restricted to the upper lid, whereas the entire excursion of the lower lid only amounts to about 1 mm. Two procedures are available based on this fact.

Morel-Fatio and Lallardrie (1964) recommend the implantation of a palpebral spring in the upper lid. A wire loop shaped like a small safety pin is introduced under slight tension into the upper lid through three small incisions using a trocar, and is fixed subcutaneously (Fig. 22.**45a–d**). This elastic wire loop maintains static closure of the lid, but the levator muscle, innervated by the oculomotor nerve, is powerful enough to overcome the tension of the wire loop and to open the lids. The ends of the wire may occasionally protrude and endanger the cornea.

Implantation of appropriately shaped magnets in the upper and lower lids carries less danger (Mühlbauer et al 1973). The lid magnets are implanted through incisions carried down through the subcutaneous tissue as far as the tarsal plate. The magnets are fixed to the cartilaginous tarsal plate with two subcutaneous sutures (Fig. 22.**46a–c**). The attraction of the individually tailored magnets is sufficient to close the lids, whereas the levator muscles can overcome the magnetic force and open the lids.

We have used this procedure on a series of patients with initially convincing results. However, the lid magnets have been rejected by some of our

Figure 22.**44a**, **b** Two stages of the Edgerton-Wolfort procedure for narrowing the palpebral fissure, **a** Incision for developing a slender flap from the subcutaneous tissue. **b** The flap is drawn through a tunnel created in the zygomatic bone, ans sutured to the periosteum under tension.

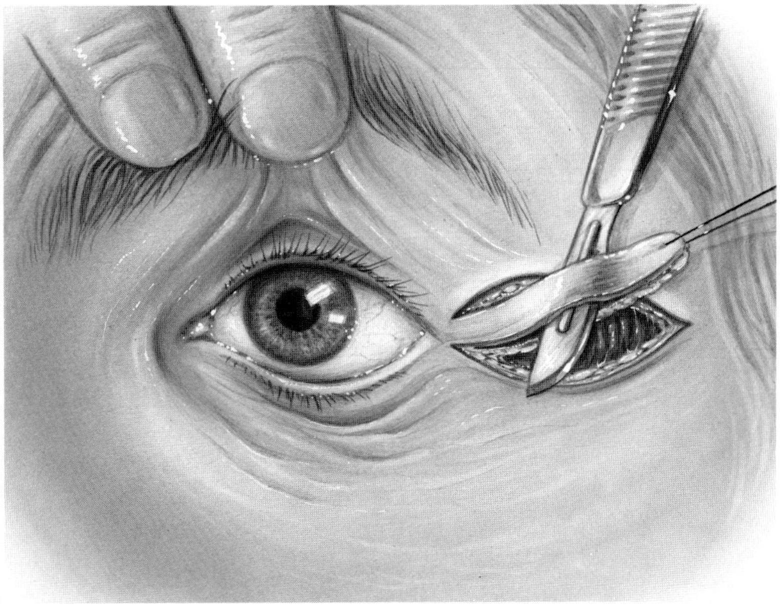

a

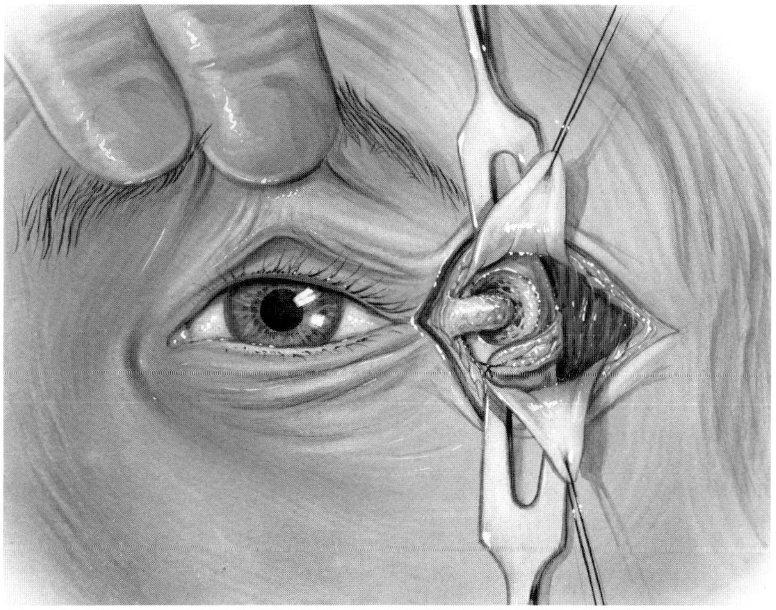

b

patients. We believe that this problem can be solved by increasing experience. The method appears to be highly satisfactory in patients with a temporary lagophthalmos who have some prospect of recovery of function after one of the methods of reconstruction of the facial nerve already described. If the function of the facial nerve recovers within several months, the magnets are removed.

Reconstitution of tone and limited voluntary movement in the oral region, an area in which paralysis is particularly noticeable, can be achieved by the nerve-muscle flap described by Johnson and Tucker (1977) and Tucker (1979). A nerve-muscle graft is prepared from the ansa cervicalis and several small muscle flaps innervated by this nerve are developed, taken from three areas:

a) The posterior wall of the anterior belly of the omohyoid muscle
b) The posterior wall of the sternothyroid muscle
c) The posterior wall of the anterior belly of the sternohyoid muscle (Fig. 22.**47a**)

The small neuromuscular island flaps are mobilized and led through a subcutaneous tunnel

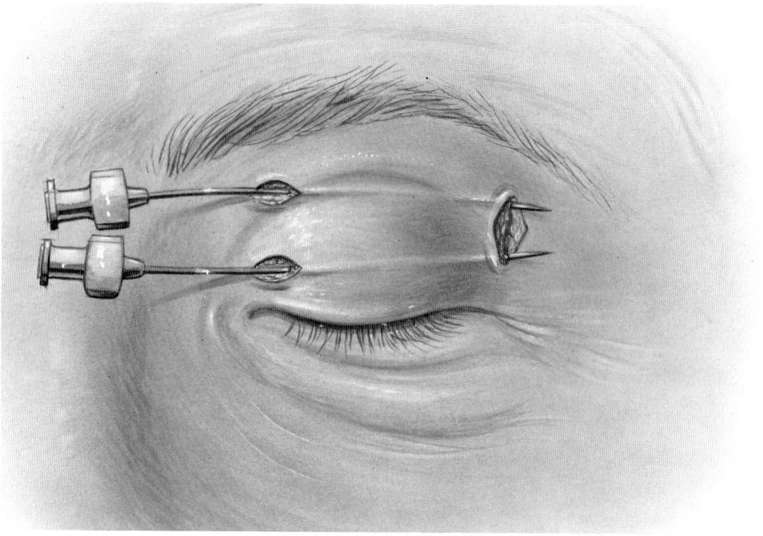

a

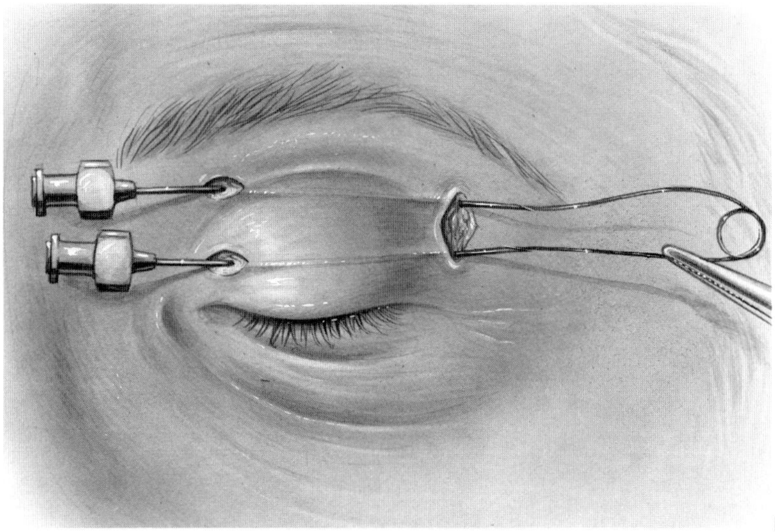

b

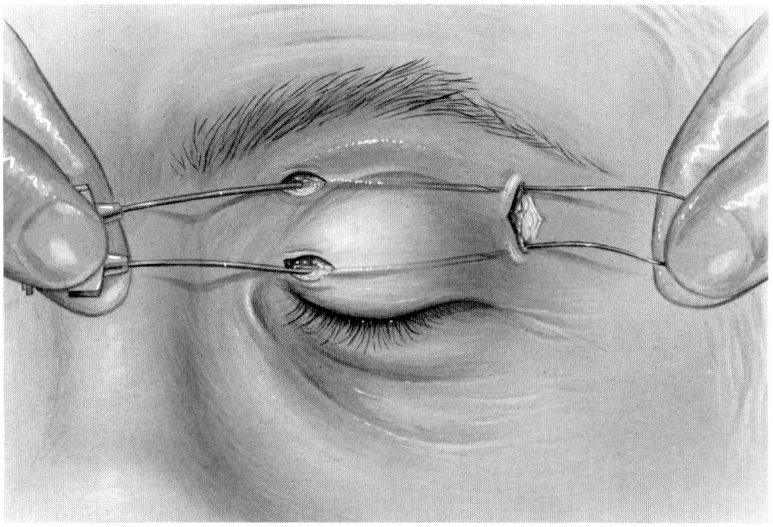

c

Figure 22.**45a-d** Palpebral spring operation.
a Introduction of two neddles into the upper lid.
b The free ends of a wire loop introduced into the needles.
c The needles together with the free ends of the wire are drawn out. The free ends of the wire are shortened and the loop is fixed with a fine suture.

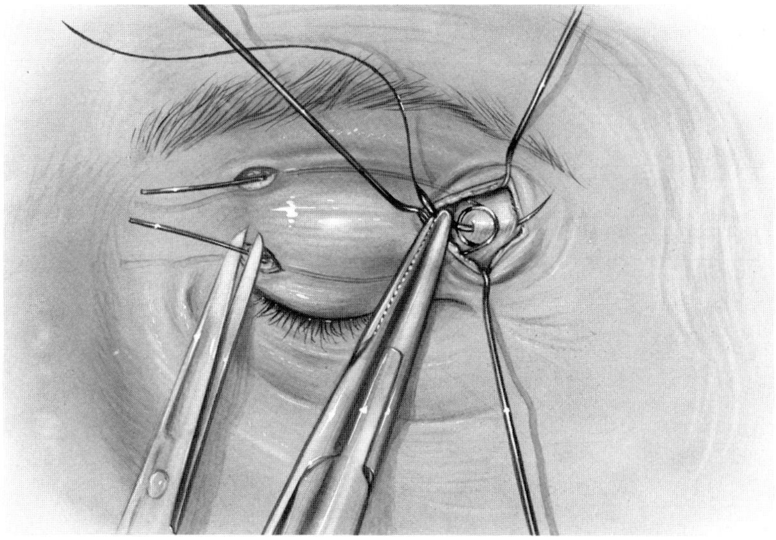

Figure 22.**45d**

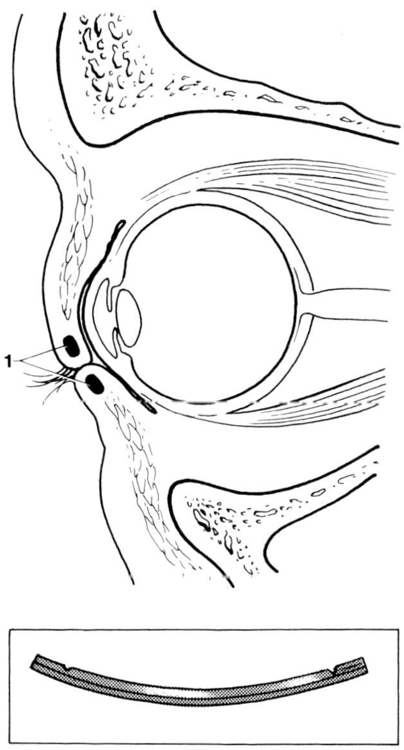

Figure 22.**46a** Implantation of lid magnets (1).

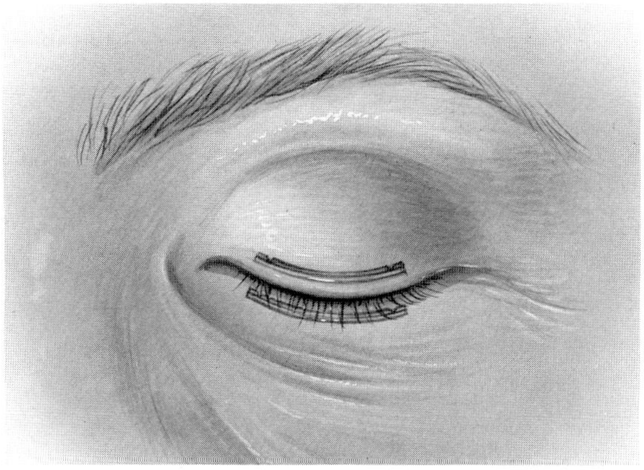

Figure 22.**46b** Lid magnets implanted in the subcutaneous tissue.

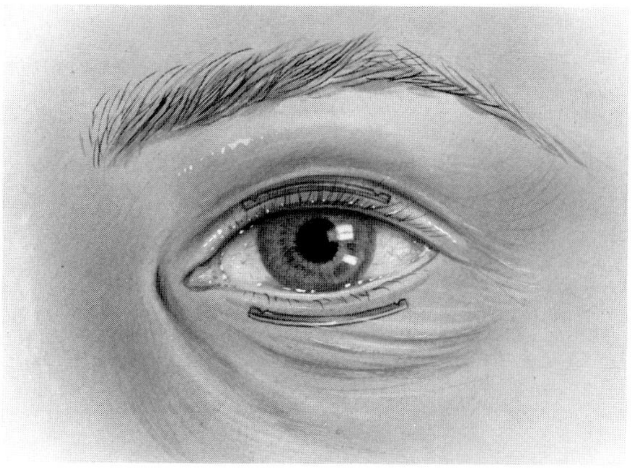

Figure 22.**46c** The upper lid can be actively opened by the retained function of the levator palpebral muscle innervated by the oculomotor nerve.

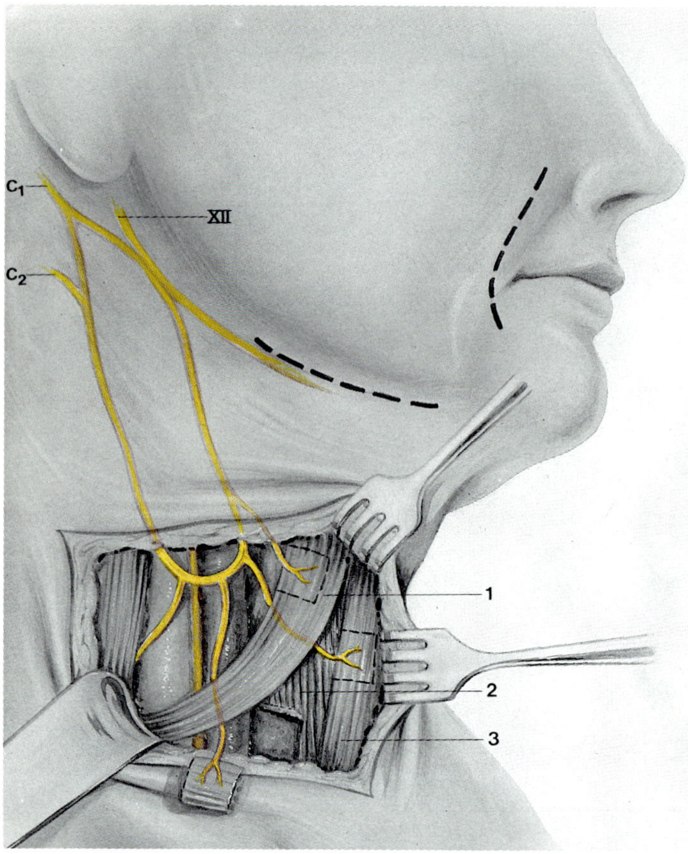

a

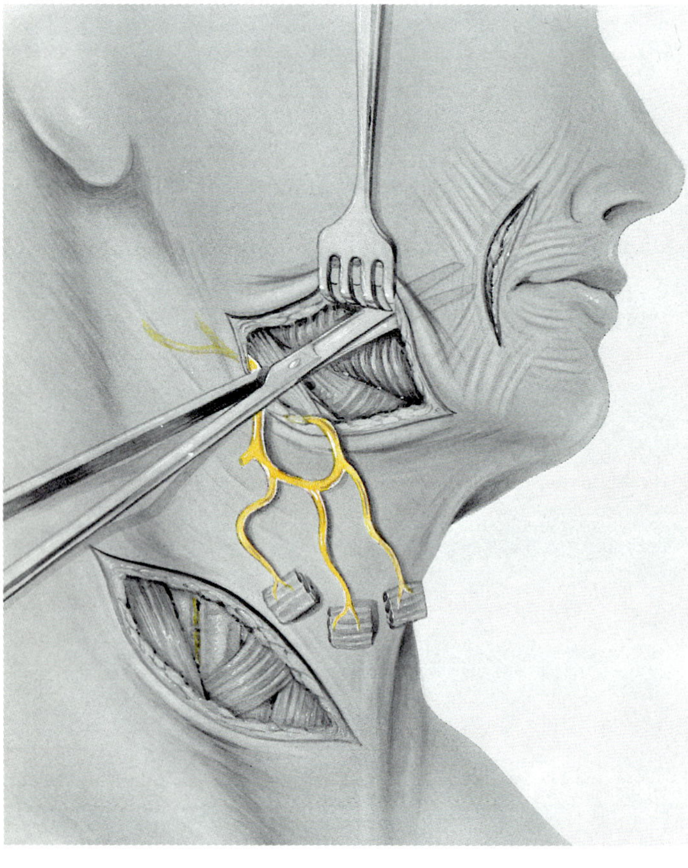

b

Figure 22.**47a**-**c** Nerve-muscle flap implantation. (Tucker & Johnson.)

a Anatomy of the ansa cervicalis and its branches to the omohyoid muscle (1 = superior belly), the sternothyroid muscle (2), and the sternohyoid muscle (3). The nerve muscle graft was removed in one block.

b Transfer of the mobilized nerve-muscle graft through a tunnel created by submandibular and nasolabial incisions to the perioral facial muscles.

c Nerve-muscle flap implanted in the zygomatic, orbicularis oris, and depressor labii inferioris muscles.

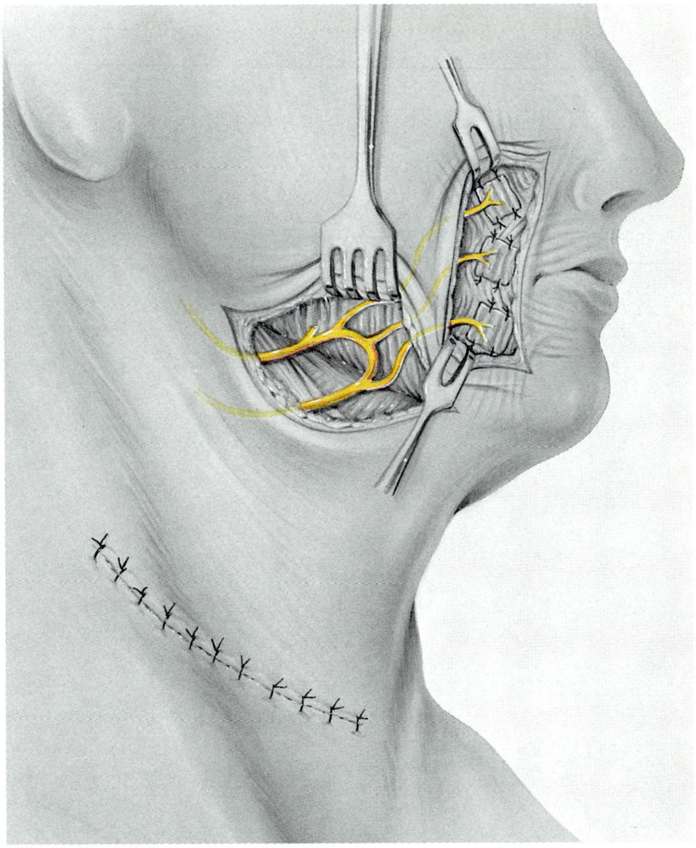

c

into the perioral region (Fig. 22.**47b**) and are sutured without tension into the zygomatic, orbicularis oris, and depressor labii inferioris muscles using fine atraumatic sutures through an incision in the nasolabial fold (Fig. 22.**47c**).

According to Tucker (1979), tone and limited voluntary movement return to the perioral area within 4 months, as can be shown by photography and electromyography.

The method appears to be a useful supplementary measure in those situations in which some degree of late correction of a paralyzed lower face is needed.

Surgery of the Submandibular Gland

Removal of the submandibular gland is often required for chronic inflammatory disease with or without stone formation. The stone generally lies in the duct. The symptoms are well known, and include severe pain, associated with swelling of the gland on eating, opaque purulent secretion from the submandibular duct or absence of saliva.

The calcium-containing stone can usually be shown by radiology, but not always. A stone may often be felt in the duct or be palpated with a probe. In the latter case the duct should be split over the probe as a preliminary measure to avoid major surgery.

Surgery is indicated for all malignant tumors of the submandibular gland. The relative frequency of adenoid cystic carcinoma of the submandibular gland must be emphasized at this point. Loss of the gland has no significance because the function has already previously been lost either in chronic inflammation or in neoplasia.

Operative Technique. A curved 5 cm skin incision is made with its convexity below. The incision begins below the angle of the jaw and runs just in front of the lateral cornu of the hyoid bone (Fig. 22.**48a**). The platysma is divided, and the facial artery and vein are identified at the lower border of the mandible. These vessels can be found on the outer surface of the mandible at the anterior border of the masseter muscle. The marginal mandibular ramus of the facial nerve is preserved by the following step:

The vessels are ligated 1 cm inferior to the edge of the mandible and divided. They are then turned

Figure 22.**48a-e** Various stages of the operation for removal of the submandibular gland.

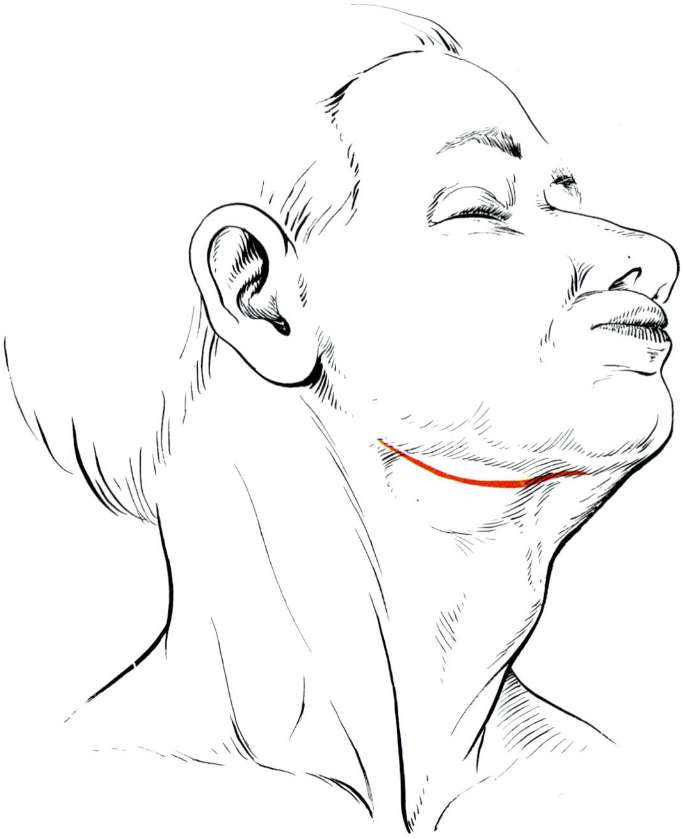

a

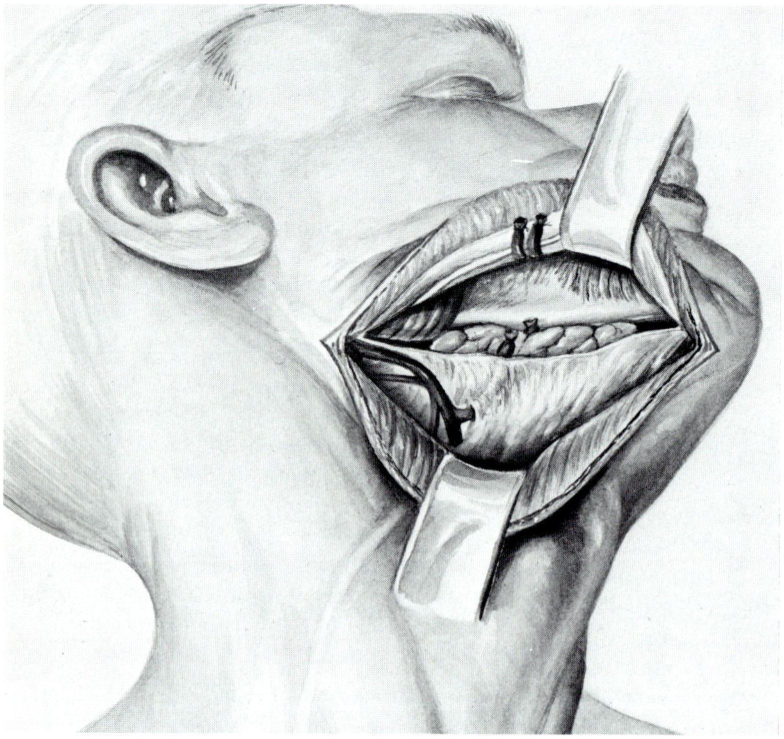

b

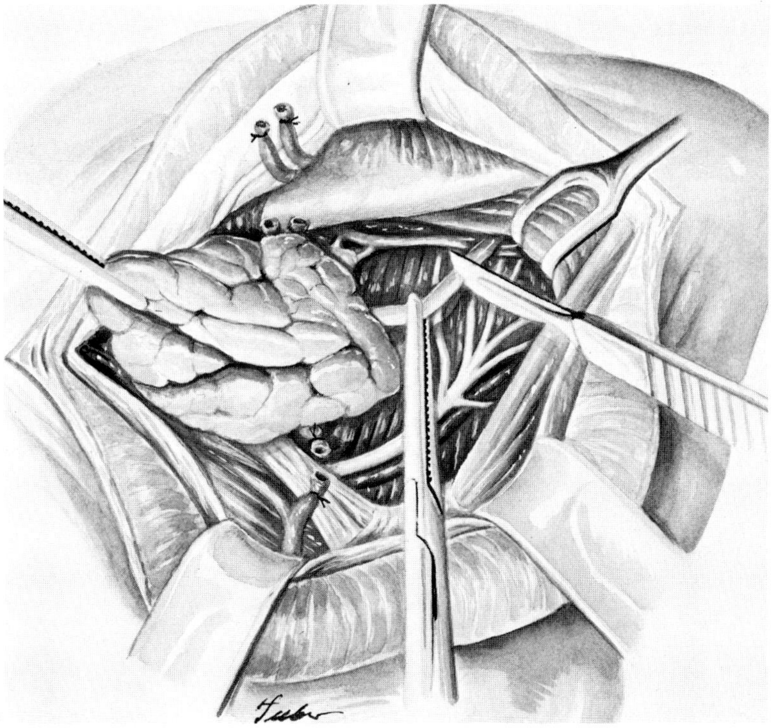

c

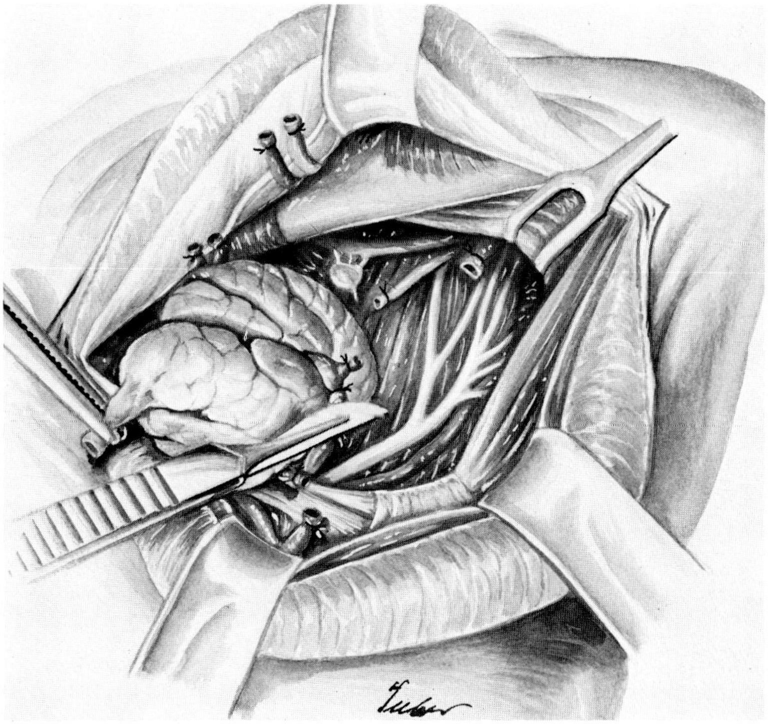

d

upward and fixed with chromic catgut sutures to the retracted soft tissues of the cheek (Fig. 22.**48b**).

The facial artery and vein cross the marginal mandibular ramus so that the nerve is retracted along with the vessels and protected from injury. The marginal mandibular ramus only anastomoses with other end branches of the facial nerve in 5–12% of subjects: it is important to preserve it, since division of this ramus causes a conspicu-

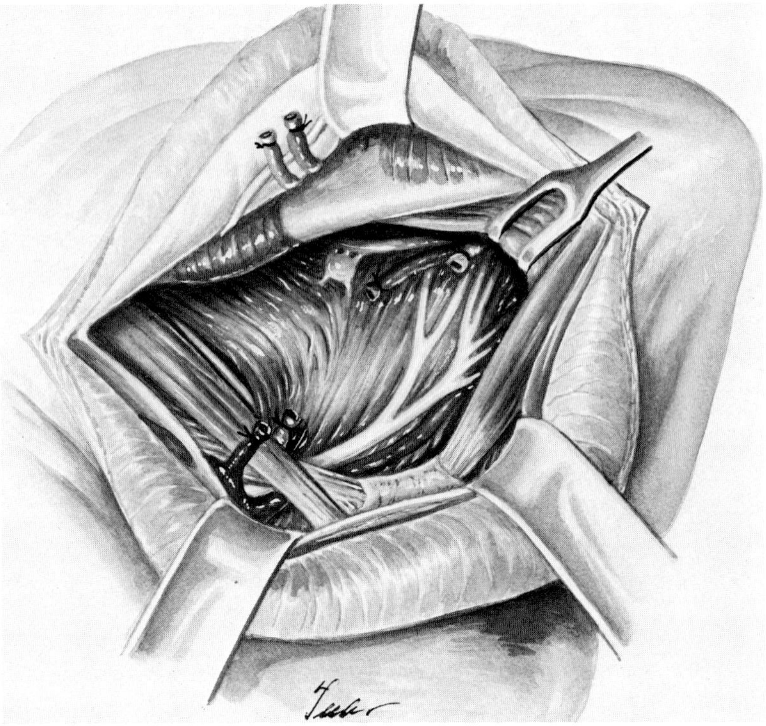

Figure 22.**48e**

ous paralysis of the lower lip. Fortunately, the marginal mandibular ramus consists of two branches in about 50% of patients.

The facial vein, unlike the facial artery, does not run deeply in the submandibular triangle, but over the body of the gland. Thus, it must be doubly ligated and divided at the inferior edge of the gland. Only now can the submandibular gland be elevated. Next, the anterior belly of the digastric muscle comes into view, and when the body of the gland is retracted posteriorly, the dorsal edge of the mylohyoid muscle can also be seen.

The mylohyoid muscle can be used as a landmark to find the hypoglossal and lingual nerves and the submandibular duct. Anterior retraction of this muscle by a double hook opens the anterior part of the submandibular triangle to such an extent that the submandibular duct can be seen running in the middle of this space, with the lingual nerve above it and the hypoglossal nerve below it.

Finally, the submandibular ganglion lying immediately inferior to the lingual nerve is demonstrated by blunt dissection of the gland capsule from the surrounding tissue (Fig. 22.**48c**). The gland is further freed by double ligature and division of the submandibular duct (Fig. 22.**48d**). The body of the gland is retracted posteriorly by retraction with forceps on the stump of the duct to expose the posterior surface of the gland, and thus the facial artery running in the depth of the wound. This vessel is also doubly ligated and divided. The submandibular gland is then removed (Figure 22.**48e** shows the appearances after removal of the gland). The operation ends with careful hemostasis, preferably using Malis's bipolar coagulation forceps, the introduction of a Penrose drain, and skin closure in layers.

Surgery of the Sublingual Gland

The sublingual gland is about one third the size of the submandibular gland. It lies beneath the mucosa of the floor of the mouth between the tongue and the mandible on the mylohyoid muscle (see Chapter 1). The best known and most frequent disease of the sublingual gland is a *ranula* (described on page 64ff).

Malignant tumors of the sublingual gland are rare. The surgery of such tumors is identical to that for excision of a malignancy of the floor of the mouth, that is, en bloc partial glossectomy, resection of the floor of the mouth, and marginal or partial mandibulectomy, if necessary with radical neck dissection. The removal of a *ranula* will be described first followed by a description of resection of the floor of the mouth (Rankow 1974).

Operative Technique. A thin silver probe is first introduced into the submandibular duct. An elliptical incision is then made through the mucosa over the cystic swelling in the floor of the mouth (Fig. 22.**49a**). The circumscribed part of the mucosa is grasped with a mosquito forceps to serve as a retractor during resection of the ranula. Figure 22.**49b** shows the mucosal layers already dissected from the cyst. A thin polyethylene catheter has been introduced into the submandibular duct. Figure 22.**49c** shows the situation from the lateral side.

The incision is now extended anteriorly and posteriorly, and the mucosal layers are freed carefully from the ranula by combined blunt and sharp dissection.

The cyst is now grasped with an Allis forceps and is dissected bluntly from the submandibular duct, freeing it from its connective tissue space and its connections with the underlying mylohyoid muscle (Fig. 22.**49d**). Small vessels are dealt with by bipolar coagulation forceps. The submandibular duct with the undamaged lingual nerve can be seen in the floor of the mouth after removal of the ranula with the sublingual gland (Figure 22.**49e**).

The mucosa is now closed with two or three catgut sutures.

The patient should take a fluid diet for several days, followed by a semisolid diet, and the mouth should be irrigated carefully with the appropriate solutions.

A *malignancy of the sublingual gland* requires resection with a wide margin, that is, partial resection of the floor of the mouth with partial glossectomy and partial mandibulectomy, if necessary combined with radical neck dissection.

A mucoperiosteal flap is cut and elevated from the medial surface of the mandible as a preliminary to marginal mandibulectomy with removal of the alveolus (Fig. 22.**50**).

Since the lymphatic pathways of the floor of the mouth run through the mucoperiosteum of the internal aspect of the mandible in 50% of cases (Polya & Navratil 1902), the inner mucoperiosteum must be excised in continuity with part of the floor of the mouth, together with the sublingual gland and a part of the lateral border of the tongue.

The floor of the mouth with the submandibular gland and the lateral border of the tongue are divided with the cutting diathermy about 2 cm from the edge of the tumor, and the dissection is carried down to the mylohyoid muscle to achieve clearance in depth. The sublingual gland is also included in the specimen. The submandibular duct is identified and its proximal stump fixed in the wound. The specimen consisting of the tumor, the tongue, the floor of the mouth, the sublingual gland, the internal mucoperiosteum, and the alveolus is removed.

The defect after marginal mandibulectomy can be closed in one of two ways:

1. The medial mucoperiosteal flap is turned over the marginal mandibular defect and sutured to the cut edge of the tongue (Fig. 22.**51a–d**).
2. The defect in the floor of the mouth and the lateral part of the tongue may be covered by a split-skin graft taken from the thigh. The graft is sutured laterally to the mucoperiosteal flap of the mandible and to the edges of the defect. The graft is fixed in place for a few days using a gauze tampon stitched in place and held with sutures (Fig. 22.**51e, f**).

References

Anderl, H.: Reconstruction of the face through cross-face-nerve transplantation in facial paralysis. Chirurg. Plast. 2 (1973) 17

Anderl, H.: Cross-face-nerve transplantation. Clin. Plast. Surg. 6 (1979) 433

Anderson, R., R. S. Flowers: Free grafts of spinal accessory nerve during radical neck-dissection. Amer. J. Surg. 188 (1969) 796

Arson, A. W., W. O. Ott: Preservation of the facial nerve in radical treatment of parotid tumors. Arch. Surg. 6 (1923) 739

Aschan, P. E.: Muskel- und Sehnentransplantation bei Facialisparese. Fortschr. Kiefer- u. Gesichtschirurg. 2 (1956) 143

Bailey, H.: Parotidectomy indications and results. Brit. med. J. 1947/I, 404

Blair, V. P.: The role of plastic surgery in the care of war injuries. Amer. Surg. 63 (1941) 697

Bocca, E.: Chirurgie der Hals-Lymph-Knoten. In Naumann, H. H.: Kopf- und Hals-Chirurgie. Thieme, Stuttgart 1972

Byars, L. T.: Preservation of the facial nerve in operations for benign conditions of parotid area. Amer. Surg. 136 (1952) 412

Chilla, R.: Types of facial nerve branching in the parotid plexus and their clinical significance. In: New Aspects in Facial Nerve Surgery. Clin. Plast. Surg. 6 (1979) 451

Conley, J. J.: Surgical treatment of tumors of the parotid gland with emphasis on immediate nerve grafting. West. J. Surg. 63 (1955a) 534

Conley, J. J.: Facial nerve grafting in treatment of parotid gland tumors; new technique. Arch. Surg. 70 (1955b) 359

Conley, J. J.: Facial rehabilitation following radical parotid gland surgery. Arch. Otolaryng. 66 (1957) 58

Conley, J. J.: Concepts in Head and Neck Surgery. Thieme, Stuttgart 1970

Conley, J. J.: Salivary Glands and the Facial Nerve. Thieme, Stuttgart 1975

Conley, J. J., D. Baker: Regional muscle transposition for rehabilitation of the paralysed face. Clin. Plast. Surg. 6 (1979) 317

Davis, R. A., B. J. Anson, J. M. Budinger, L. E. Kurth: Surgical anatomy of the facial nerve and parotid gland based upon a study of 350 cervico-facial halves. Surg. Gynec. Obstet. 102 (1956) 384

Denecke, H. J.: Zur Chirurgie des Nervus facialis im Bereich der Parotis und der Schädelbasis. Wien. klin. Wschr. 71 (1959) 180

Edgerton, M. T., F. G. Wolfort: The dermal flap canthal lift for lower eyelid support. Plast. reconstr. Surg. 43 (1969) 42

Erlacher, P.: Hyperneurotisation; muskuläre Neurotisation; freie Muskeltransplantation; experimentelle Untersuchungen. Zbl. Chir. 41 (1914) 625

Esslen, E.: Electrodiagnosis of facial palsy. In Miehlke, A.: Surgery of the Facial Nerve. Urban & Schwarzenberg, München; Saunders, Philadelphia 1973

Fisch, U.: s. Michael, E. (1973)

Gilies, H.: Plastic surgery of the face. Internat. Dent. Ars. Huntington 7 (1920) 3

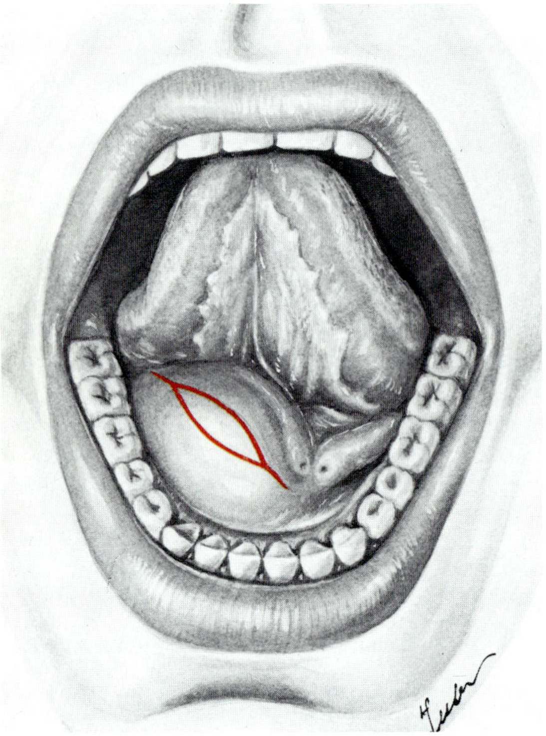

a

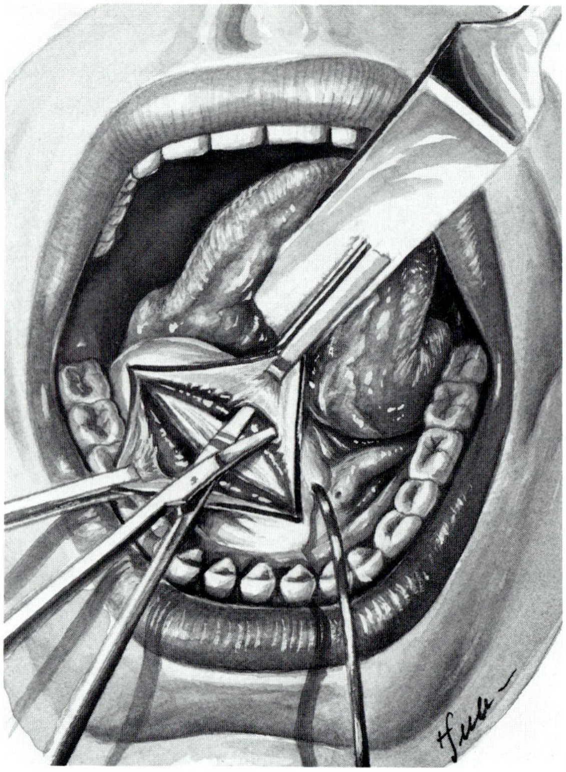

b

Figure 22.**49a–e** Various stages of the operation for the removal of a sublingual gland.

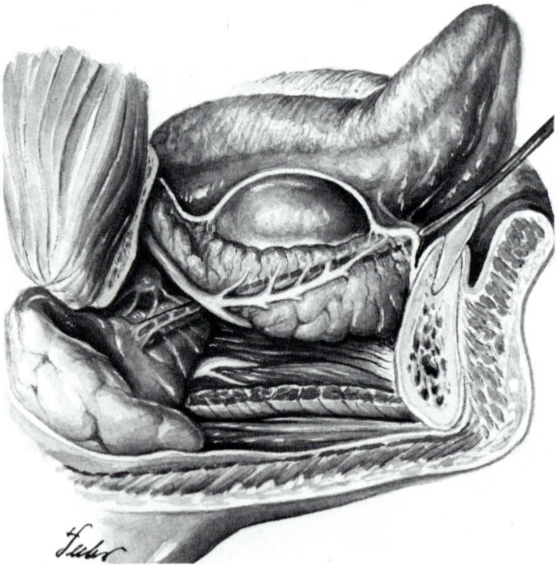

c

Gilies, H.: Experience with fascia lata-grafts in the operative treatment of facial paralysis. Proc. Roy. Soc. Med. (London) 27 (1934) 98

Gohrbandt, E.: Zur Indikation der plastisch-chirurgischen Eingriffe. In: Handbuch der plastischen Chirurgie. De Gruyter, Berlin 1972

Harries, H. H., R. R. Dickey: Nerve grafting to restore function of the trapezius muscle after radical neck-dissection. Amer. Otol. (St. Louis) 74 (1965) 880

Hogg, S. P., R. C. Kratz: Surgical exposure of the facial nerve. Arch. Otolaryng. 67 (1958) 560

Janes, R. M.: Treatment of tumors of the salivary glands by radical excision. Canad. med. Assoc. J. 43 (1940) 554

Janes, R. M.: Surgical treatment of tumors of the salivary glands. Surg. Clin. N. Amer. 23 (1943) 1429

Johnson, J., H. M. Tucker: Selective reinnervation of paralysed facial muscles: A progress report. Trans. Amer. Acad. Ophthal. Otolaryng. 84 (1977)

Jost, G., F. Legent, S. Baudelot: Le complément des dépressions résiduelles après parotidectomie par un lambeau du sternocleidomastoidien. Ann. Chir. Plast. 13 (1978) 187

Kapovits, M.: Indikation und Technik der Gesichtshautraffung bei Facialisparese. Langenbecks Arch. Klin. Chir. 298 (1961) 946

Kidd, H. A.: Complete excision of the parotid gland with preservation of the facial nerve. Brit. med. J. 1950/I, 989

Kornblut, A. D., P. Westphal, A. Miehlke: The effectiveness of a sternomastoid muscle flap in preventing post-parotidectomy occurrence of the Frey syndrome. Acta Otolaryng. (Stockh.) 77 (1974) 368

Kreutzberg, G. W., P. Schubert: Changes in axonal flow during regeneration of mammalian motor nerves. Acta Neuropatholog. (Berl.) Suppl. 5 (1971) 70

von Lanz, T., W. Wachsmuth: Praktische Anatomie, Bd. I/2: Hals. Springer, Berlin 1955

Lathrop, F. D.: Technic of exposing the facial nerve as an aid to surgery of the parotid gland. Surg. Clin. N. Amer. 29 (1949) 673

Lathrop, F. D.: Management of the facial nerve during operations on the parotid gland. Amer. Otol. (St. Louis) 72 (1963) 780

Lathrop, F. D.: Facial nerve grafting. Trans. Amer. Acad. Ophthal. Otolaryng. 68 (1964) 1060

Leicher, H., W. Becker, J. Matzker: Neck-Dissection. Z. Laryng. Rhinol. 35 (1956) 359

Lexer, E.: Die gesamte Wiederherstellungs-Chirurgie. Leipzig 1931

Marino, H.: Paralysis des N. facialis. Fortschr. Kiefer- u. Gesichts-Chir. 7 (1956) 145

Maxwell, J. H.: Repair of the facial nerve after facial lacerations. Trans. Amer. Acad. Ophthal. Otolaryng. 58 (1954a) 733

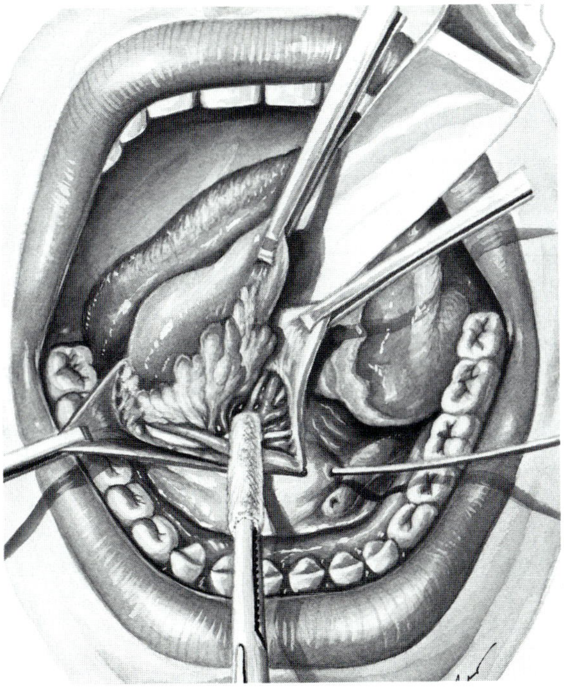

d

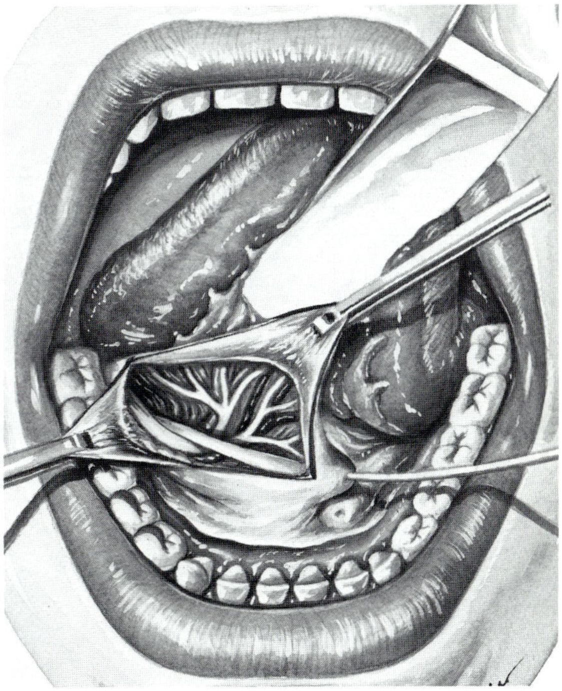

e

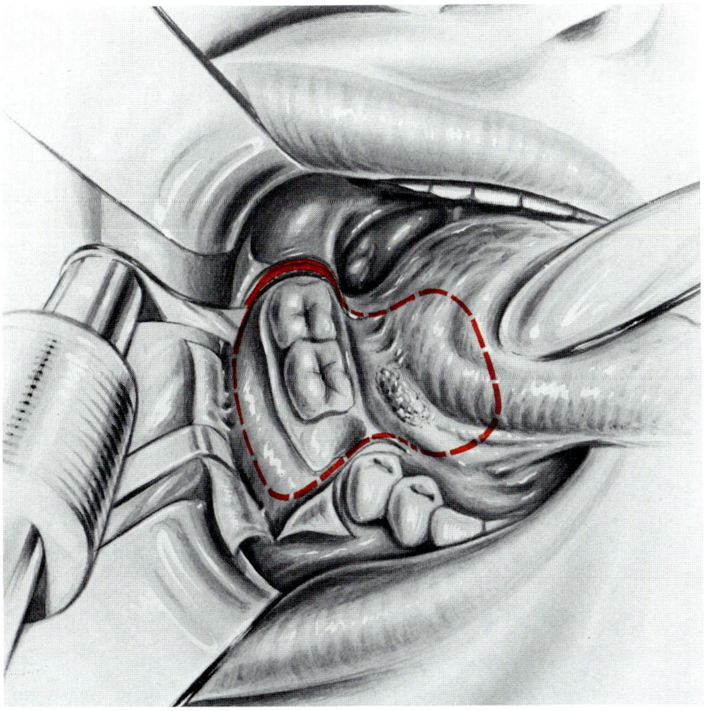

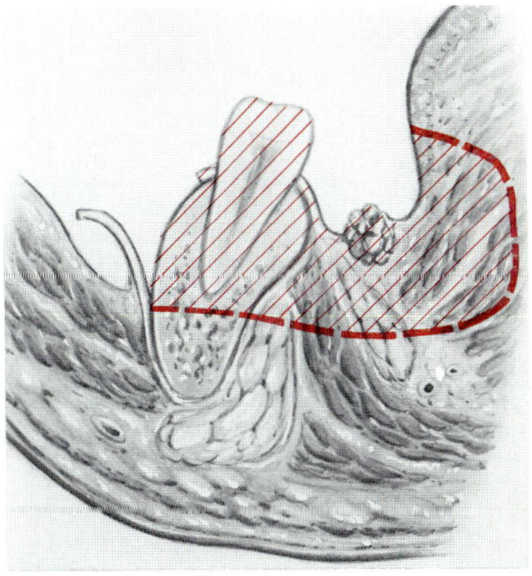

Figure 22.**50** Diagram of resection. (Naumann 1974.)

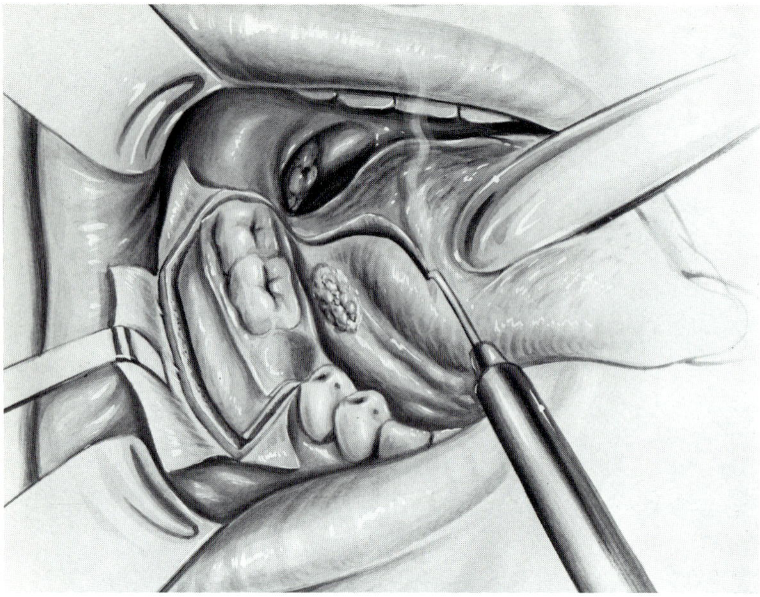

a

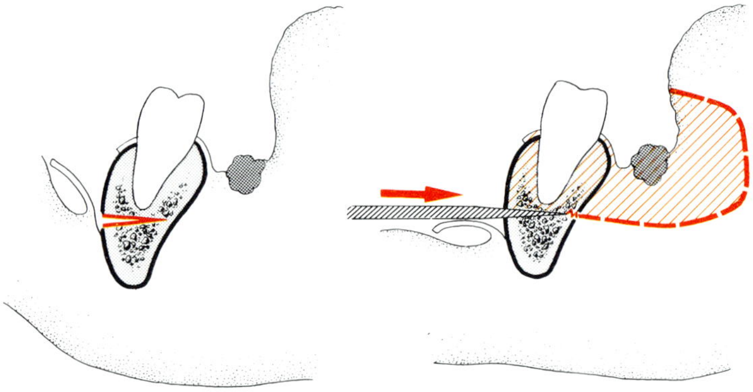

b

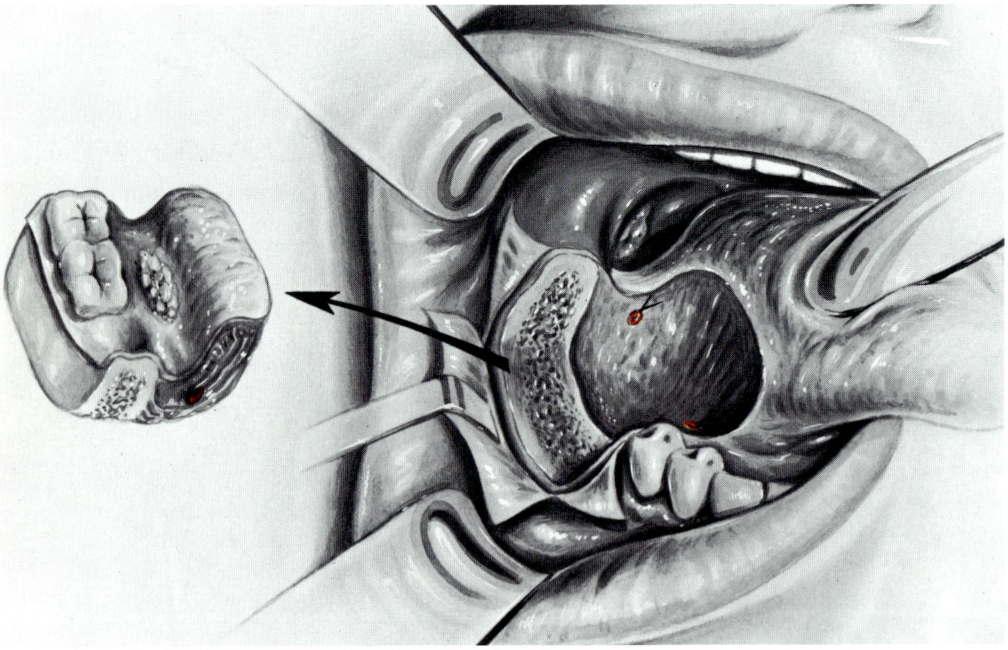

c

Figure 22.**51 a**-**d** Operative technique for the removal of a tumor of the sublingual gland. (Rankow.)
e Skin graft sutured into the defect with the sutures left long.
f The sutures are tied over a gauze bolster to fix the skin graft. (Naumann 1974.)

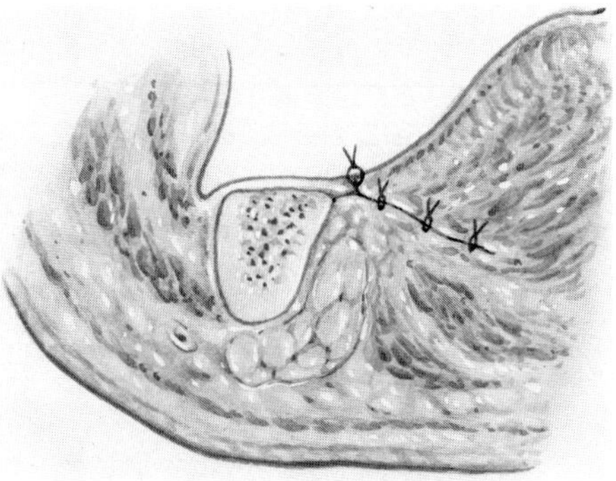

d

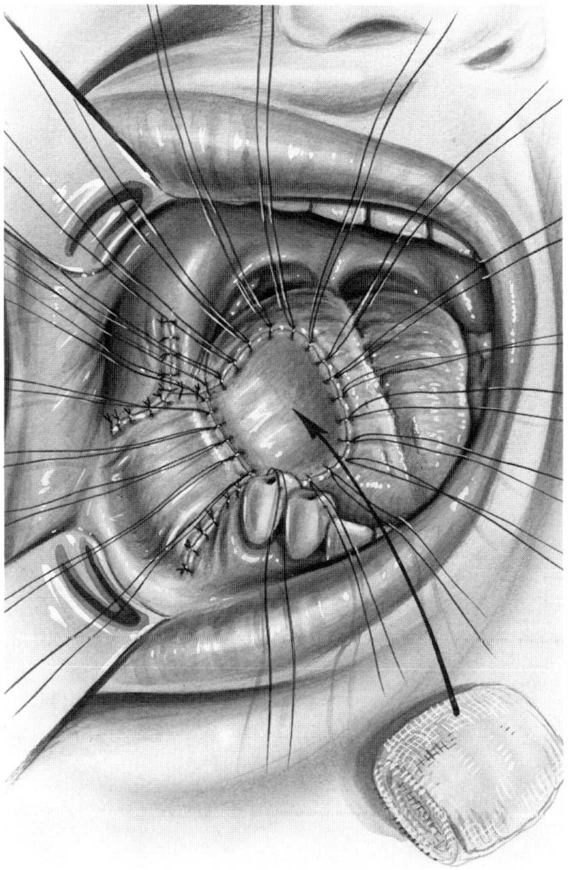

e

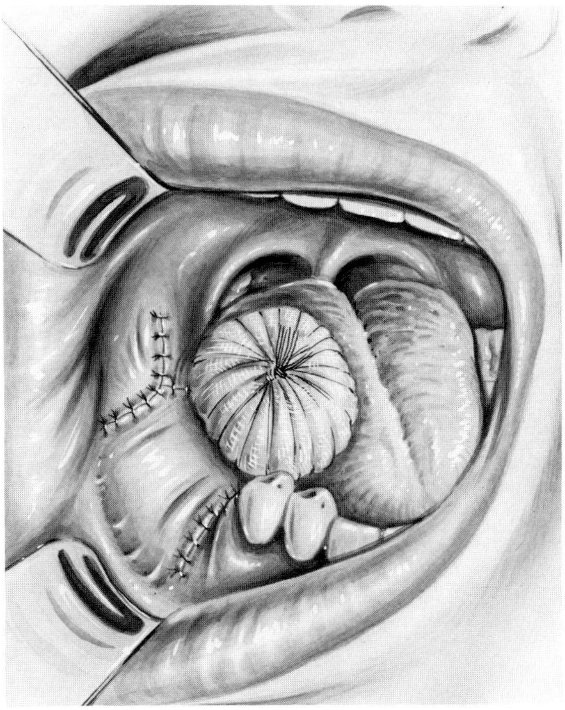

f

Maxwell, J. H.: Diseases of parotid gland. Chicago Med. Soc. Bull 56 (1954b) 733
Maxwell, J. H., R. W. Buxton, A. J. French: The surgical treatment of parotid gland tumors. Trans. Amer. Acad. Ophthal. Otolaryng. 57 (1953) 711
McLaughlin, C. R.: Surgical support in permanent facial paralysis. Plast. Reconstr. Surg. 11 (1953) 302
Michael, E.: Ergebnisse der Accessoriusplastik nach radikaler LK-Ausräumung des Halses. HNO 21 (1973) 21
Miehlke, A.: Chirurgie der Nerven; neuere Gesichtspunkte. Arch. Oto-Rhino-Laryng. 231 (1981) 464
Miehlke, A., E. Stennert, R. Arold, R. Chilla, H. Penzhold, A. Kühner, V. Sturm, J. Haubrich: Chirurgie der Nerven im HNO-Bereich (Kongreßbericht). Arch. Oto-Rhino-Laryng. 231 (1981) 89
Millesi, H.: Chirurgische Erkrankungen der peripheren Nerven. Chirurgie der Gegenwart 2 (1978) 1
Millesi, H., A. Berger, G. Meissl: Experimentelle Untersuchungen zur Heilung durchtrennter peripherer Nerven. Chir. plast. (Berl.) 1 (1972) 174
Morel-Fatio, D., J. P. Lallardrie: Palliative surgical treatment of facial paralysis – the palpebral spring. Plast. reconstr. Surg. 33 (1964) 446
Moser, F.: Zur operativen Behandlung der Parotisgeschwülste. Z. Laryng. Rhinol. 33 (1954) 195
Mühlbauer, W. D., H. Segeth, A. Viessmann: Restoration of lid function in facial palsy with permanent magnets. Chirurg. Plast. 1 (1973) 295
Nessel, E.: Die Succinyl-Kontraktur an der gelähmten Facialismuskulatur, ein neues Diagnostikum zur Beurteilung alter Lähmungen (Verh. Ber.). Arch. klin. exp. Ohr.- u. Nas.-Heilk. 196 (1970) 198
Niklison, J.: Contribution to the subject of facial paralysis. Plast. reconstr. Surg. 17 (1956) 276

Perzik, S. L.: Diagnosis and management of parotid tumors. Arch. Otolaryng. 67 (1958) 319
Pichler, H., R. Trauner: Mund- und Kieferchirurgie. Urban & Schwarzenberg, Wien 1948
Pietrantoni, L., R. Agazzi: Le problème ganglionaire dans le traitement des cancers du larynx et de l'hypopharynx. Fortschr. HNO-Heilk. 9 (1961) 275
Pollack, R. S.: Tumor Surgery of the Head and Neck. Lea & Febinger, Philadelphia 1957
Polya u. Nevratil 1902: Zit. nach Miehlke, A.: Über den heutigen Stand der Chirurgie des Zungencarcinoms. Z. Laryng. Rhinol. 38 (1959) 524
Ragnell, A.: A method for dynamic reconstruction in cases of facial paralysis. Plast. reconstr. Surg. 21 (1958) 214
Rankow, R. M.: Surgery of the Face, Mouth and Neck. Saunders, Philadelphia 1968
Rankow, R. M.: Operative Behandlung von malignen Tumoren der Zunge und des Mundbodens. In Naumann, H. H.: Kopf- und Halschirurgie, Bd. II. Thieme, Stuttgart 1974 (S. 869)
Rieske, E., W. Kreutzberg: Neurite regeneration after cell surgery with laser microbeam irradiation. Brain Res. 148 (1978) 478
Rosenthal, W.: Über die muskuläre Neurotisation bei Facialislähmung. Zbl. Chir. 43 (1916) 489
Samii, M.: Fascicular nerve repair. In "Technics of Neurosurgery". Futura, New York 1980
Scaramella, L.: Preliminary reports on facial nerve anastomosis. Third Int. Symp. on Facial Nerve Surg., Osaka 1970
Scaramella, L.: L'anastomosi tra i due nervi faciali. Arch. otol. 82 (1971) 209
Sistrunk, W. E.: Mixed tumors of the parotid gland. Minnesota Med. 4 (1921) 155
Stein, A. E.: Die kosmetische Korrektur der Facialislähmung durch freie Fascienplastik. Münchener med. Wschr. 25 (1913) 1370
Stennert, E.: Chirurgische Primärversorgung von Verletzungen der lateralen Gesichtsregion. Chirurg 53 (1982) 241
Stennert, E., C. Limberg, K. Frentrup: Paralysis and secondary defect score. In: "New Aspects in Facial Nerve Surgery". Clin. Plast. Surg. 6 (1979) 458
Struppler, A., R. Scheininger: Elektromyographische Untersuchungen zur Frage der Innervationsübernahme. Pflügers Arch. ges. Physiol. 274 (1961) 48
Tucker, H. M.: Restoration of selective facial nerve function by nerve-muscle pedicle technique. Clin. plast. Surg. 6 (1979) 301
Weiss, P., H. B. Hiscoe: Experiments on the mechanism of nerve growth. J. exp. Zool. 107 (1948) 315
Zülch, K. J.: Gedanken eines Neurologen zur konservativen und chirurgischen Behandlung der Facialislähmung. Z. Laryng. Rhinol. 40 (1961) 305

23. Medicolegal Assessment

The assessment of injuries to the facial region for estimation of reduced earning capacity must take many factors into account. Estimation of the results of an injury or a tumor operation with or without facial nerve paralysis requires assessment of the multiple functional deficits and must also take account of the patient's appearance.

For greater clarity, the assessment of the residual deficit after operations on the facial nerve will be divided into those due to absent regeneration, to incorrect regeneration, and to a dysfunction of regenerated neurones.

Absent Regeneration

Motor Paralyses at Rest

Cosmetic Problems. The angle of the mouth lies lower than normal and the nasolabial fold is lost due to failure of recovery of the zygomatic and levator labii superioris muscles. Typically, a disfiguring discrepancy is obvious between the healthy and the diseased side, particularly on laughing.

The palpebral fissure is widened, with or without an ectropion, due to failure of recovery of the orbicularis oculi muscle, and the lids cannot be closed voluntarily. The natural blink often does not recover.

An unsightly lowering of the level of the eyebrow is due to failure of recovery of the frontalis muscle.

Functional Problems. There is a danger of drying of the cornea, if lid closure is incomplete, and this danger is increased, if the secretion of tears is also reduced.

Articulation disorders, particularly for labial sounds, such as "p," and difficulties in drinking are caused by paralysis of the orbicularis oris and buccinator muscles.

Incorrect Regeneration

Synkinesia and Mass Movements

Heteromorphic reneurotization occurs after any serious injury to the nerve with partial or complete destruction of its architecture (Hiller 1949, 1951). The results are extensive false buds with crossing of the emigrating axons that enter incorrect Büngner's bands and reach the wrong motor end-plate. Voluntary contraction of individual mimic muscles is then no longer possible, and moreover synkinesia or even mass movements occur. Previously, it was hoped that it would be possible to refine the synkinetic movements by exercises in front of the mirror or by deliberate suppression (Zülch 1955) of superfluous movements, but that has not proved possible. "The functional determination of the facial motor neuron is so definitive that central relearning, even by intensive training, is obviously not possible" (Stennert et al 1977). This fact must always be taken into account when estimating the prognosis for medicolegal purposes.

The Autoparalytic Syndrome

An inevitable result of incorrect budding of regenerating axons causes the autoparalytic syndrome but in this case crossed, innervation of antagonistic mimic muscles occurs (Stennert et al 1979). From a functional point of view, this indicates that movement intentions mutually cancel each other out. For example, voluntary contraction of the zygomatic muscle leads to contraction of the orbicularis oris muscle due to crosswise innervation.

The Auriculotemporal Syndrome

This is also called Frey's syndrome and is described in detail on page 325ff.

Dysfunction of Regenerated Neurones

Secondary Hemifacial Spasm

This is of disputed origin. Recent investigations (Stennert et al 1977) suggest that spasm of the mimic muscles (for example, a tic at the angle of the mouth) synchronous with the blink are in fact a generalized blink. This fact is probably due to false budding of regenerating nerve fibers.

Contractures

There is no generally accepted explanation for this phenomenon of prominent unilateral spasm of the face. One hypothesis is that it is due to

Table 23.**1** Assessment of Clinical Grade of Facial Paralysis (Stennert), Consisting of Ten Criteria that Require a Simple Yes (plus) or No (minus). The Sum of the Plusses Indicate a Negative Finding, Giving Paresis Index

At rest					
Differences between palpebral fissures		> 3 mm		3 mm or more	
Ectropion		No		Yes	
Nasolabial fold lost		No		Yes	
Depression of angle of mouth		> 3 mm		3 mm and more	
Mobile					
Frowning		Possible		Not possible	
Open palpebral fissure	During sleep	No		Yes	
	On maximal stimulation	No		Yes	
Showing the teeth	Upper and lower canine teeth	Visible		Not visible	
	Upper second incisor	Visible		Not visible	
Shortening of the distance between the philtrum and the angle of the mouth compared with the opposite side		50% or more		> 50%	
				Paresis index	

changes in the nucleus. Contractures can resolve after several years (Miehlke), but the conditions leading to this favorable outcome are unexplained.

In addition to the three sequelae due to failure of regeneration, incorrect regeneration, and dysfunction of regenerated axons, medicolegal assessment must also take into account the cosmetic and esthetic disfigurement. In view of the complexities of the interlocking and overlapping paralysis and defective recovery, often accompanied by a serious cosmetic defect, it is obvious that a very comprehensive view should be taken in determining reduced earning capacity, and this should also take into account the effect on the patient's occupation and social life.

Feldmann (1976) and Becker et al (1982) give the following criteria for the results of injury or a tumor operation in the facial area:

Repulsive deformity: 50%
Simple deformity: 10–30%
Unilateral facial nerve paralysis: 10–30%
Bilateral facial nerve paralysis: 20–40%

Oeken (1971) came to similar conclusions for the assessment of reduced earning capacity:

Unilateral or bilateral peripheral facial nerve paralysis: 10–30%
Unilateral peripheral facial nerve paralysis with considerable irritation of the eye: 30%.

We try to achieve a refined assessment of the injury, based on two schedules. Schedule I described by Stennert (Table 23.**1**) serves for the estimation of the clinical grade of paralysis. Schedule II (Table 23.**2**) serves to assess the secondary defects of recovery.

The expert can use these two tables, and by means of a simple yes or no decision, provide the

Table 23.**2** Assessment of Secondary Deficit of Recovery (Stennert). The Five Individual Parameters are Assessed Independently, Depending on Their Functional or Cosmetic Significance. The Index of Recovery Deficit Consists of Ten Criteria Requiring a Yes or No

		No	Yes
Hyperacusis		No	Yes
Taste disorders		No	Yes
Synkinease between:	Forehead Eye Nasolabial fold Corner of the mouth Chin		
	More than 3 regions		
Generalized blinking ("secondary spasms")			
Contractures			
Secretion of tears	Less than 70% with palpebral fissure at rest		
	Less than 70%		
	0%		
Crocodile tears			
	Defective recovery index		

lawyer with a basis for his estimate. The determination of the grade of paralysis (Table 23.**1**) and the secondary recovery deficit (Table 23.**2**), plus an individually determined effect of the cosmetic deformity on the patient's occupation and social life, should then permit a comprehensible and reproducible assessment of the reduced earning capacity. The reduced earning capacity can thus be assessed even in particularly difficult cases of facial mutilation. In our experience this loss can be more than 50%.

References

Altmann, F.: Malformations of the auricle and the external auditory meatus. A critical review. Arch. Otolaryng. 54 (1951) 115

Altmann, F.: Mißbildungen des Ohres. In Berendes, J., R. Link, F. Zöllner: Handbuch der HNO-Heilkunde, Bd. III/1. Thieme, Stuttgart 1965; 2. Aufl. 1979

Arulpragasam, A. C.: On the treatment of parotid fistula. J. Laryng. Otol. 81 (1967) 633

Baron, H. C.: Surgical correction of salivary fistula. Ann. Surg. 153 (1961) 545

Beck, Ch.: Zur Chirurgie der Gehörgangsdoppelung. HNO 18 (1970) 307

Becker, W.: Erfahrungen als Gutachter bei Vorwürfen wegen mangelnder Aufklärung und Fahrlässigkeit. Z. Laryng. Rhinol. 53 (1974) 75

Becker, W., H. H. Naumann, C. R. Pfaltz: Hals-Nasen-Ohren-Heilkunde. Thieme, Stuttgart 1982

Becker, W., E. Deutsch, N. F. J. Knappen, K. Nüssen: Probleme der fachärztlichen Aufklärungspflicht. Z. Laryng. Rhinol. 54 (1975) 783 sowie HNO 24 (1976) 181

Chilla, R.: Chirurgie der Nerven im HNO-Bereich. Vegetative Hirnnervenstrukturen. Arch. Oto-Rhino-Laryng. 231 (1981) 353

Denecke, H. J.: Zur Chirurgie der Ohrmißbildungen unter Berücksichtigung des N. facialis. 43. Versammlung SW-deutscher HNO-Ärzte, Würzburg 1959

Denecke, H. J.: Die oto-rhino-laryngologischen Operationen im Mund- und Halsbereich. Springer, Berlin 1980

Deutsch, E.: Das therapeutische Privileg des Arztes: Nichtaufklärung zugunsten des Patienten. Neue Jur. Wschr. 33 (1980a) 1305

Deutsch, E.: Der Zeitpunkt der ärztlichen Aufklärung und die antezipierte Einwilligung des Patienten. Z. Laryng. Rhinol. 59 (1980b) 75

Feldmann, H.: Das Gutachten des HNO-Arztes. Thieme, Stuttgart 1976

Fishler, H. W., B. S. Pogorel: Repair of parotid fistula. Arch. Otolaryng. 61 (1955) 331

Franz, H.: Über Gehörgangsduplikaturen. Z. Laryng. Rhinol. 38 (1959) 16

Frentrup, K.: Trigemino-faciale Reflexe nach intratemporaler Facialisläsion. Habil.-Schrift, Göttingen 1977

Glascock, H., H. Glascock jun.: Repair of traumatic fistulas of Stenon's duct. Surg. Gyn. Obstet. 65 (1937) 355

Hashash, M., F. State, H. I. Dessounky: Effects of tympanic neurectomy on experimentally induced parotid fistulae. J. Laryng. Otol. 92 (1978) 399

Hiller, F.: Die Bedeutung des mesodermalen Gewebes bei der Nervenregeneration. Dtsch. Z. Nervenheilk. 160 (1949) 176

Hiller, F.: Nerve regeneration in grafts. Z. Neuropathol. Clin. Neurol. 1 (1951) 5

König, W.: Zur Kenntnis der (seltenen) congenitalen Ohr-Hals-Fisteln. HNO 6 (1957) 137

Kornblut, A. D., D. Westphal, A. Miehlke: A reevaluation of the Frey syndrome following parotid surgery. Arch. Otolaryng. 103 (1977) 258

Leriche, R.: Behandlung der permanenten Parotisfisteln durch die Entnervung der Speicheldrüse. Zbl. Chir. 41 (1914) 754

Löhr, H., H. Vieten: Die Röntgentherapie der Speicheldrüsenerkrankungen. Fortschr. Kiefer- u. Gesichtschir. 6 (1969) 266

Mandour, M. A., M. M. El-Sheikh, F. El-Garem: Tympanic neurectomy for parotid fistula. Arch. Otolaryng. 102 (1976) 327

Miehlke, A.: Die Chirurgie des N. facialis. Urban & Schwarzenberg, München 1960

Minnigerode, B., J. Haubrich: Angeborene echte Gehörgangsverdoppelung, eine seltene embryogenetische Überschußbildung. Z. Laryng. Rhinol. 44 (1965) 706

Morestin, H.: Contribution á l'étude du traitement des fistules salivaires consecutives aux blessures de guerre. Bull. Mem. Soc. Chir. (Paris) 43 (1917) 845

Muler, M.: Fistule parotidienne traitée par resection du nerf auriculo-temporal. Ann. Otolaryngol. Chir. Cervicofac. 70 (1953) 53

Oeken, F. W.: HNO-Begutachtung. VEB Thieme, Leipzig 1971

Pearson, R. S. B.: Recurrent swelling of parotid glands. Arch. Dis. Child. 10 (1953) 363

Perthes, G.: Zur operativen Behandlung der Parotis-Fisteln nach Schußverletzungen. Zbl. Chir. 44 (1917) 13

Rankow, R. M.: Surgery of the Face, Mouth and Neck. Saunders, Philadelphia 1968

Redon, H.: Chirurgie des glandes salivaires. Masson, Paris 1955

Reeves, R. J.: Roentgentherapy of bilateral parotid fistula. Ann. J. Roentgenol. 43 (1940) 425

Rehrmann, A.: Beseitigung einer Speichelfistel durch Neubildung des Ductus parotideus mit Spalthautlappen. Dtsch. Zahn- u. Kiefer-Heilkd. 28 (1958) 380

Rehrmann, A., B. Keil: Die Behandlung von Verletzungen des Ausführungsganges der Ohrspeicheldrüse. In Naumann, H. H., E. R. Kastenbauer: Plastisch-chirurgische Maßnahmen nach frischen Verletzungen. Thieme, Stuttgart 1974

Stennert, E.: Komplikationen und Rückstände nach operativen Eingriffen am N. facialis (Sekundär-Defekte), In: Chirurgie der Nerven im HNO-Bereich (Kongreßbericht). Arch. Oto-Rhino-Laryng. 231 (1981) 214

Stennert, E.: Das Autoparalytische Syndrom – ein Leitsymptom der postparetischen Fazialisfunktion. Arch. Otolaryng. 236 (1982) 110

Stennert, E., R. Arold: Der doppelte Gehörgang. HNO 21 (1973) 293

Stennert, E., C. Limberg, K. Frentrup: Parese- und Defektheilungsindex. – Ein leicht anwendbares Schema zur operativen Bewertung von Therapiefolgen bei Facialisparesen. HNO 25 (1977) 238

Stennert, E., C. Limberg, K. Frentrup: Paralysis and secondary defect score. Clin. Plast. Surg. 6 (1979) 458

Ungerecht, K.: Die Gefährdung des N. facialis bei der operativen Behandlung der angeborenen Hals-Ohr-Fistel. HNO 10 (1962) 197

Vylder, de, J., J. Carlo, G. T. Stratigos: Early recognition and treatment of the traumatically transected parotid duct. J. oral Surg. 36 (1978) 43

Work, W. P.: Newer concepts of first branchial cleft defects. Laryngoscope 82 (1972) 1581

Work, W. P., C. A. Proctor: The otologist and first branchial cleft anomalies. Ann. Orol. Rhinol. Laryngol. 72 (1963) 548

Zülch, K. J.: Kann die Nachbehandlung während der Regeneration die Wiederherstellung der Leitungssysteme beeinflussen? Zbl. Ges. Neurol. Psychiat. 133 (1955) 146

Index

B

C

D

E

F